Inflammation: Cellular and Molecular Mechanisms

Inflammation: Cellular and Molecular Mechanisms

Edited by Hazel Saunders

hayle medical

New York

Hayle Medical,
750 Third Avenue, 9th Floor,
New York, NY 10017, USA

Visit us on the World Wide Web at:
www.haylemedical.com

ISBN: 978-1-63241-809-8

The publisher's policy is to use permanent paper from mills that operate a sustainable forestry policy. Furthermore, the publisher ensures that the text paper and cover boards used have met acceptable environmental accreditation standards.

Printed in China.

Cataloging-in-Publication Data

Inflammation : cellular and molecular mechanisms / edited by Hazel Saunders.
p. cm.
Includes bibliographical references and index.
ISBN 978-1-63241-809-8
1. Inflammation. 2. Inflammation--Mediators. 3. Inflammation--Immunological aspects.
4. Cellular immunity. 5. Inflammation--Molecular aspects. I. Saunders, Hazel.
RB131 .I54 2019
617.22--dc23

Table of Contents

Preface

The part of the complex biological response of body tissues to harmful stimuli is called inflammation. It is considered to be a protective response involving the blood vessels, immune cells and molecular mediators. Its main functions involve the elimination of initial causes of cell injury, clearing out the damaged tissues and initiating tissue repair. Infection by pathogens, physical injury, burns, trauma, stress and chemical irritants are some of its primary causes. Some common inflammatory disorders are autoinflammatory diseases, colitis, acne vulgaris, rheumatic fever, vasculitis and glomerulonephritis. This book aims to shed light on some of the unexplored aspects of inflammation and the recent researches in this subject. It presents researches and studies performed by experts across the globe. Doctors, researchers and students actively engaged in this field will find this book full of crucial and unexplored concepts.

After months of intensive research and writing, this book is the end result of all who devoted their time and efforts in the initiation and progress of this book. It will surely be a source of reference in enhancing the required knowledge of the new developments in the area. During the course of developing this book, certain measures such as accuracy, authenticity and research focused analytical studies were given preference in order to produce a comprehensive book in the area of study.

This book would not have been possible without the efforts of the authors and the publisher. I extend my sincere thanks to them. Secondly, I express my gratitude to my family and well-wishers. And most importantly, I thank my students for constantly expressing their willingness and curiosity in enhancing their knowledge in the field, which encourages me to take up further research projects for the advancement of the area.

Editor

1

Distinct Lysosome Phenotypes Influence Inflammatory Function in Peritoneal and Bone Marrow-Derived Macrophages

Kassandra Weber[1,2] and Joel D. Schilling[1,2,3]

[1]*Diabetic Cardiovascular Disease Center, Washington University School of Medicine, St. Louis, MO 63110, USA*
[2]*Department of Medicine, Washington University School of Medicine, St. Louis, MO 63110, USA*
[3]*Department of Pathology and Immunology, Washington University School of Medicine, St. Louis, MO 63110, USA*

Correspondence should be addressed to Joel D. Schilling; jschilli@dom.wustl.edu

Academic Editor: B. L. Slomiany

Lysosomes play a critical role in the degradation of both extracellular and intracellular material. These dynamic organelles also contribute to nutrient sensing and cell signaling pathways. Macrophages represent a heterogeneous group of phagocytic cells that contribute to tissue homeostasis and inflammation. Recently, there has been a renewed interest in understanding the role of macrophage autophagy and lysosome function in health and disease. Thioglycollate-elicited peritoneal and bone marrow-derived macrophages are commonly used ex vivo systems to study primary macrophage function. In this study, we reveal dramatic baseline differences in the lysosome morphology and function between these macrophage populations and provide evidence that these differences can be functionally relevant. Our results provide important insights into the diversity of lysosomes in primary macrophages and illustrate the importance of accounting for this in data interpretation.

1. Introduction

The lysosome is a dynamic organelle that operates at an acidic pH and contains numerous enzymes that are critical for cellular degradation pathways. Uptake of extracellular material reaches the lysosome via the endocytic pathway, whereas intracellular cargo is delivered to the lysosome via autophagy [1]. The lysosome can also play a role in secretion, membrane repair, and cell clearance through the process of lysosomal exocytosis [2, 3]. Recently, the importance of lysosomes in cell signaling pathways and nutrient sensing has also become apparent [4, 5]. Importantly, the regulation of lysosome structure and function is cell type dependent and is regulated by environmental stimuli.

Macrophages are cells of the innate immune system that are important for organ homeostasis, inflammation, host defense, and tissue repair [6]. Recently, there has been a renewed interest in macrophage lysosome biology. The importance of macrophage autophagy in several clinically relevant diseases has helped to fuel this renaissance [7–10]. Moreover, it has also come to light that lysosomal pathways activate IL-1β release via the inflammasome in several important human diseases including atherosclerosis, gout, and Alzheimer's disease [11–13]. Also, of relevance, lipid overload and obesity can also induce "lysosomal reprogramming" in adipose tissue macrophages, which may contribute to the metabolic complications of nutrient excess [14]. Together, these and many other studies indicate that additional cellular and molecular studies of lysosome function in macrophages will be critical to understand the role of this organelle in inflammatory diseases.

Ex vivo analysis of primary macrophages will be important for mechanistic cell biology experiments investigating lysosome function in phagocytic cells. The most common sources of primary macrophages include bone marrow-derived macrophages (BMDMs) and thioglycollate-(TG-) elicited peritoneal macrophages (pMACs). Although BMDMs and pMACs are derived from very distinct environments they are often used interchangeably to model macrophage biology. pMACs are monocyte derived cells that are typically isolated from the peritoneal cavity 3–5 days after TG administration [15]. Thus, pMACs are actively involved in the process of inflammation resolution, which includes the uptake of dead cells and/or debris through efferocytosis or phagocytosis, respectively. In contrast, BMDMs are derived from a myeloid precursor cell functionally naïve and would be expected to have fewer demands on their endosomal system. Based on this, we hypothesized that the lysosomes would be phenotypically and functionally distinct in these subtypes of primary macrophages.

In the current study, we investigated lysosome content, morphology, and function in pMACs and BMDMs. Our data demonstrate that pMACs have a larger lysosome volume, increased cathepsin activity, and enhanced expression of several lysosomal genes and proteins. Moreover, using the example of the lipotoxic inflammasome, we provide evidence that these differences in the lysosomal compartment can influence macrophage inflammatory responses. Together, our results argue that the interpretation of data involving lysosome-dependent processes in primary macrophages must take the source of the cells into consideration.

2. Materials and Methods

2.1. Reagents. CAO74-ME and bafilomycin A were from Enzo Life Sciences. Lysotracker red and TMR-dextran (10,000 MW) were from Invitrogen. The cathepsin B activity assay was from Immunocytochemistry Technologies. Ultrapure *E. coli* LPS was from Invivogen. Thioglycollate was from Difco. Fatty acids were from Nu-Chek Prep. The cathepsin D and LAMP1 antibodies were from Abcam. The actin antibody was from Sigma-Aldrich. The CD107a (LAMP-1) PE conjugated antibody was from eBiosciences (cat#12-1071). The ATG5 antibody was from Novus Biologics. Ultrapure-bovine serum albumin (BSA) was from Lampire and was tested for TLR ligand contamination prior to use.

2.2. Cell Culture. Peritoneal macrophages (pMACs) were isolated from C57BL/6 mice 4 days after intraperitoneal injection of 3.85% thioglycollate and plated at a density of 0.9-1 × 10^6 cells/mL in DMEM containing 10% inactivated fetal serum (IFS), 50 U/mL penicillin G sodium, and 50 U/mL streptomycin sulfate (pen-strep), 2 mM L-glutamine, and sodium pyruvate. Stimulations were performed on the day after harvest. Bone marrow-derived macrophages (BMDMs) were prepared by harvesting bone marrow from the femurs and tibias of 8–12-week-old C57BL/6 mice. The cells were seeded in 10 cm dishes and differentiated for 6 days in DMEM media as above supplemented with 10% supernatant from CMG14.12 cells as a source of M-CSF [16]. On day 6, BMDMs were plated at 1×10^6 cells/mL in media containing 5% supernatant from CMG14.12 cells. Stimulations were performed on the day after harvest in media containing 5% CMG1.12 media. For flow cytometry experiments, macrophages were cultured on low adherence plates (Greiner Bio-One) to facilitate cell harvest. Cells were removed from the plate by washing with PBS followed by 10 minutes with Cell Stripper (GIBCO) and then 10 minutes with EDTA/trypsin (Sigma). Growth medium was supplemented with palmitate and BSA at a 2 : 1 molar ratio as described previously [17] and BSA-supplemented media were used as control. For cell stimulations, PBS or LPS (50 ng/mL) were added to BSA or free fatty acid containing media. Flow cytometry was performed on a BD Biosciences FACSCalibur machine and the data was analyzed using Flowjo software.

2.3. Mice. Wild type (WT) C57BL/6 mice were obtained from Oriental Bioscience and maintained in our mouse colony. The ATG5flox X LysM-Cre on the C57BL/6 background were kindly provided by Skip Virgin (Washington University). Mice were maintained in a pathogen-free facility on a standard chow diet ad libitum (6% fat). All animal experiments were conducted in strict accordance with NIH guidelines for humane treatment of animals and were reviewed by the Animal Studies Committee of Washington University School of Medicine.

2.4. RNA Isolation and Quantitative RT-PCR. Total cellular RNA was isolated using Qiagen RNeasy columns and reversely transcribed using a high capacity cDNA reverse transcription kit (Applied Biosystems). Real-time qRT-PCR was performed using SYBR green reagent (Applied Biosystems) on an ABI 7500 fast thermocycler. Relative gene expression was determined using the delta-delta CT method normalized to 36B4 expression. Mouse primers sequences were as follows (all 5′-3′): *36B4* (forward-ATC CCT GAC GCA CCG CCG TGA, reverse-TGC ATC TGC TTG GAG CCC ACG TT); *ctsB* (forward-GAT CAA GGA CCA CCA CAT CC, reverse-CTT AGG AGT GCA CGG GAG AG); *ctsD* (forward-GAC AGC TCC CCG TGG TAG TA, reverse-CAA CAG AAG CTG GTG GAC AA); *ctsK* (forward-TGC CGT GGC GTT ATA CAT AC, reverse-CGG CTA TAT GAC CAC TGC CT); *LAMP1* (forward-TCT TCA GTG TGC AGG TCC AG, reverse-ATG AGG ACG ATG AGG ACCAG); *LAMP2A* (forward-CCA AAT TGG GAT CCT AAC CTA, reverse-TGG TCA AGC AGT GTT TAT TAA TTC C); *LAMP2B* (forward-GGT GCT GGT CTT TCA GGC TTG ATT, reverse-ACC ACC CAA TCT AAG AGC AGG ACT): *ATP6V1H* (forward-AGA CAG CCA GCA ACA CAC TG, reverse-TCA CAG AAA CTT CGT GGC AG); *p62* (forward-GCT GCC CTA TAC CCA CAT CT, reverse-CGC CTT CAT CCG AGA AAC); *LC3* (forward-CGT CCT GGA CAA GAC CAA GT, reverse-ATT GCT GTC CCG AAT GTCTC).

2.5. Western Blotting. Total cellular protein was isolated by lysing cells in 150 mM NaCl, 10 mM Tris (pH 8), triton X-100 1%, and 1X Protease Complete. Proteins were separated on a TGX gradient gel (4–20%; Biorad) and transferred to a nitrocellulose membrane. Western blotting for cathepsin D and actin was performed using 40 μg of total cellular protein.

2.6. LAMP1 Flow Cytometry. After the indicated stimulations, pMACs were removed from the plate as described above and fixed in 4% PFA for 15 minutes in the dark at room temperature. After fixation, cells were permeabilized (PBS + 0.1% Triton X) for 15 minutes in the dark and washed with FACs buffer + 0.1% triton X. Cell were treated with Fc

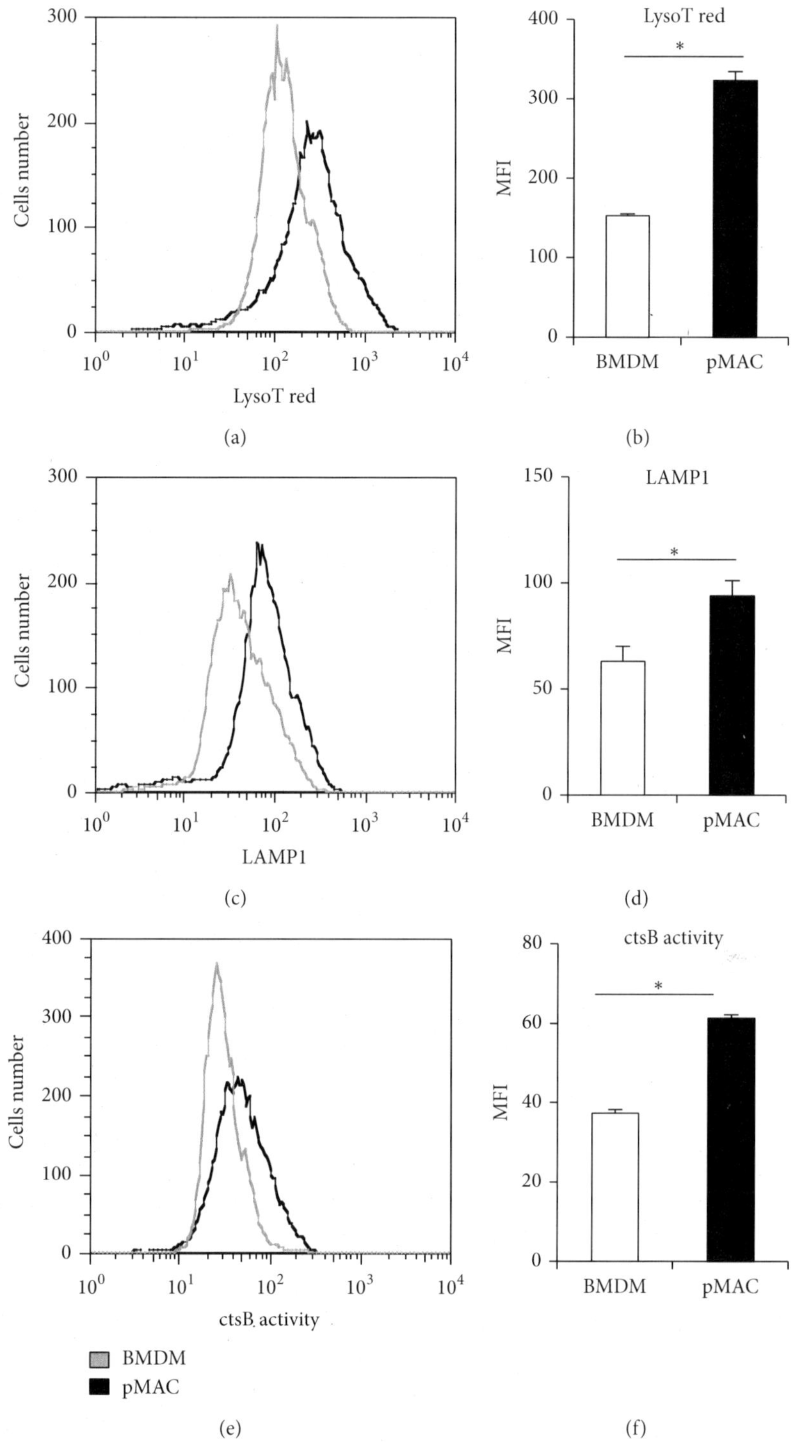

FIGURE 1: Peritoneal macrophages have increased lysosome volume and activity compared to BMDMs. (a, b) Thioglycollate-elicited peritoneal macrophages (pMACs) or bone marrow-derived macrophages (BMDMs) were stained with lysotracker red and analyzed by flow cytometry. A representative histogram (a) and FL2 mean fluorescence intensity (MFI) quantification (b) are shown. (c, d) Total LAMP1 was determined by staining fixed and permeabilized pMACs or BMDMs with a LAMP1 (CD107a) PE antibody followed by flow cytometry assessment. A representative histogram (c) and MFI quantification (d) are shown. (e, f) Cathepsin B activity was assessed using a fluorogenic cathepsin B substrate that requires cleavage to produce fluorescent signal. After incubation with substrate, pMACs and BMDMs were analyzed by flow cytometry. A representative histogram (e) and MFI quantification (f) are shown. Bar graphs report the mean ± standard error (SE) for a minimum of 3 experiments, each performed in triplicate. $^*P < 0.05$ for pMAC versus BMDM.

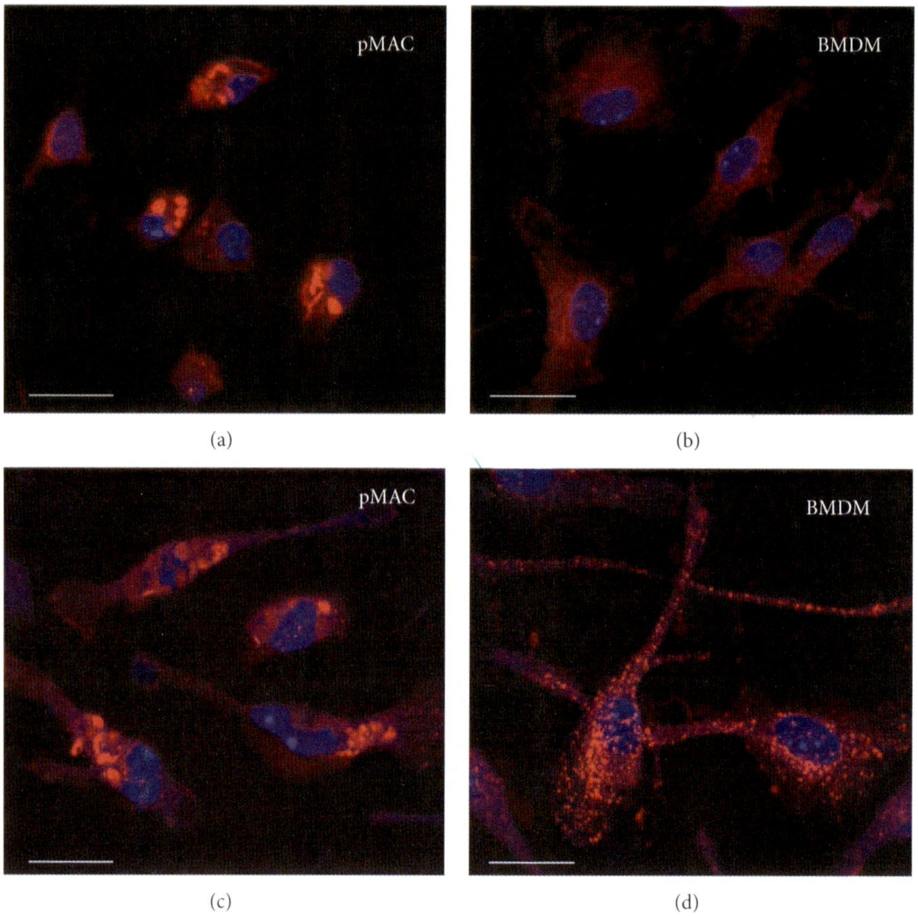

FIGURE 2: pMACs and BMDMs have distinct lysosome morphology. (a–d) pMACs (a, c) or BMDMs (b, d) were incubated with lysotracker red (a, b) or TMR-dextran (c-d) to label lysosomes. Nuclei are stained with Hoechst (blue). Representative immunofluorescent images are shown. The white bar indicates 10 microns.

receptor block (BD Pharmigen) for 5 minutes on ice followed by incubation with CD107a (LAMP1) PE antibody for 30 minutes in the dark on ice. Cells were washed in FACs buffer followed by flow cytometric analysis.

2.7. Lysosome Imaging. After the indicated stimulations, cells were removed from the plate as described above and then stained with 500 nM lysotracker red in tissue culture media for 15 minutes at 37°C. After staining, cells were washed three times with PBS, harvested as described above, and analyzed by flow cytometry. For fluorescent dextran experiments, macrophages were incubated with 500 μg/mL tetramethylrhodamine- (TMR-) dextran for 2 h in regular media. For immunofluorescence microscopy, macrophages were plated on sterile glass coverslips followed by staining. Lysotracker red or TMR-dextran stained cells were fixed for 10 minutes in 4% paraformaldehyde followed by nuclear staining with Hoechst 33342 dye. The cover slips were mounted on glass slides and imaged using a Zeiss confocal microscope.

2.8. Cathepsin B Activity Flow Cytometry. After the indicated stimulations, pMACs were removed from low adherence plates as described above. The fluorescently labeled cathepsin B substrate was reconstituted per manufacturer's instructions and diluted in DMEM+10% IFS. Macrophages were incubated in 150 μL of staining solution for 45 minutes at 37°C under 5% CO_2 with gentle mixing every 10 minutes. After the incubation, cells were washed 2 times in 1 mL of PBS and analyzed by flow cytometry (FL2).

2.9. IL-1β ELISA. Supernatants were harvested from macrophage cultures after the indicated stimulations. IL-1β was quantified using a DuoSet ELISA kit (R&D Systems) according to the manufacturer's instructions.

2.10. Statistics. Statistical analysis was performed using GraphPad Prism software. All results are expressed as means ±SE. Groups were compared by paired Student's t-test. A value of $P \leq 0.05$ was considered significant.

3. Results/Discussion

3.1. Lysosome Content and Activity Are Enhanced in pMACs Compared to BMDMs. To investigate differences in the lysosome compartment of pMACs compared to BMDMs, we

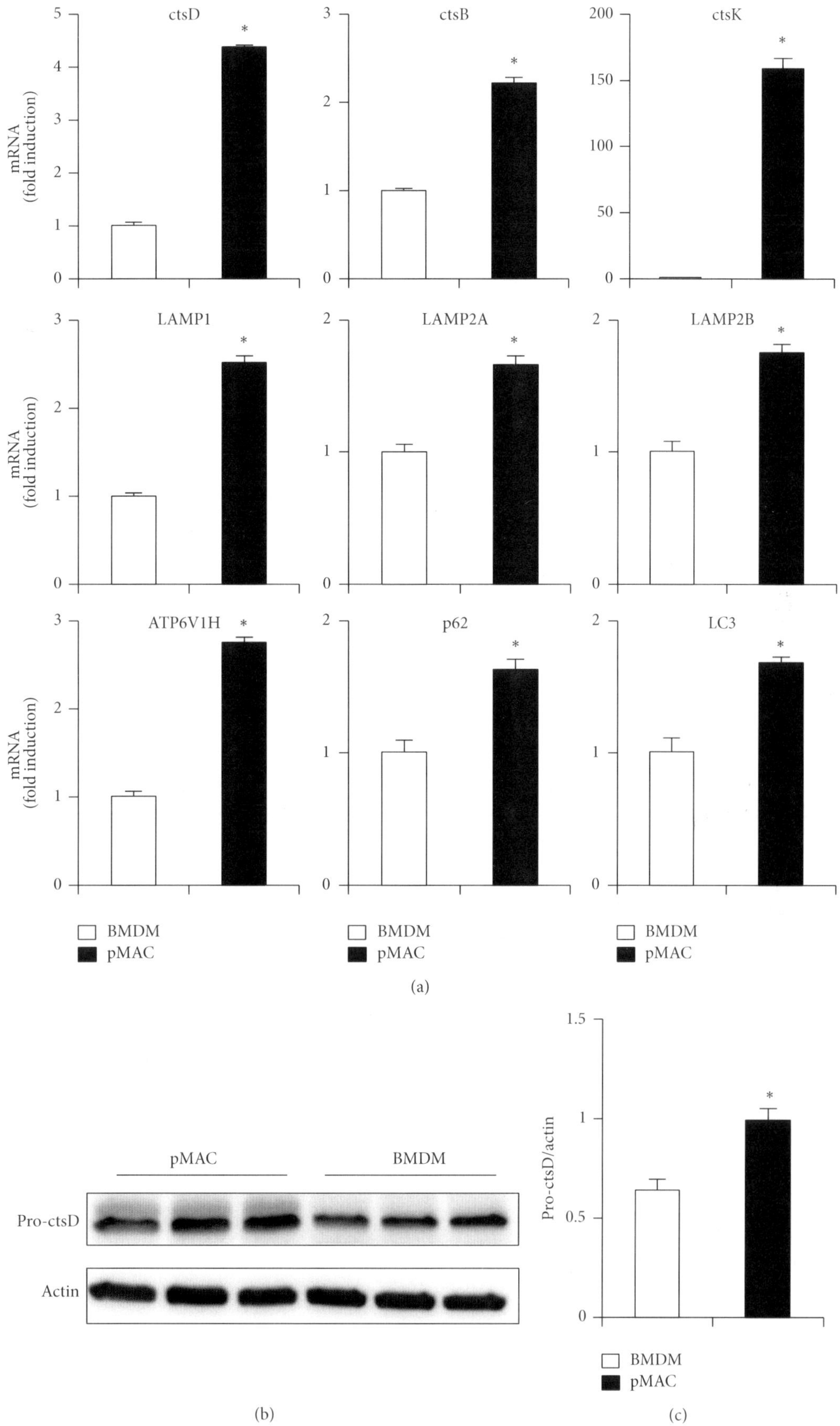

FIGURE 3: Continued.

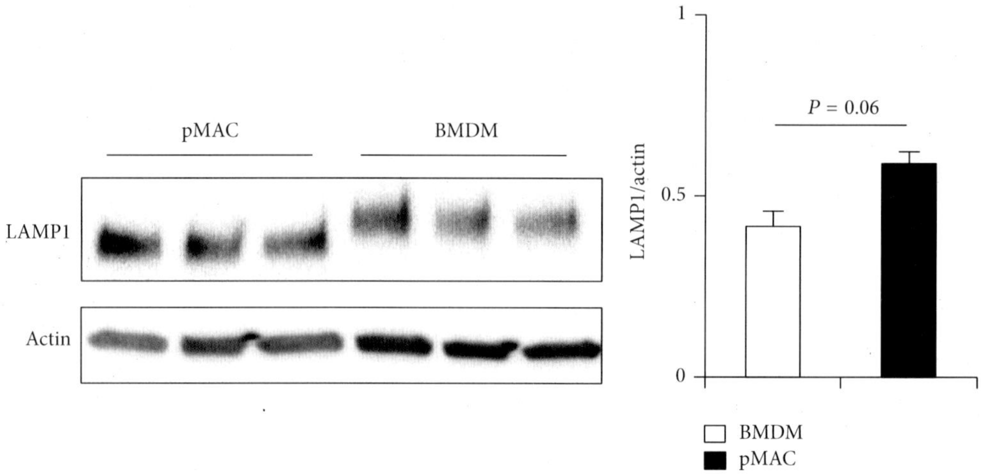

(d) (e)

Figure 3: Expression of lysosomal genes is enhanced in pMACs. (a) RNA was isolated from pMACS and BMDMs and expression of the indicated lysosome and autophagy genes was determined by qRT-PCR. Expression was normalized to 36B4. (b, d) Total cellular protein was isolated from pMACs or BMDMs and expression of pro-cathepsin D (ctsD; (b)) or LAMP1 (d) was determined by western blotting. (c, e) Quantification of pro-cstD protein (45 kD) expression (c) or LAMP1 (110–120 kD) (e) normalized to actin. Bar graphs report the mean ± SE for a minimum of 2 experiments, each performed in triplicate. $^*P < 0.05$ for pMAC versus BMDM.

quantified lysosome volume in these two sets of primary macrophages using the lysosomotropic dye lysotracker red coupled with flow cytometric analysis. Using this approach, lysosome content was significantly increased in pMACs relative to BMDMs (Figures 1(a) and 1(b)). In line with this finding, pMACs also had significantly higher levels of the lysosomal membrane protein LAMP1 compared to BMDM (Figures 1(c) and 1(d)). Together, these findings support the presence of an expanded lysosomal compartment in pMACs. To assess lysosomal protease function, we analyzed the activity of cathepsin B using the fluorogenic substrate magic red. As shown in Figures 1(e) and 1(f), cathepsin B activity was increased in pMACs when compared to BMDMs.

3.2. Distinct Lysosome Size and Morphology in pMACs Compared to BMDMs. Lysosomes have several distinct morphologic appearances that can vary based on cell type and activation status including spheroid, ovoid, or tubular. In addition, the size of lysosomes can vary dramatically [18]. To visualize lysosomes in pMACs and BMDMs, we utilized two complementary immunofluorescent approaches: (1) lysotracker red staining and (2) tetramethylrhodamine- (TMR-) dextran staining. Lysotracker red freely crosses cell membranes and is concentrated in acidic organelles whereas TMR-dextran is taken up via endocytosis and reaches lysosomes in ~30 min. Lysosome size and morphology were similar using both staining techniques (Figure 2). Strikingly, pMACs had much larger lysosomes than BMDMs. In addition, the morphology was more frequently ovoid and tubular in pMACs and spherical in BMDMs (Figures 2(a)–2(d)). Notably, pMAC lysosome morphology is similar to that described from adipose tissue macrophages during high fat feeding [14]. Stimulation of BMDMs or pMACs with LPS did not lead to a significant change in lysosome morphology (data not shown).

3.3. Lysosomal Gene and Protein Expression Are Distinct in pMACs Compared to BMDMs. Emerging data indicates that lysosome biogenesis and function are regulated in part at the transcriptional level [19]. Therefore, we compared the expression of several lysosome and autophagy related genes in BMDMs and pMACs. Consistent with the flow cytometry and imaging data, the expression of genes encoding cathepsin proteases, lysosomal membrane proteins, and the vacuolar ATPase was increased in pMACs relative to BMDMs (Figure 3(a)). In addition, the autophagy related genes LC3 and p62 were also expressed at a higher level in pMACs (Figure 3(a)). Thus, mRNA expression of lysosome and autophagy related genes is increased in pMACs, which is likely related to the expanded lysosome compartment observed in these primary macrophages. At the protein level, pro-cathepsin D protein content was increased in pMACs relative to BMDMs (Figures 3(b) and 3(c)). Similar to the flow cytometry data, LAMP1 protein content trended towards an increase in pMACs compared to BMDMs (Figures 3(d) and 3(e)). Interestingly, the molecular weight of LAMP1 was significantly greater in BMDMs suggesting a higher level of glycosylation, a finding which could further affect lysosome function and stability in these two types of primary macrophages (Figure 3(d)).

3.4. The Differences in Lysosome Phenotype Translate into Distinct Mechanisms for Activation of the Lipotoxic Inflammasome. To investigate whether the observed differences in lysosome phenotype modulate macrophage inflammatory responses, we explored the lipotoxic inflammasome as a model system. We, and others, have shown that the combination of LPS and the saturated fatty acid (SFA) palmitate triggers the release of IL-1β through an NLRP3 and caspase 1-dependent mechanism [20–22]. In prior studies using this

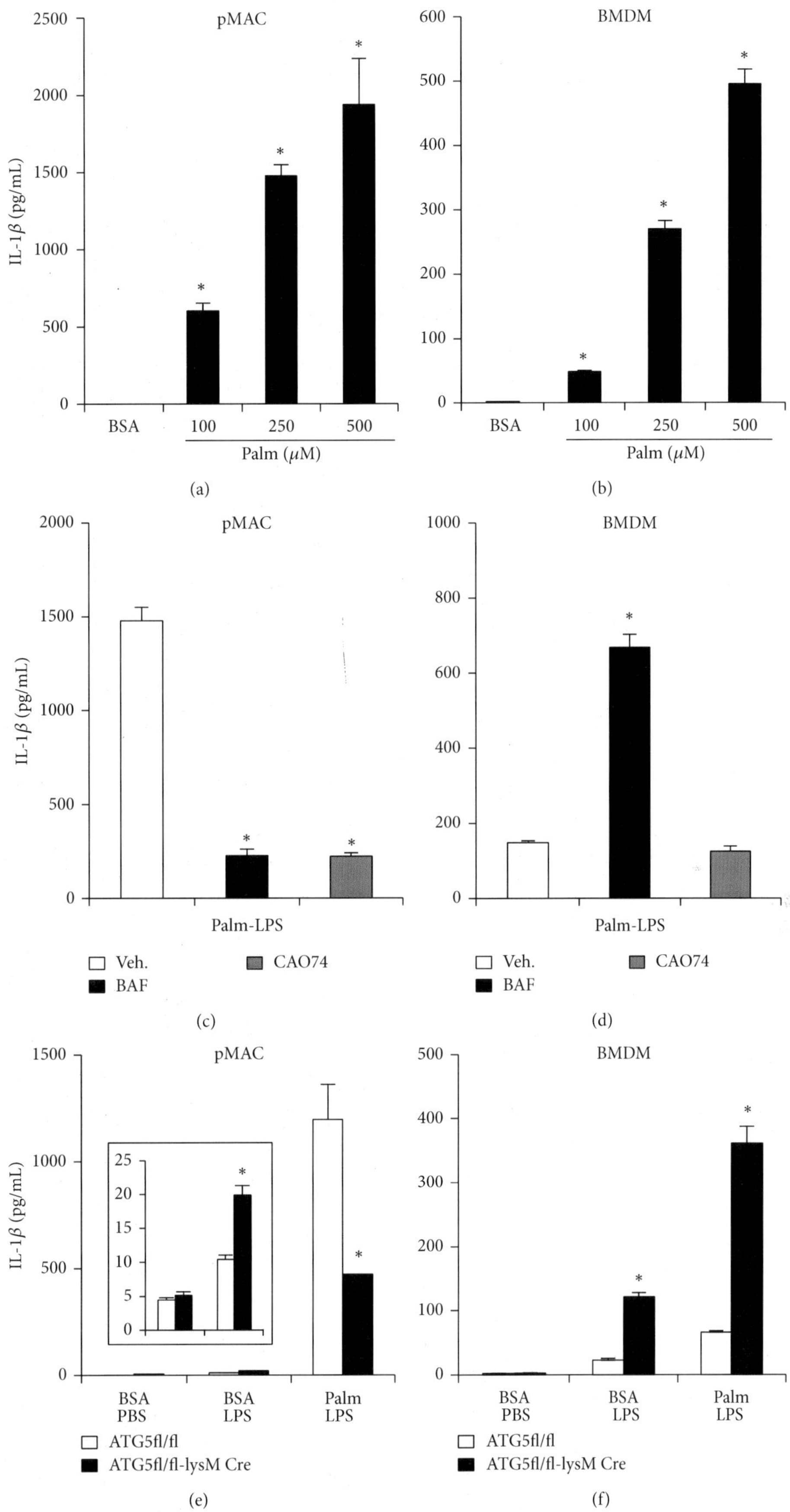

Figure 4: Continued.

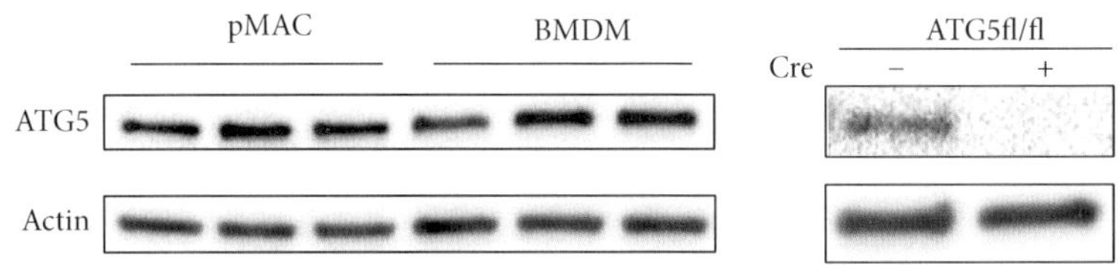

(g)

FIGURE 4: Differential role of the lysosome during activation of the lipotoxic inflammasome in pMACs compared to BMDMs. (a, b) pMACs (a) or BMDMs (b) were preloaded with the indicated doses of palmitate (palm) or with BSA for 2 h followed by BSA or palm ±50 ng/mL LPS for 20 h after which IL-1β in the supernatant was quantified by ELISA. (c, d) pMACs (c) or BMDMs (d) were stimulated with palmitate and LPS in the presence of bafilomycin (BAF, 25 nM) or CAO74-ME (10 μM) and IL-1β release at 20 h was determined by ELISA. (e, f) pMACs (e) or BMDMs (f) were prepared from WT (white bars) or ATG5KO (black bars; ATG5fl/fl X LysM-Cre) mice and were subsequently stimulated with BSA-PBS, BSA-LPS, or palm-LPS for 20 h. IL-1β release was quantified by ELISA. The inset in (e) shows data for BSA-PBS versus BSA-LPS with an adjusted scale. (g) Total cellular protein was isolated from pMACs or BMDMs and expression of ATG5 was determined by western blotting (*left panel*). As a control for the antibody, protein was also isolated from WT and ATG5KO pMACs and analyzed by western blot (*right panel*). Bar graphs report the mean ± standard error (SE) for a minimum of 3 experiments, each performed in triplicate. $^*P < 0.05$ for BSA-PBS versus palm-LPS; vehicle versus inhibitor; or WT versus KO.

system, it has been shown that IL-1β release from pMACs is dependent on lysosome damage and cathepsin proteases, whereas the role of lysosomes in BMDMs is less clear [21]. To directly compare pMACs and BMDMs using this system, we simultaneously stimulated both cell types with LPS in the presence of increasing concentrations of palmitate and the release of IL-1β was quantified. Both pMACs and BMDMs secreted IL-1β in a dose dependent fashion; however, pMACs consistently secreted 5–10 times more cytokines than BMDMs despite using a similar number of cells (Figures 4(a) and 4(b)). Importantly, FA uptake was similar between the pMACs and BMDMs (data not shown). Consistent with prior studies, IL-1β release from pMACs was almost completely prevented by the cathepsin B inhibitor, CAO74, or lysosomal acidification inhibitor, bafilomycin (BAF), in palmitate-LPS treated pMACs (Figure 4(c)). This was not the case in BMDMs where IL-1β release was unaffected by CAO74 and actually increased with BAF (Figure 4(d)). Thus, lysosome inhibitors differentially influence lipotoxic inflammasome activation in pMACs compared to BMDMs, an observation that may account for some of the discrepancies between prior publications [20–22]. More importantly, these findings argue that the baseline differences in lysosome content and function between pMACs and BMDMs can alter the response of these cells to inflammatory stimuli.

Lysosomes are also important for the degradation of autophagic cargo, which can also modulate the inflammasome response [23]. Therefore, using ATG5 KO cells, we tested the impact of autophagy deficiency on activation of the lipotoxic inflammasome in pMACs versus BMDMs. As can be seen in Figures 4(e) and 4(f), the phenotypes observed using autophagy deficient cells were different in these primary macrophage systems. In pMACs, ATG5 KO cells had a modest increase in IL-1β release after LPS treatment (Figure 4(e) *inset*), but IL-1β secretion following palmitate-LPS stimulation was reduced compared to WT cells (Figure 4(e)). In distinction, ATG5 KO BMDMs released more IL-1β in response to both LPS and palmitate-LPS treatment (Figure 4(f)). This was not related to differences in ATG5 protein expression, which was similar between the two types of macrophages (Figure 4(g)). Instead, the development of lysosome dysfunction in pMACs treated with palmitate-LPS may explain why genetic autophagy deficiency does not further enhance inflammasome activation [24]. In contrast, ATG5 KO BMDMs phenocopy cells treated with BAF, which also inhibits autophagic flux. These findings argue that genetic or pharmacologic inhibition of autophagy in BMDMs unmasks an important suppressive role for this degradative process on lipotoxic inflammasome activation. Further investigation will be necessary to evaluate the mechanisms that account for these differential phenotypes. Interestingly, recent evidence suggests that autophagy can increase lysosome activity, which could be particularly important for BMDMs as they have less active lysosomes at baseline [25, 26]. Taken together, this data suggests that pMACs and BMDMs respond to lipotoxic stimulation through fundamentally different mechanisms, and at least part of these differences is related to distinct lysosome phenotypes.

The findings presented in this paper illustrate several significant differences between lysosomes in pMACs and BMDMs. Specifically, pMACs display enhanced lysosome volume, size, and cathepsin activity. The "activated" lysosome compartment in pMACs may reflect the signals they receive in the inflammatory setting of peritonitis. In contrast, BMDMs are naïve macrophages that have not encountered "activation" signals. Using the example of the lipotoxic inflammasome, we also provide evidence that the distinct lysosome phenotypes observed in BMDMs and pMACs can influence macrophage inflammatory function. Thus, when conducting experiments of lysosome function with primary macrophages, it is critical to account for baseline lysosome phenotype to ensure appropriate interpretation of data. We would argue that the choice of BMDM versus pMAC for experimentation should be tailored to the specific research question, and a low threshold should exist for comparing multiple macrophage populations. In addition, further comparative analysis of lysosomes between pMACs, BMDMs, and other in vivo isolated macrophages will be necessary to shed additional light on the dynamic regulation of lysosomes in these important leukocytes.

Abbreviations

TG: Thioglycollate
BMDM: Bone marrow-derived macrophage
pMAC: peritoneal macrophage.

Authors' Contribution

Kassandra Weber carried out the experiments and contributed to the writing of the paper. Joel D. Schilling designed and interpreted the experiments and wrote the paper.

Acknowledgment

The authors thank Ahbinav Diwan for this critical review of this paper.

References

[1] H. Appelqvist, P. Wäster, K. Kågedal, and K. Öllinger, "The lysosome: from waste bag to potential therapeutic target," *Journal of Molecular Cell Biology*, vol. 5, no. 4, pp. 214–226, 2013.

[2] P. L. McNeil, "Repairing a torn cell surface: make way, lysosomes to the rescue," *Journal of Cell Science*, vol. 115, no. 5, pp. 873–879, 2002.

[3] D. L. Medina, A. Fraldi, V. Bouche et al., "Transcriptional activation of lysosomal exocytosis promotes cellular clearance," *Developmental Cell*, vol. 21, no. 3, pp. 421–430, 2011.

[4] C. Settembre, A. Fraldi, D. L. Medina, and A. Ballabio, "Signals from the lysosome: a control centre for cellular clearance and energy metabolism," *Nature Reviews Molecular Cell Biology*, vol. 14, no. 5, pp. 283–296, 2013.

[5] C. Settembre, R. Zoncu, D. L. Medina et al., "A lysosome-to-nucleus signalling mechanism senses and regulates the lysosome via mTOR and TFEB," *The EMBO Journal*, vol. 31, no. 5, pp. 1095–1108, 2012.

[6] D. M. Mosser and J. P. Edwards, "Exploring the full spectrum of macrophage activation," *Nature Reviews Immunology*, vol. 8, no. 12, pp. 958–969, 2008.

[7] B. Razani, C. Feng, T. Coleman et al., "Autophagy links inflammasomes to atherosclerotic progression," *Cell Metabolism*, vol. 15, no. 4, pp. 534–544, 2012.

[8] X. Liao, J. C. Sluimer, Y. Wang et al., "Macrophage autophagy plays a protective role in advanced atherosclerosis," *Cell Metabolism*, vol. 15, no. 4, pp. 545–553, 2012.

[9] C. Wang, G. R. Mendonsa, J. W. Symington et al., "Atg16L1 deficiency confers protection from uropathogenic *Escherichia coli* infection in vivo," *Proceedings of the National Academy of Sciences of the United States*, vol. 109, no. 27, pp. 11008–11013, 2012.

[10] T. Saitoh, N. Fujita, M. H. Jang et al., "Loss of the autophagy protein Atg16L1 enhances endotoxin-induced IL-1β production," *Nature*, vol. 456, no. 7219, pp. 264–268, 2008.

[11] F. Martinon, V. Pétrilli, A. Mayor, A. Tardivel, and J. Tschopp, "Gout-associated uric acid crystals activate the NALP3 inflammasome," *Nature*, vol. 440, no. 7081, pp. 237–241, 2006.

[12] P. Duewell, H. Kono, K. J. Rayner et al., "NLRP3 inflammasomes are required for atherogenesis and activated by cholesterol crystals," *Nature*, vol. 464, pp. 1357–1361, 2010.

[13] M. T. Heneka, M. P. Kummer, A. Stutz et al., "NLRP3 is activated in Alzheimer's disease and contributes to pathology in APP/PS1 mice," *Nature*, vol. 493, no. 7434, pp. 674–678, 2013.

[14] X. Xu, A. Grijalva, A. Skowronski, M. Van Eijk, M. J. Serlie, and A. W. Ferrante Jr., "Obesity activates a program of lysosomal-dependent lipid metabolism in adipose tissue macrophages independently of classic activation," *Cell Metabolism*, vol. 18, no. 6, pp. 816–830, 2013.

[15] E. L. Gautier, S. Ivanov, P. Lesnik, and G. J. Randolph, "Local apoptosis mediates clearance of macrophages from resolving inflammation in mice," *Blood*, vol. 122, no. 15, pp. 2714–2722, 2013.

[16] S. Takeshita, K. Kaji, and A. Kudo, "Identification and characterization of the new osteoclast progenitor with macrophage phenotypes being able to differentiate into mature osteoclasts," *Journal of Bone and Mineral Research*, vol. 15, no. 8, pp. 1477–1488, 2000.

[17] L. L. Listenberger, D. S. Ory, and J. E. Schaffer, "Palmitate-induced apoptosis can occur through a ceramide-independent pathway," *The Journal of Biological Chemistry*, vol. 276, no. 18, pp. 14890–14895, 2001.

[18] J. P. Luzio, P. R. Pryor, and N. A. Bright, "Lysosomes: fusion and function," *Nature Reviews Molecular Cell Biology*, vol. 8, no. 8, pp. 622–632, 2007.

[19] C. Settembre, C. Di Malta, V. A. Polito et al., "TFEB links autophagy to lysosomal biogenesis," *Science*, vol. 332, no. 6036, pp. 1429–1433, 2011.

[20] B. Vandanmagsar, Y.-H. Youm, A. Ravussin et al., "The NLRP3 inflammasome instigates obesity-induced inflammation and insulin resistance," *Nature Medicine*, vol. 17, no. 2, pp. 179–189, 2011.

[21] K. Weber and J. D. Schilling, "Lysosomes integrate metabolic-inflammatory cross-talk in primary macrophage inflammasome activation," *Journal of Biological Chemistry*, vol. 289, no. 13, pp. 9158–9171, 2014.

[22] H. Wen, D. Gris, Y. Lei et al., "Fatty acid-induced NLRP3-ASC inflammasome activation interferes with insulin signaling," *Nature Immunology*, vol. 12, no. 5, pp. 408–415, 2011.

[23] N. Mizushima, B. Levine, A. M. Cuervo, and D. J. Klionsky, "Autophagy fights disease through cellular self-digestion," *Nature*, vol. 451, no. 7182, pp. 1069–1075, 2008.

[24] J. D. Schilling, H. M. Machkovech, L. He, A. Diwan, and J. E. Schaffer, "TLR4 activation under lipotoxic conditions leads to synergistic macrophage cell death through a TRIF-dependent pathway," *Journal of Immunology*, vol. 190, no. 3, pp. 1285–1296, 2013.

[25] J. Zhou, S.-H. Tan, V. Nicolas et al., "Activation of lysosomal function in the course of autophagy via mTORC1 suppression and autophagosome-lysosome fusion," *Cell Research*, vol. 23, no. 4, pp. 508–523, 2013.

[26] H.-M. Shen and N. Mizushima, "At the end of the autophagic road: an emerging understanding of lysosomal functions in autophagy," *Trends in Biochemical Sciences*, vol. 39, no. 2, pp. 61–71, 2014.

2

Familial Mediterranean Gene (MEFV) Mutation in Parents of Children with Familial Mediterranean Fever: What Are the Exceptions?

Leila Shahbaznejad,[1,2] Sayed-Reza Raeeskarami,[3,4] Raheleh Assari,[3,4] Abbas Shakoori,[5] Hamidreza Azhideh,[5] Yahya Aghighi,[4] Fatemeh Tahghighi,[1,4] and Vahid Ziaee[3,4]

[1] *Children's Medical Center, Pediatrics Center of Excellence, Tehran, Iran*
[2] *Department of Pediatrics, Mazandaran University of Medical Sciences, Sari, Iran*
[3] *Pediatric Rheumatology Research Group, Rheumatology Research Center, Tehran University of Medical Sciences, Tehran, Iran*
[4] *Department of Pediatrics, Tehran University of Medical Sciences, Tehran, Iran*
[5] *Department of Medical Genetics, Tehran University of Medical Sciences, Tehran, Iran*

Correspondence should be addressed to Vahid Ziaee; ziaee@tums.ac.ir

Academic Editor: Jean-Marc Cavaillon

Objectives. Familial Mediterranean Fever (FMF) is one of the most prevalent periodic fever syndromes; MEFV, the responsible gene for the disease, is in the short arm of chromosome16. In the considerable count of the FMF patients, only one mutation is found in the MEFV and parents, who were the obligatory carriers for that mutation, were asymptomatic. The aim of this study was to evaluate these asymptomatic parents in regard to mutation in MEFV gene and similarity between parents and offspring patients. *Methods.* In this cross-sectional study, asymptomatic parents of FMF patients enrolled the study were referred to periodic fever clinic or pediatric rheumatology clinic of Tehran University of Medical Sciences. The patients should have at least one mutation in MEFV gene and none of them had any family history of autoinflammatory disease. Twelve mutations in MEFV gene were assessed in the parents by Vienna Lab FMF Strip Assay kit by MAS PCR/Reverse hybridization. *Results.* Forty-three patients and their parents participated in the study. Sixty-three percent (27) of patients were male. Onset of disease symptoms in 31 patients (72%) was before 4 years of old. Nine (21%) of the patients had homozygote, 16 (37%) compound heterozygote, and 17(40%) heterozygote for MEFV mutation; there was a case of complex alleles mutations (2%). M694V/M694V in 4 patients (9%) was the most homozygote genotype, and M694V/R761H in 4 (9%) and E148Q in 7 (16%) were the most compound heterozygote and heterozygote genotype, respectively. M694V, M680I, and E148Q were the most mutation in the parents. Overall, 41 patients had mutations similar to their parents' mutation, except 2 whose parents had no mutation, but a patient did. *Conclusion.* It seems that occurrence of new mutations in offspring is not prevalent among FMF patients and there are other reasons for different clinical presentation in similar mutation carriers. On the other hand, in ethnicities with high prevalence of FMF, new mutation in descendant may occur, infrequently.

1. Introduction

Familial Mediterranean fever (FMF) is one of the most frequent periodic febrile syndromes [1, 2]. Gene MEFV which was responsible for the disease was discovered in 1997, at the short arm of chromosome 16 and encode synthesis of pyrin/meranostrin [1, 2]. Today there are more than 300 variances in MEFV gene [2]. FMF is known as an autosomal recessive hereditary disease with different clinical presentation due to type of mutation, i.e., homozygote or heterozygote pattern. The other patients have not any known mutation or have only one mutation (heterozygote) [1, 2]. The patients are symptom-free between attacks, but it is notable that inflammatory reaction not only was active in each attack but also was between episodes in FMF patients. Also, in asymptomatic mutation carriers the inflammatory phenomenon has been demonstrated [3]. The most important complication of FMF is amyloidosis; when involving kidneys and other organs such as scrotum, an unfavorable prognosis is inevitable [1, 4]. The diagnosis of FMF is based on characteristic periodic complaints with fever, serositis, and a good clinical response to colchicine [1, 2].

To the best of our knowledge, there is no published study indicating mutations in the MEFV gene in asymptomatic parents of FMF patients, so we discovered MEFV gene of healthy and asymptomatic parents, who had an offspring suffering from FMF attacks and had at least one known mutation. We would like to know about mutation transmission in FMF patient population.

2. Methods and Materials

In this cross-sectional descriptive study, healthy parents of FMF patients had been evaluated about MEFV gene mutation. Each patient with two or more criteria of Yalcinkaya criteria [5] (fever, abdominal pain, chest pain, and arthritis) with exception of positive familial history of FMF in parents was included in our research. The exclusion criteria in each attack consisted of periodic oral and stomatitis aphthous lesion, periodic pharyngitis, periodic lymphadenitis (Marshal Syndrome), periodic noncharacteristic skin rashes, and CNS involvements. The patients were under observation at periodic fever clinic, children medical center (CMC), and Valiasr pediatric rheumatology clinic, Tehran University of Medical Sciences (TUMS). All of the involved patients should have at least one known mutation, and parents should not have any history for autoinflammatory disease.

At first, mutation of the present parent was evaluated; if it was negative or it was incompatible with the offspring mutation or the patient had more than one mutation, the other parent was also assessed. One milliliter of venous blood sample was needed to evaluate MEFV gene mutation with Vienna Lab FMF Strip Assay kit. The kit was equipped to assess 12 mutations in exons 2, 5, and 10 in MEFV gene, including mutations: E148Q, P369S, F479L, M680I(G/C), M680I(G/A), 1692del, M694V, M694I, K695R, V726A, A744S, and R761H. According to manufacturer's instruction, Multiplex PCR Amplification, Simultaneous Biotin Labeling, and reverse hybridization were performed, respectively. The MEFV gene assessment was done at genetic lab of cancer institute (TUMS).

The study was approved by TUMS ethics in research committee by number IR.TUMS.REC.1394.1855. All of the participants were aware of the process and free to engage the study and they should not pay any fee to the laboratory. All of them signed informed consent.

3. Results

Parents of 58 patients (116 persons) had been invited to participate in the study. Of these, parents of 11 patients refused to engage in the study; in 4 cases, one parent was assessed and MEFV gene status was not compatible with the patient, and the other parent could not participate in the study. Finally information of 43 patient and their parents was appreciable.

Of the 43 FMF patient, 27 (63%) were male. Mean age at initiation of disease symptoms was 3.4 ± 3.36 years (between 6 months to 20 years old). Eleven patients (26%) had experienced their first complaints near or before their first birthday; 20 (46%) were 1.5 to 4 years old and 7 (16%) at 5 to 7 years old and one patient was at 20 years of age at that time. In 4 cases the parent did not remember the first presentation time.

Nine patients (21%) had homozygote mutation in the MEFV gene and 16 (37%) and 17 (40%) had compound heterozygote and patients with one mutation, respectively. One patient had 3 mutations (complex allele mutations). Frequency of each genotype and mutation in the patients is shown in Table 1, as it was clear that the most homozygote mutation was M694V/M694V and compound heterozygote M694V/R761H, each of them in 4 patients (9%). The most heterozygote mutation in FMF patients was E148Q, in 7 cases (16%).

There was not any significant difference between number of mutation and age of the presentation of the symptoms.

When mutation in MEFV gene was assessed in the parents, most of them were heterozygote, except 2 mothers and 6 fathers, who had compound heterozygote and one father had complex mutations (Tables 2 and 3). Interestingly, the common mutation in nearly all of them was E148Q. Table 2 also contains mutations of patients according to each allele. It has shown that the most prevalent mutations in both study groups were M694V, E148Q, and M680I.

Fifty-six parents (66%) were of Turk ethnicity origin. The other parents were divided into different races: Turkman, Fars, Kurd, Lor, and Arab. Thirty percent of the parents (parents of 13 patients) were consanguine (second degree relatives). Most of the homozygote patients had consanguine parents (7 of nine patients).

From 43 patients who participated in the study, 41 had mutation(s) similar to their parents. In all of the cases, parents had not any symptoms or complaints regarding the FMF or any other autoinflammatory disease, at the study time or before it, but some of them recalled some nonsignificant vague abdominal pain during their childhood years. In 2 cases, MEFV gene status of patients was different from their parents. The first was a Kurdish boy who had P369S heterozygote mutation, but we could not find any mutation in MEFV gene in both parents, even after rechecking the mutation.

Another patient was a boy, from nonrelative Turk parents. His MEFV gene had compound heterozygote mutation: R761H/M694I. Mutation of father was R761H heterozygote but mother did not have any mutation. The process repeated again, but the same result had been found.

In this study, mutations in MEFV gene were compatible with mutations in fathers in 9 cases (21%), with mothers in 7 (16%), and both of them in 22 (51%). In 2 FMF patients with two mutations, one parent had one of the mutations and the other parent had not been present for assessment. As mentioned before, in two cases there were some discrepancies between the child and her parent (or parents) mutations.

Complex mutations were found if there were more than two mutations in the MEFV gene. We have found a family from north of the country (Turkman ethnicity), in which asymptomatic consanguine parents had more than one

Table 1: Frequency of different genotype in Familial Mediterranean Fever patients.

	Genotype	Frequency (percent)
Heterozygote 17(40)	E148Q	7(16)
	M694V	5(12)
	M680I(G>C)	2(5)
	P369S	1(2)
	V726A	1(2)
	M694I	1(2)
Compound heterozygote 16(37)	M694V/R761H	4(9)
	M694I/R761H	2(5)
	M680I/E148Q	2(5)
	M680I/M694V	3(7)
	P369S/E148Q	1(2)
	E148Q/M694I	1(2)
	M694V/V726A	1(2)
	M680I/R761H	1(2)
	V726A/R761H	1(2)
Homozygote 9(21)	M694V/M694V	4(9)
	M680I/M680I	3(7)
	V726A/V726A	2(5)
Complex alleles mutations	P369S/ E148Q/ E148Q	1(2)

Table 2: Frequency of mutations in Familial Mediterranean Fever patients and parents.

Mutation	Patients frequency (percent)	Parentsfrequency (percent)
M694V	21(30)	19 (25)
E148Q	13 (18)	18 (24)
M680I	14(20)	13 (17)
R761H	8 (11)	8 (11)
V726A	7 (10)	7 (9)
M694I	4(6)	4 (5)
P369S	3(4)	4 (5)
V744S		2(3)
Total number	70(100)	75(100)

mutations, E148Q/P369S and P369S/E148Q/A744S for the mother and father, respectively. The son had complex mutations: E148Q/E148Q/P369S.

Renal amyloidosis complicated a boy with heterozygote mutation of M694V; his healthy mother had the same mutation.

4. Discussion

FMF is the most monogenic autoinflammatory disease, inherited autosomal recessively. However, the heterozygote mutation and the patients with only one mutation have usually the FMF disease expressions. [6] In this study, as expected we have found similar mutation in MEFV gene in parents and their offsprings. So, we searched for some exceptions.

In some studies [3, 7], higher frequency of MEFV gene mutation in first-degree relatives of FMF patients had been reported. Lachmann and coworkers [3] reported a group of FMF patients, where 84% of them had at least two mutations and 12% had single mutation. In their study group, 92% of first-degree relatives (parents or siblings) of these patients had mutation in MEFV gene (80% had one mutation, and 12% had two mutations, without any symptoms).

To date, there is not any published article about mutation in both parents of FMF patient specifically; so, against the previous study, the highest percentages (95.3%) of the same MEFV mutation in patients and parents as the first-degree relatives were found.

In exception, the mutations of two FMF patients were not found according to their parents. The patient with single mutation P369S without any mutation in the parents has FMF disease presentation. The P369S is known as polymorphism according to frequency in general population [8], although the role of the allele in inflammatory response to environmental factor as FMF-like disease should not be missed. Also,

TABLE 3: Genotype of compound heterozygote mutations in the parents.

Father's genotype	ethnicity	Mother's genotype	Mother's ethnicity	Offspring's genotype
E148Q/M680I	Turk	NA	Fars	M680I
E148Q/M694V	Fars	NA	Fars	M694V
E148Q/P369S	Fars	NA	Fars	E148Q/P369S
E148Q/R761H	Turk	M694V	Turk	M694V/R761H
M694V/A744s	Fars	M694V	Fars	M694V/M694V
E148Q/P369S/A744S	Turkman	E148Q/P369S	Turkman	E148Q/E148Q/P369S
M694V	Turk	E148Q/M694V	Turk	M694V/M694V

NA: not assessed

cooperation between this allele and one or more unidentified modifier alleles could be presented as the typical FMF [9, 10]. So, the polymorphism of P369 and the susceptible races with their related factors such as one or more modifier allele and environmental factors could have this presentation.

The presentation of the disease is correlated with the number of mutation, the patients with more than one mutation express earlier FMF disease presentations [11]; but our study is lacking to show this relationship. This discrepancy may be due to the lower age of the participants in this study.

In this study, the most prevalent mutations in parents and patients are M694V, E148Q and M680I respectively. The result of frequency of FMF mutation in the previous studies of Iran are similar to our study. [12, 13] M694V mutation is the most common mutation in other races such as Turk [14], Jewish [15], and Armenian [16] and less common in Arabs population [17]. In spite of the other populations in the Eastern Mediterranean, E148Q mutations as the second most common mutation with FMF disease presentation have been demonstrated in our study. In Japan [18], where FMF disease is the rare disease, E148Q mutation is the most mutation.

In addition, E148Q/- was found as the most common FMF patients with one mutation. On the other hand, almost all compound heterozygote parents are E148Q/∗ with any inflammatory presentation. The roles of E148Q mutation in inflammatory presentation are controversy. Although the E148Q variant has the most distribution in the MEFV gene, certain role of this variant remains unclear [19, 20]. In some studies, The E148Q allele with high frequency in both FMF patients and general population has been recognized as polymorphism [19]. In contrast, the hypothesis supports the inflammatory role of E148Q mutation in Turkish and Greek population [21, 22]. So, our study population may have the same specialize environmental or genes.

In almost all of the cases, parents have had mutation(s) similar to their offspring, especially in heterozygote ones, but clinical symptoms are very different, and while a parent with 2 or 3 mutations did not report any symptoms, the child with the same mutation suffered periodic symptoms from early childhood. However, some parents recalled some mild and nonspecific symptoms like abdominal pain during their childhood, just after the result of mutation got clear.

Lachman et al. report higher level of acute phase protein in heterozygous carrier parents in comparison of general population [3].

As mentioned above, the E148Q mutation in almost all healthy compound heterozygous parent are present. Also, the compound heterozygous genotype with E148Q/∗ allele without any inflammatory symptoms have been reported [3, 23]. On the other hand, when parents have only one mutation E148Q is transmitted to their symptomatic offspring. So, further evaluation about the limiting role of E148Q allele in compound heterozygous genotype in nonsymptomatic population would be involved.

In addition, almost all the offsprings have not been inheriting the E148Q allele from their compound heterozygous parents (Table 3). The similar transmissions of the E148Q allele from compound heterozygous parents to their kids have been reported [7]. In FMF patients, allele may transmit as both autosomal dominant and autosomal recessive pattern. In different population, the autosomal dominant transmission has been reported [24, 25], although the "dose effect" mutation with high penetrance and low penetrance explains the differences mild to more sever presentations [26]. On the other hand, the other factors such as unidentified factor, environmental factors, and epigenetic factors may play role in the pathogenesis of FMF presentations [10]. Furthermore, further expansive evaluation should be considered.

The most of the FMF patients had one or two mutations in MEFV gene, but there are reports of patients with more than 2 mutations in different exons of this gene, so called complex alleles [27, 28]. In this study, such as the others, the combination of two or three allele located on exon 2 (E148Q, L110P) and exon 3 (P639S) can express the FMF phenotype. The cooperation of these two rare exons 2 and 3 may be presented such as exon 10 mutations. In contrast, the exon 2 and exon 3 alleles may only be the polymorphism genotype and the third mutation on exon 10 has function [8, 19]. So, further researches would evaluate this phenomenon.

The frequency of MEFV mutations in the parents of FMF patients was 88%. The exact distributions of MEFV mutation in general population are not available. In a study in Turkish population, the frequency of carrier rate of MEFV gene was 20% [29]. So, we suggest a study for evaluation of the frequency of the MEFV mutation in general population without any symptoms and positive family history of FMF. In addition, evaluation in larger population would be more valuable.

Sometimes periodic fever, aphtous stomatitis, pharyngitis, and cervical adenitis (PFAPA) syndrome mimic FMF symptoms and these patients respond to colchicine. Concurrent and FMF and PFAPA syndrome have been reported frequently [30, 31]. Evidence shows that colchicine is more efficient in PFAPA patients with underlying of MEFV mutation [32–34].

5. Conclusion

Most of the patients inherited the mutation in MEFV gen from their parents. The new onset mutation in offspring without mutation in parents is very rare. It is noted that even asymptomatic carriers of mutation in MEFV gene may have some degree of mild inflammation, and close monitoring of parents of FMF patient should be under sought.

Disclosure

A report of this study has been presented as an abstract in "Annual European congress of Rheumatology 2018, Amesterdam," and the "28th International Congress of Pediatrics 2016, Tehran."

Acknowledgments

This research was part of a fellowship thesis (of Dr. L. Shahbaznejad) and it was approved and financially supported by a grant from Tehran University of Medical Sciences (no. 93-11-46-5001) [35]. The authors would like to thank parents who participated in the study.

References

[1] C. Fonnesu, C. Cerquaglia, M. Giovinale et al., "Familial Mediterranean fever: a review for clinical management," *Joint Bone Spine*, vol. 76, no. 3, pp. 227–233, 2009.

[2] Z. Ahmadinejad, S. Mansori, V. Ziaee et al., "Periodic fever: a review on clinical, management and guideline for Iranian patients—Part I," *Iranian Journal of Pediatrics*, vol. 24, no. 1, pp. 1–13, 2014.

[3] H. J. Lachmann, B. Şengül, T. U. Yavuzşen et al., "Clinical and subclinical inflammation in patients with familial Mediterranean fever and in heterozygous carriers of MEFV mutations," *Rheumatology*, vol. 45, no. 6, pp. 746–750, 2006.

[4] R. Yilmaz and S. Ozer, "A rare presentation of familial mediterranean fever; acute scrotum and hydrocele amyloidosis," *Iranian Journal of Pediatrics*, vol. 20, no. 3, pp. 367–369, 2010.

[5] F. Yalçinkaya, S. Özen, Z. B. Özçakar et al., "A new set of criteria for the diagnosis of familial Mediterranean fever in childhood," *Rheumatology*, vol. 48, no. 4, pp. 395–398, 2009.

[6] S. Özen, E. D. Batu, and S. Demir, "Familial mediterranean fever: recent developments in pathogenesis and new recommendations for management," *Frontiers in Immunology*, vol. 8, p. 253, 2017.

[7] E. Ben-Chetrit, I. Lerer, E. Malamud, C. Domingo, and D. Abeliovich, "The E148Q mutation in the MEFV gene: is it a disease-causing mutation or a sequence variant?" *Human Mutation*, vol. 15, pp. 385-386, 2000.

[8] J. G. Ryan, S. L. Masters, M. G. Booty et al., "Clinical features and functional significance of the P369S/R408Q variant in pyrin, the familial Mediterranean fever protein," *Annals of the Rheumatic Diseases*, vol. 69, no. 7, pp. 1383–1388, 2010.

[9] P. Schaner, N. Richards, A. Wadhwa et al., "Episodic evolution of pyrin in primates: Human mutations recapitulate ancestral amino acid states," *Nature Genetics*, vol. 27, no. 3, pp. 318–321, 2001.

[10] M. G. Booty, J. C. Jae, S. L. Masters et al., "Familial Mediterranean fever with a single MEFV mutation: Where is the second hit?" *Arthritis & Rheumatology*, vol. 60, no. 6, pp. 1851–1861, 2009.

[11] M. Esfahani, A. Movahedian, M. Baranchi, and M. T. Goodarzi, "Adiponectin: an adipokine with protective features against metabolic syndrome," *Iranian Journal of Basic Medical Sciences*, vol. 18, no. 7, pp. 659–663, 2015.

[12] F. Salehzadeh, M. J. Asl, S. H. Asl, S. Jahangiri, and S. Habibzadeh, "MEFV gene profile in northwest of Iran, twelve common MEFV gene mutations analysis in 216 patients with familial mediterranean fever," *Iranian Journal of Medical Sciences*, vol. 40, no. 1, pp. 68–72, 2015.

[13] T. Sabokbar, A. malayeri, C. Azimi et al., "Spectrum of mutations of familial Mediterranean fever gene in Iranian population," *Annals of Paediatric Rheumatology*, vol. 3, no. 1, pp. 11–17, 2014.

[14] M. Tunca, S. Akar, F. Onen, H. Ozdogan, O. Kasapcopur, F. Yalcinkaya et al., "Familial Mediterranean fever (FMF) in Turkey: results of a nationwide multicenter study," *Medicine*, vol. 84, pp. 1–11, 2005.

[15] S. Padeh, Y. Shinar, E. Pras et al., "Clinical and diagnostic value of genetic testing in 216 Israeli children with familial Mediterranean fever," *The Journal of Rheumatology*, vol. 30, no. 1, pp. 185–190, 2003.

[16] M. M. Moradian, T. Sarkisian, H. Ajrapetyan, and N. Avanesian, "Genotype-phenotype studies in a large cohort of Armenian patients with familial Mediterranean fever suggest clinical disease with heterozygous MEFV mutations," *Journal of Human Genetics*, vol. 55, no. 6, pp. 389–393, 2010.

[17] H. A. Majeed, H. El-Shanti, M. S. Al-Khateeb, and Z. A. Rabaiha, "Genotype/phenotype correlations in Arab patients with familial Mediterranean fever," *Seminars in Arthritis and Rheumatism*, vol. 31, no. 6, pp. 371–376, 2002.

[18] D. Kishida, A. Nakamura, M. Yazaki, A. Tsuchiya-Suzuki, M. Matsuda, and S.-I. Ikeda, "Genotype-phenotype correlation in Japanese patients with familial Mediterranean fever: Differences in genotype and clinical features between Japanese and Mediterranean populations," *Arthritis Research & Therapy*, vol. 16, no. 5, p. 439, 2014.

[19] E. Ben-Chetrit, I. Lerer, E. Malamud, C. Domingo, and D. Abeliovich, "The E148Q mutation in the MEFV gene: is it a disease-causing mutation or a sequence variant?" *Human Mutation*, vol. 15, no. 4, pp. 385-386, 2000.

[20] S. Ozen and E. D. Batu, "The myths we believed in familial mediterranean fever: What have we learned in the past years?" *Seminars in Immunopathology*, vol. 37, no. 4, article no. A002, pp. 363–369, 2015.

[21] K. Konstantopoulos, A. Kanta, K. Lilakos, G. Papanikolaou, and I. Meletis, "Familial Mediterranean fever and E148Q pyrin gene mutation in Greece," *International Journal of Hematology*, vol. 81, no. 1, pp. 26–28, 2005.

[22] R. Topaloglu, F. Ozaltin, E. Yilmaz et al., "E148Q is a disease-causing MEFV mutation: A phenotypic evaluation in patients

with Familial Mediterranean fever," *Annals of the Rheumatic Diseases*, vol. 64, no. 5, pp. 750–752, 2005.

[23] M. Tunca, S. Akar, P. N. Hawkins et al., "The significance of paired MEFV mutations in individuals without symptoms of familial Mediterranean fever," *European Journal of Human Genetics*, vol. 10, no. 12, pp. 786–789, 2002.

[24] S. Ozen, E. Demirkaya, G. Amaryan et al., "Results from a multicentre international registry of Familial Mediterranean fever: Impact of environment on the expression of a monogenic disease in children," *Annals of the Rheumatic Diseases*, vol. 73, no. 4, pp. 662–667, 2014.

[25] D. M. Rowczenio, D. S. Iancu, H. Trojer et al., "Autosomal dominant familial Mediterranean fever in Northern European Caucasians associated with deletion of p.M694 residue-a case series and genetic exploration," *Rheumatology*, vol. 56, no. 2, pp. 209–213, 2017.

[26] S. Federici, G. Calcagno, M. Finetti et al., "Clinical impact of MEFV mutations in children with periodic fever in a prevalent western European Caucasian population," *Annals of the Rheumatic Diseases*, vol. 71, no. 12, pp. 1961–1965, 2012.

[27] F. Salehzadeh and A. Fathi, "Patient with FMF and Triple MEFV Gene Mutations," *Medical Archives*, vol. 69, no. 4, pp. 269-270, 2015.

[28] Y. Fukushima, K. Obara, H. Hirata, K. Sugiyama, T. Fukuda, and K. Takabe, "Three japanese patients (mother and two children) with familial Mediterranean fever associated with compound heterozygosity for L110p/E148Q/M694i and an autosomal true dominant inheritance pattern," *Asian Pacific Journal of Allergy and Immunology*, vol. 31, no. 4, pp. 325–329, 2013.

[29] E. Yilmaz, S. Ozen, B. Balci et al., "Mutation frequency of familial Mediterranean fever and evidence for a high carrier rate in the Turkish population," *European Journal of Human Genetics*, vol. 9, no. 7, pp. 553–555, 2001.

[30] F. F. Mehregan, V. Ziaee, Z. Ahmadinejad, F. Tahghighi, F. Sabouni, and M.-H. Moradinejad, "Periodic fever, Aphthous stomatitis, Pharyngitis and cervical adenitis (PFAPA) syndrome in Iranian children: First report of iranian periodic fever and autoinflammatory registry (IPFAIR)," *Iranian Journal of Pediatrics*, vol. 24, no. 5, pp. 598–602, 2014.

[31] F. Salehzadeh, M. Vahedi, S. Hosseini-Asl, S. Jahangiri, S. Habibzadeh, and M. Hosseini-Khotbesara, "PFAPA and 12 common MEFV gene mutations our clinical experience," *Iranian Journal of Pediatrics*, vol. 24, no. 1, pp. 64–68, 2014.

[32] M. Gunes, S. Cekic, and S. S. Kilic, "Is colchicine more effective to prevent periodic fever, aphthous stomatitis, pharyngitis and cervical adenitis episodes in Mediterranean fever gene variants?" *Pediatrics International*, vol. 59, no. 6, pp. 655–660, 2017.

[33] P. Dusser, V. Hentgen, B. Neven, and I. Koné-Paut, "Is colchicine an effective treatment in periodic fever, aphtous stomatitis, pharyngitis, cervical adenitis (PFAPA) syndrome?" *Joint Bone Spine*, vol. 83, no. 4, pp. 406–411, 2016.

[34] E. Pehlivan, A. Adrovic, S. Sahin, K. Barut, O. Kul Cınar, and O. Kasapcopur, "PFAPA syndrome in a population with endemic familial mediterranean fever," *Journal of Pediatrics*, vol. 192, pp. 253–255, 2018.

[35] L. Shahbaznejad, *Frequency of MEFV Gene mutation in healthy parents of Familial Mediterranean Fever (FMF) patients. MD (Sub-specialty of Pediatric Rheumatology dissertation in Persian)*, Tehran University of Medical Sciences, 2016, ID No: 93-11-46-5001.

3

VEGFR-2 Expression in Glioblastoma Multiforme Depends on Inflammatory Tumor Microenvironment

Jana Jaal,[1,2] Marju Kase,[1,3] Ave Minajeva,[2] Mikk Saretok,[2] Aidi Adamson,[2] Jelizaveta Junninen,[2] Tõnis Metsaots,[2] Tõnu Jõgi,[1] Madis Joonsalu,[1] Markus Vardja,[1] and Toomas Asser[2,4]

[1] *Hematology and Oncology Clinic, Department of Radiotherapy and Oncological Therapy, Tartu University Hospital, 51003 Tartu, Estonia*
[2] *Faculty of Medicine, University of Tartu, 50411 Tartu, Estonia*
[3] *East-Tallinn Central Hospital, Center of Oncology, 10138 Tallinn, Estonia*
[4] *Neurology Clinic, Department of Neurosurgery, Tartu University Hospital, 51014 Tartu, Estonia*

Correspondence should be addressed to Jana Jaal; jana.jaal@kliinikum.ee

Academic Editor: Alexander J. Steven

Glioblastoma multiforme (GBM) is one of the most angiogenic tumors. However, antiangiogenic therapy has not shown significant clinical efficacy. The aim of our study was to evaluate the impact of inflammatory tumor microenvironment on the expression of vascular endothelial growth factor receptor 2 (VEGFR-2). Surgically excised primary GBM tissues were histologically examined for overall extent of inflammation (score 1–3). After immunohistochemistry, the tissue expression of ICAM-1 (optical density), the number of VEGFR-2 positive (VEGFR-2+) blood vessels (per microscopic field), and the endothelial staining intensity of VEGFR-2 (score 0–3) were determined. In GBM, the extent of inflammation was 1.9 ± 0.7 (group mean $\pm$ SD). Mean optical density of inflammatory mediator ICAM-1 was 57.0 ± 27.1 (pixel values). The number of VEGFR-2+ blood vessels and endothelial VEGFR-2 staining intensity were 6.2 ± 2.4 and 1.2 ± 0.8, respectively. A positive association was found between endothelial VEGFR-2 staining intensity and the extent of inflammation ($p = 0.005$). Moreover, VEGFR-2 staining intensity correlated with the expression level of ICAM-1 ($p = 0.026$). The expression of VEGFR-2, one of the main targets of antiangiogenic therapy, depends on GBM microenvironment. Higher endothelial VEGFR-2 levels were seen in the presence of more pronounced inflammation. Target dependence on inflammatory tumor microenvironment has to be taken into consideration when treatment approaches that block VEGFR-2 signaling are designed.

1. Introduction

Although considered as rare tumor entity, about 27700 new primary CNS cancers are diagnosed each year in Europe [1]. Out of these, glioblastoma multiforme (GBM) is the most aggressive and lethal type of a brain tumor in adults that accounts for approximately 20% of all malignant primary CNS tumors and 82% of high grade (WHO grades III and IV) gliomas [2, 3]. The prognosis of GBM patients is extremely dismal since current standard treatment options result only in medial survival times of 14.6 months [4].

GBM is one of the most angiogenic tumors. Therefore, in recent years, the inhibition of tumor angiogenesis has been an extremely attractive and dominating experimental therapeutic strategy in neurooncology [5, 6]. A number of anticancer drugs that block formation of new blood vessels through different molecular targets and patterns of action are currently in various stages of clinical development for both newly diagnosed and recurrent GBM [7]. However, first promising results of angiogenesis inhibitors, such as high radiological response rates and apparent clinical benefit, have been replaced by prevalent disappointment. Major limitations of antiangiogenic drugs used in GBM include the modest number of durable responses and the lack of cytotoxic antitumor activity and overall survival benefit [6].

The reasons of the lack of significant clinical efficacy of antiangiogenic drugs in GBM, however, are not fully elucidated [8].

In GBM, at least five mechanisms by which tumors achieve neovascularization have been described: vascular cooption, angiogenesis, vasculogenesis, vascular mimicry, and glioblastoma-endothelial cell transdifferentiation [9]. Out of these, angiogenesis and vasculogenesis have been most extensively studied and described. During angiogenesis, blood vessels arise from sprouting and proliferation of endothelial cells from preexisting vascular network, whereas in vasculogenesis, *de novo* blood vessels are formed through colonization of circulating bone-marrow-derived endothelial progenitor cells that are recruited to the tumor [9]. Both previously mentioned mechanisms of neovascularization are largely regulated via vascular endothelial growth factor (VEGF) and its receptor 2 (VEGFR-2) [10]. It has been shown that tumor microenvironment influences glioblastoma treatment outcome [11, 12]. The aim of the current study was to evaluate the impact of tumor microenvironment, particularly inflammatory reaction, on the expression of VEGFR-2, one of the main targets of antiangiogenic drugs.

2. Materials and Methods

Study was approved by the Research Ethics Committee of the University of Tartu, Estonia.

Surgically excised primary GBM tissues ($n = 42$) were obtained after primary operation (prior to radiotherapy) from patients treated at Tartu University Hospital or North Estonian Medical Centre.

2.1. Histology. Haematoxylin and eosin stained sections (4 μm thick) were used for primary diagnosis. The diagnosis of GBM was confirmed by 2 independent pathologists. Afterwards, the overall extent of inflammatory reaction was estimated in tumor tissue by experienced pathologist. This was based on typical visual appearance of inflammation, including presence of edema and inflammatory cell infiltration. For the evaluation, an arbitrary score ranging from 1 to 3 was applied (1 = weak, 2 = moderate, and 3 = strong inflammatory reaction).

2.2. Immunohistochemistry (IHC). GBM tissues were immunohistochemically examined for ICAM-1 and VEGFR-2 expression. Sections were cut from archived paraffin blocks and stained according to standard immunohistochemistry protocol. For immunohistochemistry, primary antibodies against ICAM-1 (Santa Cruz Biotechnology, Inc., #sc-8439, dilution 1:100) and VEGFR-2 (Santa Cruz Biotechnology, Inc., #sc-6251, dilution 1:100) were applied. Diaminobenzidine was used as chromogen.

The evaluation of immunohistochemically stained slides was carried out in a blinded fashion. First, immunohistochemical expression of intercellular adhesion molecule 1 (ICAM-1) was assessed. For this, digital IHC image analysis was performed. IHC digital image analysis was carried out in 6 selected images from each slide by using the freeware program ImageJ. The brown-colored area, occupied by the immunohistochemical reaction, was selected by the color threshold filtering tool to subtract the hematoxylin-stained areas at the background. Then the images were converted to the greyscale and the optical density by the area method was measured in pixel values ranging from 0 to 255. Value 0 represents the lightest shade of the color while 255 represents the darkest shade of the color in the image. Tissue expression of ICAM-1 was determined at a magnification of ×10.

The evaluation and scoring of VEGFR-2 immunohistochemically stained slides were carried out by 2 independent researchers. For VEGFR-2 expression, two parameters were assessed. First, the number of VEGFR-2 positive (VEGFR-2+) blood vessels per microscopic field was determined. Additionally, endothelial VEGFR-2 staining intensity was evaluated using an arbitrary score ranging from 0 to 3 (0 = no staining; 1 = weak, 2 = moderate, and 3 = strong staining intensity). For individual values, both parameters were determined in 5 microscopic fields. These values were used to evaluate the correlation between the assessments of 2 independent researchers. Afterwards, the mean number of VEGFR-2+ blood vessels and VEGFR-2 staining intensity in 10 microscopic fields (2 × 5 fields) were calculated. All VEGFR-2 parameters were determined in areas with vital tumor tissue (excluding necrotic areas) at a magnification of ×40.

2.3. Statistical Analysis. The SPSS statistical software was used to calculate individual means, group mean, and standard deviation of the mean. Additionally, Pearson correlation analysis was utilized. A p value <0.05 was regarded statistically significant.

3. Results

3.1. Histology and IHC. In individual GBM samples, the extent of inflammation varied, ranging from 1.0 to 3.0 and being in the whole group 1.9 ± 0.7 (mean ± SD). Figure 1 represents GBM tissues with weak (a), moderate (b), and strong (c) visual inflammatory reaction.

Similarly, individual optical densities of ICAM-1 in GBM tissue varied, ranging from to 17.6 to 154.9 pixel values. Group mean optical density of ICAM-1 was 57.0 ± 27.1 (mean ± SD). Figure 2 illustrates GBM tissues with weak (a), moderate (b), and strong (c) optical density of ICAM-1.

VEGFR-2 parameters were determined by 2 independent researchers whose results were in good accordance ($R = 0.8$, $p < 0.0001$). In GBM tissue sections, the number of VEGFR-2+ blood vessels per microscopic field and endothelial VEGFR-2 staining intensity were 6.2 ± 2.4 (mean ± SD; range 2.8–13.5) and 1.2 ± 0.8 (mean ± SD; range 0.0–2.8), respectively. Figure 3 illustrates GBM tissues with weak (a), moderate (b), and strong (c) expression level of VEGFR-2 in tumor blood vessels.

3.2. Correlation Analysis. The results of correlation analysis are described in Table 1. A positive association was found between the extent of visual inflammation and endothelial VEGFR-2 staining intensity ($p = 0.005$). Moreover, endothelial VEGFR-2 staining intensity correlated with the

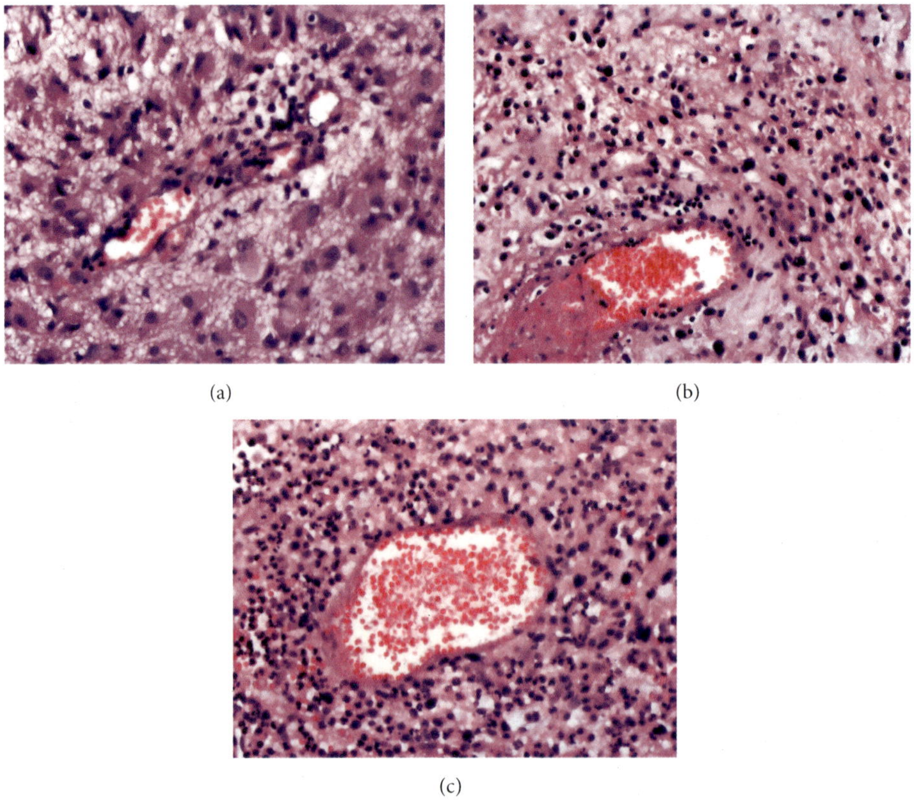

FIGURE 1: Inflammatory reaction in GBM. Photos illustrate GBM tissues with inflammatory reaction (photos represent different patients). (a) Weak (score 1) inflammation, (b) moderate (score 2) inflammation, and (c) strong (score 3) inflammation. Note the different numbers of tumor infiltrating inflammatory cells. Magnification ×40.

TABLE 1: Results of correlation analysis*.

Correlations	p value
Visual inflammatory reaction and VEGFR-2 staining intensity	$p = 0.005$
Tissue ICAM-1 expression and VEGFR-2 staining intensity	$p = 0.026$
The number of VEGFR-2+ blood vessels and VEGFR-2 staining intensity	$p = 0.065$

*Bivariate Pearson correlation test.

expression level of tissue ICAM-1 ($p = 0.026$). Additionally, there was a trend toward significant association between the number of VEGFR-2 positive blood vessels and endothelial VEGFR-2 staining intensity in GBM tissue ($p = 0.065$).

4. Discussion

Downstream effects of VEGFR-2 activation in the vascular endothelium include cell proliferation, migration, permeability, and survival, resulting in neovascularization processes, such as angiogenesis and vasculogenesis [10]. Consequently, this receptor has been very attractive target in the development of antiangiogenic drugs (e.g., bevacizumab, sunitinib, sorafenib, vatalanib, vandetanib, recentin, and cediranib) [10]. Unfortunately, a number of these antiangiogenic drugs (vandetanib, cediranib, sorafenib, and sunitinib) have failed to show clinical efficacy in different phases of clinical trials in both newly diagnosed and recurrent glioblastoma [13–17]. Moreover, the most advanced antiangiogenic drug in glioblastoma, bevacizumab, did not get approval from The European Medicines Agency Committee for Medicinal Products for Human Use (CHMP) due to the lack of clinically relevant efficacy [18, 19]. All these negative trials have caused a lot of frustration since the results do not coincide with the initial expectations. The reasons of the lack of significant clinical efficacy of antiangiogenic drugs, however, are not fully elucidated.

In the present study, we evaluated the impact of tumor microenvironment on the expression level of VEGFR-2, one of the main targets of antiangiogenic drugs. Foremost, the possible role of inflammatory reaction was assessed. Inflammatory reaction was evaluated by two means. First, visual inflammation (based on the presence of tissue edema and inflammatory cell infiltration) was estimated in hematoxylin-eosin stained sections by experienced pathologist. Afterwards, to reduce subjectivity, a digital IHC image analysis was performed in ICAM-1 stained sections. ICAM-1 was chosen as a marker of inflammation since this transmembrane glycoprotein can be induced in response to a number of stimuli, including inflammatory mediators, hormones,

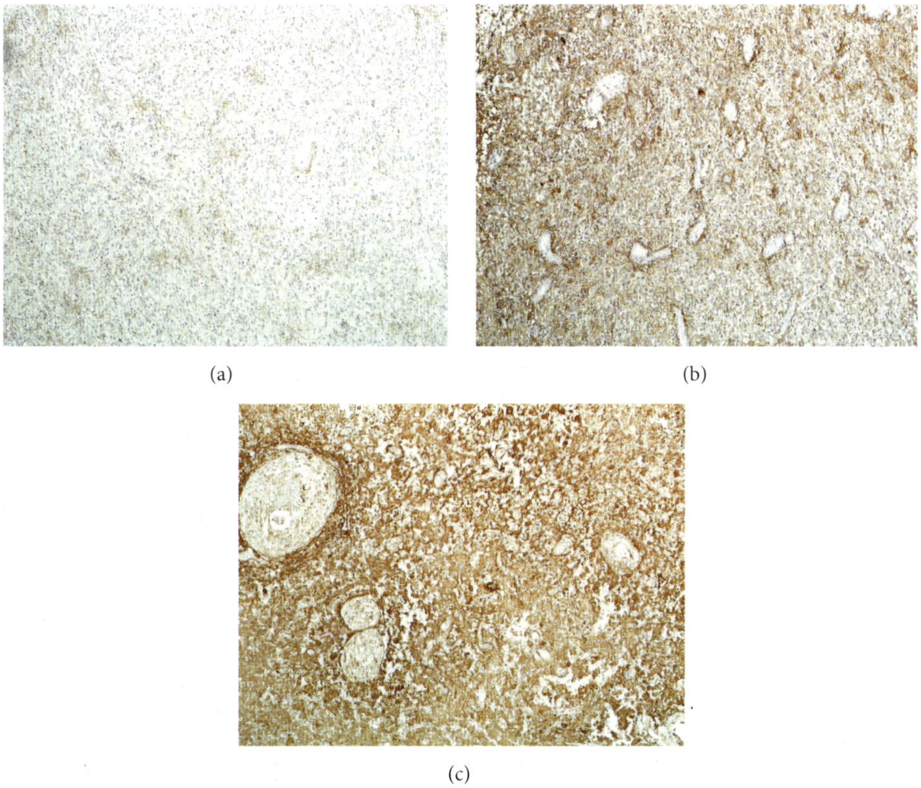

FIGURE 2: ICAM-1 expression in GBM. Photos illustrate GBM tissues with different extent of ICAM-1 expression (photos represent different patients). (a) Weak optical density, (b) moderate optical density, and (c) strong optical density. Magnification ×10.

and cellular stresses [20, 21]. Moreover, endothelial ICAM-1 is considered to represent the most important adhesion molecule for leukocyte recruitment to inflamed sites [22–24].

All glioblastoma samples showed various levels of visually confirmed inflammatory reaction. This is not surprising since inflammation is considered one of the characteristic histopathological features of glioblastoma [25]. Also, the expression of ICAM-1 was present in all digitally analyzed individual tumor samples, which is in good accordance with previous studies, where compared to peritumoral ICAM-1 expression significantly higher expression of ICAM-1 has been detected in GBM tumor areas in both gene and protein levels [26–28]. In GBM cells, ICAM-1 expression has been shown to increase following stimulation with proinflammatory cytokines, such as interleukin-1β (IL-1β), tumor necrosis factor-alpha (TNFα), and interferon-gamma (IFN-γ) [26, 29], indicating that ICAM-1 is one of the inflammatory mediators also in this type of cancer.

In GBM tissues, different numbers of VEGFR-2+ blood vessels and endothelial levels of VEGFR-2 were detected. Previous studies have shown that in normal brain, low or undetectable endothelial expression of VEGFR-2 can be found; however, in gliomas, the proportion of VEGFR-2+ vessels and endothelial VEGFR-2 expression increases with tumor grade, being the highest in GBM [30, 31]. Our study revealed that also in the most aggressive glioma—GBM—the extent of VEGFR-2 expression may vary. Additionally, present study showed that the expression of VEGFR-2 depends on inflammatory reaction in tumor tissue: the higher the endothelial VEGFR-2 expression the higher the extent of inflammation. Moreover, this association was seen for both assessments of inflammatory reaction (visual and computer software based).

Angiogenesis is a tightly controlled process that in a number of pathological conditions, including cancer and inflammation, may become aberrant [32]. Different factors produced by tissues are capable of promoting or inhibiting blood vessel proliferation, whereas in normal status, the balance between angiogenic and angiostatic factors exists. In inflammation, this balance is clearly inclined toward angiogenic factors and angiogenesis [33].

Although the link between inflammation and angiogenesis has received much attention only recently, there is a substantial body of evidence showing close association between these two processes. Previous studies have described that angiogenic factors exhibit both proangiogenic and proinflammatory effects, inflammatory cells are able to produce large quantities of proangiogenic factors, and both processes (inflammation and angiogenesis) are capable of potentiating each other [33]. For example, VEGF that exerts majority of its angiogenic effects by binding to VEGFR-2 has also been shown to induce adhesion molecules on endothelial cells during inflammation [34]. In endothelial cells, treatment with VEGF results in an increase of both ICAM-1 mRNA and protein expression [35]. Moreover, VEGF increases leukocyte

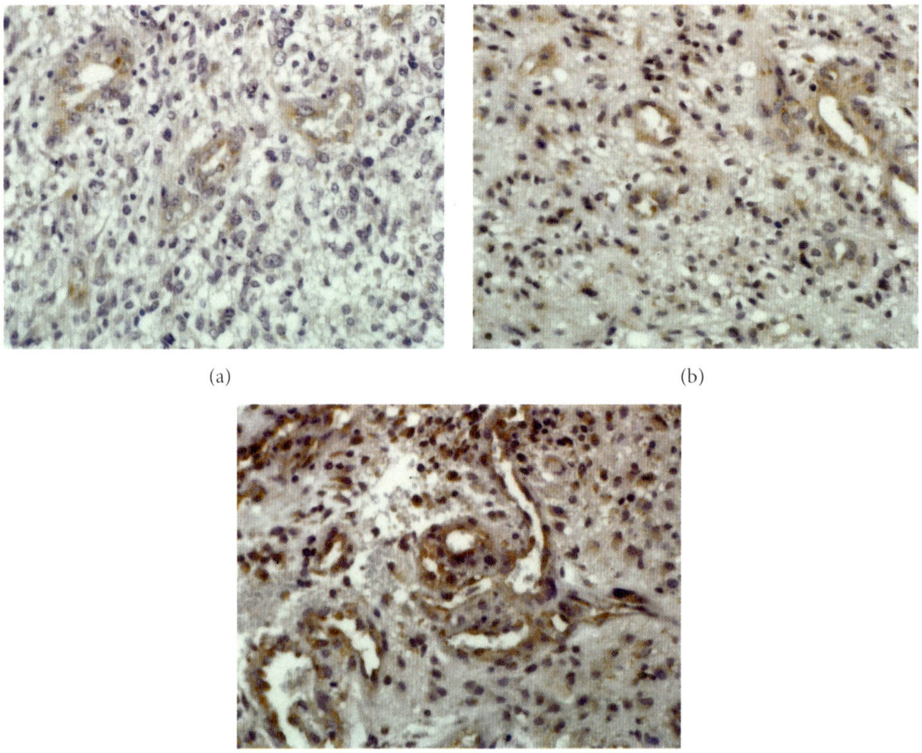

(a) (b) (c)

FIGURE 3: VEGFR-2 expression in GBM blood vessels. Photos illustrate GBM tissues with different endothelial staining intensities of VEGFR-2 in blood vessels (photos represent different patients). (a) Weak (score 1) staining intensity, (b) moderate (score 2) staining intensity, and (c) strong (score 3) staining intensity. Note also the different numbers of VEGFR-2+ blood vessels. Magnification ×40.

adhesiveness to endothelial cells, which is the first step of leukocyte trafficking into inflamed tissue [35]. Next to these effects, VEGF enhances vascular permeability and causes vasodilatation, potentiating thereby inflammation through formation of tissue edema [10, 36]. At the same time, hyperpermeability is also involved in pathological angiogenesis [36]. Additionally, inflammatory and angiogenic processes involve similar cell types. Inflammatory cells, namely, monocytes, macrophages, T lymphocytes, and neutrophils, participate in the angiogenesis by secreting cytokines that affect endothelial cell functions, proliferation, migration, and activation [37]. Macrophages, present in the inflammatory infiltrate, produce a broad array of angiogenic growth factors and cytokines, generate channels for blood flow through proteolytic mechanisms, and promote the remodeling of arterioles into arteries [32]. Inflammatory dentritic cells stimulate similarly angiogenesis by secreting angiogenic factors and cytokines, as well as by promoting proangiogenic activity of T lymphocytes [32]. Previous studies have also shown that proinflammatory cytokines, which are always present in inflamed tissue, mediate also endothelial expression of VEGFR-2 [38, 39]. Later this is also indirectly supported by our findings since positive correlation was found between the extent of VEGFR-2 expression and inflammatory response in GBM tissue.

There are several clinical situations, where inflammatory reaction in GBM may be suppressed. These particularly include the use of anti-inflammatory drugs, such as steroids and nonsteroidal anti-inflammatory drugs (NSAIDs), to manage tumor surrounding inflammation and edema [40]. Whether these very commonly used medicines influence also treatment efficacy of antiangiogenic drugs through diminishing inflammatory response and thereby the expression of VEGFR-2 remains unclear. Nevertheless, our data point toward the possibility that this association might exist. This is also supported by studies where dexamethasone, most frequently used steroid in GBM patients, has been shown to inhibit the effects of proinflammatory cytokines, VEGF mRNA expression, VEGFR-2 expression, and macrophage infiltration [39, 41, 42].

5. Conclusions

In conclusion, our study showed that the expression of VEGFR-2, one of the main targets of antiangiogenic drugs, depends on GBM microenvironment. Importantly, higher endothelial VEGFR-2 levels were seen in the presence of more pronounced inflammation, whereas in less inflamed tissues only weak expression of VEGFR-2 was found. Target dependence on inflammatory tumor microenvironment has to be taken into consideration when treatment approaches that block VEGFR-2 signaling are designed.

Acknowledgment

This work was supported by Estonian Research Council (Grant no. IUT2-4).

References

[1] E. Crocetti, A. Trama, C. Stiller et al., "Epidemiology of glial and non-glial brain tumours in Europe," *European Journal of Cancer*, vol. 48, no. 10, pp. 1532–1542, 2012.

[2] T. A. Dolecek, J. M. Propp, N. E. Stroup, and C. Kruchko, "CBTRUS statistical report: primary brain and central nervous system tumors diagnosed in the United States in 2005–2009," *Neuro-Oncology*, vol. 14, supplement 5, pp. v1–v49, 2012.

[3] C.-H. Lee, K.-W. Jung, H. Yoo, S. Park, and S. H. Lee, "Epidemiology of primary brain and central nervous system tumors in Korea," *Journal of Korean Neurosurgical Society*, vol. 48, no. 2, pp. 145–152, 2010.

[4] R. Stupp, W. P. Mason, M. J. van den Bent et al., "Radiotherapy plus concomitant and adjuvant temozolomide for glioblastoma," *The New England Journal of Medicine*, vol. 352, no. 10, pp. 987–996, 2005.

[5] A. D. Norden, J. Drappatz, and P. Y. Wen, "Antiangiogenic therapies for high-grade glioma," *Nature Reviews Neurology*, vol. 5, no. 11, pp. 610–620, 2009.

[6] K. Seystahl and M. Weller, "Is there a world beyond bevacizumab in targeting angiogenesis in glioblastoma?" *Expert Opinion on Investigational Drugs*, vol. 21, no. 5, pp. 605–617, 2012.

[7] E. Timotheadou, "New agents targeting angiogenesis in glioblastoma," *Chemotherapy Research and Practice*, vol. 2011, Article ID 878912, 8 pages, 2011.

[8] R. Rahman, S. Smith, C. Rahman, and R. Grundy, "Antiangiogenic therapy and mechanisms of tumor resistance in malignant glioma," *Journal of Oncology*, vol. 2010, Article ID 251231, 16 pages, 2010.

[9] M. E. Hardee and D. Zagzag, "Mechanisms of glioma-associated neovascularization," *The American Journal of Pathology*, vol. 181, no. 4, pp. 1126–1141, 2012.

[10] K. Holmes, O. L. Roberts, A. M. Thomas, and M. J. Cross, "Vascular endothelial growth factor receptor-2: structure, function, intracellular signalling and therapeutic inhibition," *Cellular Signalling*, vol. 19, no. 10, pp. 2003–2012, 2007.

[11] L. A. D. Cooper, D. A. Gutman, C. Chisolm et al., "The tumor microenvironment strongly impacts master transcriptional regulators and gene expression class of glioblastoma," *American Journal of Pathology*, vol. 180, no. 5, pp. 2108–2119, 2012.

[12] M. Kase, A. Adamson, M. Saretok et al., "Impact of tumor infiltrating CD63 positive cells on survival in patients with glioblastoma multiforme," *Journal of Neurosurgical Sciences*, In press.

[13] T. N. Kreisl, K. A. McNeill, J. Sul, F. M. Iwamoto, J. Shih, and H. A. Fine, "A phase I/II trial of vandetanib for patients with recurrent malignant glioma," *Neuro-Oncology*, vol. 14, no. 12, pp. 1519–1526, 2012.

[14] T. T. Batchelor, P. Mulholland, B. Neyns et al., "Phase III randomized trial comparing the efficacy of cediranib as monotherapy, and in combination with lomustine, versus lomustine alone in patients with recurrent glioblastoma," *Journal of Clinical Oncology*, vol. 31, no. 26, pp. 3212–3218, 2013.

[15] J. D. Hainsworth, T. Ervin, E. Friedman et al., "Concurrent radiotherapy and temozolomide followed by temozolomide and sorafenib in the first-line treatment of patients with glioblastoma multiforme," *Cancer*, vol. 116, no. 15, pp. 3663–3669, 2010.

[16] E. Pan, D. Yu, B. Yue et al., "A prospective phase II single-institution trial of sunitinib for recurrent malignant glioma," *Journal of Neuro-Oncology*, vol. 110, no. 1, pp. 111–118, 2012.

[17] M. Hutterer, M. Nowosielski, J. Haybaeck et al., "A single-arm phase II Austrian/German multicenter trial on continuous daily sunitinib in primary glioblastoma at first recurrence (SURGE 01-07)," *Neuro-Oncology*, vol. 16, no. 1, pp. 92–102, 2014.

[18] M. R. Gilbert, J. J. Dignam, T. S. Armstrong et al., "A randomized trial of bevacizumab for newly diagnosed glioblastoma," *The New England Journal of Medicine*, vol. 370, no. 8, pp. 699–708, 2014.

[19] O. L. Chinot, W. Wick, W. Mason et al., "Bevacizumab plus radiotherapy-temozolomide for newly diagnosed glioblastoma," *The New England Journal of Medicine*, vol. 370, no. 8, pp. 709–722, 2014.

[20] K. A. Roebuck and A. Finnegan, "Regulation of intercellular adhesion molecule-1 (CD54) gene expression," *Journal of Leukocyte Biology*, vol. 66, no. 6, pp. 876–888, 1999.

[21] C.-C. Chen, "Signal transduction pathways of inflammatory gene expressions and therapeutic implications," *Current Pharmaceutical Design*, vol. 12, no. 27, pp. 3497–3508, 2006.

[22] G. A. Koning, R. M. Schiffelers, and G. Storm, "Endothelial cells at inflammatory sites as target for therapeutic intervention," *Endothelium*, vol. 9, no. 3, pp. 161–171, 2002.

[23] S. Hua, "Targeting sites of inflammation: intercellular adhesion molecule-1 as a target for novel inflammatory therapies," *Frontiers in Pharmacology*, vol. 4, article 127, 2013.

[24] A. K. Hubbard and R. Rothlein, "Intercellular adhesion molecule-1 (ICAM-1) expression and cell signaling cascades," *Free Radical Biology and Medicine*, vol. 28, no. 9, pp. 1379–1386, 2000.

[25] C. Piperi, M. S. Themistocleous, G. A. Papavassiliou et al., "High incidence of MGMT and RARbeta promoter methylation in primary glioblastomas: association with histopathological characteristics, inflammatory mediators and clinical outcome," *Molecular Medicine*, vol. 16, no. 1-2, pp. 1–9, 2010.

[26] M. C. Kuppner, E. van Meir, M. F. Hamou, and N. de Tribolet, "Cytokine regulation of intercellular adhesion molecule-1 (ICAM-1) expression on human glioblastoma cells," *Clinical and Experimental Immunology*, vol. 81, no. 1, pp. 142–148, 1990.

[27] I. Berindan-Neagoe, R. Chiorean, C. Braicu et al., "Quantitative mRNA expression of genes involved in angiogenesis, coagulation and inflammation in multiforme glioblastoma tumoral tissue versus peritumoral brain tissue: lack of correlation with clinical data," *European Cytokine Network*, vol. 23, no. 2, pp. 45–55, 2012.

[28] M.-C. Gingras, E. Roussel, J. M. Bruner, C. D. Branch, and R. P. Moser, "Comparison of cell adhesion molecule expression between glioblastoma multiforme and autologous normal brain tissue," *Journal of Neuroimmunology*, vol. 57, no. 1-2, pp. 143–153, 1995.

[29] A. Meager, "Bioimmunoassays for proinflammatory cytokines involving cytokine-induced cellular adhesion molecule expression in human glioblastoma cell lines," *Journal of Immunological Methods*, vol. 190, no. 2, pp. 235–244, 1996.

[30] E. A. Kuczynski, S. G. Patten, and B. L. Coomber, "VEGFR2 expression and TGF-β signaling in initial and recurrent high-grade human glioma," *Oncology*, vol. 81, no. 2, pp. 126–134, 2011.

[31] H. Huang, J. Held-Feindt, R. Buhl, H. M. Mehdorn, and R. Mentlein, "Expression of VEGF and its receptors in different brain tumors," *Neurological Research*, vol. 27, no. 4, pp. 371–377, 2005.

[32] Z. M. Dong, A. C. Aplin, and R. F. Nicosia, "Regulation of angi-

ogenesis by macrophages, dendritic cells, and circulating myelomonocytic cells," *Current Pharmaceutical Design*, vol. 15, no. 4, pp. 365–379, 2009.

[33] D. N. Granger and E. Senchenkova, "Angiogenesis," in *Inflammation and the Microcirculation*, chapter 6, Morgan & Claypool Life Sciences, San Rafael, Calif, USA, 2010, http://www.ncbi.nlm.nih.gov/books/NBK53377/.

[34] M. Lohela, M. Bry, T. Tammela, and K. Alitalo, "VEGFs and receptors involved in angiogenesis versus lymphangiogenesis," *Current Opinion in Cell Biology*, vol. 21, no. 2, pp. 154–165, 2009.

[35] I. Kim, S.-O. Moon, S. H. Kim, H. J. Kim, Y. S. Koh, and G. Y. Koh, "Vascular endothelial growth factor expression of intercellular adhesion molecule 1 (ICAM-1), vascular cell adhesion molecule 1 (VCAM-1), and E-selectin through nuclear factor-kappa B activation in endothelial cells," *The Journal of Biological Chemistry*, vol. 276, no. 10, pp. 7614–7620, 2001.

[36] J. A. Nagy, L. Benjamin, H. Zeng, A. M. Dvorak, and H. F. Dvorak, "Vascular permeability, vascular hyperpermeability and angiogenesis," *Angiogenesis*, vol. 11, no. 2, pp. 109–119, 2008.

[37] A. Naldini and F. Carraro, "Role of inflammatory mediators in angiogenesis," *Current Drug Targets: Inflammation and Allergy*, vol. 4, no. 1, pp. 3–8, 2005.

[38] J. S. Yao, W. Zhai, W. L. Young, and G.-Y. Yang, "Interleukin-6 triggers human cerebral endothelial cells proliferation and migration: the role for KDR and MMP-9," *Biochemical and Biophysical Research Communications*, vol. 342, no. 4, pp. 1396–1404, 2006.

[39] A. Ristimäki, K. Narko, B. Enholm, V. Joukov, and K. Alitalo, "Proinflammatory cytokines regulate expression of the lymphatic endothelial mitogen vascular endothelial growth factor-C," *Journal of Biological Chemistry*, vol. 273, no. 14, pp. 8413–8418, 1998.

[40] P. Roth, L. Regli, M. Tonder, and M. Weller, "Tumor-associated edema in brain cancer patients: pathogenesis and management," *Expert Review of Anticancer Therapy*, vol. 13, no. 11, pp. 1319–1325, 2013.

[41] K. Narko, B. Enholm, T. Mäkinen, and A. Ristimäki, "Effect of inflammatory cytokines on the expression of the vascular endothelial growth factor-C," *International Journal of Experimental Pathology*, vol. 80, no. 3, pp. 109–112, 1999.

[42] N. Zhang, Z. Fang, P. R. Contag, A. F. Purchio, and D. B. West, "Tracking angiogenesis induced by skin wounding and contact hypersensitivity using a Vegfr2-luciferase transgenic mouse," *Blood*, vol. 103, no. 2, pp. 617–626, 2004.

4

Deciphering Asthma Biomarkers with Protein Profiling Technology

Zhizhou Kuang,[1,2,3] Jarad J. Wilson,[2] Shuhong Luo,[1,2,3] Si-Wei Zhu,[1] and Ruo-Pan Huang[1,2,3]

[1] *RayBiotech, Inc., Guangzhou 510600, China*
[2] *RayBiotech, Inc., 3607 Parkway Lane, Norcross, GA 30092, USA*
[3] *South China Biochip Research Center, Guangzhou 510600, China*

Correspondence should be addressed to Ruo-Pan Huang; rhuang@raybiotech.com

Academic Editor: G. Rogler

Asthma is a chronic inflammatory disease of the airways, resulting in bronchial hyperresponsiveness with every allergen exposure. It is now clear that asthma is not a single disease, but rather a multifaceted syndrome that results from a variety of biologic mechanisms. Asthma is further problematic given that the disease consists of many variants, each with its own etiologic and pathophysiologic factors, including different cellular responses and inflammatory phenotypes. These facets make the rapid and accurate diagnosis (not to mention treatments) of asthma extremely difficult. Protein biomarkers can serve as powerful detection tools in both clinical and basic research applications. Recent endeavors from biomedical researchers have developed technical platforms, such as cytokine antibody arrays, that have been employed and used to further the global analysis of asthma biomarker studies. In this review, we discuss potential asthma biomarkers involved in the pathophysiologic process and eventual pathogenesis of asthma, how these biomarkers are being utilized, and how further testing methods might help improve the diagnosis and treatment strain that current asthma patients suffer.

1. Introduction

1.1. Asthma. Asthma is an increasingly prevalent chronic disease of the conducting airways, affecting the lives of more than 300 million individuals worldwide. Common asthma symptoms include mucus overproduction, episodic airway obstruction, bronchial hyperreactivity (BHR), and reduced lung function. The disease has higher prevalence in wealthier communities compared to more impoverished areas, with 8–10% of adults and children being affected. This high disease prevalence leads to considerable morbidity and also causes significant economic burden on the affected families [1, 2]. This increased economic burden is estimated to cost more than $18 billion dollars annually in the US alone with regard to both direct medical bills and indirect productivity losses [3]. Given current trends in disease development, asthma could affect over 400 million people by 2025 if no further interventions are developed [1, 2].

Traditionally asthma is divided into two phenotypes based on the potential disease trigger, allergic asthma, or nonallergic asthma. Children are predominantly affected by allergic (extrinsic) asthma, while roughly 50% of adults have allergic asthma. Allergic asthma is typically characterized by high serum levels of IgE and predominantly type 2 $CD4^+$ helper T cell (Th2) response [4]. This type of asthma begins generally with itching, shortness of breath, and inflammation of the lungs, often leading to rhinitis and worse asthma symptoms over the course of many allergen exposures [5]. Instead, nonallergic (intrinsic) asthma often arises later in life and is not generally associated with high levels of antiallergen IgE. Intrinsic asthma is more associated with disease or stress factors like obesity, anxiety, strenuous exercise, and even cold air. Given the noninflammatory nature of nonallergic asthma, it is generally much more difficult to treat, as steroids and other common therapies are not as effective as they are with asthma caused by environmental and immunological triggers [6].

Recent work over the last two decades has given the community increased understanding of the pathophysiological nature of asthma, leading to better classification of the disease into groups called endotypes [7]. These endotypes are characterized by multiple disease related factors including the clinical nature of disease, genetic susceptibility, environmental risk factors, and the age of disease onset [6]. The heterogeneity of asthma is therefore increasingly suggesting that asthma itself is more of a syndrome, rather than a single disease [8]. This heterogeneous disease type, however, makes early and accurate diagnosis of asthma increasingly difficult. Currently, the main means of disease confirmation relies on tests of overall pulmonary function (spirometry), yet this method is limited as there is a high degree of variability in the extent of airway obstruction within patient groups. Furthermore, measurements of lung function can reflect the pathological seriousness of disease but may not correspond precisely with different disease endotypes, creating only a partial snapshot of the patient's disease.

Treatment for asthma generally consists of systemic steroids, a method that has been employed for over 30 years. However, not all asthmatics respond to this generalized treatment, further highlighting the nature of such a heterogeneous disease. When considering the high cost and undesired side effects of steroidal therapies, there is a need for better endotype screening that affords better targeted treatments with more improved patient outcomes [9, 10]. Protein biomarkers have recently been explored and discovered for a number of diseases, and these markers have great advantages in clinical diagnoses, disease progression prediction, and personalized treatment. Given that these markers are often isolated and detected from noninvasive means (serum, plasma, urine, etc.) which limit the need for costly operations or surgeries, they could be performed alongside more historical tests providing more complete diagnostic profile of the patient. In fact, many biomarkers are already in use for the diagnosis and treatment of cardiovascular disease and certain cancers, as well as other complex disease states. With the progress the community has made over the past 25 years in understanding the cellular and molecular mechanisms of asthma disease, more asthma biomarkers could be just around the corner.

1.2. Biomarker. As with most diseases, the early, rapid, and accurate assessment of a patient's condition drastically improves long-term prognosis and/or survival. In order to provide a more accurate assessment of an individual's disease condition/state, a comprehensive and accurate medical diagnosis is needed, and asthma is no different. Such a specific diagnostic test for asthma should allow for a more accurately defined disease phenotype, with the ultimate goal of leading to more targeted therapies and accurate prognosis. With this goal in mind, biomarkers, defined as measurable indicators that can define a biological state such as a disease, infection, or environmental exposure, have attracted huge attention in both basic research and clinical studies. There are many types of biomarkers for a variety of disease pathways, some of which are even accepted by the medical community as standard means of disease detection. Other potential biomarkers, like microRNAs, are rapidly emerging as powerful markers for disease biology [11, 12]. Currently published biomarkers include microRNAs, small biological metabolites, presence/absence of cellular populations, or levels of various molecules or enzymes within a known sample.

Given their constant variation during disease development and progression, proteins provide a rich potential biomarker pool for disease identification [13]. Proteins can even provide multiple levels of disease information as they can be differentially expressed and processed during different disease states. By measuring changes in protein levels during any biological state, we can directly compare healthy states to various disease states, gathering a wealth of information on how these proteins change over the course of disease. This unique insight can show whether increased or decreased expression levels are present or whether there is a deviation of the norm which might indicate a divergence in the patient's condition. For example, C reactive protein (CRP) is a particularly valuable biomarker of inflammation which is overexpressed during inflammatory responses caused by an infection, by autoimmune diseases like lupus and RA, or in some cancers [14].

Secondly, differential protein processing, like changes to protein folding or protein glycosylation, can deviate from normal posttranslational modifications during disease. Tau aggregation into paired helical filaments in Alzheimer's disease (AD) and other tauopathies is associated with increased Tau protein phosphorylation in the brain [15]. Similarly, the development of antibodies to self-proteins, as seen with autoantibodies against rheumatoid factor (RF) in RA, can be another molecule to identify disease development and progression. Each of these can serve or have served as valuable markers of disease states and highlight the unique insight that proteins can provide to biological pathways and for diagnostic purposes.

The application of biomarkers is not applicable solely to the clinical diagnostic and prognostic fields but is also of great interest to the basic biology of disease, as these markers can also serve to evaluate drug toxicity and efficacy. Through 2012, the FDA has approved 23 protein tumor biomarkers for clinical use, of which 9 are used in different tumor diagnosis, 6 are for monitoring disease progression, and 5 are for prediction of response to therapies. 24 biomarkers were approved in 2007 for drug evaluation and research, including various effects related to toxicity and therapeutic effect (http://www.fda.org/). Biomarker approval has slowed in recent years, however, even while preclinical research and clinic trial studies continue to identify them and put them to use. Given this decline, it has been hypothesized that the "low hanging" biomarkers have already been found. These early biomarkers were easier to find as they were single protein associated with a given disease such as RF. Biomarkers to come will more likely be more complex, with multiple proteins or other molecules involved in various disease states, rather than a single marker. This multifactorial complexity will therefore require a new tool that can simultaneously measure multiple factors within a single sample.

1.3. Cytokines. Cytokines are among the most intensely studied protein families as they possess a myriad of local and systemic functions and also offer vast potential applications in biomedicine. In addition to playing critical roles in many normal cellular events, cytokines are also noted to be involved in the initiation, development, and progression of pathologies, from the innocuous to the life-threatening. For this reason, cytokines have long been explored and studied as potential disease biomarkers.

Cytokines are secreted proteins that generate or transmit cell-cell signals. These proteins include interferons, interleukins, chemokines, growth and differentiation factors, pro- and antiangiogenic factors, adipokines, adhesive molecules, and extracellular matrix proteins. Cytokines play a critical role in a number of cellular and bodily functions, from homeostasis, growth, and wound healing to inflammation, immunity, and angiogenesis [16–23]. Given their wide ranging role in the body, it is no surprise that cytokines have been associated with cancer, diabetes, and autoimmune and infectious diseases. It has been suggested that chronic inflammation plays a key role in neurodegenerative diseases, such as Alzheimer's and Parkinson's diseases, insulin resistance and type 2 diabetes, atherosclerosis, and other cardiovascular diseases [16, 24–27].

Typically, cytokines function as a complex network of specifically controlled signaling pathways. Their individual and even global signals are modulated by each other through cytokine specific receptors. Many cytokines are pleiotropic, meaning that a single cytokine may induce a wide range of effects in various cell and tissue types [28]. Interleukin-6 (IL-6), for example, acts as proinflammatory factor to stimulate macrophages and generate a Type 1 helper T cell response but can also act as an anti-inflammatory cytokine through its inhibitory effects on levels of TNF-alpha, IL-1, and its activation of IL-1ra and IL-10 [29]. This pleiotropic nature often leads as well to cytokine redundancy, wherein multiple cytokines have similar effects on a single cell type. For example, IL-4, IL-5, and IL-13 have similar activities to induce the differentiation of Th2 cells [28]. Some of the redundant nature of cytokines and their signaling events are due to the homology within the protein sequences or the use of the same or similar receptor types, each generating the same signaling pathways upon cytokine binding. However, other cytokines share minimal sequence homology but still result in similar downstream signaling events, possibly due to converging signaling pathways or differential distribution of cellular receptors on the target cells [30].

A number of approved disease treatments actually work via specific cytokine pathways, either targeting cytokines directly for activation/blockade or through the use of recombinant cytokines in an effort to create a specific response within the patient. These treatments include growth factors like epithelial growth factor receptor (EGFR) which is overexpressed in many tumors [31], tumor necrosis factor alpha (TNFα) which is a key proinflammatory protein in many autoimmune diseases [32], interferon-alpha (IFNα) which is used to treat chronic viral hepatitis [33], and AIDS-related Kaposi's Sarcoma [34], to name a few. Because of the complexity of cytokine biology, single cytokine analysis and evaluation is becoming limiting for its ability to diagnose, evaluate, and treat diseases, requiring more multiplex cytokine platforms to be used to consider the complexity of disease involving multiple cytokine perturbations.

2. Biomarker Discovery in Asthma

Typically during an asthmatic response, inflammation in the airway epithelium plays a central role in disease symptoms and progression. This lining acts as the primary interface between host and any environmental stimulus causing the allergic hyperresponsiveness, be it from microbes, particles, pollutants, and oxidants. These environmental insults trigger pathogen recognition receptors and/or already generated specific antibodies, stimulating the production of inflammatory cytokines and chemokines. Pollutants and oxidants on the other hand generally stimulate an inflammatory response via their direct impact on cells or the function of proteins, lipids, and nucleic acids, together resulting in cellular stress and injury [35–38]. In patients with asthma, persistent inflammatory stimuli modulate the functions of the airway epithelium, with both the innate and adaptive immune systems, further augmenting the development of a chronic allergic response. Once advanced enough, bronchial hyperreactivity (BHR) (the tendency of smooth muscle cells in people with asthma to react to nonspecific stimuli such as cold air and exercise), mucus overproduction, airway wall remodeling, and airway narrowing develop over the course of chronic exposure [39].

The immunohistopathologic features of asthma include epithelial injury and the infiltration of inflammatory cells, generally the eosinophils, mast cells, and lymphocytes into the lung. The adaptive immune response that develops is typically polarized to a Th2 $CD4^+$ T cell response, characterized by elevated expression of IL-4, IL-8, and IL-10. This T cell polarization preferentially promotes B cell activation and antibody production favoring the allergic IgE and IgG isotypes. The resulting elevation in serum IgE and corresponding increases in infiltrating eosinophils, basophils, and mast cells are all prototypical hallmarks of atopic asthmatics [3, 39]. However, since heightened serum IgE levels are also seen in nonasthma related hypersensitivities, sera IgE levels may not be a suitable asthma biomarker when considered alone [40]. Therefore, it is necessary to look for surrogate biomarkers of this asthma endotype. As outlined in Table 1, cytokines released by the epithelium and the populations and numbers of activated inflammatory cells are of most interest (in terms of biomarkers) for asthma studies, because they recruit inflammatory cells to the airways and alter the activation state of airway resident cells [41].

Data collected from people with asthma and also in mouse models of asthma driven by inhalation of the model antigen ovalbumin (OVA) have shown that IL-4, IL-5, and

Table 1: Cytokines as biomarkers in asthma explored in these years.

Cytokine targets	Typical physiologic functions	Potential application	Sample source
IL-4	Activating Th2 immunity; priming the vessel wall for eosinophil extravasations	Diagnosis, therapeutic	Tissue, sputum, BALF, serum
IL-5	Promoting eosinophilia	Diagnosis, therapeutic	Tissue, sputum, BALF, serum
IL-13	Mounting BHR, goblet cell metaplasia	Diagnosis, therapeutic	Tissue, sputum, BALF, serum
IL-25	Activating innate lymphoid cells	Diagnosis, therapeutic	Tissue, sputum, BALF, serum
IL-33	Activating innate lymphoid cells	Diagnosis, therapeutic	Tissue, sputum, BALF, serum
TSLP	Activating dendritic cells and promoting Th2 immunity	Diagnosis, therapeutic	Tissue, serum
Eotaxin-1/CCL11	Eosinophil chemotaxis	Diagnosis, prediction	Tissue, sputum, BALF
Eotaxin-2/CCL24	Eosinophil chemotaxis	Diagnosis	Tissue, sputum, BALF
Eotaxin-3/CCL26	Eosinophil chemotaxis	Diagnosis	Blood, tissue
MCP-4/CCL13	Chemoattractant for eosinophils, monocytes, lymphocytes, and basophils	Diagnosis, prediction	Sputum, BALF, plasma
IL-9	Promoting IL-4-driven antibody, inducing goblet cell metaplasia	Diagnosis, therapeutic	Tissue, serum
CCL17	Recruitment of Th2 cells	Diagnosis, prediction	Sputum, serum

IL-13 have potential to serve as an allergic asthma biomarker profile. Pulmonary Th2 polarization has long been considered as a typical characteristic of allergic asthma, which has been supported by studies with bronchoalveolar lavage (BAL) fluid, bronchial biopsies, and sputum from asthmatic patients [42–45]. Patients with mild-to-moderate asthma present with elevated levels of IL-4 and IL-5 in BAL fluid, and pulmonary isolates found elevated numbers of CD4+ T cells and a high degree of airway eosinophilia [46]. Careful enumeration of the levels of IL-4, IL-5, and IL-13 together and the levels of eosinophils in serum and tissue can classify asthma endotypes into $Th2^{hi}$ and $Th2^{lo}$ subsets [40, 47].

Mouse models of asthma support the roles of IL-4, IL-5, and IL-13 in disease development, as knockout mice for these cytokines show reduction in overall asthma symptoms [48]. In mice, IL-4 is necessary for the development of Th2 CD4 T cell response, the resulting IgG1 and IgE antibodies to OVA (the allergen stimulus), and also for priming the vessel wall for eosinophil extravasation [48, 49]. IL-4 also results in the priming and activation of basophils and mast cells, resulting in further release of inflammatory histamines and leukotrienes, further exacerbating and extending the chronic disease.

IL-13 has been reported to play an indispensable role in mounting bronchial hyperreactivity (BHR) and goblet cell hyperplasia, caused by elevated expression of the mucin proteins MUC5AC and MUC5B, leading ultimately to mucus overproduction and airway obstruction [50, 51]. In moderate-to-severe asthmatic patients with a high level of hematic eosinophilia, treatment with a monoclonal therapy that modulates the signaling of IL-4 receptor (dupilumab; Regeneron Pharmaceuticals), lung function was dramatically improved. With this treatment, the frequency of atopic dermatitis exacerbations was also reduced significantly, so that the drug received Breakthrough Therapy Designation from the FDA in 2014 [52]. Similar effects were seen from lebrikizumab (Genentech), an antibody blocking IL-13 in humans with $Th2^{hi}$ endotype asthma [53]. Lastly, IL-5 promotes trafficking and maintenance of eosinophils within the lung tissue by directly recruiting eosinophils from the circulation and also promoting eosinophil differentiation from the bone marrow. A humanized monoclonal antibody that blocks IL-5 from signaling its receptor (mepolizumab; GlaxoSmithKline) has completed Phase III trials and is awaiting FDA and European clearance for patients with severe eosinophilic asthma [54]. When IL-5 was blocked, improvements in airway remodeling were seen and this improvement occurred alongside decreased eosinophils accumulation, further implying an exacerbating role for both IL-5 and the levels of eosinophils in the lungs [55].

Eosinophil induces BHR directly through eosinophil peroxidase and the resulting increases in inflammatory chloride and bromide ions, both significantly affecting airway remodeling during allergen exposures. Together with the antigen presenting nature of dendritic cells, the adaptive immune response is primed to respond to repeat antigen insult and airway hyperreactivity ensues. Eosinophil knockout mouse models of asthma have confirmed this cell population's role in contributing to airway wall remodeling and subepithelial membrane thickening [56, 57]. Eosinophilia in lung tissue is driven partially by the recruitment of eosinophils to the lung mucosa and interstitium due to airway produced IL-5, as well as production of eotaxin (CCL11), eotaxin-2 (CCL24), and eotaxin-3 (CCL26) [58, 59]. Eotaxins are CC chemokine with high specificity for eosinophils populations given this cell types preferential expression of eotaxin receptors, CCR2, CCR3, and CCR5. Eotaxins were first discovered from the purification of BAL fluid taken from allergen-challenged, sensitized guinea pigs, and, after their discovery, they were quickly identified in mouse and humans as well [60, 61].

In animal models of pulmonary allergic inflammation, eosinophil accumulation correlates with local eotaxin generation and differentiation, increased recruitment of eosinophils from circulation, and the rapid proliferation of eosinophils within the bone marrow [62, 63]. Increased expression of eotaxin at sites of allergic inflammation has been observed in both atopic asthmatics and nonatopic asthmatics and is also seen at increased levels in patient sputum [64–67]. Even in occupational asthmatics, increased eotaxin mRNA levels have been reported in sputum leukocytes, and Nakamura et al. have reported a correlation between eotaxin levels and compromised lung function in asthmatic patients [68, 69]. Similarly, patients with acute asthma are reported to display significantly higher plasma eotaxin levels compared to those with stable asthma [70].

There are also two functional homologues of eotaxin, eotaxin-2, and eotaxin-3, which show 40% homology to eotaxin at the amino acid level and also possess similar eosinophil-selective properties via CCR3 signaling [71, 72]. In assays of eosinophil chemotaxis, eotaxin and eotaxin-2 exhibit similar potencies in their ability to recruit eosinophils. Increased eotaxin-2 mRNA levels have been reported in bronchial biopsies taken from atopic and nonatopic asthmatics [65]. The chemotactic role of eotaxin-3 is less clear as there are contradictory results between various studies. In one investigation, eotaxin-3 shows only around 10% of the activity as eotaxin [72]; however, a more recent study by Provost et al. found that eotaxin-3 is a more effective chemoattractant than eotaxin and eotaxin-2 for eosinophils, specifically in asthmatics when compared to healthy volunteers [73]. Individually or collectively, these eosinophil chemokines could prove to be potential biomarkers for diagnosis and prognosis of asthmatic featured with eosinophilia, especially if eotaxin profiles between asthmatic patient groups can be identified.

Allergen induced expression of monocyte chemoattractant protein-4 (MCP-4; CCL-1) within asthmatic airways has also been shown recently as a potential biomarker [74]. MCP-4 signals through several receptors, including CCR2, CCR-3, and CCR5 and is a potent chemoattractant for asthma related cell populations including eosinophils, monocytes, and basophils [65, 75, 76]. MCP-4 signaling induces the release of histamine from IL-3-primed basophils and activates eosinophil respiratory burst. During allergic inflammation, MCP-4 levels are significantly elevated in asthmatic sputum, BAL fluid, and respiratory epithelium and within the cells that line the airways [77, 78]. Following allergen induced challenge, TNFα and IL-1β trigger the release of MCP-4 from the epithelium and endothelial cells that are inflamed, which in turn facilitates the recruitment of other types of asthma inducing inflammatory cells and the cytokines they produce.

The exacerbating role of MCP-4 expression in asthma has recently been supported by a large scale asthma study. Using 240 normal subjects, 356 chronic-stable asthma patients, and 30 patients who required emergency asthma treatments, the study found that plasma levels of MCP-4 in chronic-stable asthma patients compared to normal patients were significantly higher (399 pg/mL versus 307 pg/mL) [74]. Additionally, MCP-4 levels > 218 pg/mL marked a patient group at increased risk of developing asthma ($P < 0.001$ odds ratio). In acute asthma patients, MCP-4 levels were even higher during an exacerbation event when compared to chronic but stable asthma sufferers (513 versus 355 pg/mL). In conclusion, systemic levels of MCP-4 could prove an excellent asthma biomarker that can predict susceptibility to asthma, the severity of asthma exacerbations, and therefore potentially the efficacy of asthma control medicines.

Another potent cytokine which is released by inflamed epithelium and has been linked with asthma exacerbations is thymic stromal lymphopoietin (TSLP). TSLP is required to mount a normal CD4 T cell response where it acts directly on naive, but not, memory CD4 T cells, promoting their proliferation in response to cognate antigen [79]. However, TSLP's interaction with dendritic cell populations favors the polarization of primed CD4 T cells into Th2 phenotype [80, 81]. TSLP induces key changes in dendritic cells, such that, during antigen ligation to cognate T cells, DCs also are promoted to express the chemokine ligands 17 (CCL17) and CCL22, as well as inducing surface expression of OX40 12 ligand [81, 82]. In concert with other epithelial-derived inflammatory cytokines, such as TNFα and IL-1β, TSLP also activates mast cells which in turn can produce cytokines that increase the preferentially progression of Th2 polarization [41]. In mice genetically lacking the TSLP receptor, Th1 responses are elevated, including cytokine increases in levels of interleukin- (IL-) 12, interferon-γ, and immunoglobulin G2a (IgG2a), and also show lower expression of Th2 cytokines like IL-4, IL-5, IL-10, and IL-13. Furthermore, TSLPR KO mice challenged with inhaled antigen exhibit reduced pulmonary inflammation, a result that could be restored if wild type CD4 T cells were added back [80]. Reversion of pulmonary inflammation suggests that TSLP also can act directly on CD4 T cells during an inflammatory response. Collectively TSLP seems to play an important role in the development of allergic airway responses, and monitoring its levels in patient samples could provide another disease biomarker [83].

While IgE levels in atopic asthmatics can be a valuable disease indicator, IL-25 and IL-33 may be better surrogate biomarkers of both asthmatic disease and even disease stratification. In response to airway injury or allergen stimulation, epithelial cells can produce IL-25 and IL-33, which in turn can act on nearby innate lymphoid cells [84]. The innate populations receive these signals and can initiate degranulation of their cytokine and chemokine loaded granules, releasing additional allergen exacerbating factors. These cytokines include TSLP, IL-4, IL-5, and IL-9, all classical Th2 polarizing cytokines, and all cytokines that significantly affect the development of pulmonary inflammation. Interestingly, this same population is capable of producing these same Th2 cytokines (IL-5, IL-9, and IL-13) in response to mice infected with helminthes, promoting an eosinophilic gut response and enhanced mucus production [85]. These derived innate lymphoid cells resemble Th2 polarized CD4 T cells but do not express an antigen specific receptor [86–88]. It may be these cells that are responsible for the ability of RAG KO mice (i.e., mice lacking T and B cells) to generate a potent Th2-like allergic response and eosinophilia independent of any adaptive immune response. Data suggests that these cells originally develop from common lymphoid progenitors, and, following their initial allergen exposure, they can rapidly be activated to induce the features of atopic asthma following antigen reexposure [89].

IL-9 has also been recently evaluated for its use as an asthma biomarker given its heightened expression in the lungs of asthmatic patients. IL-9 functions in multiple potential asthmatic roles, from promoting mast cell growth and development to initiating IL-4 expression and subsequent B cell production of allergic antibodies [90, 91]. Mouse models of asthma have highlighted the role of IL-9, as treatment of asthmatic mice with neutralizing antibodies to IL-9 significantly alleviates symptoms [92, 93]. This blockade treatment also reduced the levels of airway remodeling which occurs during chronic asthma and also reduced the levels of infiltrating mast cells into the inflamed tissue [90]. Recent evidence suggests that IL-9 may arise from the aforementioned innate lymphoid cell population, and not directly from T cells [94, 95]. However, the contribution(s) of IL-9 to asthmatic disease, either from the innate or adaptive cell populations, remains to be determined. While the alleviation seen in mouse models of anti-IL-9 treatment provides a glimpse of promise for potential treatments and disease monitoring, this therapeutic effect has not yet been fully evaluated in asthmatic patients [96].

Many other novel biomarkers for asthma are potentially available from the current literature, as well as ongoing studies. For example, CCL-17 (TARC) is a dendritic and epithelial cell derived cytokine that is initially released upon allergen contact. CCL-17 is a potent chemoattractant for CCR4 expressing Th2 cells which then feed forward into the allergen derived inflammatory response. Recent studies found that CCL-17 levels were significantly elevated in asthmatic patient sputum and also were elevated in serum samples from children suffering from asthma [97, 98]. Interestingly CCL-17 could also serve as an indicator of treatment efficacy, as its levels significantly decline following steroidal treatment [98].

Cytokine biomarkers therefore hold significant promise for their potential ability to predict, diagnose, and monitor asthmatic disease. Because of the underlying heterogeneity of the asthmatic phenotypes and the general complexity of cytokine biology, examination of a single biomarker, or even a small handful of molecules, to detect and/or treat asthmatic patients is unrealistic. With their ability to be quantified in noninvasive sample types, like serum, sputum, or even exhaled breath condensates, cytokines could complement current diagnostic and monitoring measures to give a more complete profile of patient disease. Combining these two methods of patient analysis, comparisons between healthy and diseased patients may better help stratify potential biomarkers to their respective disease states.

3. New Discovery in Asthma by Antibody Array Technology

3.1. Antibody Arrays Technology. Traditionally, the measurement of cytokine/protein mediators involves the use of bioassays, enzyme assays, or immunoassays. Since these are single target assays where simultaneous detection of other targets is not possible, the use of these assays requires a sizeable amount of sample and/or budget. Also, the investigator must already have a fairly specific hypothesized protein biomarker to evaluate. This makes true discovery of the unknown increasingly difficult. If the initially chosen markers are not differentially present in established sample groups (especially small sample groups), entire sample sets or experiments may be abandoned, all while some combination of these markers with others may remain undiscovered.

In the past twenty years, the discovery, characterization, and application of biomarkers in clinical and the basic research fields have exploded with a number of critical advancements and findings. Through the availability of DNA sequencing technologies, the completion of the Human Genome Project, and genetic sequencing platforms, the comprehensive and rapid detection of genes in a sample is now possible. High-throughput gene microarray technology has greatly expanded the ability to define nucleic acid biomarkers of disease within a single sample, and the same is now coming true with protein biomarkers. Protein microarrays have been adapted from DNA microarray platforms and now offer the ability to do multiplex protein biomarker discovery and to do so in a high-throughput manner. These protein arrays, also known as antibody arrays or antibody microarrays, are one of the most promising platforms to break through the single biomarker bottleneck that the field is currently stuck in.

The design principle of antibody arrays is usually based on either a sandwich based ELISA immunoassay or a direct-labeling of target proteins approach. Similar to common single target sandwich ELISA platforms, multiplex antibody array platforms utilize an antibody pair, where a capture antibody is immobilized on the surface of glass slides or nitrocellulose membranes and is paired with a labeled target specific detection antibody in solution (Figure 1(a)). This method has the advantages of excellent specificity and sensitivity given the dual binding requirements for target signal detection. The capture antibody is specific for one region of the target protein, while the detection antibody recognizes a different region of the target, combining to remove almost all potential for epitope cross-reactivity. However, the combinations and the number of protein targets to be measured in each array are limited because of cross-reactivity between detection antibodies within a single array. To overcome this restriction, multiple independent arrays with panels of nonoverlapping and cross-reactivity compatible antibody pairs can be employed to allow increasing numbers of cytokines to be measured [99].

Alternatively, label-based strategies can be employed to remove the need for a detection antibody and to dramatically increase the size of the potential array [100]. In the label based method, the sample itself is directly labeled with some substrate that can later be measured (biotin for example), while the capture antibody is still arrayed onto the solid surface (Figure 1(b)). In this case, there is an increase in sensitivity, as the dual binding requirement is removed, but there is a simultaneous loss in some of the specificity seen with a standard detection pair from a sandwich ELISA format. With only a single antibody required for target

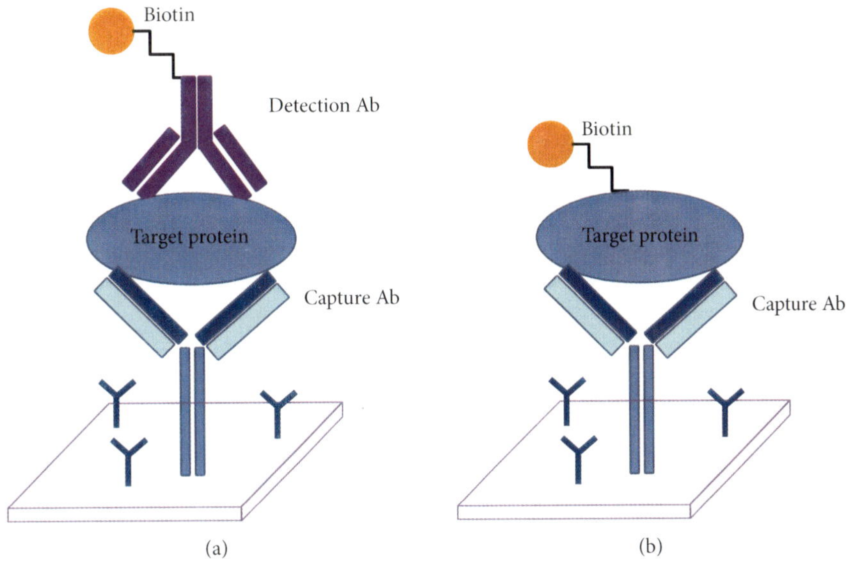

FIGURE 1: The principle employed in most antibody arrays. (a) The sandwich method which requires an immobilized capture antibody and a labeled detection antibody. (b) Direct-label method with capture antibody and labeled analyte.

detection, label based techniques are especially useful for small peptides/molecules or for more novel proteins for which an antibody pair may not be available. Both of these platform types have been extensively published in the discovery and analysis of disease biomarkers and offer the largest simultaneous arrays available on the market [101, 102].

Glass slide based arrays provide several advantages in comparison with membrane based or 96-well based multiplex platforms. The capability to spot the target antibody with a diameter of <200 μm allows glass based antibody arrays to be much smaller in size and require less sample for target detection, while also allowing them to be robotically printed in mass quantities suitable for high-throughput analysis [103]. Another advantage of the glass slide support format is the use of fluorescence as a signal readout. Fluorescence detection affords a much larger linear range of signal detection and superior signal stability over the long term when compared to chemiluminescent detection technologies [103–105]. This platform is being promoted and explored by a number of companies including RayBiotech, Abcam, Sigma-Aldrich, R&D Systems, Full Moon Biosystems, Gentel, Whatman, Aushon, MesoScale, and Quansys. These powerful platforms have been extensively published in recent years since their development in the early 2000s and have also been comprehensively applied in preclinical and basic research for biomarker discovery [106–109].

3.2. New Discovery of Asthma Biomarkers by Antibody Array Technology. The application of antibody arrays in biomarker discovery has allowed significant progress on a number of disease fronts, including cancer, neurodegeneration, cardiovascular disease, as well as in asthma. As previously described, the complex biology of asthma syndrome has linked a number of cytokines and chemokines as potential disease biomarkers. Additional asthma biomarker limitations are due to a number of single target cytokine biomarker studies that have been of limited use or yielded incomplete definition of disease after further evaluation. This is where multiplex analysis has such a broad appeal as it affords a large nonbiased look at large numbers of proteins within a sample and can include a broad array of protein factors. Published biomarkers that have been explored and/or discovered with antibody arrays have been partially compiled in Table 2. It is of note that antibody arrays have both confirmed the previously suggested biomarkers in a number of studies and also unveiled a number of novel biomarkers as well.

Recently, Patil et al. used antibody arrays to study the serological profiles from nonsmokers with moderate and severe persistent asthma to sera of nonasthmatic healthy controls. Using a 50-target protein multiplex array which included detection of cytokines, chemokines, and growth factors, this group found that several proteins could serve as potential disease biomarkers (notably, FGF, HGF, and SCGFβ) for the moderate and severe asthma groups. Furthermore, these same biomarkers in addition to IL-18 were found to positively correlate with poor asthmatic control and were associated negatively with quality of life scores [110]. With the hopes of identifying critically important inflammatory molecules in COPD and asthma, Kim et al. analyzed asthma sputum samples with a 79 target multiplex array. Among the tested cytokines, asthmatic patient sputum displayed significantly elevated levels of CXCL1, eotaxin-2, and CCL18. Interestingly, the levels of CCL18 correlated significantly with the overall levels of eosinophils in the sputum sample, which is a significant marker of underlying disease [111]. This might allow for a noninvasive and novel diagnostic measurement of patient disease from a simple sputum sample and also further highlights a role of CCL18 in asthmatic disease.

Given the influx of inflammatory cells into the lungs during asthmatic exacerbations, noninvasive sputum samples could allow for biomarker detection of the underlying

TABLE 2: Cytokine biomarkers in asthma explored by using antibody array technology.

Authors [reference]	Cytokine panels	Potential application	Sample source
Patil et al. [110]	Interleukin-18, FGF, HGF, and SCGFβ	Diagnosis, prediction	Serum
Kim et al. [111]	GROα/CXCL1, Eotaxin-2/CCL24, and PARC/CCL18	Diagnosis, therapeutic	Sputum
Hastie et al. [112]	BDNF, IL-1b, and MCP 3a/CCL20	Prediction	Sputum
Matsunaga et al. [113, 114]	RANTES/CCL5, TNFα and TGFβ1	Therapeutic evaluation	Exhaled breath condensate (EBC)
Nakamura et al. [115]	TNF-α and RANTES	Diagnosis	BALF
Matsunaga et al. [116]	IL-4 and RANTES	Diagnosis, prediction	Exhaled breath condensate (EBC)
Simcock et al. [117]	Angiogenin, VEGF, and MCP-1	Diagnosis, therapeutic	BALF

inflammation within the lungs. This hypothesis was tested by Hastie et al. using inflammatory antibody arrays in a cohort of asthma patients in the Severe Asthma Research Program. Sputum samples indicated that elevated levels of eosinophil and neutrophil counts were associated with decreased lung function and elevated cytokine levels of brain-derived neurotrophic factor, IL-1b, and macrophage inflammatory protein 3a/CCL20 were associated with increased disease severity and were also linked to the increased neutrophil counts [112]. Similarly Matsunaga et al. have also shown a strong correlation between RANTES (CCL5) levels and FEV_1, as well as expression levels of TNFα and TGFβ1 with BHR [113, 114]. In addition, the expression level of these cytokines was also positively and specifically correlated with the disease symptoms and disease severity in asthmatic patients.

A very unique study and sample type was recently undertaken by Nakamura et al. Using exhaled breath condensates (EBC), this group compared this novel sample type to the invasive BAL fluid samples taken from asthmatic patients [115]. They found that levels of cytokines in the EBC, including TNF-α and RANTES, significantly correlate with those presented in the patient's BAL fluid. BAL collection in patients is an extremely unpleasant and invasive procedure requiring the flushing of patient's lungs with fluid. However, EBC could afford a nontraumatic sample type that is much more easily obtained and also more economically viable for patient disease monitoring. The authors also noted a correlation of the levels of TNF-α and RANTES in EBC samples with the levels of lymphocytes eventually extracted from the BAL isolates. Lung lymphocyte counts are one of the critical indicators associated with asthmatic disease states, so EBC measurements might allow yet another option for diagnostic disease monitoring.

Along these same experimental lines, Matusunaga's group also used a large antibody array to monitor the cytokine profiles of asthmatic patients undergoing corticosteroid treatment [116]. Patients treated with corticosteroids showed decreased levels of CXCL10 and increased levels of IL-4 and RANTES compared to untreated controls, and these changes correlated to improved FEV_1 and overall airway obstruction. These findings strongly suggest that IL-4 and RANTES levels in EBC could not only be applied as predictive biomarkers for the success of steroidal therapies but also mark cytokines with potential as therapeutic targets during disease intervention and monitoring.

Like applications in other diseases, inflammatory antibody arrays have also been explored during the evaluation of drugs for disease efficacy and other disease indicators. Antibody arrays have even been used to study homeopathic remedies against asthmatic disease, like in the case of the antiasthmatic effect of mangiferin. Mangiferin is a major bioactive ingredient in *Mangifera indica* Linn. leaves and is currently used as an indigenous remedy for respiratory diseases in traditional Chinese medicine. To study mangiferin's effects, the authors used a mouse allergen model (Ova model) to evaluate the levels of Th1/Th2 cytokine profiles during disease. Mangiferin treatment reduced the inflammatory cell influx of eosinophils, reduced the BAL fluid levels of PGD2, and reduced the levels of serum ovalbumin specific IgE [118]. Antibody array analysis confirmed the downregulation of Th2 related cytokines (IL-4, IL-5, and IL-13), and even the upregulation of Th1 promoting cytokines like IFN-γ, IL-2, and IL-12 during mangiferin treatment. These results suggest mangiferin's potential as an antiasthmatic therapy and might also suggest its potential route of action, since the treatment resulted in conversion of allergic Th2 response into a more nonallergenic Th1 type response. These inflammatory array panels, or even more broad panels, could be used to monitor other antiasthmatic drugs for disease outcome, progression, and efficacy.

While targeted inflammatory antibody arrays may seem to be the most obvious candidates for asthmatic disease analysis, other arrays also have shown promise in asthma biomarker studies. Several studies have shown that asthmatic airways have an increased number and size of vascular structures, which contribute to airflow obstruction and hyperresponsiveness [119–121]. Therefore evaluation of angiogenic markers in a multiplex array might prove of great utility in monitoring patient airway remodeling. Using this hypothesis, BAL samples from atopic asthma patients were found to contain significantly elevated levels of angiogenic growth factors including angiogenenin, VEGF, and MCP-1 when compared to nonatopic healthy controls. Healthy controls conversely showed no change in the levels of common antiangiogenic factors. This proangiogenic effect was confirmed in vitro when the same group found that BAL taken from asthmatic patients could support tubule vessel formation in a coculture of human endothelial and dermal fibroblasts. This vessel formation capability arose primarily due to the presence of VEGF in the BAL sample. This observation suggests that a panel of angiogenic markers, like angiogenin, VEGF, and MCP-1, could serve as a novel diagnostic panel to monitor vascular disease modeling and may be a good companion study to other traditional diagnostic measures [117].

4. Conclusion

Over the past few years there have been numerous publications providing a substantial body of information collectively revealing the multitude of biological pathways involved in the pathogenesis of asthma. More recently the heterogeneous nature of asthmatic disease has been identified and has suggested the presence of many disease endotypes that warrant special diagnostic measures and even specific treatments for the best disease outcomes. Multiple aspects of host immunity are involved in the development, exacerbations, and eventual chronic nature of asthma. The major reasons for allergic disease development include common allergens, environmental triggers, and even respiratory viruses. These sensitizing agents create specific disease outcomes, and our current understanding of the disease implies that each may need a specific disease treatment. Understanding these individual disease cohorts and their underlying causes is critical to making the best outcome for disease possible.

Diagnostic measures currently revolve around visual inspection and spirometry, but a growing field of research is finding that these two methodologies are insufficient for the best classification of asthmatic disease. There are extensive endeavors currently underway in discovering protein biomarkers that could be used in asthma diagnosis, prognosis, and serving as therapeutic targets. No single protein target is likely to be effective for all diseases, especially one of such complexity, but targeted cytokine panels may provide hope for the multiprotein detection panels needed for future basic research and clinical trials for this debilitating syndrome.

Cytokine antibody arrays have gained popularity over the past several years with hundreds of publications in scientific journals. Their popularity is owed to their ability to approach a sample in a nonbiased way and detect a wide range and large number of cytokines simultaneously. This broad view allows the best chance at discovering the vast network of complex interactions occurring in disease states. As more and more cytokines are evaluated for any disease state and more and more samples probed, there is no doubt that we can uncover complex and in-depth molecular pathways involved in disease outcomes, disease progression, and disease therapies and cures.

Abbreviations

AIDS: Acquired immunodeficiency syndrome
AD: Alzheimer's disease
BAL: Bronchoalveolar lavage fluid
BHR: Bronchial hyperreactivity
CCL: CC chemokine ligand
CRP: C reactive protein
CSF: Cerebrospinal fluid
CT-1: Cardiotrophin-1
CXCL: CXC chemokine ligand
EBC: Exhaled breath condensate
EGFR: Epithelial growth factor receptor
ELISA: Enzyme-linked immunosorbent assay
FEV_1: Forced expiratory volume in 1 second
FGF: Fibroblast growth factor
GRO: Growth-regulated oncogene
HGF: Hepatocyte growth factor
IBD: Inflammatory bowel disease
IFN: Interferon
IL: Interleukin
IL-2Rα: Interleukin 2 receptor alpha
ILCs: Innate lymphoid cells
MAb: Monoclonal antibody
MCP-1: Monocyte chemotactic protein 1
MCP-4: Monocyte chemotactic protein 4
OVA: Ovalbumin
PARC: Pulmonary and activation-regulated chemokine
RA: Rheumatoid arthritis
RANTES: Regulated upon activation normal T cell expressed and secreted
SCGFβ: Stem cell growth factor beta
TGFβ1: Transforming growth factor beta-1
Th1: $CD4^+$ type 1 helper T cells
Th2: $CD4^+$ type 2 helper T cells
TLR: Toll-like receptor
TNF: Tumor necrosis factor
TSLP: Thymic stromal lymphopoietin
VEGF: Vascular endothelial growth factor.

Acknowledgments

The authors would like to express their thanks for the support of RayBiotech Innovative Research Fund, Guangdong Innovative Research Team Program (201001s0104659419), UK-China (Guangzhou) Healthtech Open Innovation (2012Q-P182), Guangzhou Municipal Innovation Fund (2013J4400170), Foundation of Enterprise University Research Institute Cooperation of Guangdong Province and Ministry of Education of China (2012B090600021), Special Program for the Development of Technology Business Incubators in Guangzhou (2013J4200016), and Foundation of Enterprise University Research Institute Cooperation of Guangdong Province and Ministry of Education of China (2012B091000145), National High Technology Research and Development Program 863 (2014AA020905), "Five-twelfth" National Science and Technology Support Program (2012EP001000), and UK-China (Guangzhou) Healthtech Open Innovation (2014Q-P037).

References

[1] GINA, "Global Strategy for Asthma Management and Prevention," Global Initiative for Asthma, 2004, http://www.ginasthma.org/.

[2] M. Masoli, D. Fabian, S. Holt, and R. Beasley, "The global burden of asthma: executive summary of the GINA Dissemination Committee Report," *Allergy*, vol. 59, no. 5, pp. 469–478, 2004.

[3] B. N. Lambrecht and H. Hammad, "The immunology of asthma," *Nature Immunology*, vol. 16, no. 1, pp. 45–56, 2014.

[4] J. M. Spergel and A. S. Paller, "Atopic dermatitis and the atopic march," *Journal of Allergy and Clinical Immunology*, vol. 112, no. 6, pp. S118–S127, 2003.

[5] A. Simpson, V. Y. F. Tan, J. Winn et al., "Beyond atopy: multiple patterns of sensitization in relation to asthma in a birth cohort study," *The American Journal of Respiratory and Critical Care Medicine*, vol. 181, no. 11, pp. 1200–1206, 2010.

[6] W. Wu, E. Bleecker, W. Moore et al., "Unsupervised phenotyping of Severe Asthma Research Program participants using expanded lung data," *Journal of Allergy and Clinical Immunology*, vol. 133, no. 5, pp. 1280–1288, 2014.

[7] J. Lötvall, C. A. Akdis, L. B. Bacharier et al., "Asthma endotypes: a new approach to classification of disease entities within the asthma syndrome," *Journal of Allergy and Clinical Immunology*, vol. 127, no. 2, pp. 355–360, 2011.

[8] S. E. Wenzel, "Asthma phenotypes: the evolution from clinical to molecular approaches," *Nature Medicine*, vol. 18, no. 5, pp. 716–725, 2012.

[9] A. J. Apter, "Advances in adult asthma diagnosis and treatment in 2013," *Journal of Allergy and Clinical Immunology*, vol. 133, no. 1, pp. 49–56, 2014.

[10] A. Bush, "Diagnosis of asthma in children under five," *Primary Care Respiratory Journal*, vol. 16, no. 1, pp. 7–15, 2007.

[11] H. S. Soifer, J. J. Rossi, and P. Sætrom, "MicroRNAs in disease and potential therapeutic applications," *Molecular Therapy*, vol. 15, no. 12, pp. 2070–2079, 2007.

[12] V. Rottiers and A. M. Näär, "MicroRNAs in metabolism and metabolic disorders," *Nature Reviews Molecular Cell Biology*, vol. 13, no. 4, pp. 239–250, 2012.

[13] K. Novak, "Taking out the trash," *Nature Reviews Drug Discovery*, vol. 5, no. 2, pp. 104–105, 2006.

[14] B. Clyne and J. S. Olshaker, "The C-reactive protein," *The Journal of Emergency Medicine*, vol. 17, no. 6, pp. 1019–1025, 1999.

[15] C.-X. Gong, F. Liu, I. Grundke-Iqbal, and K. Iqbal, "Post-translational modifications of tau protein in Alzheimer's disease," *Journal of Neural Transmission*, vol. 112, no. 6, pp. 813–838, 2005.

[16] G. K. Hansson, "Inflammation, atherosclerosis, and coronary artery disease," *The New England Journal of Medicine*, vol. 352, no. 16, pp. 1626–1695, 2005.

[17] G. Trinchieri, "Interleukin-12: a proinflammatory cytokine with immunoregulatory functions that bridge innate resistance and antigen-specific adaptive immunity," *Annual Review of Immunology*, vol. 13, no. 1, pp. 251–276, 1995.

[18] L. Van Parijs and A. K. Abbas, "Homeostasis and self-tolerance in the immune system: turning lymphocytes off," *Science*, vol. 280, no. 5361, pp. 243–248, 1998.

[19] B. Moser, M. Wolf, A. Walz, and P. Loetscher, "Chemokines: multiple levels of leukocyte migration control," *Trends in Immunology*, vol. 25, no. 2, pp. 75–84, 2004.

[20] J. A. Belperio, M. P. Keane, D. A. Arenberg et al., "CXC chemokines in angiogenesis," *Journal of Leukocyte Biology*, vol. 68, no. 1, pp. 1–8, 2000.

[21] O. A. MacDougald and S. Mandrup, "Adipogenesis: forces that tip the scales," *Trends in Endocrinology & Metabolism*, vol. 13, no. 1, pp. 5–11, 2002.

[22] K. A. Janes, J. G. Albeck, S. Gaudet, P. K. Sorger, D. A. Lauffenburger, and M. B. Yaffe, "Cell signaling: a systems model of signaling identifies a molecular basis set for cytokine-induced apoptosis," *Science*, vol. 310, no. 5754, pp. 1646–1653, 2005.

[23] S. Werner and R. Grose, "Regulation of wound healing by growth factors and cytokines," *Physiological Reviews*, vol. 83, no. 3, pp. 835–870, 2003.

[24] H. Akiyama, S. Barger, S. Barnum et al., "Inflammation and Alzheimer's disease," *Neurobiology of Aging*, vol. 21, no. 3, pp. 383–421, 2000.

[25] E. C. Hirsch and S. Hunot, "Neuroinflammation in Parkinson's disease: a target for neuroprotection?" *The Lancet Neurology*, vol. 8, no. 4, pp. 382–397, 2009.

[26] K. E. Wellen and G. S. Hotamisligil, "Inflammation, stress, and diabetes," *The Journal of Clinical Investigation*, vol. 115, no. 5, pp. 1111–1119, 2005.

[27] J. S. Ross and J. A. Fletcher, "The HER-2/neu oncogene in breast cancer: prognostic factor, predictive factor, and target for therapy," *Stem Cells*, vol. 16, no. 6, pp. 413–428, 1998.

[28] K. Ozaki and W. J. Leonard, "Cytokine and cytokine receptor pleiotropy and redundancy," *The Journal of Biological Chemistry*, vol. 277, no. 33, pp. 29355–29358, 2002.

[29] T. Kishimoto, S. Akira, M. Narazaki, and T. Taga, "Interleukin-6 family of cytokines and gp130," *Blood*, vol. 86, no. 4, pp. 1243–1254, 1995.

[30] J. Audet, "Adventures in time and space: nonlinearity and complexity of cytokine effects on stem cell fate decisions," *Biotechnology and Bioengineering*, vol. 106, no. 2, pp. 173–182, 2010.

[31] J. Mendelsohn and J. Baselga, "Status of epidermal growth factor receptor antagonists in the biology and treatment of cancer," *Journal of Clinical Oncology*, vol. 21, no. 14, pp. 2787–2799, 2003.

[32] M. Feldmann and R. N. Maini, "TNF defined as a therapeutic target for rheumatoid arthritis and other autoimmune diseases," *Nature Medicine*, vol. 9, no. 10, pp. 1245–1250, 2003.

[33] J. H. Hoofnagle, "Therapy of acute and chronic viral hepatitis," *Advances in Internal Medicine*, vol. 39, pp. 241–275, 1994.

[34] H. C. Lane, J. Feinberg, V. Davey et al., "Anti-retroviral effects of interferon-alpha in AIDS-associated Kaposi's sarcoma," *The Lancet*, vol. 332, no. 8622, pp. 1218–1222, 1988.

[35] R. P. Schleimer, A. Kato, R. Kern, D. Kuperman, and P. C. Avila, "Epithelium: at the interface of innate and adaptive immune responses," *Journal of Allergy and Clinical Immunology*, vol. 120, no. 6, pp. 1279–1284, 2007.

[36] R. P. Schleimer, A. Kato, A. Peters et al., "Epithelium, inflammation, and immunity in the upper airways of humans: studies in chronic rhinosinusitis," *Proceedings of the American Thoracic Society*, vol. 6, no. 3, pp. 288–294, 2009.

[37] A. Kato and R. P. Schleimer, "Beyond inflammation: airway epithelial cells are at the interface of innate and adaptive immunity," *Current Opinion in Immunology*, vol. 19, no. 6, pp. 711–720, 2007.

[38] J. Ciencewicki, S. Trivedi, and S. R. Kleeberger, "Oxidants and the pathogenesis of lung diseases," *Journal of Allergy and Clinical Immunology*, vol. 122, no. 3, pp. 456–468, 2008.

[39] F. T. Ishmael, "The inflammatory response in the pathogenesis of asthma," *The Journal of the American Osteopathic Association*, vol. 111, no. 11, pp. S11–S17, 2011.

[40] P. G. Woodruff, B. Modrek, D. F. Choy et al., "T-helper type 2-driven inflammation defines major subphenotypes of asthma," *American Journal of Respiratory and Critical Care Medicine*, vol. 180, no. 5, pp. 388–395, 2009.

[41] P. J. Barnes, "The cytokine network in asthma and chronic obstructive pulmonary disease," *The Journal of Clinical Investigation*, vol. 118, no. 11, pp. 3546–3556, 2008.

[42] J. G. R. de Monchy, H. F. Kauffman, P. Venge et al., "Bronchoalveolar eosinophilia during allergen-induced late asthmatic reactions," *American Review of Respiratory Disease*, vol. 131, no. 3, pp. 373–376, 1985.

[43] D. C. Webb, A. N. J. McKenzie, A. M. L. Koskinen, M. Yang, J. Mattes, and P. S. Foster, "Integrated signals between IL-13, IL-4, and IL-5 regulate airways hyperreactivity," *The Journal of Immunology*, vol. 165, no. 1, pp. 108–113, 2000.

[44] M. Wills-Karp, "Interleukin-13 in asthma pathogenesis," *Immunological Reviews*, vol. 202, no. 1, pp. 175–190, 2004.

[45] K. Minton, "Allergy and Asthma: what 'drives' IL-4 versus IL-13 signalling?" *Nature Reviews Immunology*, vol. 8, no. 3, pp. 166–167, 2008.

[46] D. S. Robinson, Q. Hamid, S. Ying et al., "Predominant TH2-like bronchoalveolar T-lymphocyte population in atopic asthma," *The New England Journal of Medicine*, vol. 326, no. 5, pp. 298–304, 1992.

[47] P. G. Woodruff, H. A. Boushey, G. M. Dolganov et al., "Genome-wide profiling identifies epithelial cell genes associated with asthma and with treatment response to corticosteroids," *Proceedings of the National Academy of Sciences of the United States of America*, vol. 104, no. 40, pp. 15858–15863, 2007.

[48] M. T. Kasaian, K. Marquette, S. Fish et al., "An IL-4/IL-13 dual antagonist reduces lung inflammation, airway hyperresponsiveness, and IgE production in mice," *The American Journal of Respiratory Cell and Molecular Biology*, vol. 49, no. 1, pp. 37–46, 2013.

[49] D. B. Corry, H. G. Folkesson, M. L. Warnock et al., "Interleukin 4, but not interleukin 5 or eosinophils, is required in a murine model of acute airway hyperreactivity," *The Journal of Experimental Medicine*, vol. 183, no. 1, pp. 109–117, 1996.

[50] M. Wills-Karp, J. Luyimbazi, X. Xu et al., "Interleukin-13: central mediator of allergic asthma," *Science*, vol. 282, no. 5397, pp. 2258–2261, 1998.

[51] G. Grünig, D. B. Corry, J. Reibman, and M. Wills-Karp, "Interleukin 13 and the evolution of asthma therapy," *American Journal of Clinical and Experimental Immunology*, vol. 1, no. 1, pp. 20–27, 2012.

[52] S. Wenzel, L. Ford, D. Pearlman et al., "Dupilumab in persistent asthma with elevated eosinophil levels," *The New England Journal of Medicine*, vol. 368, no. 26, pp. 2455–2466, 2013.

[53] J. Corren, R. F. Lemanske Jr., N. A. Hanania et al., "Lebrikizumab treatment in adults with asthma," *The New England Journal of Medicine*, vol. 365, no. 12, pp. 1088–1098, 2011.

[54] H. G. Ortega, M. C. Liu, I. D. Pavord et al., "Mepolizumab treatment in patients with severe eosinophilic asthma," *The New England Journal of Medicine*, vol. 371, no. 13, pp. 1198–1207, 2014.

[55] P. Flood-Page, A. Menzies-Gow, S. Phipps et al., "Anti-IL-5 treatment reduces deposition of ECM proteins in the bronchial subepithelial basement membrane of mild atopic asthmatics," *The Journal of Clinical Investigation*, vol. 112, no. 7, pp. 1029–1036, 2003.

[56] D. J. Song, J. Y. Cho, S. Y. Lee et al., "Anti-siglec-F antibody reduces allergen-induced eosinophilic inflammation and airway remodeling," *The Journal of Immunology*, vol. 183, no. 8, pp. 5333–5341, 2009.

[57] R. Fattouh, A. Al-Garawi, M. Fattouh et al., "Eosinophils are dispensable for allergic remodeling and immunity in a model of house dust mite-induced airway disease," *American Journal of Respiratory and Critical Care Medicine*, vol. 183, no. 2, pp. 179–188, 2011.

[58] A. J. Coyle, S. J. Ackerman, R. Burch, D. Proud, and C. G. Irvin, "Human eosinophil-granule major basic protein and synthetic polycations induce airway hyperresponsiveness in vivo dependent on bradykinin generation," *The Journal of Clinical Investigation*, vol. 95, no. 4, pp. 1735–1740, 1995.

[59] D. K. Chu, R. Jimenez-Saiz, C. P. Verschoor et al., "Indigenous enteric eosinophils control DCs to initiate a primary Th2 immune response in vivo," *The Journal of Experimental Medicine*, vol. 211, no. 8, pp. 1657–1672, 2014.

[60] P. D. Ponath, S. Qin, D. J. Ringler et al., "Cloning of the human eosinophil chemoattractant, eotaxin. Expression, receptor binding and functional properties suggest a mechanism for the selective recruitment of eosinophils," *The Journal of Clinical Investigation*, vol. 97, no. 3, pp. 604–612, 1996.

[61] M. E. Rothenberg, A. D. Luster, and P. Leder, "Murine eotaxin: An eosinophil chemoattractant inducible in endothelial cells and in interleukin 4-induced tumor suppression," *Proceedings of the National Academy of Sciences of the United States of America*, vol. 92, no. 19, pp. 8960–8964, 1995.

[62] P. C. Fulkerson, C. A. Fischetti, M. L. McBride, L. M. Hassman, S. P. Hogan, and M. E. Rothenberg, "A central regulatory role for eosinophils and the eotaxin/CCR3 axis in chronic experimental allergic airway inflammation," *Proceedings of the National Academy of Sciences of the United States of America*, vol. 103, no. 44, pp. 16418–16423, 2006.

[63] S. M. Pope, N. Zimmermann, K. F. Stringer, M. L. Karow, and M. E. Rothenberg, "The eotaxin chemokines and CCR3 are fundamental regulators of allergen-induced pulmonary eosinophilia," *Journal of Immunology*, vol. 175, no. 8, pp. 5341–5350, 2005.

[64] D. Wu, J. Zhou, H. Bi et al., "CCL11 as a potential diagnostic marker for asthma?" *Journal of Asthma*, vol. 51, no. 8, pp. 847–854, 2014.

[65] S. Ying, Q. Meng, K. Zeibecoglou et al., "Eosinophil chemotactic chemokines (eotaxin, eotaxin-2, RANTES, monocyte chemoattractant protein-3 (MCP-3), and MCP-4), and CC chemokine receptor 3 expression in bronchial biopsies from atopic and nonatopic (Intrinsic) asthmatics," *The Journal of Immunology*, vol. 163, no. 11, pp. 6321–6329, 1999.

[66] N. Bhardwaj and G. Ghaffari, "Biomarkers for eosinophilic esophagitis: a review," *Annals of Allergy, Asthma and Immunology*, vol. 109, no. 3, pp. 155–159, 2012.

[67] H. Yamada, M. Yamaguchi, K. Yamamoto et al., "Eotaxin in induced sputum of asthmatics: relationship with eosinophils and eosinophil cationic protein in sputum," *Allergy*, vol. 55, no. 4, pp. 392–397, 2000.

[68] C. Lemière, S. Chaboilliez, C. Trudeau et al., "Characterization of airway inflammation after repeated exposures to occupational agents," *Journal of Allergy and Clinical Immunology*, vol. 106, no. 6, pp. 1163–1170, 2000.

[69] H. Nakamura, S. T. Weiss, E. Israel, A. D. Luster, J. M. Drazen, and C. M. Lilly, "Eotaxin and impaired lung function in asthma," *American Journal of Respiratory and Critical Care Medicine*, vol. 160, no. 6, pp. 1952–1956, 1999.

[70] C. M. Lilly, P. G. Woodruff, C. A. Camargo Jr. et al., "Elevated plasma eotaxin levels in patients with acute asthma," *Journal of Allergy and Clinical Immunology*, vol. 104, no. 4, pp. 786–790, 1999.

[71] M. E. Scheicher, M. M. Teixeira, F. Q. Cunha et al., "Eotaxin-2 in sputum cell culture to evaluate asthma inflammation," *European Respiratory Journal*, vol. 29, no. 3, pp. 489–495, 2007.

[72] J. M. Coleman, C. Naik, F. Holguin et al., "Epithelial eotaxin-2 and eotaxin-3 expression: relation to asthma severity, luminal eosinophilia and age at onset," *Thorax*, vol. 67, no. 12, pp. 1061–1066, 2012.

[73] V. Provost, M.-C. Larose, A. Langlois, M. Rola-Pleszczynski, N. Flamand, and M. Laviolette, "CCL26/eotaxin-3 is more effective to induce the migration of eosinophils of asthmatics than CCL11/eotaxin-1 and CCL24/eotaxin-2," *Journal of Leukocyte Biology*, vol. 94, no. 2, pp. 213–222, 2013.

[74] O. Kalayci, L. A. Sonna, P. G. Woodruff, C. A. Camargo Jr., A. D. Luster, and C. M. Lilly, "Monocyte chemotactic protein-4 (MCP-4; CCL-13): a biomarker of asthma," *Journal of Asthma*, vol. 41, no. 1, pp. 27–33, 2004.

[75] C. Stellato, P. Collins, P. D. Ponath et al., "Production of the novel C-C chemokine MCP-4 by airway cells and comparison of its biological activity to other C-C chemokines," *The Journal of Clinical Investigation*, vol. 99, no. 5, pp. 926–936, 1997.

[76] H. Petering, R. Höchstetter, D. Kimmig, R. Smolarski, A. Kapp, and J. Elsner, "Detection of MCP-4 in dermal fibroblasts and its activation of the respiratory burst in human eosinophils," *The Journal of Immunology*, vol. 160, no. 2, pp. 555–558, 1998.

[77] B. Lamkhioued, E. A. Garcia-Zepeda, S. Abi-Younes et al., "Monocyte chemoattractant protein (MCP)-4 expression in the airways of patients with asthma. Induction in epithelial cells and mononuclear cells by proinflammatory cytokines," *The American Journal of Respiratory and Critical Care Medicine*, vol. 162, no. 2, pp. 723–732, 2000.

[78] R. A. Taha, S. Laberge, Q. Hamid, and R. Olivenstein, "Increased expression of the chemoattractant cytokines eotaxin, monocyte chemotactic protein-4, and interleukin-16 in induced sputum in asthmatic patients," *Chest*, vol. 120, no. 2, pp. 595–601, 2001.

[79] A. Al-Shami, R. Spolski, J. Kelly, A. Keane-Myers, and W. J. Leonard, "A role for TSLP in the development of inflammation in an asthma model," *The Journal of Experimental Medicine*, vol. 202, no. 6, pp. 829–839, 2005.

[80] V. Soumelis, P. A. Reche, H. Kanzler et al., "Human epithelial cells trigger dendritic cell-mediated allergic inflammation by producing TSLP," *Nature Immunology*, vol. 3, no. 7, pp. 673–680, 2002.

[81] T. Ito, Y.-H. Wang, O. Duramad et al., "TSLP-activated dendritic cells induce an inflammatory T helper type 2 cell response through OX40 ligand," *The Journal of Experimental Medicine*, vol. 202, no. 9, pp. 1213–1223, 2005.

[82] N. Watanabe, S. Hanabuchi, V. Soumelis et al., "Human thymic stromal lymphopoietin promotes dendritic cell-mediated $CD4^+$ T cell homeostatic expansion," *Nature Immunology*, vol. 5, no. 4, pp. 426–434, 2004.

[83] A. Al-Shami, R. Spolski, J. Kelly et al., "A role for thymic stromal lymphopoietin in $CD4^+$ T cell development," *The Journal of Experimental Medicine*, vol. 200, no. 2, pp. 159–168, 2004.

[84] D. Cheng, Z. Xue, L. Yi et al., "Epithelial interleukin-25 is a key mediator in Th2-high, corticosteroid-responsive asthma," *American Journal of Respiratory and Critical Care Medicine*, vol. 190, no. 6, pp. 639–648, 2014.

[85] J. A. Walker, J. L. Barlow, and A. N. J. McKenzie, "Innate lymphoid cells-how did we miss them?" *Nature Reviews Immunology*, vol. 13, no. 2, pp. 75–87, 2013.

[86] P. G. Fallon, S. J. Ballantyne, N. E. Mangan et al., "Identification of an interleukin (IL)-25–dependent cell population that provides IL-4, IL-5, and IL-13 at the onset of helminth expulsion," *The Journal of Experimental Medicine*, vol. 203, no. 4, pp. 1105–1116, 2006.

[87] M. M. Fort, J. Cheung, D. Yen et al., "IL-25 Induces IL-4, IL-5, and IL-13 and Th2-associated pathologies in vivo," *Immunity*, vol. 15, no. 6, pp. 985–995, 2001.

[88] Z. Kang, S. Swaidani, W. Yin et al., "Epithelial cell-specific Act1 adaptor mediates interleukin-25-dependent helminth expulsion through expansion of Lin^- $c\text{-}Kit^+$ innate cell population," *Immunity*, vol. 36, no. 5, pp. 821–833, 2012.

[89] K. R. Bartemes, K. Iijima, T. Kobayashi et al., "IL-33-responsive $lineage^-CD25^+$ $CD44^{hi}$ lymphoid cells mediate innate type 2 immunity and allergic inflammation in the lungs," *The Journal of Immunology*, vol. 188, no. 3, pp. 1503–1513, 2012.

[90] J. Kearley, J. S. Erjefalt, C. Andersson et al., "IL-9 governs allergen-induced mast cell numbers in the lung and chronic remodeling of the airways," *The American Journal of Respiratory and Critical Care Medicine*, vol. 183, no. 7, pp. 865–875, 2011.

[91] V. J. Erpenbeck, J. M. Hohlfeld, B. Volkmann et al., "Segmental allergen challenge in patients with atopic asthma leads to increased IL-9 expression in bronchoalveolar lavage fluid lymphocytes," *Journal of Allergy and Clinical Immunology*, vol. 111, no. 6, pp. 1319–1327, 2003.

[92] V. Staudt, E. Bothur, M. Klein et al., "Interferon-regulatory factor 4 is essential for the developmental program of T helper 9 cells," *Immunity*, vol. 33, no. 2, pp. 192–202, 2010.

[93] J. Kerzerho, H. Maazi, A. O. Speak et al., "Programmed cell death ligand 2 regulates TH9 differentiation and induction of chronic airway hyperreactivity," *The Journal of Allergy and Clinical Immunology*, vol. 131, no. 4, pp. 1048.e2–1057.e2, 2013.

[94] C. Wilhelm, K. Hirota, B. Stieglitz et al., "An IL-9 fate reporter demonstrates the induction of an innate IL-9 response in lung inflammation," *Nature Immunology*, vol. 12, no. 11, pp. 1071–1077, 2011.

[95] J.-E. Turner, P. J. Morrison, C. Wilhelm et al., "IL-9-mediated survival of type 2 innate lymphoid cells promotes damage control in helminth-induced lung inflammation," *The Journal of Experimental Medicine*, vol. 210, no. 13, pp. 2951–2965, 2013.

[96] J. M. Parker, C. K. Oh, C. LaForce et al., "Safety profile and clinical activity of multiple subcutaneous doses of MEDI-528, a humanized anti-interleukin-9 monoclonal antibody, in two randomized phase 2a studies in subjects with asthma," *BMC Pulmonary Medicine*, vol. 11, no. 1, article 14, 2011.

[97] T. Sekiya, H. Yamada, M. Yamaguchi et al., "Increased levels of a TH2-type CC chemokine thymus and activation-regulated chemokine (TARC) in serum and induced sputum of asthmatics," *Allergy*, vol. 57, no. 2, pp. 173–177, 2002.

[98] T.-F. Leung, C.-K. Wong, I. H. S. Chan, W.-K. Ip, C. W. K. Lam, and G. W. K. Wong, "Plasma concentration of thymus and activation-regulated chemokine is elevated in childhood asthma," *Journal of Allergy and Clinical Immunology*, vol. 110, no. 3, pp. 404–409, 2002.

[99] H.-Y. Hsu, S. Wittemann, and T. O. Joos, "Miniaturized paral-

lelized sandwich immunoassays," *Methods in Molecular Biology*, vol. 428, pp. 247–261, 2007.

[100] W. Kusnezow, V. Banzon, C. Schröder et al., "Antibody microarray-based profiling of complex specimens: systematic evaluation of labeling strategies," *Proteomics*, vol. 7, no. 11, pp. 1786–1799, 2007.

[101] R. Huang, W. Jiang, J. Yang et al., "A biotin label-based antibody array for high-content profiling of protein expression," *Cancer Genomics and Proteomics*, vol. 7, no. 3, pp. 129–141, 2010.

[102] S. Ray, M. Britschgi, C. Herbert et al., "Classification and prediction of clinical Alzheimer's diagnosis based on plasma signaling proteins," *Nature Medicine*, vol. 13, no. 11, pp. 1359–1362, 2007.

[103] H. Chandra, P. J. Reddy, and S. Srivastava, "Protein microarrays and novel detection platforms," *Expert Review of Proteomics*, vol. 8, no. 1, pp. 61–79, 2011.

[104] C. Wingren and C. A. K. Borrebaeck, "Antibody-based microarrays," *Microchip Methods in Diagnostics*, vol. 509, pp. 57–84, 2009.

[105] C. A. K. Borrebaeck and C. Wingren, "High-throughput proteomics using antibody microarrays: an update," *Expert Review of Molecular Diagnostics*, vol. 7, no. 5, pp. 673–686, 2007.

[106] A. Vazquez-martin, R. Colomer, and J. A. Menendez, "Protein array technology to detect HER2 (erbB-2)-induced 'cytokine signature' in breast cancer," *European Journal of Cancer*, vol. 43, no. 7, pp. 1117–1124, 2007.

[107] J. L. Perez-Gracia, C. Prior, F. Guillén-Grima et al., "Identification of TNF-α and MMP-9 as potential baseline predictive serum markers of sunitinib activity in patients with renal cell carcinoma using a human cytokine array," *British Journal of Cancer*, vol. 101, no. 11, pp. 1876–1883, 2009.

[108] M.-Y. Kim, T. Oskarsson, S. Acharyya et al., "Tumor self-seeding by circulating cancer cells," *Cell*, vol. 139, no. 7, pp. 1315–1326, 2009.

[109] T. Deuse, X. Hua, D. Wang et al., "Dichloroacetate prevents restenosis in preclinical animal models of vessel injury," *Nature*, vol. 509, no. 7502, pp. 641–644, 2014.

[110] S. P. Patil, J. P. Wisnivesky, P. J. Busse, E. A. Halm, and X.-M. Li, "Detection of immunological biomarkers correlated with asthma control and quality of life measurements in sera from chronic asthmatic patients," *Annals of Allergy, Asthma and Immunology*, vol. 106, no. 3, pp. 205–213, 2011.

[111] H.-B. Kim, C.-K. Kim, K. Iijima, T. Kobayashi, and H. Kita, "Protein microarray analysis in patients with asthma: elevation of the chemokine PARC/CCL18 in sputum," *Chest*, vol. 135, no. 2, pp. 295–302, 2009.

[112] A. T. Hastie, W. C. Moore, D. A. Meyers et al., "Analyses of asthma severity phenotypes and inflammatory proteins in subjects stratified by sputum granulocytes," *Journal of Allergy and Clinical Immunology*, vol. 125, no. 5, pp. 1028.e13–1036.e13, 2010.

[113] K. Matsunaga, S. Yanagisawa, T. Ichikawa et al., "Airway cytokine expression measured by means of protein array in exhaled breath condensate: correlation with physiologic properties in asthmatic patients," *Journal of Allergy and Clinical Immunology*, vol. 118, no. 1, pp. 84–90, 2006.

[114] T. Ichikawa, K. Matsunaga, Y. Minakata et al., "Possible impact of salivary influence on cytokine analysis in exhaled breath condensate," *Analytical Chemistry Insights*, vol. 2, pp. 85–92, 2007.

[115] K. Nakamura, M. Mikuniya, S. Takanashi et al., "Is analysis of exhaled breath condensate equivalent to that of bronchoalveolar lavage fluid?" *European Respiratory Journal*, vol. 38, supplement 55, p. 476, 2011.

[116] K. Matsunaga, T. Ichikawa, S. Yanagisawa et al., "Clinical application of exhaled breath condensate analysis in asthma: prediction of FEV1 improvement by steroid therapy," *Respiration*, vol. 78, no. 4, pp. 393–398, 2009.

[117] D. E. Simcock, V. Kanabar, G. W. Clarke, B. J. O'Connor, T. H. Lee, and S. J. Hirst, "Proangiogenic activity in bronchoalveolar lavage fluid from patients with asthma," *American Journal of Respiratory and Critical Care Medicine*, vol. 176, no. 2, pp. 146–153, 2007.

[118] H.-W. Guo, C.-X. Yun, G.-H. Hou et al., "Mangiferin attenuates Th1/Th2 cytokine imbalance in an ovalbumin-induced asthmatic mouse model," *PLoS ONE*, vol. 9, no. 6, Article ID e100394, 2014.

[119] A. Chetta, A. Zanini, A. Foresi et al., "Vascular component of airway remodeling in asthma is reduced by high dose of fluticasone," *American Journal of Respiratory and Critical Care Medicine*, vol. 167, no. 5, pp. 751–757, 2003.

[120] A. Grigoras, I. D. Caruntu, C. C. Grigoras et al., "Relationship between immunohistochemical assessment of bronchial mucosa microvascularization and clinical stage in asthma," *Romanian Journal of Morphology and Embryology*, vol. 53, no. 3, pp. 485–490, 2012.

[121] M. Hashimoto and Y. Hatanaka, "Post-biotinylation of photocrosslinking by staudinger-bertozzi ligation of preinstalled alkylazide tag," *Chemical and Pharmaceutical Bulletin*, vol. 53, no. 11, pp. 1510–1512, 2005.

5

Identification of a Novel Alternatively Spliced Form of Inflammatory Regulator SWAP-70-Like Adapter of T Cells

Marie Hashimoto,[1,2] Jun-ichi Nagao,[1] Shojiro Ikezaki,[1] Sonoko Tasaki,[1] Ken-ichi Arita-Morioka,[3] Yuka Narita,[1] Tamaki Cho,[1] Kenji Yuasa,[2] Amnon Altman,[4] and Yoshihiko Tanaka[1,3]

[1]*Section of Infection Biology, Department of Functional Bioscience, Fukuoka Dental College, Fukuoka 814-0193, Japan*
[2]*Section of Image Diagnosis, Department of Diagnostics and General Care, Fukuoka Dental College, Fukuoka 814-0193, Japan*
[3]*Advanced Science Research Center, Fukuoka Dental College, Fukuoka 814-0193, Japan*
[4]*Division of Cell Biology, La Jolla Institute for Allergy and Immunology, La Jolla, CA 92037, USA*

Correspondence should be addressed to Yoshihiko Tanaka; tanakayo@college.fdcnet.ac.jp

Academic Editor: Istvan Boldogh

Activation of naive $CD4^+$ T cells results in the development of several distinct subsets of effector Th cells, including Th2 cells that play a pivotal role in allergic inflammation and helminthic infections. SWAP-70-like adapter of T cells (SLAT), also known as Def6 or IBP, is a guanine nucleotide exchange factor for small GTPases, which regulates $CD4^+$ T cell inflammatory responses by controlling Ca^{2+}/NFAT signaling. In this study, we have identified a novel alternatively spliced isoform of SLAT, named SLAT2, which lacks the region encoded by exons 2–7 of the *Def6* gene. SLAT2 was selectively expressed in differentiated Th2 cells after the second round of in vitro stimulation, but not in differentiated Th1, Th17, or regulatory T (Treg) cells. Functional assays revealed that SLAT2 shared with SLAT the ability to enhance T cell receptor- (TCR-) mediated activation of NFAT and production of IL-4 but was unable to enhance TCR-induced adhesion to ICAM-1. Ectopic expression of SLAT2 or SLAT in Jurkat T cells resulted in the expression of distinct forms of filopodia, namely, short versus long ones, respectively. These results demonstrate that modulating either SLAT2 or SLAT protein expression could play critical roles in cytokine production and actin reorganization during inflammatory immune responses.

1. Introduction

During inflammatory immune responses under local cytokine environment, naive $CD4^+$ T cells differentiate into distinct lineages including T helper 1 (Th1), Th2, Th17, and regulatory T (Treg) cells [1]. Both TCR-derived signals and the cytokine environment at the site of inflammatory immune responses play an important role in the fate decisions of Th subsets, and several TCR-proximal signaling intermediates can regulate Th subset differentiation [2]. Each Th cell subset expresses a unique set of transcription factors and produces hallmark cytokines [2], with Th2 cells being controlled by the master transcription factor, GATA3. Differentiated Th2 cells secrete IL-4, IL-5, and IL-13, which are important in inflammatory asthma and atopy, and constitute a defense against extracellular pathogens during inflammation. However, little information exists with regard to TCR-proximal signaling events that are unique to the differentiated Th2 subset.

We have previously isolated and characterized a TCR-regulated signaling protein termed SWAP-70-like adapter of T cells (SLAT) [3] encoded by the *Def6* gene and found it to share homology with SWAP-70, which is involved in B and mast cell activation [4–6] and to be expressed predominantly in Th cells and thymocytes. SLAT, also known as Def6 [7] or IBP [8], displays a guanine nucleotide exchange factor (GEF) activity for the Cdc42 and Rac1 small GTPases [9–14]. The human homolog of SLAT, termed IRF-4-binding protein (IBP), was independently isolated by another group [8]. Structurally, SLAT contains, beginning at its N terminus, a Ca^{2+}-binding EF-hand domain [15], an immunoreceptor tyrosine-based activation motif- (ITAM-) like sequence, a phosphatidylinositol 3,4,5-trisphosphate-binding pleckstrin homology (PH) domain [3], and a catalytic Dbl homology (DH) domain [9–14, 16]. Our previous study of *Def6*-deficient mice revealed SLAT to be a critical selective regulator of the TCR-coupled Ca^{2+}/NFAT signaling pathway, controlling positively $CD4^+$ Th cell activation and differentiation, as evidenced by its critical role in the development of T cell-dependent inflammatory diseases such as allergic lung inflammation [17] and experimental autoimmune encephalomyelitis [18].

Alternative splicing is a critical mechanism that regulates gene expression at the posttranscriptional level. A number of genes exhibit significant changes in isoform expression during inflammatory immune responses, including several instances, in which alternative splicing changes are known to impact Th cell function [19]. Differential pre-mRNA splicing generates structural and functional diversities that contribute to various physiological processes such as differentiation into distinct lineages of Th cells.

In this study, we report the identification and characterization of a novel alternatively spliced isoform of SLAT, named SLAT2, which lacks the region encoded by exons 2–7 of the *Def6* gene. SLAT2 protein was expressed in differentiated Th2 cells after two rounds of in vitro stimulation, but not in differentiated Th1, Th17, and Treg cells. Similar to SLAT, SLAT2 enhanced TCR-mediated activation of NFAT and production of IL-4, but unlike SLAT [16] it was not required for TCR-induced adhesion to intercellular adhesion molecule-1 (ICAM-1). Ectopic expression of SLAT2 or SLAT in Jurkat T cells resulted in the expression of distinct forms of filopodia, namely, short versus long ones, respectively. Thus, SLAT2 in differentiated Th2 cells appears to exhibit distinct biological properties by comparison with SLAT. Differential expression of SLAT2 or SLAT protein could thus play critical roles in cytokine production and actin reorganization during inflammatory immune responses, leading to altered functional activities of these regulators.

2. Materials and Methods

2.1. Mice. OT-II TCR-transgenic mice (The Jackson Laboratory, Bar Harbor, ME) and C57BL/6N (B6) mice (Kyudo, Saga, Japan) were purchased and kept under specific pathogen-free conditions in the animal facility of Fukuoka Dental College. 6- to 8-week-old mice were used in all experiments. All experiments were performed in accordance with the guidelines of the committee of Ethics of Animal Experiments of Fukuoka Dental College.

2.2. Cell Culture and Stimulation. $CD4^+$ T cells were purified from lymph node and spleen cells by magnetic sorting using Dynabeads Mouse CD4 followed by treatment with DETACHaBEAD Mouse CD4 (both from Invitrogen). Splenic antigen-presenting cells (APCs) from B6 mice were prepared by depletion of T cells through the use of CD90.2 MicroBeads Mouse (Miltenyi Biotec) and were treated with mitomycin C before use. $CD4^+$ T cells (5×10^5 per well) from OT-II or B6 mice were cultured in a 24-well plate with T cell-depleted, mitomycin C-treated B6 spleen cells (5×10^6 per well) in a total volume of 2 mL in the presence of 1 μg/mL ovalbumin $(OVA)_{323-339}$ peptide or 1 μg/mL anti-CD3 antibody (Ab) (145-2C11; BD), respectively. Th1 cells were cultured by the addition of 10 μg/mL anti-IL-4 Ab (11B11; BD) and 10 U/mL recombinant murine IL-12 (Peprotech). Th2 cells were initiated by the addition of 10 μg/mL anti-IL-12 Ab (C17.8; BD), 10 μg/mL anti-IFNγ Ab (XMG1.2; BD), and 100 U/mL recombinant murine IL-4 (Peprotech). Th17 or Treg cells were differentiated in the presence of 2 ng/mL recombinant human TGF-β1 (R&D system) and 20 ng/mL recombinant murine IL-6 (Peprotech), or in the presence of 2 ng/mL recombinant human TGF-β1 and 2 ng/mL recombinant murine IL-2 (Peprotech), respectively. After 5 days, differentiated T cells subsets (1×10^6 per well) were washed and restimulated using 1 μg/mL anti-CD3 Ab- plus 1 μg/mL anti-CD28 Ab (37.51; BD)-coated plates.

2.3. Cloning of the Gene Encoding SLAT2. $CD4^+$ T cells from B6 mice were cultured under Th2-inducing conditions and then restimulated with plate-bound anti-CD3 Ab (1 μg/mL) and anti-CD28 Ab (1 μg/mL) for 2 days. The cells were harvested and total RNA was isolated using an RNeasy Kit (Qiagen). The RNA was reverse-transcribed into cDNA by oligo (dT) priming with the SuperScript III reverse transcriptase (Invitrogen). RT-PCR was performed with the primers 5′-ATGGCCCTGCGCAAGGAGCT-3′ and 5′-CTAATTCCCTGGTGCTGGAT-3′ and the amplified fragment having ~750 bp was cloned into the pGEM-T easy vector (Promega).

2.4. Plasmid Constructs. SLAT cDNA was cloned into the pEF-Myc-HisA vector (empty vector), resulting in the pEF-SLAT-Myc plasmid, as described previously [3]. SLAT2 cDNA was cloned into the *EcoRI* and *NotI* sites of pEF-Myc-HisA vector, giving rise to the pEF-SLAT2-Myc plasmid. A DNA fragment encoding the FLAG epitope (DYKDDDDK) was cloned into the *XhoI* and *XbaI* sites of pcDNA4/V5His-A, resulting in the pcDNA-FLAG plasmid. SLAT and SLAT2 cDNAs were PCR-amplified and cloned into the *SalI* and *NotI* sites of pcDNA-FLAG, fused in frame with the FLAG tag at their 3′ termini, yielding the plasmids pcDNA-SLAT-FLAG and pcDNA-SLAT2-FLAG, respectively. A PCR-amplified enhanced GFP (eGFP) gene was cloned into the *NheI* and *SalI* sites of the pSI vector to result in the plasmid pSI-EGFP. DNA fragments encoding SLAT-FLAG and SLAT2-FLAG were PCR-amplified from plasmids pcDNA-SLAT-FLAG and pcDNA-SLAT2-FLAG, respectively, and cloned into the *SalI* and *NotI* sites of pSI-EGFP, giving rise to the plasmids pSI-EGFP-SLAT-FLAG and pSI-EGFP-SLAT2-FLAG, respectively. SLAT cDNA was cloned into the retroviral vector pMIG, resulting in a pMIG-SLAT plasmid, as described previously [3]. SLAT2 cDNA was cloned into the *BglII* site of pMIG vector, resulting in plasmid pMIG-SLAT2.

2.5. Cell Transfection and Western Blotting Analysis. SV40 large T antigen-transfected human leukemic Jurkat T cells (Jurkat-TAg) in logarithmic growth phase were transfected with plasmid DNAs by electroporation using NEPA21 Super Electroporator (NEPAGENE, Japan). For detection of SLAT and SLAT2 proteins, the samples were separated by 11% SDS-PAGE, transferred to a PVDF membrane, and immunoblotted with anti-SLAT antisera prepared as described [3], anti-Myc Ab (9E10; Sigma), anti-GFP Ab (sc-9996; Santa Cruz Biotechnology), or anti-actin Ab (sc-1616; Santa Cruz Biotechnology). The signal intensity of SLAT and SLAT2 was quantified relative to the actin control using ImageJ software.

2.6. Luciferase Reporter Assay. Jurkat-TAg cells were transfected with an NFAT-luciferase plasmid plus a β-galactosidase (β-gal) reporter plasmid as described [20, 21]. After washing twice with phosphate-buffered saline (PBS), transfected cells were lysed in 100 μL of lysis buffer (pH 7.8, 0.5% Triton X-100, 1 mM DTT, and 100 mM KPO_4) for 10 min at room temperature. The lysate were centrifuged (12,000 ×g) for 10 min at 4°C. After centrifugation, 20 μL of the supernatants was added with 50 μL of Luciferase Assay Substrate (Promega). Luciferase activity was determined in a luminometer (GloMax 20/20 Single Tube Luminometer, Promega). Each group of luciferase activity was normalized to the cotransfected β-gal reporter activity.

2.7. Retroviral Transduction and Intracellular Cytokine Staining. Retroviral transduction was performed as described [22]. Briefly, Th2 cells were differentiated under Th2-inducing conditions by culture with T cell-depleted, mitomycin C-treated B6 spleen cells (5×10^6) in the presence of 1 μg/mL anti-CD3 for 5 days. The plasmids (10 μg) were transfected into Platinum-E packaging cells using X-tremeGENE 9 DNA transfection reagent (Roche). The retroviral supernatants were harvested 48 h after transfection, supplemented with 4 ng/mL recombinant murine IL-2 (Peprotech) and 5 μg/mL Polybrene (Sigma-Aldrich), and used to infect the differentiated Th2 cells that had been stimulated with plate-coated anti-CD3 plus -CD28 monoclonal antibodies (mAbs) (1 μg/mL each) for 18 h after depletion of dead cells by Lympholyte-M (Cedarlane). After centrifugation for 1 h (800 ×g, room temperature), plates were incubated for 8 h at 32°C and for 16 h at 37°C. Two additional retroviral infections were carried out at daily intervals. One day after the last retroviral infection (day 4), IL-4 producing cells were analyzed by intracellular cytokine staining (ICS). ICS was performed as described [3]. Briefly, Th2 cells were restimulated with plate-bound anti-CD3 plus -CD28 mAbs (1 μg/mL each) for 8 h in the presence of 10 μg/mL brefeldin A (Sigma-Aldrich) during the final 2 h of culture. The stimulated cells were fixed in 3.7% paraformaldehyde (Wako) for 10 min at room temperature. The fixed cells were permeabilized with PBS containing 0.5% bovine serum albumin (BSA) plus 0.5% saponin (Sigma-Aldrich) and stained with PE-conjugated anti-IL-4 Ab (11B11; BD) for 30 min. After washing twice with PBS containing 0.5% BSA and 0.5% saponin, the stained cells were analyzed using a FACSCalibur (BD). Data were analyzed with FlowJo software.

2.8. Adhesion Assay. Adhesion to ICAM-1 was performed as described [16] with slight modification. Briefly, 5 μg/mL goat anti-human-IgG (Fc) Ab (Jackson ImmunoResearch)-immobilized plates were coated with 1 μg/mL fusion protein (Fc-ICAM-1) of recombinant mouse ICAM-1 and human IgG1 Fc fragment (R&D Systems) overnight at 4°C. The coated plates were blocked with 1% BSA in PBS for 1 h at room temperature. Transfected cells were labeled with 2.5 μM Calcein-AM (DOJINDO) for 30 min at 37°C in Phenol-Red-free Hanks' balanced salt solution, washed twice, and incubated (1×10^5) on Fc-ICAM-1-coated plates, in the absence or presence of 10 μg/mL anti-CD3 Ab (OKT3; Biolegend). Obtained specific adhesion was expressed as a percentage of output fluorescence divided by input fluorescence.

2.9. Confocal Microscopy. Transfected Jurkat-TAg cells were placed on poly-L-lysine-coated coverslips with or without 2 μg/mL anti-CD3 Ab (OKT3; Biolegend) for 30 min at 37°C, fixed in 4% paraformaldehyde for 10 min at room temperature, and stained with Alexa Fluor 546 phalloidin (Thermo Fisher Scientific) and 4′,6′-diamidino-2-phenylindole (DAPI) (DOJINDO) for 40 min at room temperature. Images were captured with a LSM710 confocal laser scanning microscope (Carl Zeiss, Germany) with a 100x/1.40 Oil DIC objective.

2.10. Statistical Analysis. Statistical analysis was performed by using two-tailed Student's t-test.

3. Results

3.1. Identification of a Novel SLAT Splice Variant. To examine the expression of SLAT during Th2 differentiation, B6 naive $CD4^+$ T cells were activated in vitro under Th2-inducing conditions. Western blotting analysis using an anti-SLAT Ab revealed an unexpected smaller size SLAT-related molecule in differentiated Th2 cells, but not in differentiated Th1 cells, two days after the second round of in vitro stimulation (Figure 1(a)). To better characterize this gene product, we performed an RT-PCR on cDNA derived from Th2 cells two days after the second round of stimulation using primers designed to amplify the entire SLAT open reading frame (ORF). This resulted in amplification of a ~750 bp product revealed after a short (10 s) extension reaction, at which time the PCR product corresponding to the full length SLAT cDNA was not evident (Figure 1(b)). The ~750 bp PCR product was subcloned and sequenced, revealing a previously unreported *Def6* ORF, in which exons 2–7 were absent and exon 1 was directly spliced to exon 8 without frameshifts. This ORF potentially encodes a mature peptide comprising 257 amino acids. Western blotting analysis revealed that Jurkat-TAg cells transfected with the alternatively spliced SLAT cDNA expressed, as expected, a protein with a molecular mass of ~35 kDa, designated as SLAT2, in primary differentiated Th2 cells after the second round of stimulation.

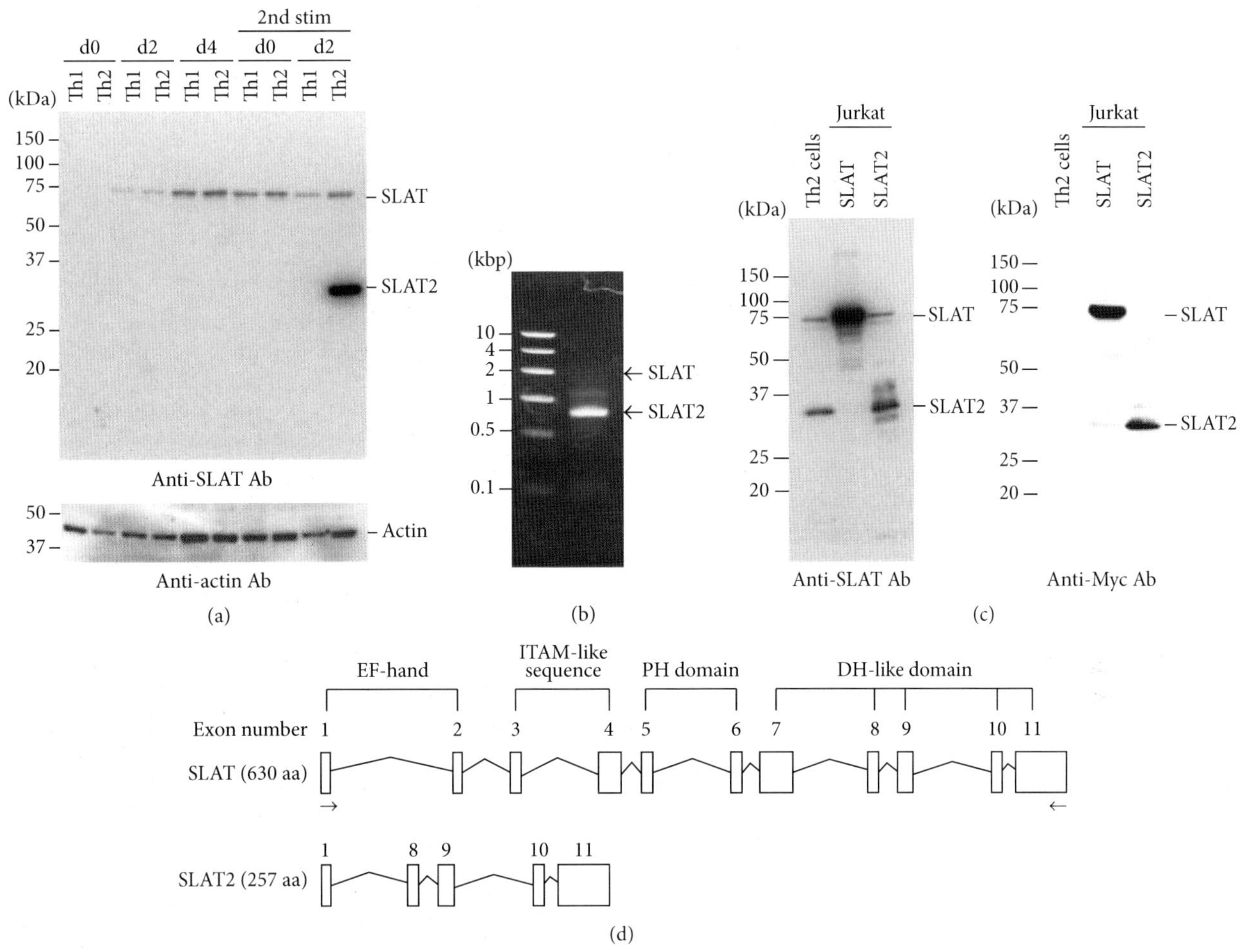

FIGURE 1: Identification of SLAT2, a novel SLAT splice variant. (a) $CD4^+$ T cells from B6 mice were differentiated under Th1- or Th2-inducing conditions with spleen-derived APCs and anti-CD3 Ab for 5 days, and the cells were then restimulated with plate-bound anti-CD3 plus -CD28 mAbs. Cell lysates were prepared at the indicated days and analyzed by Western blotting using anti-SLAT Ab. Data are representative of three independent experiments. (b) Gel electrophoresis of RT-PCR products amplified from Th2 cells two days after the second round of stimulation using primers spanning the entire SLAT open reading frame. Arrows indicate the position of SLAT2 (lower) or a predictable full length SLAT (upper). (c) Expression of SLAT and SLAT2 proteins in differentiated Th2 cells and Jurkat-TAg cells transfected with pEF-SLAT or pEF-SLAT2. Differentiated Th2 cells from B6 mice were restimulated with plate-bound anti-CD3 plus -CD28 mAbs for 4 days. Cell lysates were analyzed by anti-SLAT or anti-Myc immunoblotting. Data are representative of three independent experiments. (d) Genomic structure of SLAT and the alternatively spliced isoform SLAT2. Primers used for PCR amplification are indicated with arrows. Exons and introns are shown as open boxes and lines, respectively. SLAT2 contains the DH-like domain but lacks the part of EF-hand and the entire ITAM-like sequence and PH domain.

In contrast, SLAT-transfected cells expressed a protein of ~75 kDa (Figure 1(c)). Residues 33–257 are identical to the DH domain of SLAT. Primary structures of SLAT and SLAT2 are shown in Figure 1(d).

3.2. Expression and Regulation of SLAT2. To determine the kinetics of SLAT2 protein expression, B6 naive $CD4^+$ T cells differentiated under Th2- or Th1-inducing conditions were restimulated on day 5 with plate-coated anti-CD3 plus -CD28 mAbs under neutral culture conditions (Figure 2(a)). Prior to restimulation (day 0), SLAT2 was not expressed in either Th2 or Th1 cells, while SLAT was expressed in Th2, but not (or substantially less) in Th1 cells. Importantly, restimulation led to a substantial upregulation of SLAT2 protein expression on day 2 in Th2 cells, but not in Th1 cells. This upregulation was sustained on day 4 and decreased by day 6. In contrast, upregulation of SLAT was not observed on day 2 but was evident on days 4 and 6 in Th2 cells. To evaluate the expression of SLAT2 and SLAT under conditions of specific antigen stimulation, we obtained naive $CD4^+$ T cells from OT-II TCR-transgenic mice, which express an OVA-specific TCR, and cultured the cells with a low dose of OVA peptide and splenic APCs from B6 mice under Th2- or Th1-inducing conditions. Similar to B6 Th cells, SLAT2 was not expressed during the initial round of OVA stimulation (data not shown). However, following the second round of stimulation, the expression of SLAT2 was induced within one day reaching a maximum on day 2, with no SLAT2 detected

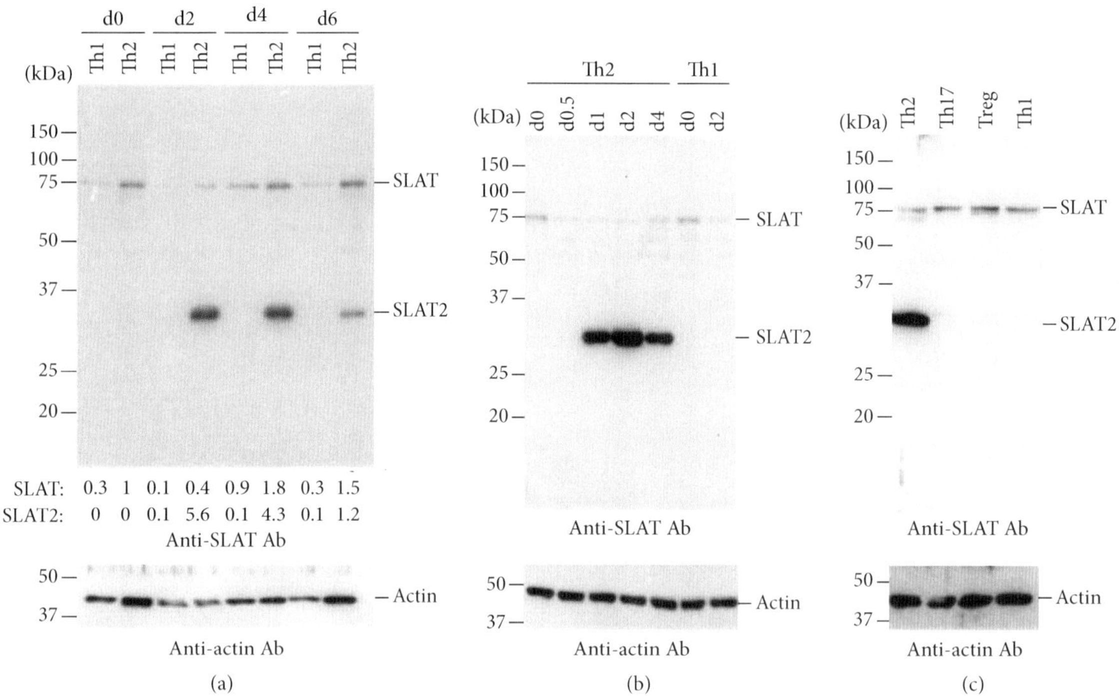

FIGURE 2: Kinetics of SLAT2 expression in differentiated Th cells. (a) $CD4^+$ T cells from B6 mice were differentiated under Th1- and Th2-inducing conditions as in Figure 1. Cell lysates were prepared at the indicated days and analyzed by Western blotting using anti-SLAT Ab. Numbers under the SLAT blot indicate intensity of SLAT and SLAT2 signals relative to SLAT signal of Th2 cells on day 0 (=1) after normalization to the actin signal. (b) $CD4^+$ T cells from OT-II mice were differentiated under Th1- or Th2-inducing conditions with splenic APCs and 1 μg/mL $OVA_{323-339}$ peptide for 5 days, and the cells were further restimulated with plate-bound anti-CD3 plus -CD28 mAbs. Cell lysates were prepared at the indicated days and analyzed as in (a). (c) $CD4^+$ T cells from B6 mice were differentiated into the indicated Th cell subset and restimulated with splenic APCs and anti-CD3 Ab for 4 days. Cell lysates were analyzed by Western blotting as in (a). Data are representative of at least two independent experiments.

after 0.5 days of stimulation (Figure 2(b)). Next, we examined the expression of SLAT2 in other subsets of differentiated Th cells, namely, Th17 and Treg cells. SLAT2 was observed in restimulated Th2 cells, but not in differentiated Th1, Th17, or Treg cells (Figure 2(c)). In contrast, SLAT was expressed in all subsets of differentiated Th cells. These results indicate that the expression of SLAT2 in differentiated and restimulated T cells is unique to the Th2 subset.

3.3. SLAT2 Enhances TCR-Induced NFAT Activity and IL-4 Expression. SLAT promotes Th1 and Th2 cell differentiation by controlling NFAT activation in $CD4^+$ T cells [17] and enhances TCR-induced NFAT activity [11]. To understand the function of SLAT2, we examined the effect of ectopic SLAT2 versus SLAT expression on the TCR-induced activation of an NFAT-luciferase reporter gene in Jurkat-TAg cells. Similar to SLAT and as previously shown [11], SLAT2 induced a dose-dependent increase in NFAT activity relative to empty vector-transfected cells (Figure 3(a)). Thus, SLAT2 can enhance the TCR-induced NFAT activity, just like SLAT. Next, we determined whether additional SLAT2 expression enhanced SLAT-mediated NFAT activity under TCR stimulation. Importantly, SLAT2 had an additive effect combined with SLAT on the TCR-induced NFAT activity (Figure 3(b)). These results suggest that the activation of TCR-induced NFAT is enhanced by SLAT2 and/or SLAT in Jurkat T cells.

NFAT activation promotes the expression of IL-4 in Th2 cells [23, 24]. To explore whether SLAT2 can regulate the production of IL-4, we generated a retroviral SLAT2 expression vector (Figure 3(c)), which was used to infect differentiated Th2 cells, resulting in a transduction efficiency of 25%–45% (data not shown). We have previously shown that transduction of differentiated Th2 cells with SLAT increases the fraction of IL-4-producing cells in the GFP^+ population [3]. Importantly, under the same conditions SLAT2 increased the fraction of IL-4-producing cells, *that is*, from ~39% to ~55% $IL\text{-}4^+$ cells (Figure 3(d)), even though SLAT minimally increased the fraction of IL-4-producing cells from ~39% to ~43% (Figure 3(d)). These results indicate that SLAT2 increases the level of IL-4-producing cells by differentiated Th2 cells.

3.4. SLAT2 Is Not Required for TCR-Induced Adhesion to ICAM-1. SLAT promotes the TCR-induced adhesion of T cells to ICAM-1 via leukocyte function-associated antigen-1 (LFA-1) activation [16]. To explore the role of SLAT2 in regulating LFA-1 function following TCR engagement, we examined the effect of ectopic SLAT2 expression on the TCR-mediated adhesion to ICAM-1. SLAT-transfected Jurkat-TAg

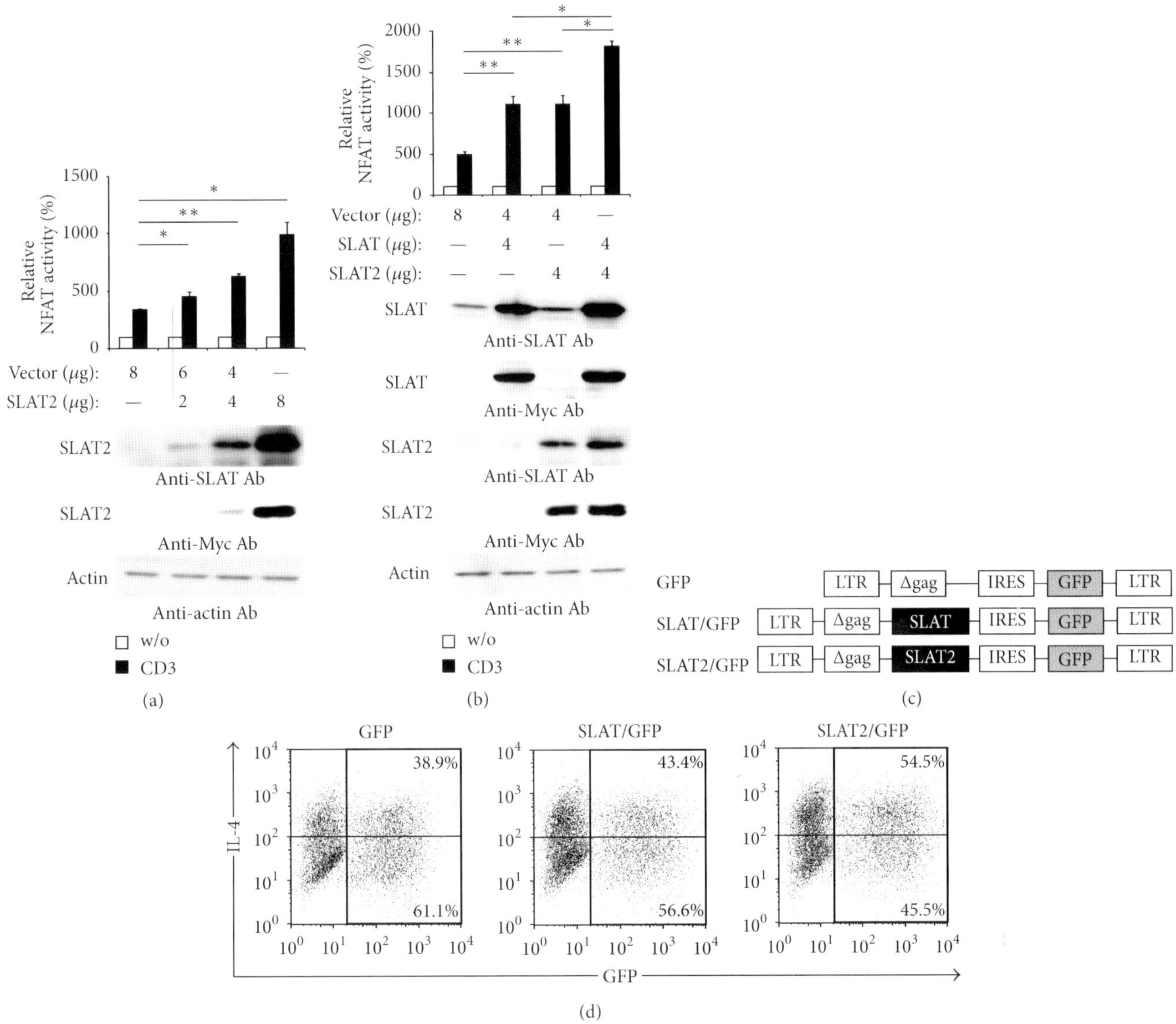

FIGURE 3: SLAT2 enhances TCR-induced NFAT activity and IL-4 expression. (a and b) Jurkat-TAg cells (5×10^6) were cotransfected with the indicated plasmid cDNA amounts of empty vector or SLAT and/or SLAT2 together with NFAT-Luc (5 μg) and β-galactosidase (β-gal) (5 μg) reporter plasmids. The cells were left unstimulated or were stimulated with 2 μg/mL anti-CD3 Ab (OKT3) for 6 h at 37°C. Luciferase activity was normalized to the activity of β-gal and data are displayed as % NFAT activity relative to basal activity in unstimulated cells (=100%). Data represent means of triplicates, and graphs show means ± SD. Statistical analysis was performed using Student's t-test ($^{*}P < 0.01$; $^{**}P < 0.001$). Expression of transfected SLAT and SLAT2 or endogenous actin proteins was detected by Western blotting (bottom panels). Data are representative of three independent experiments. (c) Schematic diagram of retroviral SLAT and SLAT2 constructs in the pMIG vector. (d) Five-day differentiated Th2 cells were restimulated with anti-CD3 plus -CD28 mAbs and infected with the indicated retroviruses. Cells were harvested on day 9 (4 days after second stimulation), restimulated with anti-CD3 plus -CD28 mAbs, and IL-4-producing cells were enumerated by intracellular cytokine staining. Data are representative of two independent experiments.

cells showed an increase in TCR-induced adhesion to ICAM-1 relative to control transfectants, as previously shown [16]. In contrast, SLAT2 had no effect on TCR-induced adhesion to ICAM-1 (Figure 4(a)). Thus, unlike SLAT, SLAT2 does not appear to enhance TCR-induced adhesion to ICAM-1 in T cells. These results suggest that SLAT2 may function in a manner different from SLAT during TCR-mediated T cell activation.

3.5. SLAT2 Localizes within Cytoplasm and Induces Short Filopodia. It is known that SLAT localizes to the plasma membrane and spreads diffusely throughout the cytoplasm in COS-7 cells [10, 13, 25]. To determine the cellular distribution of SLAT2, GFP-tagged SLAT2 or SLAT was expressed with Alexa Fluor 546-labeled phalloidin in Jurkat-TAg cells. The intracellular location of the proteins was determined by confocal microscopy. GFP-SLAT was found to colocalize

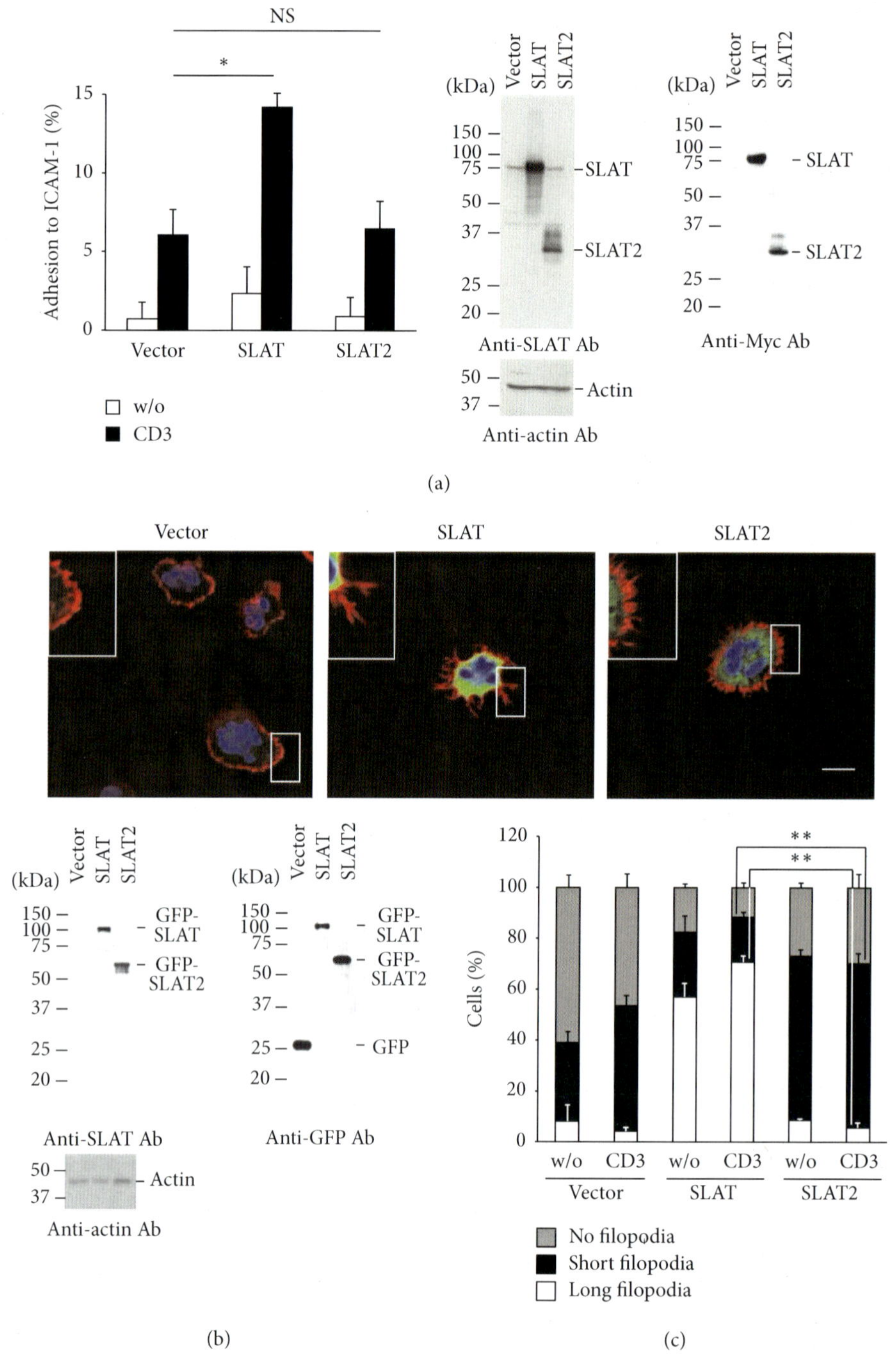

FIGURE 4: Effect of SLAT2 expression on T cell adhesion and filopodia formation. (a) Jurkat-TAg cells (5×10^6) were transfected with empty vector, pEF-SLAT or pEF-SLAT2 (8 μg each). The cells were either left unstimulated or stimulated with 10 μg/mL anti-CD3 Ab (OKT3) for 45 min and subsequently analyzed for adhesion to plate-bound Fc-ICAM-1. Data represent means of triplicates, and graphs show means ± SD (left). Expression of transfected proteins was detected with an anti-SLAT Ab or anti-Myc Ab (right). Statistical analysis was performed using Student's t-test ($^*P < 0.01$; NS, not significant). (b) Jurkat-TAg cells (5×10^6) were transfected with pSI-EGFP vector, pSI-EGFP-SLAT, or pSI-EGFP-SLAT2 (8 μg each). The cells were stimulated with 2 μg/mL anti-CD3 Ab (OKT3), immobilized on poly-L-lysine-coated coverslips, and fixed and stained with Alexa Fluor 546 Phalloidin and DAPI. Representative confocal images of stimulated cells imaged in each group are shown (upper). Scale bar, 10 μm. Expression of transfected proteins was detected with an anti-SLAT Ab or anti-GFP Ab (lower). (c) Quantitative analysis of the imaging data in panel (b). Cells were categorized into three groups, namely, long filopodia, short filopodia, or no filopodia. Long filopodia are defined as having a length ~5 times longer than short filopodia [43]. The percentage of cells in each class is shown. >100 cells were counted in each group. Data represent means of triplicates, and graphs show means ± SD. Statistical analysis was performed using Student's t-test ($^{**}P < 0.001$). Scale bar, 10 μm. Data are representative of three independent experiments.

with F-actin at the plasma membrane with or without TCR stimulation and, furthermore, compared to the empty vector-transfected cells, GFP-SLAT expression resulted in an apparent formation of long filopodia in Jurkat T cells in unstimulated T cells, and anti-CD3 stimulation caused a further increase (Figure 4(b), middle panel). In contrast, GFP-SLAT2 localized within the cytoplasm but did not colocalize with F-actin near the plasma membrane. Furthermore, GFP-SLAT2 mostly induced short filopodia formation in Jurkat T cells in either the absence or presence of TCR stimulation (Figure 4(b), right panel). In the control cells, faint short filopodia formation was observed in some GFP-transfected Jurkat-TAg cells. Quantitation of filopodia formation in the transfected T cells (Figure 4(c)) revealed that ectopic GFP-SLAT2 protein increased short filopodia formation in TCR-stimulated cells (17.3% ± 2.1% in GFP-SLAT-transfected cells versus 64.7% ± 3.5% in GFP-SLAT2-transfected cells; $P < 0.001$). In contrast to SLAT2, GFP-SLAT preferentially mediated long filopodia formation (70.7% ± 2.5% in GFP-SLAT-transfected cells versus 5.7% ± 2.1% in GFP-SLAT2-transfected cells; $P < 0.001$). These results indicate that, unlike SLAT, SLAT2 expression augments short filopodia formation at the expense of long filopodia in stimulated T cells.

4. Discussion

Alternative splicing is an important mechanism for controlling gene expression and increasing protein diversity from a single primary transcript. In the immune system, alternative splicing allows large proteomic complexity from a limited number of genes in inflammatory immune regulation network. Indeed, a few recent notable examples of alternative splicing, in $CD4^+$ T cell-expressed mucosa-associated lymphoid tissue protein 1 (MALT1) [26] and Foxp3 [27], have been demonstrated to regulate T cell responses to antigen [19]. In the present study, we have identified a new alternatively spliced product, termed SLAT2, of the murine *Def6* gene in differentiated Th2 cells after the second round of stimulation. SLAT2 mRNA is generated by the splicing of exons 2–7 that results in a partial deletion of Ca^{2+}-binding EF-hand and in the complete deletion of the ITAM-like sequence and the PH domain, generating a correct reading frame and a translated product that contains the C-terminal DH domain. The selective and transient upregulation of SLAT2 induced in differentiated Th2 cells by TCR restimulation suggests that SLAT2 may play a role in Th2-mediated immune responses, *for example*, allergic lung inflammation.

NFAT, a major regulator of T cell activation, is critical for IL-4 production and Th2 differentiation [23, 24]. Increasing evidence indicates that SLAT, which is predominantly expressed in T cells, plays important roles in TCR-mediated signaling by linking actin cytoskeleton reorganization and Cdc42 activation to the Ca^{2+}-NFAT signaling pathway and consequently to Th cell differentiation during inflammation [11, 12, 17, 28]. Our recent study demonstrated that the N-terminal EF-hand domain and the PH domain of SLAT interact with inositol 1,4,5-triphosphate receptor type 1 and that this interaction is important for TCR-mediated Ca^{2+}-NFAT signaling [15]. Interestingly, SLAT2 still possessed the ability to enhance NFAT activation, and coexpression of SLAT2 with SLAT resulted in further enhancement of TCR-induced NFAT activation despite the fact that SLAT2 lacks the ITAM-like sequence and PH domain, which were previously shown to contribute to the Ca^{2+}-NFAT signaling function of SLAT [11]. In addition, confocal microscopy analysis showed that SLAT2 did not translocate to the plasma membrane upon TCR stimulation. We therefore propose that cytosolic SLAT2 can enhance Ca^{2+}-NFAT signaling in a different way from SLAT or it may be able to act additively to SLAT in this pathway. We have also provided evidence that ectopic SLAT2 expression enhances the production of IL-4, in differentiated Th2 cells. Thus, the enhancement of NFAT activation induced by SLAT2 could account for the increased IL-4 expression by SLAT2-transduced Th2 cells.

SLAT2 expression was transiently and selectively upregulated in differentiated Th2 cells within one day of the second TCR stimulation, reached a maximum after two days, and declined by the sixth day, even though upregulation of SLAT2 was not observed during the first stimulation at all. SLAT2 is therefore expressed at a relatively late stage of Th cell differentiation, suggesting that it may not contribute to early Th2 cell differentiation per se, but may function during the effector phase of Th2 cell function. Differentiated Th2 cells transcribe *Il4* as early as 1 day after TCR restimulation (data not shown), a time when SLAT2 was already substantially upregulated. Further work should be aimed at defining the precise mechanisms that regulate the enhanced IL-4 expression by SLAT2 in differentiated Th2 cells, including in vivo, during inflammation.

Some of SLAT functions were not observed in SLAT2, including adhesion to ICAM-1 that reflects LFA-1 activation, and long filopodia formation in Jurkat T cell. SLAT is involved in TCR-induced adhesion through interaction of its PH domain with Rap1 GTPase, which was required for T cell adhesion to ICAM-1 [16]. Therefore, the deletion of the PH domain in SLAT2 likely explains the inability of SLAT2 to promote adhesion to ICAM-1. Thus, the functions of SLAT2 seem to be distinct from those of SLAT in TCR-mediated activation. SLAT is expressed and functions not only in Th cells but also in other types of cells, such as macrophages [29, 30], osteoclasts [31], and cancer cells [32–35]. Thus, it would be interesting to determine whether SLAT2 is expressed and functions in these other cell types.

Cdc42 member of the Rho family of small GTPases is cytosol in its GDP-bound resting form. Cdc42 functions as a molecular switch by cycling between GDP-bound inactive and GTP-bound active states and is recruited to membranes where its GDP is exchanged for GTP through the action of several GEFs with known reactivity toward Rho family GTPases [36]. Dbl family proteins, which possess a catalytic DH domain followed by a PH domain, constitute the largest subgroup of Rho-specific GEFs, followed by the dedicator of cytokinesis (DOCK) family, whose members possess a DOCK homology region 2 (DHR2) instead of a DH domain. The smallest subgroup of SWAP-70 subfamily includes SWAP-70 and SLAT, which contain a DH-like domain but neither a DH nor a DHR2 domain. Some of these Rho GEFs, *that is*, Vav [22] and βPIX [37] (Dbl subfamily), DOCK8 [38] (DOCK subfamily), and SLAT [3, 9–14, 39–42] (SWAP-70 subfamily), participate in TCR signaling and Th cell differentiation and are known to mediate GEF activity on Cdc42. The SLAT DH-like domain possesses TCR-mediated, plasma membrane-residing GEF activity toward Cdc42 that controls dynamics of the actin cytoskeleton and leads to long filopodia formation [10]. Additionally, the TCR-induced tyrosine phosphorylation of the ITAM-like sequence in SLAT is required for its translocation to the plasma membrane and immunological synapse [11]. We observed lack of membrane localization of SLAT2, which correlated with reduced long filopodia formation in SLAT2-transfected T cells compared to SLAT-transfected cells. Instead, SLAT2 increased formation of short, rather than long, filopodia in TCR-stimulated cells. Therefore, the differential localization and function of the two SLAT proteins and, potentially, differences in their reactivity toward Cdc42 might play an important role in regulating the formation of filopodia at the site of inflammatory immune responses.

5. Conclusions

Collectively, our results suggest that alternative splicing of SLAT may exhibit differential biological activities upon TCR-mediated stimulation and that modulating either SLAT2 or SLAT protein expression could play critical roles in cytokine production and actin reorganization during inflammatory immune responses, leading to altered functional activities of these regulators. Precise understanding of the mechanism through which SLAT2 modulates TCR-mediated signaling and Th2 cell function awaits future studies.

Acknowledgments

This work was supported in part by Japan Society for the Promotion of Science KAKENHI (Grant nos. 16J09588 to Marie Hashimoto and 26293393, 16K15792, and 26670822 to Yoshihiko Tanaka); Futaba Electronics Memorial Foundation, the NOVARTIS Foundation (Japan) for the Promotion of Science, Astellas Foundation for Research on Metabolic Disorders, SENSHIN Medical Research Foundation, and Takeda Science Foundation (to Yoshihiko Tanaka); and NIH (Grant AI068320 to Amnon Altman). The authors thank M. Matsumoto, K. I. Nakayama, and Y. Fukui for helpful comments, and this work was partly performed in the Cooperative Research Project Program of the Medical Institute of Bioregulation, Kyushu University.

References

[1] K. Hirahara and T. Nakayama, "CD4+ T-cell subsets in inflammatory diseases: beyond the Th1/Th2 paradigm," *International Immunology*, vol. 28, no. 4, pp. 163–171, 2016.

[2] H. Yamane and W. E. Paul, "Early signaling events that underlie fate decisions of naive CD4+ T cells toward distinct T-helper cell subsets," *Immunological Reviews*, vol. 252, no. 1, pp. 12–23, 2013.

[3] Y. Tanaka, K. Bi, R. Kitamura et al., "SWAP-70-like adapter of T Cells, an adapter protein that regulates early TCR-initiated signaling in Th2 lineage cells," *Immunity*, vol. 18, no. 3, pp. 403–414, 2003.

[4] M. Shinohara, Y. Terada, A. Iwamatsu et al., "SWAP-70 is a guanine-nucleotide-exchange factor that mediates signalling of membrane ruffling," *Nature*, vol. 416, no. 6882, pp. 759–763, 2002.

[5] B. Gross, T. Borggrefe, M. Wabl et al., "SWAP-70-deficient mast cells are impaired in development and IgE-mediated degranulation," *European Journal of Immunology*, vol. 32, no. 4, pp. 1121–1128, 2002.

[6] R. R. Sivalenka and R. Jessberger, "SWAP-70 regulates c-kit-induced mast cell activation, cell-cell adhesion, and migration," *Molecular and Cellular Biology*, vol. 24, no. 23, pp. 10277–10288, 2004.

[7] M. Hotfilder, S. Baxendale, M. A. Cross, and F. Sablitzky, "Def-2, -3, -6 and -8, novel mouse genes differentially expressed in the haemopoietic system," *British Journal of Haematology*, vol. 106, no. 2, pp. 335–344, 1999.

[8] S. Gupta, A. Lee, C. Hu et al., "Molecular cloning of IBP, a SWAP-70 homologous GEF, which is highly expressed in the immune system," *Human Immunology*, vol. 64, no. 4, pp. 389–401, 2003.

[9] S. Gupta, J. C. Fanzo, C. Hu et al., "T cell receptor engagement leads to the recruitment of IBP, a novel guanine nucleotide exchange factor, to the immunological synapse," *Journal of Biological Chemistry*, vol. 278, no. 44, pp. 43541–43549, 2003.

[10] K. J. Mavrakis, K. J. McKinlay, P. Jones, and F. Sablitzky, "DEF6, a novel PH-DH-like domain protein, is an upstream activator of the Rho GTPases Rac1, Cdc42, and RhoA," *Experimental Cell Research*, vol. 294, no. 2, pp. 335–344, 2004.

[11] S. Bécart, A. J. Canonigo Balancio, C. Charvet, S. Feau, C. E. Sedwick, and A. Altman, "Tyrosine-phosphorylation-dependent translocation of the SLAT protein to the immunological synapse is required for NFAT transcription factor activation," *Immunity*, vol. 29, no. 5, pp. 704–719, 2008.

[12] K. L. Singleton, M. Gosh, R. D. Dandekar et al., "Itk controls the spatiotemporal organization of T cell activation," *Science Signaling*, vol. 4, no. 193, p. ra66, 2011.

[13] F. Hey, N. Czyzewicz, P. Jones, and F. Sablitzky, "DEF6, a novel substrate for the tec kinase ITK, contains a glutamine-rich aggregation-prone region and forms cytoplasmic granules that co-localize with P-bodies," *Journal of Biological Chemistry*, vol. 287, no. 37, pp. 31073–31084, 2012.

[14] S. Feau, S. P. Schoenberger, A. Altman, and S. Bécart, "SLAT regulates CD8+ T cell clonal expansion in a Cdc42- and NFAT1-dependent manner," *Journal of Immunology*, vol. 190, no. 1, pp. 174–183, 2013.

[15] C. Fos, S. Bécart, A. J. Canonigo Balancio, D. Boehning, and A. Altman, "Association of the EF-hand and PH domains of the guanine nucleotide exchange factor SLAT with IP_3 receptor 1 promotes Ca^{2+} signaling in T cells," *Science Signaling*, vol. 7, no. 345, p. ra93, 2014.

[16] M. Côte, C. Fos, A. J. Canonigo-Balancio, K. Ley, S. Bécart, and A. Altman, "SLAT promotes TCR-mediated, Rap1-dependent LFA-1 activation and adhesion through interaction of its PH domain with Rap1," *Journal of Cell Science*, vol. 128, no. 23, pp. 4341–4352, 2015.

[17] S. Bécart, C. Charvet, A. J. Canonigo Balancio et al., "SLAT regulates Th1 and Th2 inflammatory responses by controlling Ca^{2+}/NFAT signaling," *Journal of Clinical Investigation*, vol. 117, no. 8, pp. 2164–2175, 2007.

[18] A. J. Canonigo-Balancio, C. Fos, T. Prod'homme, S. Bécart, and A. Altman, "SLAT/Def6 plays a critical role in the development of Th17 cell-mediated experimental autoimmune encephalomyelitis," *Journal of Immunology*, vol. 183, no. 11, pp. 7259–7267, 2009.

[19] N. M. Martinez and K. W. Lynch, "Control of alternative splicing in immune responses: many regulators, many predictions, much still to learn," *Immunological Reviews*, vol. 253, no. 1, pp. 216–236, 2013.

[20] M. Villalba, N. Coudronniere, M. Deckert, E. Teixeiro, P. Mas, and A. Altman, "A novel functional interaction between Vav and PKCθ is required for TCR-induced T cell activation," *Immunity*, vol. 12, no. 2, pp. 151–160, 2000.

[21] M. Villalba, S. Kasibhatla, L. Genestier, A. Mahboubi, D. R. Green, and A. Altman, "Protein kinase Cθ cooperates with calcineurin to induce Fas ligand expression during activation-induced T cell death," *Journal of Immunology*, vol. 163, no. 11, pp. 5813–5819, 1999.

[22] Y. Tanaka, T. So, S. Lebedeva, M. Croft, and A. Altman, "Impaired IL-4 and c-Maf expression and enhanced Th1-cell development in Vav1-deficient mice," *Blood*, vol. 106, no. 4, pp. 1286–1295, 2005.

[23] A. M. Ranger, M. R. Hodge, E. M. Gravallese et al., "Delayed lymphoid repopulation with defects in IL-4-driven responses produced by inactivation of NF-ATc," *Immunity*, vol. 8, no. 1, pp. 125–134, 1998.

[24] H. Yoshida, H. Nishina, H. Takimoto et al., "The transcription factor NF-ATc1 regulates lymphocyte proliferation and Th2 cytokine production," *Immunity*, vol. 8, no. 1, pp. 115–124, 1998.

[25] T. Oka, S. Ihara, and Y. Fukui, "Cooperation of DEF6 with activated Rac in regulating cell morphology," *Journal of Biological Chemistry*, vol. 282, no. 3, pp. 2011–2018, 2007.

[26] I. Meininger, R. A. Griesbach, D. Hu et al., "Alternative splicing of MALT1 controls signalling and activation of $CD4^{+}$ T cells," *Nature Communications*, vol. 7, Article ID 11292, 2016.

[27] V. De Rosa, M. Galgani, A. Porcellini et al., "Glycolysis controls the induction of human regulatory T cells by modulating the expression of FOXP3 exon 2 splicing variants," *Nature Immunology*, vol. 16, no. 11, pp. 1174–1184, 2015.

[28] S. Bécart and A. Altman, "SWAP-70-like adapter of T cells: a novel Lck-regulated guanine nucleotide exchange factor coordinating actin cytoskeleton reorganization and Ca^{2+} signaling in T cells," *Immunological Reviews*, vol. 232, no. 1, pp. 319–333, 2009.

[29] H. Mehta, M. Glogauer, S. Bécart, A. Altman, and K. M. Coggeshall, "Adaptor protein SLAT modulates Fcγ receptor-mediated phagocytosis in murine macrophages," *Journal of Biological Chemistry*, vol. 284, no. 18, pp. 11882–11891, 2009.

[30] Q. Chen, S. Gupta, and A. B. Pernis, "Regulation of TLR4-mediated signaling by IBP/Def6, a novel activator of Rho GTPases," *Journal of Leukocyte Biology*, vol. 85, no. 3, pp. 539–543, 2009.

[31] B. U. Youn, K. Kim, J. H. Kim et al., "SLAT negatively regulates RANKL-induced osteoclast differentiation," *Molecules and Cells*, vol. 36, no. 3, pp. 252–257, 2013.

[32] P. Li, Z. Zhang, Q. Wang et al., "The ectopic expression of IFN regulatory factor 4-binding protein is correlated with the malignant behavior of human breast cancer cells," *International Immunopharmacology*, vol. 9, no. 7-8, pp. 1002–1009, 2009.

[33] Z. Zhang, Q. Wang, P. Li et al., "Overexpression of the Interferon regulatory factor 4-binding protein in human colorectal cancer and its clinical significance," *Cancer Epidemiology*, vol. 33, no. 2, pp. 130–136, 2009.

[34] M. Yang, F. Yuan, P. Li et al., "Interferon regulatory factor 4 binding protein is a novel p53 target gene and suppresses cisplatin-induced apoptosis of breast cancer cells," *Molecular Cancer*, vol. 11, article 54, 2012.

[35] C.-X. Jian, M.-Z. Yang, P. Li et al., "Ectopically expressed IBP promotes cell proliferation in oral squamous cell carcinoma," *Cancer Investigation*, vol. 30, no. 10, pp. 748–756, 2012.

[36] V. L. J. Tybulewicz and R. B. Henderson, "Rho family GTPases and their regulators in lymphocytes," *Nature Reviews Immunology*, vol. 9, no. 9, pp. 630–644, 2009.

[37] G. M. Ku, D. Yablonski, E. Manser, L. Lim, and A. Weiss, "A PAK1-PIX-PKL complex is activated by the T-cell receptor independent of Nck, Slp-76 and LAT," *EMBO Journal*, vol. 20, no. 3, pp. 457–465, 2001.

[38] X. Xu, L. Han, G. Zhao et al., "LRCH1 interferes with DOCK8-Cdc42-induced T cell migration and ameliorates experimental autoimmune encephalomyelitis," *The Journal of Experimental Medicine*, vol. 214, no. 1, pp. 209–226, 2017.

[39] J. C. Fanzo, W. Yang, S. Y. Jang et al., "Loss of IRF-4-binding protein leads to the spontaneous development of systemic autoimmunity," *Journal of Clinical Investigation*, vol. 116, no. 3, pp. 703–714, 2006.

[40] Q. Chen, W. Yang, S. Gupta et al., "IRF-4-binding protein inhibits interleukin-17 and interleukin-21 production by controlling the activity of IRF-4 transcription factor," *Immunity*, vol. 29, no. 6, pp. 899–911, 2008.

[41] P. S. Biswas, G. Bhagat, and A. B. Pernis, "IRF4 and its regulators: evolving insights into the pathogenesis of inflammatory arthritis?" *Immunological Reviews*, vol. 233, no. 1, pp. 79–96, 2010.

[42] P. S. Biswas, S. Gupta, E. Chang et al., "Phosphorylation of IRF4 by ROCK2 regulates IL-17 and IL-21 production and the development of autoimmunity in mice," *Journal of Clinical Investigation*, vol. 120, no. 9, pp. 3280–3295, 2010.

[43] G. A. Murphy, P. A. Solski, S. A. Jillian et al., "Cellular functions of TC10, a Rho family GTPase: regulation of morphology, signal transduction and cell growth," *Oncogene*, vol. 18, no. 26, pp. 3831–3845, 1999.

6

CCR7 Receptor Expression in Mono-MAC-1 Cells: Modulation by Liver X Receptor α Activation and Prostaglandin E_2

Bérengère Tanné, Stéphane Bernier, and Nancy Dumais

Département de Biologie, Faculté des Sciences, Université de Sherbrooke, Sherbrooke, QC, Canada J1K 2R1

Correspondence should be addressed to Nancy Dumais; nancy.dumais@usherbrooke.ca

Academic Editor: G. Rogler

Cell migration via chemokine receptor CCR7 expression is an essential function of the immune system. We previously showed that prostaglandin E_2 (PGE_2), an important immunomodulatory molecule, increases CCR7 expression and function in monocytes. Here, we explore the role of the liver X receptor α (LXRα) activation on CCR7 expression in Mono-Mac-1 (MM-1) cells in the presence of PGE_2. To do this, MM-1 cells were stimulated with the LXRα synthetic agonist T0901317 in the presence or absence of PGE_2. *CCR7* mRNA transcription was measured using quantitative RT-PCR and protein expression was examined using flow cytometry. CCR7 function was analyzed using migration assays in response to CCL19/CCL21, which are natural ligands for CCR7. Our results show that agonist-mediated activation of LXRα in the presence of PGE_2 increases CCR7 mRNA transcription and MM-1 cell migratory capacity in response to CCL19/21. In addition, our results demonstrate that engagement of the E-prostanoids 2 and 4 (EP_2/EP_4) receptors present on MM-1 cells is responsible for the observed increase in *CCR7* mRNA expression and function during LXRα activation. Examination of monocyte migration in response to lipid derivatives such as PGE_2 and oxysterols that are produced at sites of chronic inflammation would contribute to understanding the excessive monocyte migration that characterizes atherosclerosis.

1. Introduction

Inflammatory monocytes are rapidly recruited to sites of inflammation, but their excessive and/or prolonged recruitment hinders the resolution of inflammation and is a hallmark of numerous diseases. Chemokines CCL19 and CCL21, which are important for cellular migration, are expressed by lymphatic endothelia as well as within lymph nodes by stromal cells, endothelial cells, and dendritic cells (DCs) [1–4]. These chemokines are the natural ligands of CCR7, which is expressed in DCs [5], T and B cells [6], and monocytes [7]. Mice deficient in CCL19, CCL21, or CCR7 demonstrate defective DC trafficking and altered immune responses [8, 9].

PGE_2 modulates immune responses both *in vitro* and *in vivo* [10]. A marked increase in PGE_2 production (as high as 10^{-4} M) is generated in response to a variety of immunological stimuli and infections with different pathogens (reviewed in [11]). The immunomodulatory molecule PGE_2 appears to have a dual role in DC migration by regulating CCR7 expression and activity. Maturation-induced upregulation of CCR7 surface expression is not sufficient for monocyte-derived DCs (MoDCs) to migrate toward CCL19 and CCL21 [12, 13]. Indeed, MoDC migration toward CCL19 and CCL21 was readily observed upon maturation in the presence of the proinflammatory mediator PGE_2. However, PGE_2 did not alter expression levels of CCR7 on mature DCs [12, 13]. In human monocytes, PGE_2 affects *CCR7* mRNA expression and function [6, 14].

In macrophages as well as in DCs, oxysterol-mediated activation of the nuclear liver X receptor (LXR) has been shown to modulate innate immunity and tumor growth (reviewed in [15]). LXRβ is expressed ubiquitously, whereas LXRα is expressed in the liver, adipose tissue, adrenal glands, intestine, lungs, and cells of the myelomonocytic lineage [16]. Interestingly, it has been demonstrated that LXR-dependent effects in DCs regulate CCR7-dependent migration. Indeed, LXRα and LXRβ, which are oxysterol-activated transcription factors, prevent TLR-induced CCR7 upregulation in MoDCs

Table 1: Primers used in real-time qPCR assays.

Target	$MgCl_2$	Forward primer	Reverse primer
LXR	3.5 mM	5′-GCTGCAAGTGGAATTCATCAACC-3′	5′-ATATGTGTGCTGCAGCCTCTCCA-3′
CCR7	2 mM	5′-GTGGTGGCTCTCCTTGTCAT-3′	5′-TGTGGTGTTGTCTCCGATGT-3′
ABCG1	2 mM	5′-CACCAGCCGACTGTTCTGCAT-3′	5′-TGTACCGGGGAAAAGTCTGC-3′
B2M	2 mM	5′-GAGTATGCCTGCCGTGTGAA-3′	5′-TGCGGCATCTTCAAACCTCC-3′
hOGG1	3.5 mM	5′-TGGAAGAACAGGGCGGGCTA-3′	5′-ATGGACATCCACGGGCACAG-3′

[17] and interfere with CCR7 expression on mature DCs, resulting in a dampened antitumor immune response [18]. Moreover, a recent study showed that PGE_2 interferes with LXR activation, downregulates LXRα expression, and rescues the migratory ability of DCs to migrate toward CCR7 ligands [19]. Therefore, because lipid derivatives such as oxysterols and prostaglandins are important in DC migration, we examined whether PGE_2 and LXR activation can modify CCR7-dependent migration of human monocytes.

Our results show that PGE_2 and synthetic LXRα ligand, T0901317, strongly increase MM-1 cell migratory capacity in response to CCL19/21. Examination of monocyte migration in response to lipid derivatives, produced during chronic inflammation, would contribute to understanding the excessive monocyte migration that characterizes atherosclerosis.

2. Materials and Methods

2.1. Reagents. Prostaglandin E_2 and the LXR agonist T0901317 were purchased from Sigma-Aldrich (St. Louis, MO, USA). The MEK kinase inhibitor PD98059 was purchased from Enzo Life Sciences (Farmingdale, NY, USA). The EP agonists butaprost, 11-deoxy-PGE_1, and 17-phenyl-trinor-PGE_2, as well as the phosphatidylinositol 3-kinase (PI3K) inhibitor LY294002 and PKA inhibitor H-89 were obtained from Cayman Chemical (Ann Arbor, MI, USA). The blocking antibody against human CCR7 and chemokines CCL19/CCL21 were purchased from R&D Systems (Minneapolis, MN, USA).

2.2. Cell Culture. Mono-Mac-1 cells (MM-1; ACC 252), an acute peripheral monoblastic leukemia derived cell line (German Collection of Microorganisms and Cell Cultures, Braunschweig, Germany), were cultured in RPMI 1640 media (Sigma-Aldrich) supplemented with 10% heat-inactivated fetal bovine serum (FBS), nonessential amino acids (NEAA), 1 mM sodium pyruvate, 100 I.U. penicillin G, and 100 μg/mL streptomycin (all were obtained from Wisent, St-Bruno, QC, Canada).

2.3. Blood Monocyte Isolation. Total blood mononuclear cells were isolated from the blood of healthy donors using lymphocyte separation Medium 1077 (Sigma) and washed twice in Hank's balanced salt solution (Wisent). Cells were cultured in RPMI 1640 medium, 20% heat-inactivated FBS, and 10% heat-inactivated human serum for 2 h before use. Monocytes were washed from nonadherent cells with phosphate-buffered saline (PBS). Monocytes were then enriched from peripheral blood mononuclear cells using the MACS Monocyte Isolation Kit II and MACS LS Columns (Miltenyi Biotec, Auburn, CA, USA), yielding an average purity of 98%. The purity was assessed by flow cytometric analyses as recommend by the manufacturer, and isolated monocytes were fluorescently stained with CD14-FITC and anti-Biotin-PE that labeled nonmonocytes. Blood monocytes were stimulated for the indicated times using 1 μM PGE_2 and/or 1 μM T0901317.

2.4. Real-Time Quantitative Polymerase Chain Reaction (qPCR) Analyses. MM-1 cells were incubated with stimulants for the indicated times, and total RNA was extracted using Nucleospin RNA columns (Macherey-Nagel, BioLynx, Brockville, ON, Canada) according to the manufacturer's instructions. RNA (2 μg) was reverse-transcribed into cDNA in the presence of 0.5 μg of oligonucleotide $d(T)_{15}$, 200 units of M-MLV RT (Promega, Madison, WI, USA), and 250 μM deoxyribonucleotide triphosphates (dNTPs) at 42°C for 1 h. Amplification of human *NR1H3* (*LXRα*), *CCR7*, and *ABCG1* was performed using the SYBR Green I nucleic acid gel stain (Invitrogen, Burlington, ON, Canada) on a CFX Connect Real Time System (BIO-RAD, Mississauga, ON, Canada). Results were analyzed using the software BIO-RAD CFX Manager. qPCR reactions contained 0.25 μM forward and reverse primers (Table 1), 0.1 mM dNTPs, 2 mM or 3.5 mM $MgCl_2$, and 1.25 units of Omni Klentaq (Enzymatics, Beverly, MA, USA). In each reaction, we used 8 μL of a 1 : 2 dilution of each cDNA (dilutions were performed using molecular grade sterile water (Wisent)). PCR cycling conditions consisted of an initial denaturation at 95°C for 3 minutes and 40 cycles of 95°C for 10 sec, 60°C for 40 sec, 72°C for 40 sec, and a melting curve at 95°C for 10 sec, 65°C for 5 sec, and 95°C for 5 sec.

2.5. Chemotaxis Assays. MM-1 cell chemotaxis was measured by migration through a polycarbonate filter (5 μm pore size) in a 96-well transwell chambers (Millipore, Nepean, ON, Canada). The lower chamber contained either 150 μL of a 300 ng/mL dilution of chemokine CCL19/CCL21 in RPMI 1640 media without FBS, NEAA, and sodium pyruvate, but complemented with 0.25% BSA, or media alone as a spontaneous migration control. The upper chamber contained 2.5 $\times 10^5$ cells in 75 μL of medium. Chambers containing MM-1 cells were incubated for 4 h at 37°C. An aliquot (150 μL) of cells that migrated to the bottom chamber was mixed with 1x PBS (150 μL) and counted using a BD FACSCalibur flow cytometer (BD Biosciences, San Jose, CA, USA) by acquiring events for a fixed period of 60 seconds using CellQuest

Software (BD Biosciences). The percentage of migrated cells was calculated as follows: the number of migrated cells in response to media only was subtracted from the number of migrated cells in response to CCL19/CCL21. This number was normalized to the total input of cells. Each experiment was performed in triplicate and repeated at least three times.

2.6. Flow Cytometry Analyses. MM-1 cells were collected and washed twice with PBS supplemented with 3% bovine serum albumin (BSA). Fc receptors were blocked for 15 minutes at room temperature using 100 μL of human serum (diluted 1:5 in 1x PBS) for 1×10^6 cells. Cells were then washed twice in PBS plus 3% BSA. Cells were labeled with an anti-CCR7 antibody conjugated with allophycocyanin (APC), or corresponding isotypes as a negative control, for 45 minutes on ice in the dark. Cells were then washed twice with PBS plus 3% BSA and centrifuged 5 minutes at 10 g at 4°C. For intracellular experiments, cells were collected and washed with buffer (1x PBS plus 1% BSA and 0.02% sodium azide). Fc receptors were blocked using 100 μL human serum for 15 minutes at room temperature and washed with wash buffer. Cells were fixed with 200 μL 4% paraformaldehyde for 15 minutes at 4°C and again washed with wash buffer. Cells were permeabilized by adding 200 μL of 1% saponin to the wash buffer and then incubated for 45 minutes on ice with anti-CCR7 coupled with APC (Abcam, San Francisco, CA, USA) or the corresponding isotype controls. Cells were then washed twice with wash buffer. Fluorescence was read using a BD FACSCalibur flow cytometer (BD Biosciences) and results were analyzed using CellQuest software (BD Biosciences).

2.7. Statistical Analyses. Each experiment was performed at least three times. Statistically significant differences between experimental groups were evaluated using paired t-tests and $p < 0.05$ was considered statistically significant. Computations were performed using GraphPad PRISM version 6.0 statistical software (GraphPad, San Diego, CA, USA).

3. Results

3.1. PGE_2 and LXRα Activation Upregulate CCR7 mRNA Production and Function without Affecting CCR7 Surface Expression in MM-1 Cells. MM-1 is a human cell line with the properties of blood monocytes that can be used as a model system to study monocytic functions *in vitro* [20]. We first used real-time qPCR to examine whether PGE_2 and LXRα activation could modulate *CCR7* transcription in MM-1 cells. MM-1 cells were treated with 1 μM PGE_2 and 1 μM T0901317, a synthetic LXRα agonist, for 8 or 24 h (Figure 1(a)). As previously observed, PGE_2 induces *CCR7* mRNA expression with a maximal effect after stimulation for 8 h [7]. Treatment of MM-1 cells with T0901317 alone does not modify the expression of *CCR7* mRNA. Interestingly, we found that cells treated with a combination of PGE_2 and T0901317 showed significantly upregulated *CCR7* mRNA transcription.

Next, we determined whether MM-1 cells can autoregulate LXRα expression as previously demonstrated in macrophages [21]. *LXRα* transcripts were measured using real-time qPCR following stimulation with 1 μM PGE_2 and 1 μM T0901317 (Figure 1(b)). We observed an increase in *LXRα* levels following treatment with PGE_2 or T0901317 alone. mRNA production plateaued after 8 h of stimulation with PGE_2 or T0901317 alone. However, MM-1 cells that were stimulated with a combination of PGE_2 and T0901317 showed increased levels of *LXRα* mRNA after 24 h compared to cells stimulated with PGE_2 or T0901317 alone.

We also investigated whether PGE_2 in combination with T0901317 affects the expression of one LXRα target gene, *ABCG1* (Figure 1(c)). As expected, *ABCG1* mRNA levels were augmented when cells were treated with T0901317 alone. PGE_2 had no effect on *ABCG1* transcription. However, MM-1 cells treated with a combination of PGE_2 and T0901317 showed significantly reduced levels of *ABCG1* transcription.

We next established whether increased mRNA production correlates with CCR7 receptor function in MM-1 cells. MM-1 cells were treated with the stimulants for 24 or 48 h before migration through polycarbonate filters (5 μm pore size) for 4 h. The chemotaxis assay results showed that PGE_2 increases MM-1 cell migration to both CCR7 natural ligands CCL19 (Figure 2(a)) and CCL21 (Figure 2(b)) after treatment for 24 h. Although the migratory capacity of MM-1 cells is sustained in response to CCL21 after 48 h, migration in response to CCL19 appears transient. The LXR agonist alone did not affect the migratory capacity of MM-1 cells in response to CCL19 whereas 24 h treatment with T0901317 significantly increased migration in response to CCL21. In contrast, migration of MM-1 cells treated with PGE_2 and T0901317 for 48 h was increased compared to untreated cells or cells treated with PGE_2 alone. For all chemotaxis assays, we confirmed the specificity of migration by incubating PGE_2- and T0901317-stimulated cells with a blocking antibody against human CCR7 for 10 min prior to migration assays. Blockade of CCR7 at the MM-1 cell surface completely abolished specific migration to CCL19 and CCL21 (data not shown). To further investigate the effects of PGE_2 and T0901317 on CCR7 expression, we repeated migration assays with freshly isolated human blood monocytes. Results showed that monocyte migration toward CCL19 and CCL21 is increased following treatment of blood monocytes with PGE_2 and T0901317 (Figure 3).

We aimed at establishing whether the CCR7 receptor is expressed at the cell surface of PGE_2- and T0901317-stimulated MM-1 cells. Cells were incubated in the presence or absence of PGE_2 and T0901317 for 24 and 48 h. Surface expression of CCR7 was analyzed using flow cytometry. Our results showed that MM-1 cells basally express CCR7 (13.57% with a MFI (mean fluorescence intensity) of 4.94). However, after 24 h, CCR7 cell surface expression was upregulated by 1 μM PGE_2 (31.66% with a MFI of 7.82) but not by T0901317 (13.11% with a MFI of 4.83) (Figure 4(a), upper panel). Similar results were observed after 48 h (Figure 4(b), lower panel). Statistics for CCR7 cell surface expression are presented in Table 2. Because CCR7 cell surface expression was not upregulated following the addition of PGE_2 and T0901317, we performed intracellular flow cytometry assays after 24 h (Figure 4(b), upper panel) and 48 h (Figure 4(b), lower panel)

TABLE 2: Statistical analyses of CCR7 surface expression in MM-1 cells.

	Mean % of positive cells	SD	p value	Mean MFI	SD	p value
24 h						
Untreated	16,04	2,21		4,32	0,54	
PGE_2	36,40	5,67	0.0044	9,24	1,55	0.0066
T0901317	11,32	1,86	0.047	4,76	0,72	0.45
PGE_2 + T0901317	26,83	2,06	0.0038	6,68	1,18	0.035
48 h						
Untreated	6,11	2,04		3,32	0,76	
PGE_2	17,81	3,99	0.011	7,59	2,13	0.030
T0901317	5,07	2,49	0.61	3,71	0,88	0.57
PGE_2 + T0901317	20,11	2,48	0.0016	8,06	1,69	0.011

Data represent mean ± standard deviation (SD) of three independent flow cytometry experiments after 24 or 48 h of treatment with 1 μM PGE_2 and/or 1 μM T0901317.

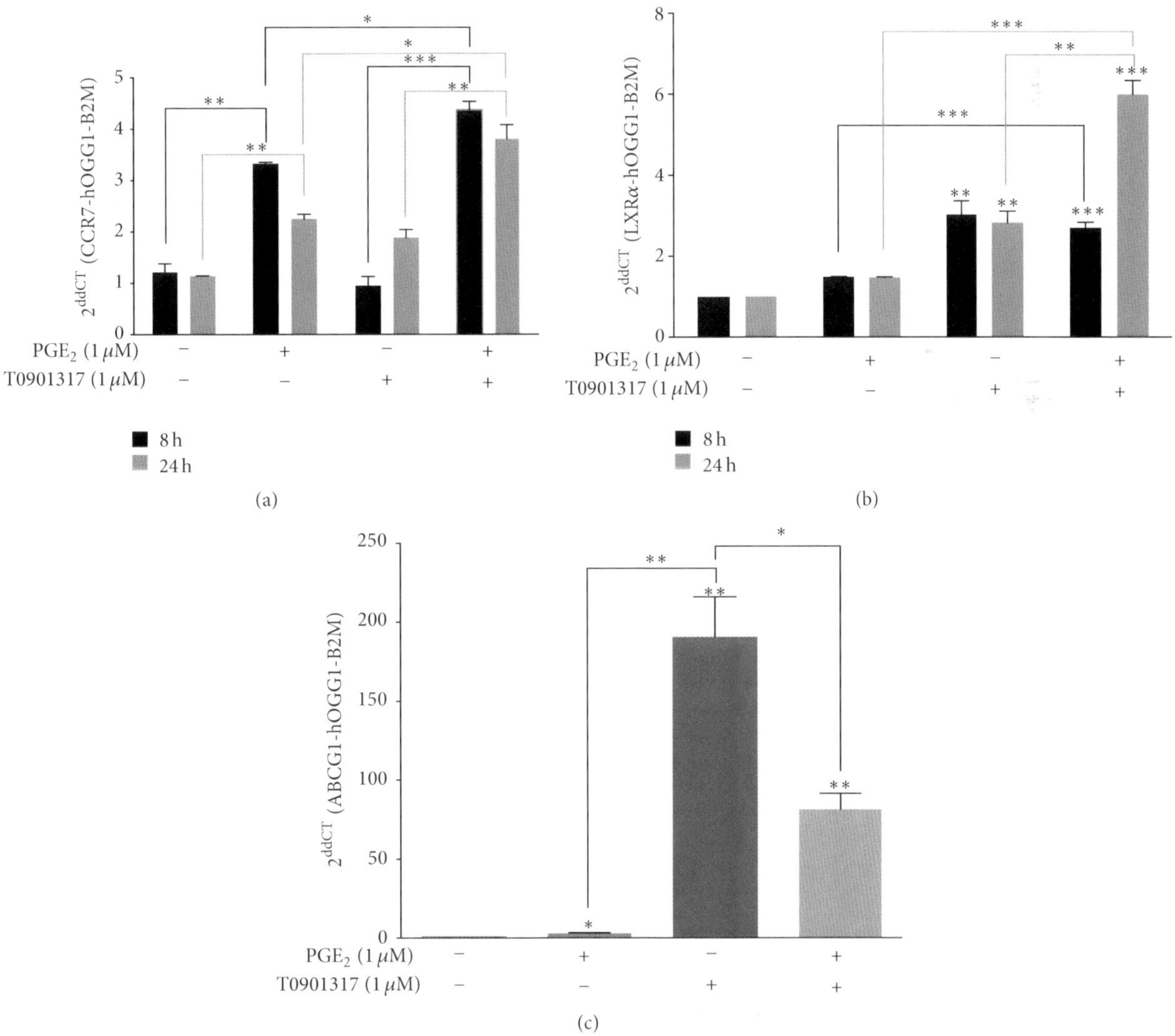

FIGURE 1: Effects of PGE_2 and T0901317 on *CCR7*, *ABCG1*, and *LXRα* transcription in MM-1 cells. MM-1 cells were stimulated for 8 h and 24 h with 1 μM PGE_2 and 1 μM T0901317. Total RNA was extracted and examined using real-time quantitative PCR to detect *CCR7* (a), *ABCG1* (b), and *LXRα* (c) mRNA levels. Data represent mean ± standard deviation (SD) of three independent experiments. $^{*}p < 0.05$, $^{**}p < 0.01$, and $^{***}p < 0.001$.

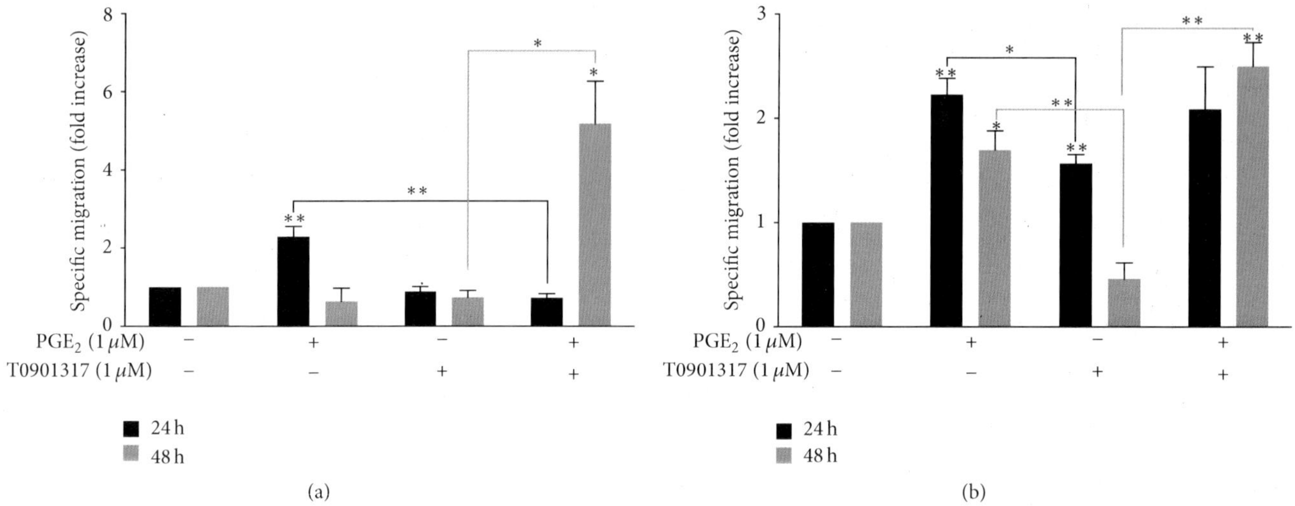

FIGURE 2: PGE_2 alone and in combination with T0901317 induces functional CCR7-specific migration of MM-1 cells. Chemotaxis assays in response to 300 ng/mL CCL19 (a) or CCL21 (b) were performed in MM-1 cells stimulated for 24 h (filled black) or 48 h (filled gray) with 1 μM PGE_2 and 1 μM T0901317. The mean number of spontaneously migrating cells (that migrated to media alone) was subtracted from the number of cells that migrated in response to CCL19 or CCL21. Data represent mean ± SD of three independent experiments. $^{*}p < 0.05$, $^{**}p < 0.01$.

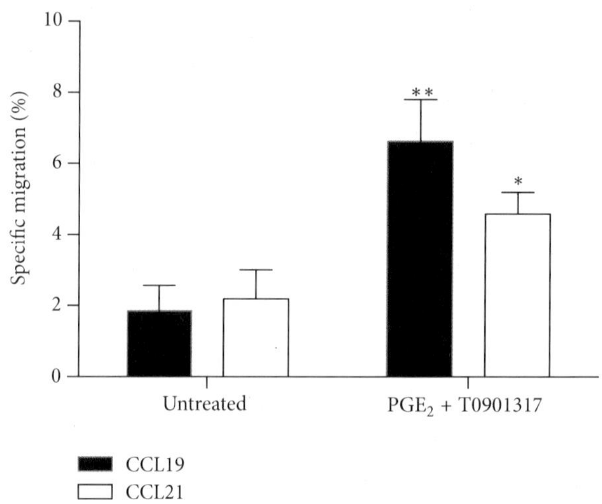

FIGURE 3: Freshly isolated monocytes migrate toward the CCR7-specific ligands CCL19 and CCL21. Chemotaxis assays using 300 ng/mL CCL19 and CCL21 were performed using human monocytes incubated in the presence or absence of 1 μM PGE_2 and 1 μM T0901317 for 48 h. Data represent the means of three different experiments. Data represent mean ± SD of three independent experiments. $^{*}p < 0.05$, $^{**}p < 0.01$ compared to untreated cells.

to determine whether CCR7 receptors are trapped internally. We observed that, after 24 h, the basal level of CCR7 is higher than the surface levels (20.87% with a MFI of 9.96), which is similar with PGE_2 treatment (27.72% with a MFI of 12.21). However, there is no variation between treatments: In addition, there is no variation internal CCR7 expression between MM-1 cells treated with PGE_2 (24.20% with a MFI of 10.84) or with PGE_2 in combination with T0901317 (20.77% with a MFI of 10.07). When MM-1 cells are treated for 48 h, decreased levels of CCR7 are observed compared with 24 h treatment: untreated (3.09% with a MFI of 3.71), PGE_2 (6.04% with a MFI of 3.34), T0901317 (5.04% with a MFI of 3.25), and PGE_2 in combination with T0901317 (5.76% with a MFI of 4.18).

3.2. The EP_2 and EP_4 Receptors Are Involved in LXRα Activation and PGE_2-Induced CCR7 Transcription and Functional Migration. We previously showed that monocytes primarily express two PGE_2 receptors, EP_2 and EP_4 [7]. Moreover, we demonstrated that both receptors are implicated in PGE_2-induced CCR7 upregulation in MM-1 cells [7]. Thus, using pharmacological agonists for PGE_2 receptors, we next determined whether EP_2 and/or EP_4 play a role in PGE_2- and T0901317-induced CCR7 migration (Figure 5). Treatment of MM-1 cells with the EP_2 and EP_4 agonist 11-deoxy-PGE_1 increased *CCR7* mRNA levels compared to untreated cells (Figure 5(a)). Although 17-PT-PGE_2 is described as an EP_1/EP_3 (EP_1 > EP_3) agonist, at high doses, 17-PT-PGE_2 also activates EP_4 receptor (Ki = 1 μM) [22, 23]. Our

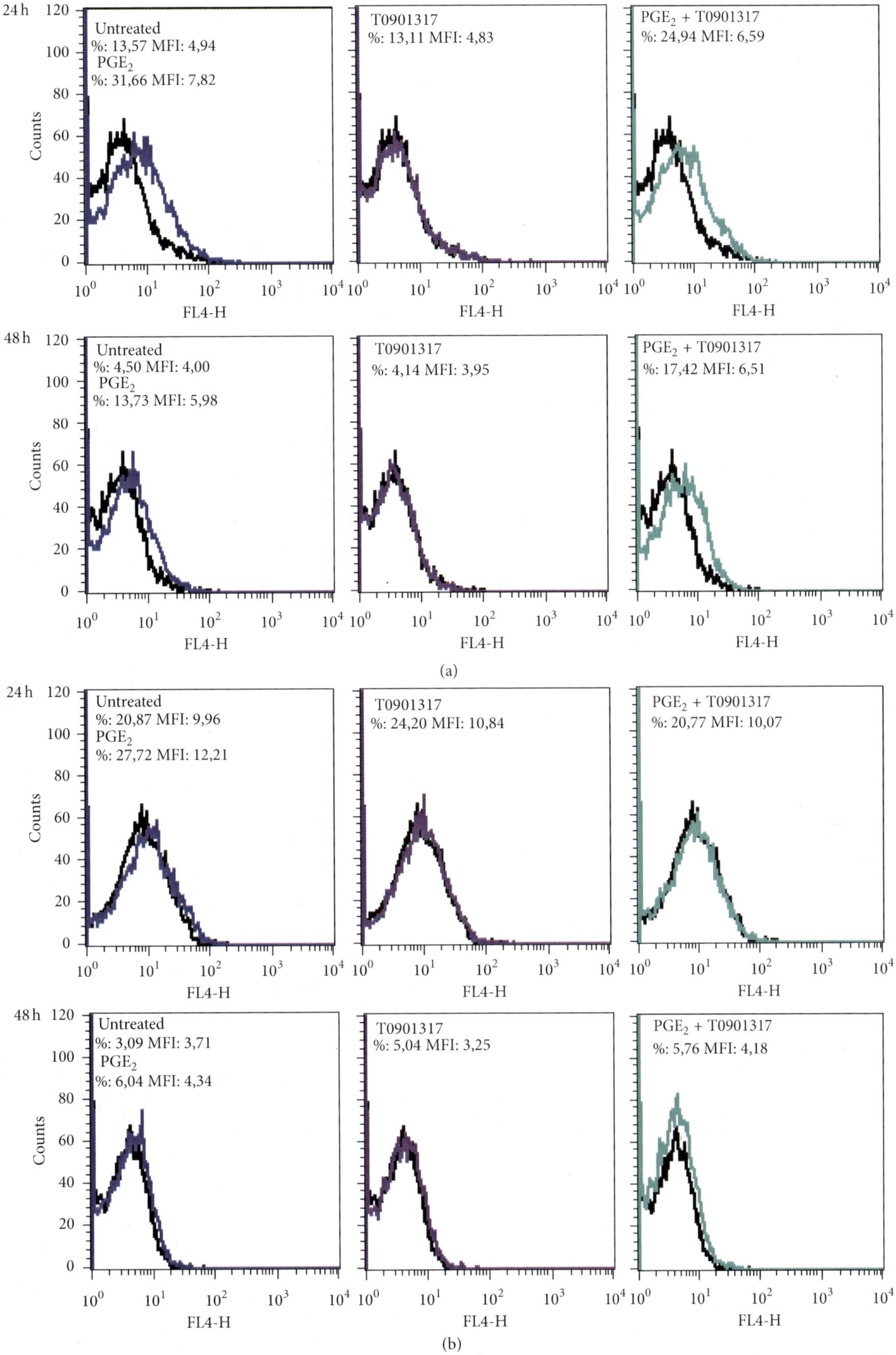

Figure 4: Cell surface and intracellular expression of CCR7 in MM-1 cells. CCR7 surface expression (a) or intracellular expression (b) was evaluated by flow cytometry after treatment with 1 μM PGE_2 and/or 1 μM T0901317 for 24 h or 48 h. Data shown are from one of three representative experiments.

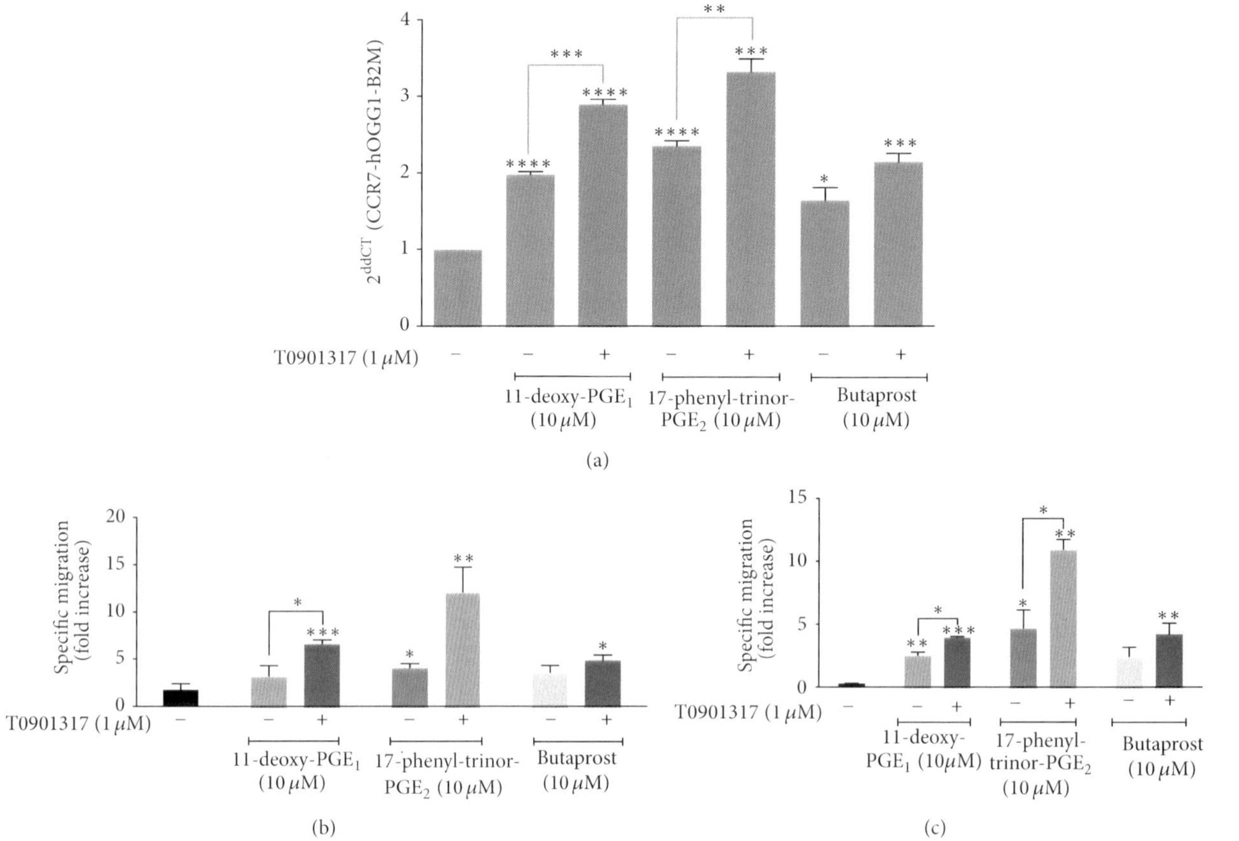

FIGURE 5: Functional migration in response to PGE_2 and T0901317 is dependent on EP_2 and EP_4 receptors in MM-1 cells. (a) MM-1 cells were treated for 8 h (filled black) and 24 h (filled gray) with the indicated concentrations of 11-deoxy-PGE_1, 17-phenyl-trinor-PGE_2, and butaprost. Total RNA was extracted and *CCR7* transcripts were detected using real-time qPCR. Data represent mean ± SD of three independent experiments. Chemotaxis assays in response to 300 ng/mL CCL19 (b) or CCL21 (c) were performed using MM-1 cells stimulated for 48 h with 1 μM T0901317. The mean number of spontaneously migrating cells (that migrated to media alone) was subtracted from the number of cells that migrated in response to CCL19. Data represent mean ± SD of three independent experiments. $^{*}p < 0.05$, $^{**}p < 0.01$, $^{***}p < 0.001$, and $^{****}p < 0.0001$.

results showed that 17-PT-PGE_2 significantly enhanced *CCR7* expression whereas butaprost alone or in combination with T0901317 slightly increased *CCR7* RNA levels compared to control. To determine which PGE_2 receptors regulate the migratory response of T0901317-treated monocytes to CCL19 and CCL21, chemotaxis assays were performed on MM-1 cells in response to CCL19 (Figure 5(b)) or CCL21 (Figure 5(c)). Our results indicated that MM-1 cells migrated efficiently toward CCL19 or CCL21 when butaprost, 11-deoxy-PGE_1, and 17-PT-PGE_2 were added to the milieu. However, the most remarkable migration occurred when PGE_2-treated MM-1 cells were cultivated in the presence of T0901317.

Because EP_2 and EP_4 receptors activate adenylate cyclase (AC), which then increases intracellular cAMP levels [23], we next assessed whether forskolin, a pharmacological activator of AC, contributed to the observed induction of *CCR7* mRNA (Figure 6(a)). MM-1 cells were stimulated with 100 μM forskolin for 8 h or 24 h in the presence or absence of T0901317. We found that forskolin alone increases *CCR7* mRNA transcription whereas forskolin combined with T0901317 did not affect *CCR7* expression. AC activation did not modulate *CCR7* mRNA production in T0901317-treated MM-1 cells. Thus, we searched for alternative signaling pathways. MM-1 cells were treated with H-89 (a PKA inhibitor), LY294002 (a PI3K inhibitor), or PD98059 (a MEK inhibitor) before the addition of PGE_2 and T0901317 for 48 h. Cells were used in migration assays in response to CCL19 or CCL21 (Figure 6(b)). The results showed that selective inhibition of PKA and MEK did not affect CCR7-dependent migration of MM-1 cells in response to CCL19 or 21. In contrast, inhibition of PI3K further enhanced MM-1 cell migration mediated by PGE_2 and T0901317.

4. Discussion

In addition to modulating cholesterol homeostasis, LXRs have emerged as important regulators of inflammatory gene expression and innate immunity [21]. In inflammation, PGE_2 is of particular interest because its deregulation is associated with the pathogenesis of various diseases and numerous tumor types [11, 24]. In this study, we showed for the first time that PGE_2 in combination with LXRα activation strongly

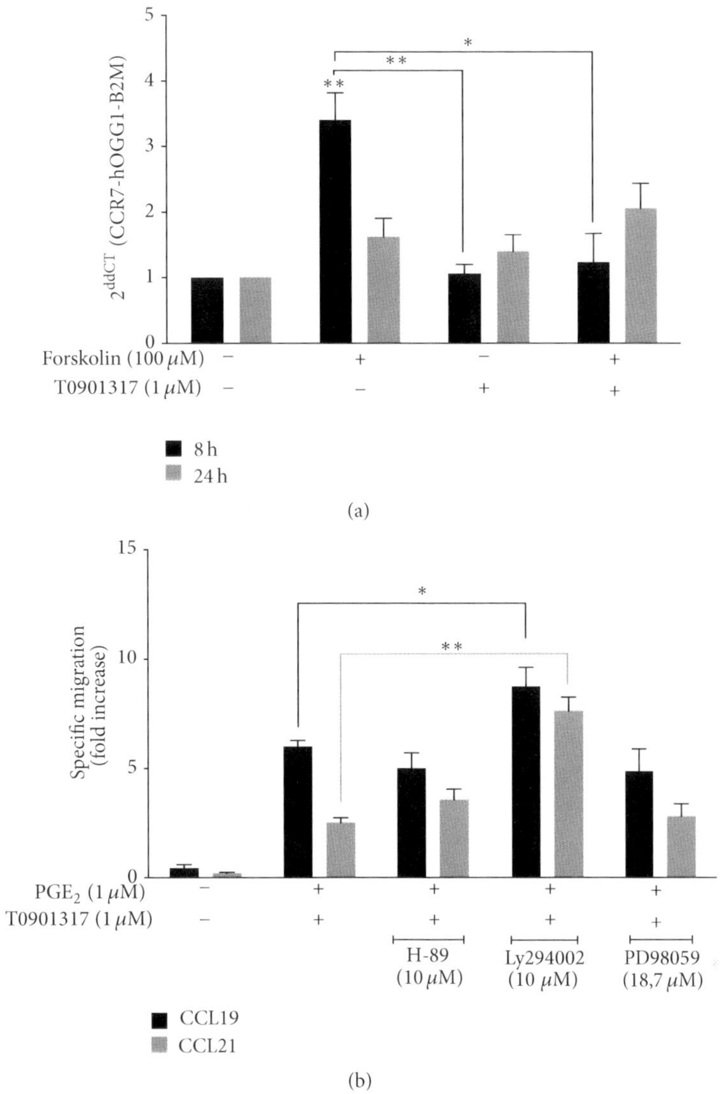

FIGURE 6: The role of cAMP and alternative EP_2/EP_4 signaling pathways in PGE_2- and T0901317-induced *CCR7* mRNA expression and function. (a) MM-1 cells were treated for 8 h (filled black) and 24 h (filled gray) with 100 μM forskolin alone or in combination with 1 μM T0901317. Total RNA was extracted and *CCR7* transcripts were detected using real-time qPCR. (b) Chemotaxis assays in response to 300 ng/mL CCL19 (filled black) or CCL21 (filled gray) were performed in MM-1 cells treated with the indicated concentrations of H-89, Ly294002, and PD98059 before the addition of 1 μM PGE_2 and T0901317 for 48 h. The mean number of spontaneously migrating cells (that migrated to media alone) was subtracted from the number of cells that migrated in response to CCL19 or CCL21. Data represent mean ± SD of three independent experiments. $^{*}p < 0.05$, $^{**}p < 0.01$.

increased the CCR7-dependent migratory capacity of MM-1 cells, a monocytoid cell line. We showed that although *CCR7* mRNA levels are upregulated following treatment with PGE_2 and T0901317, there was no change in CCR7 cell surface expression. In addition, our results indicate that EP_2 and EP_4 receptors are implicated in PGE_2-mediated *CCR7* transcription required for upregulating the migratory capacity of MM-1 cells in response to CCL19 and CCL21.

In mature DCs, it has been previously shown that activation of LXRs interferes with CCR7 expression, resulting in a dampened antitumor immune response [18]. Recently, Bruckner et al. [19] demonstrated that PGE_2 rescues the migratory capacity of DCs cultivated in the presence of LXR ligands to migrate toward CCR7 ligands. In contrast to these results, LXR activation in MM-1 cells by the synthetic ligand T0901317 does not modify *CCR7* expression (Figure 1(a)) or CCR7-dependent migration in response to CCL19 (Figure 2(a)) or CCL21 (Figure 2(b)). However, the combination of PGE_2 and T0901317 significantly increased *CCR7* mRNA production and MM-1 cell migration compared to cells treated with PGE_2 or T0901317 alone. In addition, blood monocytes treated PGE_2 and T0901317 migrate in response to CCR7 specific ligands compared to untreated monocytes (Figure 3). Importantly, MM-1 surface expression of CCR7 (Figure 4(a)) did not correlate with migration efficiency (Figure 2). Indeed, other studies have shown

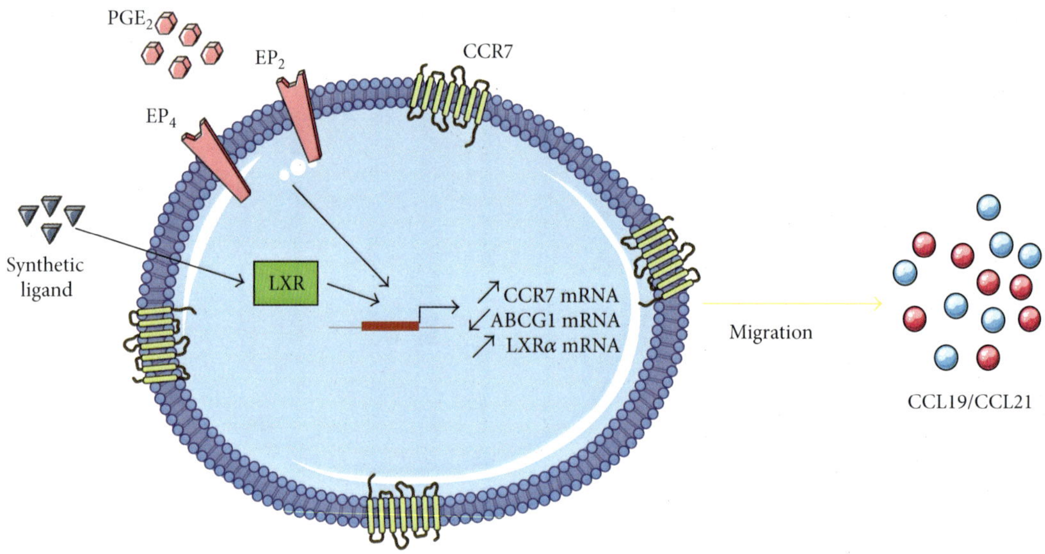

FIGURE 7: Schematic depicting effects of PGE_2 and LXR activation on CCR7 functionality in MM-1 cells.

that PGE_2 significantly enhances DC migration through an unknown mechanism that does not depend on the magnitude of CCR7 expression [12, 25, 26]. This phenomenon is also observed with MoDCs matured in the presence of both PGE_2 and T0901317 [19]. Thus, our results in monocytes are consistent with those observed by other groups in DCs. In addition, flow cytometry analyses were also performed to detect intracellular changes in CCR7 protein expression (Figure 4(b)). However, no changes in expression were detectable. Together, our results demonstrate that LXR activation and PGE_2 stimulation of MM-1 cells profoundly affect monocyte migration in response to CCL19 and CCL21. Further studies are required to examine the effect of LXR activation in the presence of PGE_2 on CCR7-dependent migration of freshly isolated blood monocytes from healthy donors.

In macrophages, LXR activation results in the synthesis of the cholesterol efflux transporter ABCG1 as well as of LXRα itself through an autoregulatory mechanism [21]. In DCs, PGE_2 downregulated basal expression of *LXRα* but also inhibited T0901317-mediated autoinduction of *LXRα* [19]. In addition, T0901317-mediated ABCG1 induction was also significantly reduced in MoDCs matured in the presence of PGE_2 [19]. In our study, we observed that PGE_2 did not modulate *ABCG1* mRNA production whereas T0901317 alone significantly affected transcription (Figure 1(b)). In contrast, in MM-1 cells stimulated with PGE_2 and T0901317 for 24 h, we observed significantly reduced *ABCG1* mRNA production. In MM-1 cells, LXRα activation upregulated *LXRα* mRNA expression but PGE_2 had no effect. In contrast to results observed in DCs [19], 24 h treatment with PGE_2 and T0901317 strongly increased *LXRα* mRNA transcription. Our results demonstrated that the addition of PGE_2 to T0901317-treated MM-1 cells reduced *ABCG1* mRNA production. Because *LXRα* expression was increased after MM-1 cells were treated with PGE_2 and T0901317 (Figure 1(c)), the effect on *ABCG1* is likely LXRα-independent. It has been shown that ABCG1 and ABCG4 act in concert with ABCA1 to maximize removal of excess cholesterol from cells [27]. Taken together, our results suggest that the presence of PGE_2 and oxysterols negatively impacts cholesterol efflux in monocytes. Moreover, the presence of these two lipids derivatives may favor intracellular cholesterol accumulation, thereby leading to deregulation of cholesterol homeostasis in monocytes. However, further studies are needed to clarify the mechanisms underlying the observed modulation of *ABCG1* by PGE_2 and LXRα ligands in monocytes.

The EP_2 and EP_4 receptors were previously shown to be important for CCR7 expression in mature MoDCs [13, 19, 25] and monocytes [7]. Here, our results showed that PGE_2 binding to the EP_4 receptor subtype, and to a lesser extent EP_2, triggered signals that led to *CCR7* mRNA expression and CCR7-dependent migration of MM-1 cells cultivated in the presence of the LXRα synthetic ligand (Figure 5). Interestingly, our data showed that PGE_2- and T0901317-upregulation of CCR7 expression and function is independent of the cAMP/PKA or MEK branches of EP_2/EP_4 signaling (Figure 6). However, we showed that inhibition of the PI3K pathway is responsible for enhanced CCR7-dependent MM-1 cell migration. Thus, our results suggest the contribution of other signaling pathways.

In summary, our results demonstrate that PGE_2, in combination with LXRα activation, increased CCR7-dependent migration of MM-1 cells (Figure 7). Lipid derivatives, including PGE_2 and oxysterols, may also favor cholesterol accumulation in monocytes. Therefore, our results may have important implications regarding the mechanisms that contribute to atherosclerosis. However, further studies are needed to better understand the role of lipid derivatives produced during inflammation.

Acknowledgment

This study was supported by the Canadian Institutes of Health Research (Funding Reference no. 123681).

References

[1] M. D. Gunn, K. Tangemann, C. Tam, J. G. Cyster, S. D. Rosen, and L. T. Williams, "A chemokine expressed in lymphoid high endothelial venules promotes the adhesion and chemotaxis of naive T lymphocytes," *Proceedings of the National Academy of Sciences of the United States of America*, vol. 95, no. 1, pp. 258–263, 1998.

[2] S. A. Luther, H. L. Tang, P. L. Hyman, A. G. Farr, and J. G. Cyster, "Coexpression of the chemokines ELC and SLC by T zone stromal cells and deletion of the ELC gene in the plt/plt mouse," *Proceedings of the National Academy of Sciences of the United States of America*, vol. 97, no. 23, pp. 12694–12699, 2000.

[3] V. N. Ngo, H. L. Tang, and J. G. Cyster, "Epstein-Barr virus-induced molecule 1 ligand chemokine is expressed by dendritic cells in lymphoid tissues and strongly attracts naive T cells and activated B cells," *The Journal of Experimental Medicine*, vol. 188, no. 1, pp. 181–191, 1998.

[4] J. V. Stein, A. Rot, Y. Luo et al., "The CC chemokine thymus-derived chemotactic agent 4 (TCA-4, secondary lymphoid tissue chemokine, 6Ckine, exodus-2) triggers lymphocyte function-associated antigen 1-mediated arrest of rolling T lymphocytes in peripheral lymph node high endothelial venules," *The Journal of Experimental Medicine*, vol. 191, pp. 61–76, 2000.

[5] H. Saeki, A. M. Moore, M. J. Brown, and S. T. Hwang, "Cutting edge: secondary lymphoid-tissue chemokine (SLC) and CC chemokine receptor 7 (CCR7) participate in the emigration pathway of mature dendritic cells from the skin to regional lymph nodes," *Journal of Immunology*, vol. 162, no. 5, pp. 2472–2475, 1999.

[6] R. A. Warnock, J. J. Campbell, M. E. Dorf, A. Matsuzawa, L. M. McEvoy, and E. C. Butcher, "The role of chemokines in the microenvironmental control of T versus B cell arrest in Peyer's patch high endothelial venules," *The Journal of Experimental Medicine*, vol. 191, no. 1, pp. 77–88, 2000.

[7] S. C. Côté, S. Pasvanis, S. Bounou, and N. Dumais, "CCR7-specific migration to CCL19 and CCL21 is induced by PGE_2 stimulation in human monocytes: involvement of EP_2/EP_4 receptors activation," *Molecular Immunology*, vol. 46, no. 13, pp. 2682–2693, 2009.

[8] R. Förster, A. Schubel, D. Breitfeld et al., "CCR7 coordinates the primary immune response by establishing functional microenvironments in secondary lymphoid organs," *Cell*, vol. 99, no. 1, pp. 23–33, 1999.

[9] M. D. Gunn, S. Kyuwa, C. Tam et al., "Mice lacking expression of secondary lymphoid organ chemokine have defects in lymphocyte homing and dendritic cell localization," *The Journal of Experimental Medicine*, vol. 189, no. 3, pp. 451–460, 1999.

[10] J. S. Goodwin and D. R. Webb, "Regulation of the immune response by prostaglandins," *Clinical Immunology and Immunopathology*, vol. 15, no. 1, pp. 106–122, 1980.

[11] B. Rocca and G. A. FitzGerald, "Cyclooxygenases and prostaglandins: shaping up the immune response," *International Immunopharmacology*, vol. 2, no. 5, pp. 603–630, 2002.

[12] E. Scandella, Y. Men, S. Gillessen, R. Förster, and M. Groettrup, "Prostaglandin E2 is a key factor for CCR7 surface expression and migration of monocyte-derived dendritic cells," *Blood*, vol. 100, no. 4, pp. 1354–1361, 2002.

[13] T. Luft, M. Jefford, P. Luetjens et al., "Functionally distinct dendritic cell (DC) populations induced by physiologic stimuli: prostaglandin E_2 regulates the migratory capacity of specific DC subsets," *Blood*, vol. 100, no. 4, pp. 1362–1372, 2002.

[14] M.-A. Allaire and N. Dumais, "Involvement of the MAPK and RhoA/ROCK pathways in PGE_2-mediated CCR7-dependent monocyte migration," *Immunology Letters*, vol. 146, no. 1-2, pp. 70–73, 2012.

[15] C. Traversari, S. Sozzani, K. R. Steffensen, and V. Russo, "LXR-dependent and -independent effects of oxysterols on immunity and tumor growth," *European Journal of Immunology*, vol. 44, no. 7, pp. 1896–1903, 2014.

[16] N. Y. Kalaany and D. J. Mangelsdorf, "LXRs and FXR: the yin and yang of cholesterol and fat metabolism," *Annual Review of Physiology*, vol. 68, pp. 159–191, 2006.

[17] T. M. Hanley, W. B. Puryear, S. Gummuluru, and G. A. Viglianti, "PPARγ and LXR signaling inhibit dendritic cell-mediated HIV-1 capture and trans-infection," *PLoS Pathogens*, vol. 6, no. 7, Article ID e1000981, 2010.

[18] E. J. Villablanca, L. Raccosta, D. Zhou et al., "Tumor-mediated liver X receptor-α activation inhibits CC chemokine receptor-7 expression on dendritic cells and dampens antitumor responses," *Nature Medicine*, vol. 16, no. 1, pp. 98–105, 2010.

[19] M. Bruckner, D. Dickel, E. Singer, and D. F. Legler, "Converse regulation of CCR7-driven human dendritic cell migration by prostaglandin E_2 and liver X receptor activation," *European Journal of Immunology*, vol. 42, no. 11, pp. 2949–2958, 2012.

[20] K. G. Steube, D. D. Teepe, C. Meyer, M. Zaborski, and H. G. Drexler, "A model system in haematology and immunology: the human monocytic cell line MONO-MAC-1," *Leukemia Research*, vol. 21, no. 4, pp. 327–335, 1997.

[21] S. J. Bensinger and P. Tontonoz, "Integration of metabolism and inflammation by lipid-activated nuclear receptors," *Nature*, vol. 454, no. 7203, pp. 470–477, 2008.

[22] S. Gerlo, P. Verdood, B. Gellersen, E. L. Hooghe-Peters, and R. Kooijman, "Mechanism of prostaglandin (PG)E2-induced prolactin expression in human T cells: cooperation of two PGE2 receptor subtypes, E-prostanoid (EP) 3 and EP4, via calcium- and cyclic adenosine 5′-monophosphate-mediated signaling pathways," *Journal of Immunology*, vol. 173, no. 10, pp. 5952–5962, 2004.

[23] S. Narumiya, Y. Sugimoto, and F. Ushikubi, "Prostanoid receptors: structures, properties, and functions," *Physiological Reviews*, vol. 79, no. 4, pp. 1193–1226, 1999.

[24] S. G. Harris, J. Padilla, L. Koumas, D. Ray, and R. P. Phipps, "Prostaglandins as modulators of immunity," *Trends in Immunology*, vol. 23, no. 3, pp. 144–150, 2002.

[25] D. F. Legler, P. Krause, E. Scandella, E. Singer, and M. Groettrup, "Prostaglandin E_2 is generally required for human dendritic cell migration and exerts its effect via EP2 and EP4 receptors," *The Journal of Immunology*, vol. 176, no. 2, pp. 966–973, 2006.

[26] R. Muthuswamy, J. Mueller-Berghaus, U. Haberkorn, T. A. Reinhart, D. Schadendorf, and P. Kalinski, "PGE2 transiently enhances DC expression of CCR7 but inhibits the ability of DCs to produce CCL19 and attract naive T cells," *Blood*, vol. 116, no. 9, pp. 1454–1459, 2010.

[27] A. M. Vaughan and J. F. Oram, "ABCA1 and ABCG1 or ABCG4 act sequentially to remove cellular cholesterol and generate cholesterol-rich HDL," *Journal of Lipid Research*, vol. 47, no. 11, pp. 2433–2443, 2006.

7

Impaired Inflammatory Response to LPS in Type 2 Diabetes Mellitus

Lusine Khondkaryan,[1] Sona Margaryan,[2,3] David Poghosyan,[2] and Gayane Manukyan[2,3]

[1]*Group of Cell Technologies, Institute of Molecular Biology, National Academy of Sciences, Yerevan, Armenia*
[2]*Laboratory of Molecular and Cellular Immunology, Institute of Molecular Biology, National Academy of Sciences, Yerevan, Armenia*
[3]*Russian-Armenian (Slavonic) University, Yerevan, Armenia*

Correspondence should be addressed to Gayane Manukyan; gaya.manukyan@gmail.com

Academic Editor: B. L. Slomiany

Type 2 diabetes mellitus (T2DM) is a severe health problem worldwide, reaching epidemic levels. High susceptibility to infections of T2DM patients indicates dysregulated immune responses to pathogens. However, innate immune responses, including monocyte functions, in T2DM are poorly investigated. Therefore, in this study we aimed to assess lipopolysaccharide- (LPS-) induced immune responses of circulating monocytes from T2DM patients. The results showed that monocytes from T2DM were hyporesponsive to LPS challenge as reflected by significantly suppressed secretion of TNFα ($p < 0.01$) and expression of CD11b ($p < 0.001$) and TLR4 ($p < 0.001$) compared to those in monocytes from healthy subjects. Furthermore, LPS-induced IL-10 levels were similar in diabetic and healthy supernatants, while expression levels of CD163 were found to be downregulated on monocytes from T2DM ($p < 0.001$) suggesting impaired ability of monocytes to switch their phenotype to anti-inflammatory. Taken together, our results suggest compromised function of monocytes in T2DM, which may explain, at least partly, high incidence of infection in these patients.

1. Introduction

Type 2 diabetes mellitus (T2DM) represents a global public health concern with rapidly increasing prevalence worldwide [1]. It is a chronic metabolic disease characterized by a loss of insulin sensitivity by many cell types and progressive pancreatic β-cell dysfunction as a consequence of a hyperglycemia [2]. It has long been appreciated that chronic activation of the innate immune system is associated with T2DM. Growing evidence supports the involvement of inflammatory processes with an abnormal production of cytokines and activation of inflammatory signaling pathways in the development of this metabolic disease [3, 4]. Despite underlying chronic inflammation, high incidence of community-acquired and nosocomial infectious diseases in T2DM [5, 6] may indicate dysfunctions in innate immune response in these patients. Indeed, studies in T2DM subjects have revealed impaired phagocytic, chemotactic activity of monocytes and neutrophils [7–11], decreased natural killer cells and dendritic cell functions [12, 13], and so on. The presence of microbiota is associated with increased exposure of the host to microbe-derived products such as lipopolysaccharide (LPS). It was shown that a shift in the complex microbial system resulted in higher LPS levels in serum [14] and directly associated with the degree of insulin resistance [15].

Monocytes are the main cells of innate immunity that play central role in the initiation and resolution of inflammatory response to pathogens [16]. Recognition of LPS by its receptor TLR4 results in production of a broad range of molecules, including proinflammatory cytokines, chemokines, reactive oxygen species, and upregulation of adhesion and costimulatory receptors [17]. At the same time upregulation of anti-inflammatory mediators ensures successful resolution of the inflammatory response. A delicate balance between pro- and anti-inflammatory responses is required to prevent the progression from nonresolving acute inflammation to persistent chronic inflammation. Although monocytes are the main

TABLE 1: Participant characteristics.

	Healthy donors ($n = 7$)	Type 2 diabetes ($n = 10$)	p value
Gender (F/M)	4/3	8/2	
Age	41.8 ± 12	53.2 ± 7.8	NS
BMI (kg/m^2)	20.9 ± 2.2	31.2 ± 4.7	0.001
Fasting blood glucose (mmol/L)	4.9 ± 0.77	8.3 ± 3.1	0.001

Data are means ± SD. p values correspond to the differences between healthy subjects and patients with T2DM.

cells producing proinflammatory cytokines in norm, controversial results have been obtained concerning their potential role in inflammatory processes during T2DM [18–21]. Given the fact that LPS may abnormally activate monocytes, we aimed to determine whether circulating monocytes from T2DM patients exhibit differential features of activation after LPS challenge. For this, we assessed expression of surface markers TLR4, CD11b, and CD163 on circulating monocytes as well as production of TNFα and IL-10 by whole blood cells in the presence and absence of LPS.

2. Materials and Methods

2.1. Subjects. Peripheral blood samples were obtained from 10 patients with T2DM (mean age 53.2) and 7 healthy volunteers (mean age 41.8). Mean diabetes duration is 5.2 years. Patients were diagnosed at the "Surb Astvatsamayr" Medical Center (Yerevan, Armenia) based on criteria established by an expert committee on the diagnosis and classification of diabetes mellitus (1): (i) random venous plasma glucose ≥ 11.1 mmol/L, (ii) fasting plasma glucose ≥ 7 mmol/L, (iii) laboratory HbA1c > 48 mmol/mol (6.5%). All the patients with T2DM were treated with diet therapy and oral hypoglycemic agents. No patients received insulin therapy. None of healthy volunteers reported presence of diabetes or a family history of this disease, obesity, or chronic diseases. Study participant characteristics are given in Table 1. All participants in this study had provided written informed consent. The study was approved by the Ethics Committee of the Institute of Molecular Biology of the NAS RA (IRB IORG0003427).

2.2. Blood Sampling and Ex Vivo Stimulation of Whole Blood. The strategy for the whole blood assay was chosen to preserve physiological environment and avoid possible artificial stimulation of monocytes arising from mononuclear cell separation. Blood samples from all study participants were taken upon 12 h fasting, between 9:00 and 10:00 am. Venous blood was collected by venipuncture into a sterile tubes containing EDTA (Vacuette, Greiner Bio-One) and proceed within two hours. Aliquots of whole blood were diluted 1 : 3 in RPMI 1640 supplemented with 10% FBS, L-glutamine (2 mmol/l), and penicillin (100 U/ml) and cultured in the presence or absence of 100 ng/ml LPS (*Escherichia coli* 026:B6; Sigma) at 37°C for 24 hours. Afterwards supernatants were collected and stored at −70°C until assayed, while cells were harvested for the surface marker expression analysis.

2.3. Flow Cytometry. After stimulation, cells were harvested and contaminating red blood cells removed with lysis buffer. Remaining cells were washed with phosphate buffered saline (PBS) and incubated with following fluorescent monoclonal antibodies: CD14 PE-Cy7, TLR4 FITC, CD163 PE, and CD11b (activated) PE (BioLegend, UK) for 30 minutes in dark at room temperature. Appropriate mouse FITC, PE, and PE-Cy7-conjugated IgG subclasses were used as negative controls. Labeled cells after further washing with PBS supplemented with 0.5% BSA were fixed by the addition of fixation buffer (BioLegend, UK) and kept at 4°C until acquisition within 24 hours.

Samples were measured on BD FACScan flow cytometer (Becton Dickinson, San Jose, CA, USA) and at least 10000 events were obtained. The data was analyzed using FlowJo version 10.1 (Ashland, OR, USA). The monocyte population was determined as CD14 positive cells and back gated on FSC/SSC dot plot. The median fluorescent intensity (MFI) of TLR4, CD11b, and CD163 positive cells within monocytes population was estimated.

2.4. ELISA. The concentrations of TNFα and IL-10 in culture supernatants were measured by ELISA kits (Biolegend, UK), according to manufacturer's instructions. The detection limits were 7.8 and 3.9 pg/ml for TNFα and IL-10, respectively.

2.5. Statistical Analysis. Data analysis was performed with GraphPad Prism 5.01 (GraphPad Software, USA). Statistical significance between treatments (unstimulated versus stimulated) was analyzed by Wilcoxon matched-pairs test. Between-group differences were evaluated by Mann–Whitney U test. Significance was defined at the level of $p < 0.05$.

3. Results

3.1. LPS-Induced Surface Expression of Monocytes Markers. To evaluate the effect of LPS administration on expression of monocytes' surface receptors, whole blood was incubated with 100 ng/ml LPS for 24 hours and the median fluorescence intensity (MFI) of CD11b, TLR4, and CD163 were determined by flow cytometry. LPS treatment resulted in upregulation of CD11b expression on monocytes from both T2DM and healthy subjects ($p < 0.01$, Figure 1). However, the induction of CD11b was markedly decreased on diabetic cells, not reaching the expression levels on monocytes from healthy subjects ($p < 0.001$). Similarly, suppressed levels of CD11b were found on monocytes from T2DM patients cultured in medium alone ($p < 0.01$).

As shown in Figure 1, stimulation with LPS did not alter the expression levels of TLR4 in both studied groups.

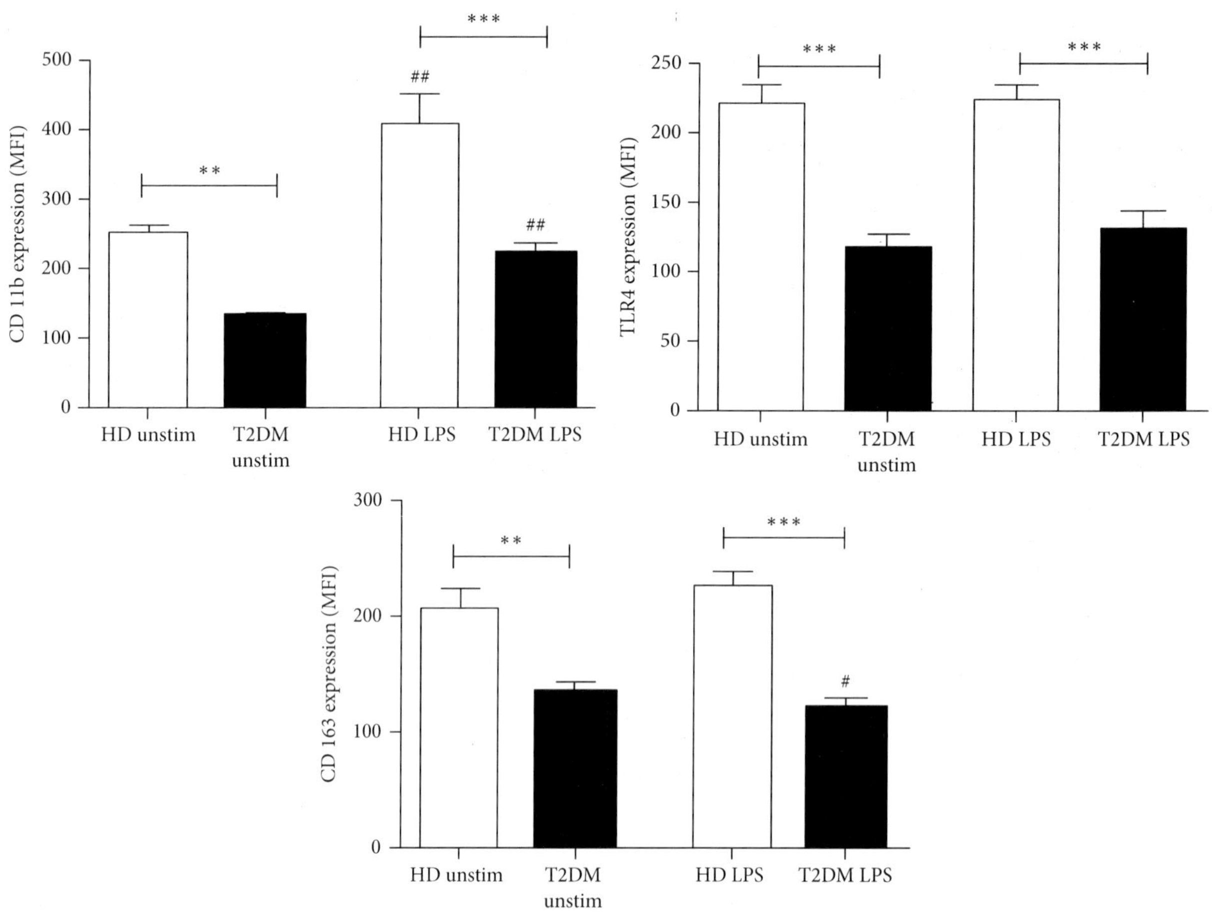

FIGURE 1: Surface expression of CD11b, CD163, and TLR4 on monocytes after cultivation of whole blood from healthy donors (HD, white bars) and type 2 diabetic (T2DM, black bars) patients with medium alone (unstimulated) or 100 ng/ml LPS for 24 hours. Data are given as median fluorescent intensity (MFI). Results are presented as mean ± SE. $^{\#}p < 0.05$; $^{\#\#}p < 0.01$ versus unstimulated cultures; $^{**}p < 0.01$; $^{***}p < 0.001$ versus healthy donors.

However, TLR4 expression was significantly reduced on both LPS-treated and unstimulated T2DM monocytes compared to respective cells from healthy donors ($p < 0.001$).

In order to evaluate the ability of diabetic monocytes to switch from proinflammatory towards anti-inflammatory phenotype, we measured the surface expression of CD163. LPS treatment resulted in decreased CD163 expression on monocytes from T2DM patients compared to unstimulated cells ($p < 0.05$, Figure 1). In contrast, monocytes from healthy donors slightly upregulated CD163 in response to LPS, though this increase did not reach statistical significance ($p = 0.07$). Respectively, the difference between LPS-treated CD163 was significantly lower in patients with T2DM as compared to healthy donors ($p < 0.001$).

3.2. LPS-Induced Cytokine Secretion. Next, we studied TNFα and IL-10 production capacity by whole blood cultures of healthy and diseased subjects in response to LPS (Figure 2). LPS exposure resulted in significant increase in the secretion of TNFα and IL-10 in both groups as compared to unstimulated cultures ($p < 0.01$, Figure 2). Whereas concentrations of LPS-induced TNFα in T2DM were significantly lower than in healthy donors ($p < 0.01$), no differences in levels of IL-10 were found.

4. Discussion

Although chronic inflammation is one of the characteristics of T2DM, high incidence of infections in these patients may be partially attributed to disturbances in innate immune responses. In the present study, we clearly demonstrated dysregulation of peripheral blood monocytes in patients with T2DM. Monocytes from T2DM subjects exhibited initially impaired immune response as reflected by lower levels of phenotypic markers on the cells cultured in medium alone. Despite the fact that LPS exposure of monocytes from T2DM patients resulted in increased expression of CD11b and TNFα production, their levels were significantly lower than those in healthy controls. Observed "refractory state" of monocytes appeared to be a result of impaired LPS recognition, which is supported by the lower TLR4 expression on these cells. Failure of LPS to properly activate monocytes from T2DM patients in our study accounts for the endotoxin tolerance. This concept is further supported by the fact that low TNFα

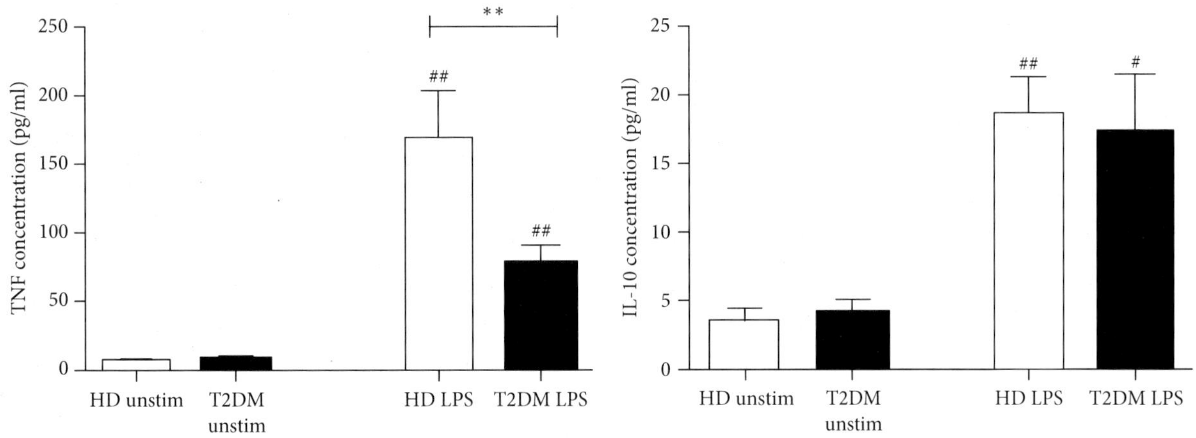

FIGURE 2: Concentrations of TNFα and IL-10 in supernatants after cultivation of whole blood from healthy donors (HD, white bars) and type 2 diabetic (T2DM, black bars) subjects with medium alone (unstimulated) or 100 ng/ml LPS for 24 hours. Results are presented as mean ± SE. $^{\#}p < 0.05$; $^{\#\#}p < 0.01$ versus unstimulated cultures; $^{**}p < 0.01$ versus healthy donors.

secretion was not counterbalanced by IL-10. It is likely that diabetic monocytes were primed by the low-dose *in vivo* LPS challenge, resulting in a reduced response of TNFα after *ex vivo* LPS stimulation. Indeed, recent evidences suggest that LPS play an important role in metabolic perturbations and might be a triggering factor for the onset of insulin resistance [15]. Low-grade increase in plasma LPS termed "metabolic endotoxemia" is a well-known feature of T2DM [22, 23]. On the other hand, T2DM is characterized as a state of hyperglycemia and hyperinsulinemia. Insulin has been shown to decrease monocyte TLR4 mRNA levels in T2DM [24], while high glucose levels have been reported to increase its membrane expression levels [25]. In parallel, it has been suggested that attenuated inflammatory response in T2DM is a direct consequence of hyperglycemia [26]. Taken together, hyperglycemia, hyperinsulinemia, and metabolic endotoxemia may affect monocytes functions in a complex manner. In contrast to our study, previous studies have demonstrated either increased or comparable levels of CD11b baseline expression in monocytes derived from T2DM patients [27–29]. Similarly, increased expression of TLR4 has been found in diabetic monocytes [25]. Intriguingly, Gupta et al. found suppressed TLR4 gene expression in diabetic patients with long disease duration and poor glycaemic control [30]. Methodological differences among studies that characterize the immune response may contribute to the discrepant findings.

Priming of innate immune cells by the endotoxin through TLR4 receptor enables the immune system to arise inflammatory response against potential pathogens. Fine-tuned regulation of excessive inflammation serves as an important mechanism for host protection against endotoxin shock [31, 32]. One of the classic examples of such protective mechanism is endotoxin tolerance [33]. However, when uncontrolled, this protective mechanism can become a serious clinical problem, increasing the risk for infection [34]. LPS-induced immune responses in T2DM have been a subject of considerable controversy. Attenuated, pronounced, or normal cytokine secretion in LPS-treated cells has been found in diabetic patients [18, 35–39]. *Ex vivo* whole blood stimulation revealed conflicting results as well. No difference between diabetic and healthy subjects in the production of TNFα and IL-10 upon LPS treatment have been found [36, 40], while in study by Geerlings et al. [41] a tendency towards decreased secretion of TNFα has been reported. These discrepancies may be attributed to the differences in demographic and metabolic characteristics of studied participants. In our study lean healthy individuals were enrolled as a control group; however higher BMI in our patients could have diminished immune response [42].

In parallel, we analyzed the anti-inflammatory potential of diabetic monocytes by analyzing surface expression of CD163. Previously it has been shown that LPS treatment resulted in a rapid shedding of CD163 from monocyte surface (within 1 hour), followed by its upregulation (24 hour later) [43]. CD163 upregulation is a marker of switching from proinflammatory towards anti-inflammatory profile and IL-10 is one of the most potent stimulators of this process [43, 44]. Our results suggest that the ability of monocytes to change their phenotype towards anti-inflammatory is impaired in T2DM patients. Respectively, we observed decreased expression of CD163 on diabetic monocytes upon LPS exposure, while slight (albeit not significant) upregulation was observed on healthy cells. At the same time, IL-10 levels were comparable between groups, which suggest that monocytes from T2DM patients may be hyporesponsive to IL-10. Our data in an agreement with the study by Barry et al. [40] who showed that immunosuppressive effect of IL-10 is a result of impaired downstream IL10 signaling under hyperglycemic conditions. Contradictory results have been reported on the expression levels of CD163 on endotoxin-tolerant monocytes. While some studies suggested that upregulated CD163 on monocytes is a marker of endotoxin tolerance [45], the others found no association between expression levels and tolerant state [46]. Decreased expression of anti-inflammatory CD163 by monocytes in T2DM provides additional evidence that innate immune response in these patients is disturbed. Thus, impaired LPS-induced expression of the markers with apparent opposing functions could indicate exhausted phenotype of circulating monocytes as a result of their persistent activation.

The limitations of this study include small sample size and the fact that studied patients were treated with oral hypoglycemic agents which may interfere and affect results. Second, we showed only weakened response of monocytes to LPS in T2DM; however the direct association of this state with endotoxin dysfunction in an inflammatory environment has yet to be established. Our future research aims to address these limitations.

5. Conclusion

Our data suggest that monocyte function is impaired in T2DM patients, a finding which could alter inflammatory response during common infection. Failure to mount an adequate inflammatory response may represent a state of immunosuppression in these patients. Our results raise the question about the role of monocytes in pathogenesis and maintenance of low-grade inflammation in T2DM.

Acknowledgments

This work was supported by Russian-Armenian University within the framework of the grant of the Ministry of Education and Science of the Russian Federation.

References

[1] L. Guariguata, D. Whiting, I. Hambleton, J. Beagley, U. Linnenkamp, and J. Shaw, "Global estimates of diabetes prevalence for 2013 and projections for 2035," *Diabetes Research and Clinical Practice*, vol. 103, no. 2, pp. 137–149, 2014.

[2] F. M. Ashcroft and P. Rorsman, "Diabetes mellitus and the β cell: the last ten years," *Cell*, vol. 148, no. 6, pp. 1160–1171, 2012.

[3] K. E. Wellen and G. S. Hotamisligil, "Inflammation, stress, and diabetes," *The Journal of Clinical Investigation*, vol. 115, no. 5, pp. 1111–1119, 2005.

[4] M. Y. Donath and S. E. Shoelson, "Type 2 diabetes as an inflammatory disease," *Nature Reviews Immunology*, vol. 11, no. 2, pp. 98–107, 2011.

[5] L. M. A. J. Muller, K. J. Gorter, E. Hak et al., "Increased risk of common infections in patients with type 1 and type 2 diabetes mellitus," *Clinical Infectious Diseases*, vol. 41, no. 3, pp. 281–288, 2005.

[6] A. Y. Peleg, T. Weerarathna, J. S. McCarthy, and T. M. E. Davis, "Common infections in diabetes: pathogenesis, management and relationship to glycaemic control," *Diabetes/Metabolism Research and Reviews*, vol. 23, no. 1, pp. 3–13, 2007.

[7] A. Lecube, G. Pachón, J. Petriz, C. Hernández, and R. Simó, "Phagocytic activity is impaired in type 2 diabetes mellitus and increases after metabolic improvement," *PLoS ONE*, vol. 6, no. 8, Article ID e23366, 2011.

[8] S. Chanchamroen, C. Kewcharoenwong, W. Susaengrat, M. Ato, and G. Lertmemongkolchai, "Human polymorphonuclear neutrophil responses to *Burkholderia pseudomallei* in healthy and diabetic subjects," *Infection and Immunity*, vol. 77, no. 1, pp. 456–463, 2009.

[9] D. Riyapa, S. Buddhisa, S. Korbsrisate et al., "Neutrophil extracellular traps exhibit antibacterial activity against Burkholderia pseudomallei and are influenced by bacterial and host factors," *Infection and Immunity*, vol. 80, no. 11, pp. 3921–3929, 2012.

[10] B. I. Restrepo, M. Twahirwa, M. H. Rahbar, and L. S. Schlesinger, "Phagocytosis via complement or Fc-gamma receptors is compromised in monocytes from type 2 diabetes patients with chronic hyperglycemia," *PLoS ONE*, vol. 9, no. 3, Article ID e92977, 2014.

[11] M. Delamaire, D. Maugendre, M. Moreno, M.-C. Le Goff, H. Allannic, and B. Genetet, "Impaired leucocyte functions in diabetic patients," *Diabetic Medicine*, vol. 14, no. 1, pp. 29–34, 1997.

[12] P. Piątkiewicz, T. Miłek, M. Bernat-Karpińska, M. Ohams, A. Czech, and P. Ciostek, "The dysfunction of nk cells in patients with type 2 diabetes and colon cancer," *Archivum Immunologiae et Therapia Experimentalis*, vol. 61, no. 3, pp. 245–253, 2013.

[13] K. L. Summers, A. M. Marleau, J. L. Mahon, R. McManus, I. Hramiak, and B. Singh, "Reduced IFN-α secretion by blood dendritic cells in human diabetes," *Clinical Immunology*, vol. 121, no. 1, pp. 81–89, 2006.

[14] P. D. Cani, R. Bibiloni, C. Knauf et al., "Changes in gut microbiota control metabolic endotoxemia-induced inflammation in high-fat diet-induced obesity and diabetes in mice," *Diabetes*, vol. 57, no. 6, pp. 1470–1481, 2008.

[15] P. D. Cani, J. Amar, M. A. Iglesias et al., "Metabolic endotoxemia initiates obesity and insulin resistance," *Diabetes*, vol. 56, no. 7, pp. 1761–1772, 2007.

[16] C. Auffray, M. H. Sieweke, and F. Geissmann, "Blood monocytes: development, heterogeneity, and relationship with dendritic cells," *Annual Review of Immunology*, vol. 27, pp. 669–692, 2009.

[17] S. Akira, S. Uematsu, and O. Takeuchi, "Pathogen recognition and innate immunity," *Cell*, vol. 124, no. 4, pp. 783–801, 2006.

[18] E. Hatanaka, P. T. Monteagudo, M. S. M. Marrocos, and A. Campa, "Neutrophils and monocytes as potentially important sources of proinflammatory cytokines in diabetes," *Clinical & Experimental Immunology*, vol. 146, no. 3, pp. 443–447, 2006.

[19] R. L. Baldeón, K. Weigelt, H. De Wit et al., "Type 2 diabetes monocyte microrna and mrna expression: dyslipidemia associates with increased differentiation-related genes but not inflammatory activation," *PLoS ONE*, vol. 10, no. 6, Article ID e0129421, 2015.

[20] M. Gacka, T. Dobosz, S. Szymaniec, D. Bednarska-Chabowska, R. Adamiec, and A. Sadakierska-Chudy, "Proinflammatory and atherogenic activity of monocytes in Type 2 diabetes," *Journal of Diabetes and its Complications*, vol. 24, no. 1, pp. 1–8, 2010.

[21] A. Giulietti, E. van Etten, L. Overbergh, K. Stoffels, R. Bouillon, and C. Mathieu, "Monocytes from type 2 diabetic patients have a pro-inflammatory profile. 1,25-Dihydroxyvitamin D3 works as anti-inflammatory," *Diabetes Research and Clinical Practice*, vol. 77, no. 1, pp. 47–57, 2007.

[22] S. J. Creely, P. G. McTernan, C. M. Kusminski et al., "Lipopolysaccharide activates an innate immune system response in human adipose tissue in obesity and type 2 diabetes," *American Journal of Physiology—Endocrinology and Metabolism*, vol. 292, no. 3, pp. E740–E747, 2007.

[23] B. Jayashree, Y. S. Bibin, D. Prabhu et al., "Increased circulatory levels of lipopolysaccharide (LPS) and zonulin signify

novel biomarkers of proinflammation in patients with type 2 diabetes," *Molecular and Cellular Biochemistry*, vol. 388, no. 1-2, pp. 203–210, 2014.

[24] H. Ghanim, P. Mohanty, R. Deopurkar et al., "Acute modulation of toll-like receptors by insulin," *Diabetes Care*, vol. 31, no. 9, pp. 1827–1831, 2008.

[25] M. R. Dasu, S. Devaraj, L. Zhao, D. H. Hwang, and I. Jialal, "High glucose induces toll-like receptor expression in human monocytes: mechanism of activation," *Diabetes*, vol. 57, no. 11, pp. 3090–3098, 2008.

[26] K. S. Tan, K. O. Lee, K. C. Low et al., "Glutathione deficiency in type 2 diabetes impairs cytokine responses and control of intracellular bacteria," *The Journal of Clinical Investigation*, vol. 122, no. 6, pp. 2289–2300, 2012.

[27] M. J. Sampson, I. R. Davies, J. C. Brown, K. Ivory, and D. A. Hughes, "Monocyte and neutrophil adhesion molecule expression during acute hyperglycemia and after antioxidant treatment in type 2 diabetes and control patients," *Arteriosclerosis, Thrombosis, and Vascular Biology*, vol. 22, no. 7, pp. 1187–1193, 2002.

[28] A. J. van Oostrom, J. P. van Wijk, T. P. Sijmonsma, T. J. Rabelink, and M. Castro Cabezas, "Increased expression of activation markers on monocytes and neutrophils in type 2 diabetes," *The Netherlands Journal of Medicine*, vol. 62, no. 9, pp. 320–325, 2004.

[29] M. A. de Vries, A. Alipour, B. Klop et al., "Glucose-dependent leukocyte activation in patients with type 2 diabetes mellitus, familial combined hyperlipidemia and healthy controls," *Metabolism*, vol. 64, no. 2, pp. 213–217, 2015.

[30] S. Gupta, A. Maratha, J. Siednienko et al., "Analysis of inflammatory cytokine and TLR expression levels in Type 2 Diabetes with complications," *Scientific Reports*, vol. 7, article 7633, 2017.

[31] R. Medzhitov and T. Horng, "Transcriptional control of the inflammatory response," *Nature Reviews Immunology*, vol. 9, no. 10, pp. 692–703, 2009.

[32] C. Nathan and A. Ding, "Nonresolving inflammation," *Cell*, vol. 140, no. 6, pp. 871–882, 2010.

[33] H. Fan and J. A. Cook, "Molecular mechanism of endotoxin tolerance," *Journal of Endotoxin Research*, vol. 10, no. 2, pp. 71–84, 2004.

[34] E. López-Collazo and C. del Fresno, "Pathophysiology of endotoxin tolerance: mechanisms and clinical consequences," *Critical Care*, vol. 17, no. 6, article 242, 2013.

[35] S. E. Geerlings and A. I. M. Hoepelman, "Immune dysfunction in patients with diabetes mellitus (DM)," *FEMS Immunology & Medical Microbiology*, vol. 26, no. 3-4, pp. 259–265, 1999.

[36] J. C. Pickup, G. D. Chusney, S. M. Thomas, and D. Burt, "Plasma interleukin-6, tumour necrosis factor α and blood cytokine production in type 2 diabetes," *Life Sciences*, vol. 67, no. 3, pp. 291–300, 2000.

[37] M. C. Foss-Freitas, N. T. Foss, E. A. Donadi, and M. C. Foss, "In vitro TNF-a and IL-6 production by adherent peripheral blood mononuclear cells obtained from type 1 and type 2 diabetic patients evaluated according to the metabolic control," *Annals of the New York Academy of Sciences*, vol. 1079, pp. 177–180, 2006.

[38] M. R. Chacón, J. Vendrell, M. Miranda et al., "Different TNFα expression elicited by glucose in monocytes from type 2 diabetes mellitus patients," *Atherosclerosis*, vol. 194, no. 2, pp. e18–e25, 2007.

[39] A. S. Andreasen, T. Pedersen-Skovsgaard, R. M. G. Berg et al., "Type 2 diabetes mellitus is associated with impaired cytokine response and adhesion molecule expression in human endotoxemia," *Intensive Care Medicine*, vol. 36, no. 9, pp. 1548–1555, 2010.

[40] J. C. Barry, S. Shakibakho, C. Durrer et al., "Hyporesponsiveness to the anti-inflammatory action of interleukin-10 in type 2 diabetes," *Scientific Reports*, vol. 6, Article ID 21244, 2016.

[41] S. E. Geerlings, E. C. Brouwer, K. C. P. M. Van Kessel, W. Gaastra, R. P. Stolk, and A. I. M. Hoepelman, "Cytokine secretion is impaired in women with diabetes mellitus," *European Journal of Clinical Investigation*, vol. 30, no. 11, pp. 995–1001, 2000.

[42] E. F. Devêvre, M. Renovato-Martins, K. Clément, C. Sautès-Fridman, I. Cremer, and C. Poitou, "Profiling of the three circulating monocyte subpopulations in human obesity," *The Journal of Immunology*, vol. 194, no. 8, pp. 3917–3923, 2015.

[43] L. K. Weaver, P. A. Pioli, K. Wardwell, S. N. Vogel, and P. M. Guyre, "Up-regulation of human monocyte CD163 upon activation of cell-surface Toll-like receptors," *Journal of Leukocyte Biology*, vol. 81, no. 3, pp. 663–671, 2007.

[44] T. H. Sulahian, P. Högger, A. E. Wahner et al., "Human monocytes express CD163, which is upregulated by IL-10 and identical to p155," *Cytokine*, vol. 12, no. 9, pp. 1312–1321, 2000.

[45] O. M. Pena, J. Pistolic, D. Raj, C. D. Fjell, and R. E. W. Hancock, "Endotoxin tolerance represents a distinctive state of alternative polarization (M2) in human mononuclear cells," *The Journal of Immunology*, vol. 186, no. 12, pp. 7243–7254, 2011.

[46] A. B. Alves-Januzzi, M. K. Brunialti, and R. Salomao, "CD163 and CD206 expression does not correlate with tolerance and cytokine production in LPS-tolerant human monocytes," *Cytometry Part B: Clinical Cytometry*, vol. 92, no. 3, pp. 192–199, 2017.

8

Contradictory Immune Response in Post Liver Transplantation Hepatitis B and C

Akinobu Takaki,[1] Takahito Yagi,[2] and Kazuhide Yamamoto[1]

[1] *Department of Gastroenterology and Hepatology, Okayama University Graduate School of Medicine, Dentistry, and Pharmaceutical Sciences, 2-5-1 Shikata-cho, Kita-ku, Okayama 700-8558, Japan*
[2] *Department of Gastroenterological Surgery Transplant and Surgical Oncology, Okayama University Graduate School of Medicine, Dentistry, and Pharmaceutical Sciences, 2-5-1 Shikata-cho, Kita-ku, Okayama 700-8558, Japan*

Correspondence should be addressed to Akinobu Takaki; akitaka@md.okayama-u.ac.jp

Academic Editor: Asif Jilani Iqbal

Hepatitis B and C often progress to decompensated liver cirrhosis requiring orthotopic liver transplantation (OLT). After OLT, hepatitis B recurrence is clinically controlled with a combination of hepatitis B immunoglobulin (HBIG) and nucleos(t)ide analogues. Another approach is to induce self-producing anti-hepatitis B virus (HBV) antibodies using a HBV envelope antigen vaccine. Patients who had not been HBV carriers such as acutely infected liver failure or who received liver from HBV self-limited donor are good candidate. For chronic HBV carrier patients, a successful response can only be achieved in selected patients such as those treated with experimentally reduced immunosuppression protocols or received an anti-HBV adaptive memory carrying donor liver. Hepatitis C virus (HCV) reinfects transplanted livers at a rate of >90%. HCV reinfected patients show different severities of hepatitis, from mild and slowly progressing to severe and rapidly progressing, possibly resulting from different adaptive immune responses. More than half the patients require interferon treatment, although the success rate is low and carries risks for leukocytopenia and rejection. Managing the immune response has an important role in controlling recurrent hepatitis C. This study aimed to review the adaptive immune response in post-OLT hepatitis B and C.

1. Introduction

Hepatitis B virus (HBV) infection and hepatitis C virus (HCV) infection are the main causes of end-stage liver disease requiring orthotopic liver transplantation (OLT). However, the post-OLT course is quite different between the two types of hepatitis. The post-OLT hepatitis B recurrence rate is >80% without any prevention, while >90% of recurrent infections can be controlled with a combination of hepatitis B immunoglobulin (HBIG) and nucleos(t)ide analogues (NAs) [1]. Non-OLT chronic hepatitis B patients are treated with antiviral proliferative NA agents, with >90% long-term control with minute side effects. The first commercially available NA, lamivudine (LAM), produced a rapid and definite short-term antiviral response, but 15–20% of the patients experienced annual recurrence of resistant virus and 70% of them did so after 5 years [2]. Fewer than 3% of patients treated with newer NAs such as entecavir (ETV) or tenofovir (TDF) experience resistant virus; these newer NAs are accepted as first-line and long-term treatment [3, 4].

After OLT, more than half of the patients become reinfected. It is difficult to eradicate the virus once these patients become reinfected [5].

The mechanism for controlling HBV viral recurrence is direct viral replication control by a combination of NAs and HBIG as passive immunoprophylaxis [6]. As HBIG combination therapy has important roles, the B-cell-related adaptive immune response appears to play a role in controlling HBV after OLT. However, as HBV-induced hepatitis is characterized by T-cell immune response, both B- and T-cell adaptive immune responses have vital roles [7]. When active immunization of patients with HBV vaccine is performed, HBV-specific and non-HBV-specific immune responses can be obtained.

HCV reinfects >90% of patients, with more than half of these patients developing chronic hepatitis requiring interferon- (IFN-) based antiviral treatment [8]. Non-OLT chronic hepatitis C patients have been treated with IFN-based immune reaction-related treatment. Recently, pegylated IFN (Peg-IFN) has been used in combination with ribavirin and, more recently, with the addition of a direct-acting antiviral agent (DAA) targeting the HCV nonstructural protein (NS) 3/4A protease [9]. Single Peg-IFN resulted in only 30% of patients experiencing sustained viral response (SVR), representing undetectable HCV-RNA longer than 24 weeks after finishing IFN [10]. This demonstrated >99% viral eradication, while the Peg-IFN and ribavirin combination resulted in 50% SVR [10, 11]. Peg-IFN plus ribavirin and telaprevir or simeprevir resulted in >80% SVR for patients with genotype 1, which is the more difficult-to-treat genotype of HCV [12]. All-oral, IFN-free regimens are expected to become commercially available in the near future [13].

HCV-related liver cirrhosis is a common indication for OLT [14]. However, HCV persists in almost all post-OLT patients. Graft reinfection is universal after OLT [15], leading to high-titer HCV viremia, with cirrhosis developing within 5 years of transplantation in approximately 20% of patients and within 10 years in 50% [16]. Thus, HCV infection after OLT differs completely from chronic hepatitis C (CHC) without transplantation. However, the mechanisms underlying accelerated HCV-induced liver damage after OLT are poorly understood. Several factors appear to be involved in the risk of hepatitis C recurrence, particularly those related to viral and immune responses. Immunosuppressive therapy is a likely cause for the severe accelerated course of HCV-related hepatitis after OLT [16, 17]. In particular, high-dose steroids, immunosuppressive drug combinations, powerful induction treatments, and acute rejection can worsen patient outcomes [18]. The pathology of HCV-related disease reflects immune reactions to virus-infected hepatocytes [7]. In post-OLT settings, immunosuppressive drugs definitely affect the clinical course. The effects of interferon-based treatment are limited to 30–50% of patients, with especially poorer results in post-OLT patients, and also carry the possibility of inducing mortal chronic rejection that should be avoided [19].

In this review, we summarize the aberrant immune system in HBV- and HCV-related hepatitis, together with the changes in these diseases after OLT.

2. Immune Mechanisms in Non-OLT HBV- and HCV-Related Hepatitis

2.1. Immune Mechanisms in HBV-Related Hepatitis. After infecting a patient once, HBV persists in the liver for the rest of a person's life, even after the patient achieves a clinically cured condition with seroclearance of HBV envelope antigen (hepatitis B surface antigen, HBsAg) and emergence of HBs antibody (HBsAb) [20]. In controlling viral replication, immune function has been revealed to be important, as immunosuppressive treatment for cancer chemotherapy or organ transplantation can induce viral replication even in HBsAg negative with HBsAb positive clinically cured patients and organ transplant recipients [21, 22]. HBV is an enveloped DNA virus containing a relaxed circular DNA genome, which is converted into a covalently closed circular (CCC) DNA that persists in the nucleus of infected cells as minichromosomes [23].

Natural killer (NK) cells work as the innate immune modulator to induce the death of microbial-infected cells with strong cytotoxic activity and the production of high levels of certain cytokines and chemokines in a nonmajor histocompatibility complex- (MHC-) restricted manner distinct from T and B cells [24]. Upon HBV infection, NK cells migrate to the liver, with a decrease in their numbers in the spleen and bone marrow, suggesting the recruitment of NK cells from these organs [24]. As hepatocytes normally express little MHC class I, NK cells may play a more important role in the early defense against HBV infection before the MHC class I expression is upregulated after viral replication in hepatocytes [25].

Antigen-presenting cells (APCs), such as Kupffer cells (liver resident macrophages) and dendritic cells, have important roles in intermediating the innate to adaptive immune responses [26]. Kupffer cells or macrophages behave in both an immunostimulatory and immunoregulatory fashion upon HBV exposure. The addition of HBV particles and HBsAg induces the production of proinflammatory cytokines interleukin- (IL-) 1β, IL-6, CXCL-8, and tumor necrosis factor (TNF)-α by human CD68$^+$ macrophage-enriched cells via NF-κB (nuclear factor kappa-light-chain-enhancer of activated B cells) activation [27]. However, another study reported no such cytokine production with immunoregulatory cytokine transforming growth factor- (TGF-) β production [28]. The immune system activates Kupffer cells to eradicate HBV, while HBV evades the Kupffer cell-related pathway to reduce the inflammatory pathway and change the environment to be favorable for survival. Pretreatment of nonparenchymal cells, including Kupffer cells, with HBsAg or HBV virion, abrogates the Toll-like receptor- (TLR-) related antiviral response such as IFN-β, interferon-stimulated gene (ISG), or NF-κB. In the liver biopsy specimens of patients with active hepatitis B, Kupffer cells have been revealed to possess higher expression of galectin-9, which is an immunoregulatory molecule [29]. Kupffer cells accumulate around injured hepatic loci and produce several cytotoxic and fibrosis progression-related molecules [30]. However, they also have an important function in scavenging apoptotic hepatocytes, which could function as a bait for inflammation, and depletion of Kupffer cells could induce worsening of hepatitis [31, 32]. Kupffer cells function as both proinflammatory and anti-inflammatory and profibrotic and antifibrotic cells in their environment. Both the hepatitis state and Kupffer cell polarity are needed to understand the immunological pathogenesis in HBV-related hepatitis.

Strong HBV-specific CD8$^+$ T-cell responses have been shown to correlate with viral and hepatitis control during acute infection [33]. In chronically infected patients, HBV-specific CD8$^+$ T-cell responses are weak and occur with low frequency, while patients with low viral load exhibit multispecific strong responses [34]. The epitopes targeted by the $CD8^+$ T cells have been deeply analyzed in HLA-A and -B restricted epitopes, as these have been believed to have antiviral impact [35, 36]. However, a recently characterized HLA-C restricted epitope has also been revealed to have a clinical impact and is an especially frequent allele in patients who live in Southeast Asia [37]. Several factors have been suggested to explain this phenomenon. In HBV-specific $CD8^+$ T cells, proapoptotic protein Bcl2-interacting mediator (BIM) is upregulated, naïve T-cell phenotypes such as CD45RA, CD27, CD28, and CCR7 are highly expressed, and immune regulatory molecules such as programmed death-1 (PD-1), cytotoxic lymphocyte antigen 4 (CTLA-4), and T-cell immunoglobulin mucin-3 (TIM-3) are also highly expressed [29, 38–41]. Several experimental trials that were conducted to block such immunoregulatory exhaustion molecules showed reversal of these immunoregulatory conditions [41, 42].

Similar to the $CD8^+$ T cells, $CD4^+$ T cells have also been found to exhibit a lower response in the acute phase of infection in patients who developed chronic hepatitis later [43]. The $CD4^+$ T-cell response in patients who recovered was found to be more frequent, stronger, and more multispecific than that observed later in patients with chronic hepatitis [40]. The IFN-γ producing antiviral Th1 response against HBV core has been revealed to be stronger in patients with resolved infection even several years after infection [44].

The humoral immune response has been acknowledged as an avenue for understanding the clinical course of acute and chronic hepatitis B [45]. The antibody responds against viral structural antigens such as the core antigen (HBcAg) and the envelope antigen (HBsAg). Anti-HBcAg IgM antibody (IgM-HBcAb) is accepted as the earliest and most diagnostic marker of acute infection. Anti-HBc IgG antibody (IgG-HBcAb) develops during acute infection and remains positive for the duration of the patient's life [46]. HBsAg emerges in serum from the acute phase of infection and remains when the patient exhibits chronic hepatitis B, while in patients who experience an acute self-limiting course HBsAg could be cleared. Anti-HBs antibody (HBsAb) is a virus-neutralizing antibody recognized as having lower viral and disease activities. The lack of anti-HBs in chronic infection can be attributed to a selective exhaustion of B cells and IL-10 secreting immunoregulatory B-cell expansion [45, 46].

2.2. Immune Mechanisms in HCV-Related Hepatitis. Since HCV is not also a cytopathic virus, immune reactions play a central role in the development of chronic hepatitis (Figure 1) [47, 48]. Innate antiviral responses constitute the first-line defense system against infected virus. HCV disables some innate antiviral systems to escape from the immune pressure [48]. The lack of a strong Th1-type helper T-cell response and cytotoxic T-cell response against HCV leads to chronic infection with this virus [49–51]. High-magnitude, broad, polyfunctional, and sustained T-cell responses correlate with spontaneous recovery [35, 49, 52], but these responses are not correlated with interferon-induced viral clearance [53].

The role of NK cells in chronic hepatitis C is not completely understood. However, as NK cells are the first immunological walls against HCV, much evidence has been uncovered. An NK-cell activating and inhibitory receptor gene polymorphism has been discovered to have roles in the course of HCV infection [54, 55]. As IFN-α is the basic treatment for chronic hepatitis C, IFN-producing NK cells have been defined as key immune cells. NK cells can produce IFN-α, IFN-γ, and TNF-α and induce dendritic cell activation and support innate to adaptive immune response bridging [56]. NK cells can also lyse HCV-infected hepatocytes, T cells, and APCs and modulate immune responses [57]. However, HCV itself has been revealed to have a role in the potential inhibition of NK cell function, resulting in chronic hepatitis [58].

Antigen presenting cells such as Kupffer cells, macrophages, or dendritic cells (DCs) behave in both an immunostimulatory and immunoregulatory manner upon HCV exposure, as in HBV [26]. In chronic hepatitis C patients, Kupffer cells are increased and activated as the higher expression markers CD163 and CD33 [59, 60]. *In vitro* analysis has revealed that HCV core and NS3-affected Kupffer cells secrete proinflammatory cytokines such as IL-1β, IL-6, and TNF-α and also immunosuppressive cytokine IL-10 [61]. Proinflammatory cytokine release might explain the induction and persistent inflammation in chronic hepatitis C, while immunosuppressive cytokine release explains the difficulty in the eradication of HCV-infected hepatocytes. The direct effects of HCV on the inflammatory signal in Kupffer cells have been revealed to upregulate the immunoregulatory molecule PD-L1 [62]. Probably, HCV interferes with Kupffer cell-related antiviral activities but induces strong enough inflammatory cytokines to result in chronic inflammation. The effects of Kupffer cells on liver fibrosis progression are similar to those in HBV infection. The Kupffer cells accumulate around inflammatory foci and express cytotoxic molecules such as granzyme B, perforin, and reactive oxygen species to induce inflammation and fibrosis [63].

There are a minimum of two subsets of DCs. Myeloid DCs (mDCs) produce a large amount of IL-12 upon stimulation, while plasmacytoid DCs (pDCs) produce a large amount of IFN-α in viral infection [64]. DC function has been reported as broadly impaired in CHC patients [65–68]. However, several reports have indicated contradictory results that DC function is not impaired in CHC patients [69–73]. Most of these reports are studies with mDCs; however, pDCs are also reportedly functionally impaired and reduced by increased apoptosis [74]. Since culture conditions and chronic hepatitis conditions in the patient may change the phenotype of immune cells, functional differences in DCs during chronic HCV infection remain contentious. *In vitro* transfection or the addition of HCV proteins such as core, NS3, or NS4 has been reported to result in reduced function of DCs [75]. Because of the scarcity of *in vitro* culture systems for HCV, these experimental results are also contentious. With the recent establishment of infectious cell culture-produced HCV, impaired pDC functions have been revealed [64].

The role of the humoral immune response in the clearance of HCV is not well understood. After viral clearance, most

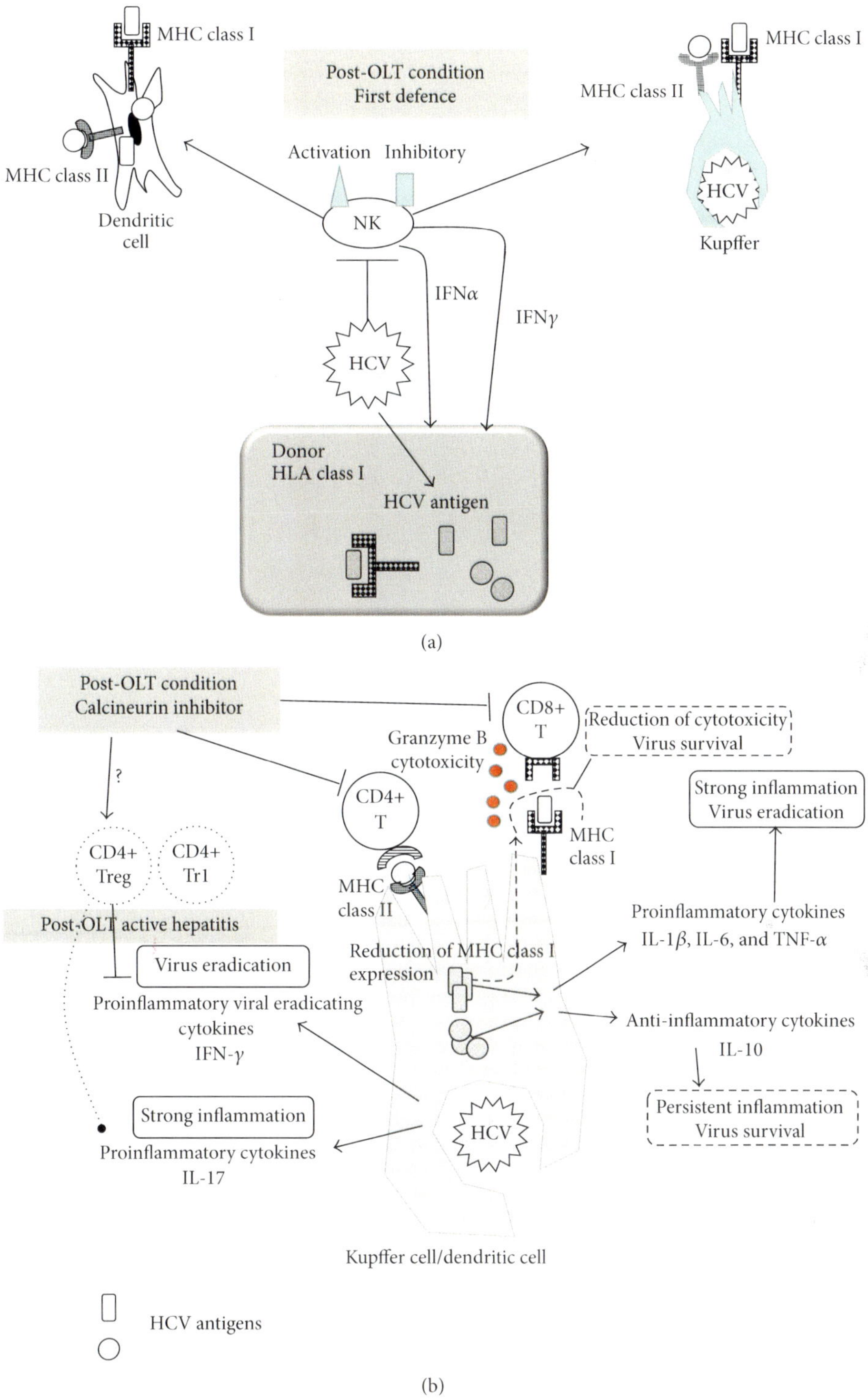

Figure 1: Immune status in chronic hepatitis C and postorthotopic liver transplantation (OLT) hepatitis C. (a) NK cells are the first immunological defense system from hepatitis C virus (HCV). The phenotype defined with the activation or inhibitory receptor gene polymorphism affects the chronic hepatitis C activity and the post-OLT hepatitis activity. The interferon producing function is decreased by HCV proteins. (b) Kupffer cells or dendritic cells (DCs) have important roles in bridging innate and adaptive immune responses. These cells show proinflammatory and anti-inflammatory functions when infected with HCV. These cytokines' balance is well controlled for viral persistence and chronic inflammatory state by viral antigens. After OLT, regulatory T cells might affect to reduce antiviral defence but not to reduce inflammatory cytokines resulting in severer chronic hepatitis. The type 1 regulatory T cells (Tr1) may induce severe hepatitis, while a lower frequency of Tr1 is correlated with hepatitis control with HCV positive status. NK: natural killer cell, OLT: orthotopic liver transplantation, HCV: hepatitis C virus, MHC: major histocompatibility complex, IFN: interferon, Treg: regulatory T cell, and Tr1: type 1 regulatory T cell.

antibody titers wane despite the persistent T-cell response [35]. A neutralizing antibody response is detectable, even in chronic hepatitis C patients [76]. The target of the response is placed in and around the envelop proteins E1 and E2 and the hypervariable region near the amino terminus of E2 [77]. Neutralization epitopes have been revealed to be masked by extensive glycosylation and by virions covered with lipid droplets and might not be effectively targeted [78, 79]. In addition, as the RNA-dependent RNA polymerase of HCV lacks proofreading activity, it is easy for HCV-RNA to mutate and escape from the host immune pressures [80]. Although 20–30% of infected patients recover from the infection with strong T-cell response memory and possible neutralization antibody B-cell response, they could be reinfected with the virus, indicating difficulties in producing disease-controlling vaccines [81].

Strong HCV-specific $CD4^+$ T-cell and $CD8^+$ T-cell responses have been shown to be evident in HCV patients with resolved infection, while diminished in patients with chronic hepatitis C [7]. To recognize viral-infected hepatocytes or APCs, viral epitopes should be expressed on the MHC. Interferon upregulates MHC class I expression; however, replicating HCV-RNA reduces that expression [82]. Interferon is released from NK cells and DCs during an early phase of viral infection and has important roles in eradicating HCV, as this is the key drug for treatment [83]. This HCV interference with MHC expression must be one reason why CHC patients show reduced $CD8^+$ T-cell responses.

Recent attention has focused on regulatory T cells (Tregs) and their contribution to CHC. Their mechanism of immunosuppression depends on both cell-cell contact and immunosuppressive cytokine secretion [84]. A subpopulation of Tregs that express CD18 and also CD49b-expressing type 1 regulatory T (Tr1) cells have also attracted attention [85], because they produce large amounts of immunosuppressive cytokines such as IL-10 and TGF-β, with which they inhibit type 1 and 2 helper responses [86]. Tregs and Tr1 cells may contribute to HCV persistence by suppressing HCV-specific T-cell responses [87–89]. Treg frequencies and activities are apparently higher in CHC patients than in those who have achieved viral clearance [90]. Recently discovered T-cell regulatory molecules such as PD-1, 2B4, and TIM-3 have been revealed to be coexpressed in intrahepatic HCV-specific CD8 T cells, indicating that HCV-induced T-cell functional exhaustion represses viral eradication [91].

Strong innate and adaptive immune responses are responsible for HCV clearance; however, the virus itself affects many sites of the immune system, ameliorating the effective antiviral immune functions. To control NK, Kupffer cells, B cells, or T cells might be difficult as they act in different ways in different CHC conditions.

3. Immune Responses in Post-OLT HBV Recurrence Control

3.1. Overview of Post-OLT HBV Control with Nucleos(t)ide Analogues and Hepatitis B Immunoglobulin. A multicenter study in Europe in 1993 identified the risk of post-OLT HBV recurrence [92]. The risk was low in patients with acute liver failure who were intolerant of HBV. However, the recurrence rate in patients with liver cirrhosis, especially with high serum HBV-DNA at OLT, was >80% [92]. As the immune system is repressed with steroids and calcineurin inhibitors, recurrent hepatitis B produces severe hepatitis with a high incidence of mortal liver failure. However, present protocols that use NA in combination with long-term HBIG have resulted in >90% control of HBV recurrence [1].

The first trial of long-term HBIG combined with the first-generation NA lamivudine (LAM) was conducted in 1998. Monthly HBIG administration with LAM resulted in all patients surviving for 1 year after OLT without serum HBV-DNA positivity [93]. Subsequent reports also described successful control of HBV recurrence with this combination [94]. The historical progression of controlling post-OLT HBV recurrence is summarized in Table 1. As patients with positive HBV-DNA before OLT were more likely to later have HBV recurrence, to maintain anti-HBs antibody titers >500 IU/L was recommended. If HBV-DNA was negative before OLT, the anti-HBs antibody titer could be reduced to 100–150 IU/L with or without LAM. From the standpoint of cost savings, the HBIG dose requirement was able to be decreased as clinical data accumulated [95–97]. Currently, HBIG is administered as required only when anti-HBs antibody titers fall below target levels. Some reports indicate that only a short duration of HBIG administration is required and that it can be withdrawn several months after OLT [98]. If HBV-DNA was negative at the time of OLT, HBIG could be withdrawn at several months after OLT. For acute liver failure patients who had been infected with the virus shortly before hepatitis development, HBIG could also be withdrawn. Of course, strict monitoring of HBV-DNA and HBV surface antigen (HBsAg) titers should be continued throughout the patient's life.

The mechanism of protection against HBV reactivation by the combination of drugs is not well defined. The cccDNA episome is the transcriptional template for HBV messenger RNA transcripts that encode viral structural and NS proteins and the pregenomic RNA template for reverse transcription and synthesis of the viral genome [5]. NAs inhibit the reverse transcription of pregenomic RNA, resulting in a rapid decrease in serum HBV-DNA, but cannot eliminate the cccDNA reservoir [99]. HBIG contains high-titer antibodies against HBsAg, which is the major component of the envelope of the HBV virion.

The possible mechanisms through which HBIG prevents HBV transmission are that it neutralizes circulating virus by immune complex formation, protects naïve hepatocytes against HBV released from extrahepatic sites through blocking the putative HBV receptor, or anti-HBs antibody internalizes into hepatocytes, interacts with HBsAg, and inhibits HBsAg secretion from cells [100]. To protect against HBV infection of naïve hepatocytes might be difficult, since recent studies have revealed that intrahepatic HBV-DNA is detectable in >50% of even well-controlled patients after OLT [5]. The HBV virion released from the infected cells could be blocked with anti-HBs antibody. In an *in vitro* assay, the internalized antibody was seen to induce the accumulation

TABLE 1: Recent post-OLT HBV prophylaxis with nucleos(t)ide analogue and/or HBIG combination.

	HBV-DNA recurrence (%)	Followup (months)	Reference number	Reported year
Lamivudine + HBIG				
HBIG IV 10000 IU/month	0	13	[93]	1998
HBIG IV to maintain HBsAb >200 IU/L	9.5	21 (2.4–49.1)	[96]	2001
HBIG to maintain HBsAb >70 IU/L	0	16 (9–22)	[97]	2004
HBIG IV to maintain HBsAb >10 IU/L	0	30 (7–73)	[6]	2007
Short course (1 month) HBIG	7	18	[98]	2003
Entecavir + HBIG				
HBIG; IM to maintain HBsAb >100 IU/L	0	41.2 (33–54)	[107]	2012
One year HBIG IM; 2000 IU/month Lamivudine + adefovir or tenofovir, tenofovir, entecavir	0	24 (6–40) post HBIG withdrawal	[106]	2012
One year HBIG IV; dose not specified	3.8	24	[105]	2013
HBIG free with newer nucleos(t)ide analogues regimen				
Lamivudine + adefovir (no HBIG when HBV-DNA below 3 log(10)IU/mL)	0	22 (10–58)	[103]	2013
Entecavir, lamivudine + adefovir, tenofovir, entecavir + tenofovir (no HBIG when HBV-DNA below 3.3 log(10)IU/mL)	8 (5/6 withdrawn NAs)	21 (1–83)	[110]	2013

OLT; orthotopic liver transplantation, HBV: hepatitis B virus, HBIG; hepatitis B immunoglobulin, HBV-DNA: hepatitis B virus DNA, IV: intravenous administration, IM: intramuscular administration, IU: international unit, HBsAb: anti-hepatitis B s antibody, and NAs: nucleos(t)ide analogues.

of intracellular viral particles even after the antibody was removed from the cell culture supernatant [101].

Several new NAs such as adefovir dipivoxil (ADV), entecavir (ETV), telbivudine (LdT), and tenofovir (TDF) have become commercially available [102]. Because of the risk of developing resistance, LAM is no longer recommended as a first-line treatment for hepatitis B. The currently recommended first-line agents are ETV and TDF, which have resulted in a very low emergence of resistance [3, 4]. Such newer NAs are very effective when combined with HBIG even during short duration, post-OLT HBV control [103–109]. Because of low resistance and the powerful antiviral response evoked by ETV and TDF or a combination of NAs, several institutions have developed successful HBIG-free protocols if the HBV-DNA titer is low enough at the time of OLT [103, 110].

As the strong NAs are very effective in HBV control, immune cell-related treatments are not administered, although hepatitis B infection is an immune mediated disease [1].

3.2. Adaptive Immune System to Get Anti-HBs Antibody Response with HBV Vaccine. The practice of active immunization of post-OLT recipients with HBV vaccine is emerging. For a successful vaccine response, the immune system has important roles. Most studies report low response rates, even with doubled concentrations or prolonged injections of vaccines (Table 2) [111–115]. Patients who had not been HBV carriers (such as adult patients with acute liver failure due to sexual transmission and nonchronic HBV carriers with anti-HBc antibody-positive donor livers) are good candidates for vaccine administration [112, 116–121]. Patients with acute HBV infection who undergo OLT are often positive for anti-HBs antibody even before OLT and have powerful immune responses. Such patients should respond well to vaccination since they have not developed tolerance to HBV, unlike chronic carriers. However, some HBV carriers have responded to vaccination.

Since noncarriers respond well to HBV vaccination, even under prednisolone and calcineurin inhibitor usage, immune tolerance is expected to play a large role in this process. In non-OLT HBV patients, analysis has revealed that HBsAg-positive newborns had higher regulatory T-cell frequencies and dysfunctional CD8 T cells, which represent immune tolerant status [122]. However, another report analyzing the immunological characteristics of HBsAg-positive young carriers and aged patients with active hepatitis revealed comparable peripheral T-cell proinflammatory cytokine production capacity and HBV-specific IFN-γ responses [123]. These findings indicate that tolerant carriers can react with HBV antigens and can show active immunity against HBV vaccination, if regulatory T-cell function diminishes. With good responses to newer NAs after OLT, HBV-DNA decreases even in the liver, and this might recover compressed HBV-specific T cells to react with HBV.

Chronic HBV carrier recipients, including patients with positive HBV-DNA at OLT, do not respond well to HBs-antigen-containing vaccine, with response rates being mostly <30% [114, 115, 119, 124, 125]. Tahara et al. reported 64.7% positive responses to experimentally minimized immunosuppressant treatment [118]. The immune status of these patients was evaluated by a mixed lymphocyte reaction (MLR) assay in response to antidonor and anti-third-party allostimulation using an intracellular carboxyfluorescein diacetate succinimidyl ester- (CFSE-) labeling technique. "Third-party" refers to healthy volunteers with the same blood type as the patients. The autologous lymphocytes, the donor lymphocytes, and the third-party lymphocytes were irradiated and used as the stimulator cells, and the recipients' lymphocytes were used as the responder cells in MLR. The investigators minimized immunosuppression until the donor lymphocytes showed no response as autologous lymphocytes, but third-party lymphocytes showed a positive response. The investigators found that vaccination was successful in patients showing a donor-specific MLR hyporesponse, with a well-maintained response to the third-party stimulus. The vaccine was not successful in patients showing hyporesponse to both the donor and the third party. These results provide encouragement that even immune tolerant liver cirrhosis patients can react with HBV vaccines under lower immunosuppressant protocols after OLT.

Another protocol of repeated vaccine administration resulted in successful immunization in 40% of patients with post-OLT liver cirrhosis [117]. The donors to good responders were the spouses of recipients and had high anti-HBs antibody titers before donation. The spouses with high-titer anti-HBs antibodies were probably infected with HBV by the recipients after marriage, resulting in the anti-HBs antibody boost. The immune systems of these donors should not have developed tolerance to the virus [126]. The adoptive immune transfer of the HBV-specific immune response could be achieved [127].

To successfully transfer immune memory to recipients, the anti-HBs antibody titer of the donors should be high. Luo et al. have shown that a high anti-HBs antibody titer (>1000 IU/L) in donors is essential for adoptive transfer [128]. These results suggest that pre-OLT HBV vaccination for candidate living donors might facilitate improved post-OLT vaccine responses in recipients with liver cirrhosis. Several experimental adjuvant vaccines have also been tried with up to 44.8% success rates [111, 119, 129].

The vaccine response depends on immune tolerance to the virus in both recipients and donors. The liver is the largest immune organ in the abdomen; therefore, it plays a critical role in immune responses. Multiple populations of nonhematopoietic liver cells, including sinusoidal endothelial cells, stellate cells located in the subendothelial space, and liver parenchymal cells, can function as APCs [130]. The viral-specific immune competence of the grafted liver might overcome general immune tolerance to the virus in chronic HBV carriers.

3.3. Adaptive Immune System to Get Anti-HBs Antibody Response with HBV Vaccine in HBV Naïve Recipients Who Received Livers from Anti-HBc Antibody Positive Donors. As a shortage of donor organs is a universal problem, anti-HBc

Table 2: Post-OLT HBV vaccine administration trials.

	Methods	Definition of success	Success rate (%)	Reference number	Reported year
Liver cirrhosis	10–20 μg monthly with experimentally minimized immunosuppressant	HBsAb >100 IU/L without HBIG	64	[118]	2009
	20 μg monthly	HBsAb >100 IU/L 6 months without HBIG	40	[117]	2013
	20 μg monthly	HBsAb >100 IU/L 3 months without HBIG	0	[112]	2011
	40 μg 0, 1, 2, 6, 7, and 8 months	HBsAb >100 IU/L without HBIG	0	[114]	2009
	40 μg 0, 1, and 6 months	HBsAb >10 IU/L without HBIG	82	[113]	2000
	20–40 μg 0, 1, and 6 months	HBsAb >10 IU/L 16 months without HBIG	0	[115]	2010
	20 μg with MPL adjuvant 12 monthly	HBsAb >100 IU/L 18 months without HBIG	44.8	[129]	2010
	Experimental adjuvant vaccine 0, 1, 2, 6, and 12 months	HBsAb >500 IU/L 18 months without HBIG	25	[119]	2005
Acute liver failure	20 μg monthly	HBsAb >100 IU/L 6 months without HBIG	100	[117]	2013
	Experimental adjuvant vaccine 0, 1, 2, 6, and 12 months	HBsAb >500 IU/L 18 months without HBIG	100	[119]	2005
	10–20 μg monthly	HBsAb >100 IU/L without HBIG	66	[118]	2009
Non-HBV-related patients with HBcAb positive donors	20 μg monthly	HBsAb >100 IU/L 3 months without HBIG	83	[112]	2011
	Infant 20–40 μg according to body weight 2–4 times/year	HBsAb >100 IU/L without HBIG	75	[121]	2007
	20 μg 0, 1, and 6 months	HBsAb >100 IU/L 6 months without HBIG	50	[120]	2007

OLT: orthotopic liver transplantation, HBV: hepatitis B virus, HBIG: hepatitis B immunoglobulin, IU: international unit, and HBsAb: anti-hepatitis B s antibody.

positive healthy carriers could be candidate donors. With regard to the above vaccination protocols, non-HBV-related patients who received anti-HBc antibody positive donor livers have fared quite favorably. The post-OLT incidence of *de novo* hepatitis B occurring in anti-HBc antibody-positive donors without prophylaxis is high (33–100%) [22, 131, 132]. These HBV-naïve patients are good candidates for the HBV vaccine because 50–80% tend to respond well [112, 120, 121]. Pre-OLT vaccination is also possible if patients have sufficient time before undergoing OLT. In countries with universal vaccination programs, the recipients might already have anti-HBs antibody and could be boosted with additional vaccination before OLT, resulting in 78% of prospective recipients having a high titer of anti-HBs antibody (>1000 IU/L) [133]. In pediatric patients, the vaccination responses were observed to be good in recipients with higher anti-HBs titers at the time of OLT and lower tacrolimus levels at the time of vaccination [134].

4. Adaptive Immune Responses in Post-OLT Hepatitis C Recurrence Control

4.1. Overview of Post-OLT Hepatitis C Recurrence and Treatment. As HCV recurrence is observed in almost all the patients who receive OLT, HCV eradication before OLT has been tried, although with unsuccessful outcomes [135, 136].

Post-OLT IFN administration is the only way to achieve better outcomes. HCV genotypes 1b and 4 seem to be negative predictive factors for recurrence because of a lower response to pegylated interferon (Peg-IFN) and ribavirin combination therapy [136]. The host and donor factors associated with poorer outcomes are female gender, older donor age, steatosis of the graft, and the IL-28B single nucleotide polymorphism (SNP) [137–140]. A human genomewide association study recently uncovered many disease-susceptible genes or drug sensitivity-related genes. In CHC patients, the IL-28B gene SNP was found to be related to spontaneous clearance and susceptibility to treatment with Peg-IFN plus ribavirin [141–143]. The combination of recipient and donor IL-28B genetic polymorphism has been revealed to be important in post-OLT HCV treatment outcomes [137].

Recently, direct-acting antivirals such as NS3 protease inhibitors or NS5 polymerase inhibitors or a combination of them have come to represent a new highly effective treatment strategy [144]. The triple combination therapy of Peg-IFN, ribavirin, and a protease inhibitor (telaprevir) has been accepted as a highly effective treatment for non-OLT CHC, producing >75% sustained virological response (SVR) [145]. However, as telaprevir inhibits cytochrome P450 3A4 and reduces the metabolism of calcineurin inhibitors, the trough levels of cyclosporine A (CyA) increase to 4.6-fold and FK 506 (FK) to 70-fold [146]. This phenomenon requires that triple therapy be used with strict care. The second generation protease inhibitor simeprevir very weakly inhibits cytochrome P450 3A4 and is safer than telaprevir. Triple therapy including simeprevir is safer than triple therapy with telaprevir and is currently recommended [147].

4.2. Adaptive Immune Responses in Hepatitis C Recurrence. In post-OLT settings, T-cell activities are affected by immunosuppressive therapy [148]. Although the T-cell response is repressed with calcineurin inhibitors, post-OLT CHC patients often show severe hepatitis recurrence with high viral load [14]. In post-OLT CHC patients, the importance of immune reaction has been accepted. Several reports have mentioned that HCV-specific immune responses correlate with post-OLT hepatitis C progression [149, 150]. The frequency of HCV-specific IL-17-secreting $CD4^+$ T cells was shown to be increased in severe inflammation in liver fibrosis patients [150]. The serum cytokine profile of these patients with severe recurrence exhibited higher inflammatory cytokines (IL-17, IL-1β, IL-6, IL-8, and monocyte chemoattractant protein [MCP]-1), decreased antiviral cytokine IFN-γ, and increased IFN-γ reducing cytokine IL-10, suggesting the presence of the inflammatory phenotype with repressed antiviral immune response.

Several studies have demonstrated that Tregs induce allograft tolerance [151, 152]. Moreover, Tregs and Tr1 cells are overexpressed in patients with severe hepatitis C recurrence compared with patients with no or minor recurrence [86, 153]. These results suggest that Tregs and Tr1 cells are involved in HCV recurrence after OLT. Because the strength of immunosuppressive therapy and the viral load would be changed after OLT, the time course of the immune response has important roles. Recently, we have shown that Tr1 frequency was repressed in 40 days after OLT under the condition of persistently normal alanine aminotransferase (ALT), even at 3 years after OLT [8]. Tr1, which has a strong IL-10 production capacity, may reduce HCV-specific T-cell responses and induce active hepatitis with ALT elevation. Monitoring Tr1 frequency might be a way to determine which patients would develop active hepatitis. However, HCV-specific $CD4^+$ T-cell IFN-γ production, which was higher in patients with persistently normal ALT until 3 years after OLT, was found to diminish after 3 years (Tsuzaki R. et al. accepted manuscript for Acta Med Okayama, 2014). This result indicates that, although the adaptive immune response could control hepatitis, the strength of the response might diminish over time. These results from our experience indicate that IFN-based anti-HCV therapy could be applied for patients with higher Tr1 after OLT, who might show active hepatitis until 3 years after OLT. Whether the Tr1 reduction treatment will become the next treatment strategy is not clear, as selective reduction of Tr1 might be difficult. However, as calcineurin inhibitors reduce regulatory T cells, minimum usage of calcineurin inhibitors might be the way this can be accomplished now [154].

4.3. Innate Immune Responses in Hepatitis C Recurrence. Innate immune responses have also been identified as HCV targets and could be depressed with respect to their functions. Dendritic cells (DCs) and NK cells are thought to play a central role in the interplay between the innate and adaptive immune responses. Kupffer cells are also involved in post-OLT hepatitis C recurrence, as NF-κB was highly expressed in patients with post-OLT HCV recurrence. However, the specificity for the disease state is not well characterized [155].

In post-OLT settings, blood pDCs decreased after OLT and the pDC product IFN-α also decreased. These decreases might affect the recurrence of post-OLT hepatitis C [156].

NK cells have also been deeply investigated with respect to their activities in HCV infection and hepatitis. NK cells are implicated in various viral infections, including HCV and front-line anticancer immune responses. The HCV-E2 protein has been revealed to bind the NK CD81 receptor and decrease the release of IFN-γ, resulting in noneffective antiviral responses [157]. Another NK cell receptor, the killer immunoglobulin receptor (KIR), which displays an inhibitory function, has been revealed to be correlated with post-OLT hepatitis C. The KIR-ligand mismatch and recipient KIR2L3 haplotype have been shown to correlate with recurrent hepatitis C [55]. IFN treatment susceptibility of post-OLT HCV recurrence has also been shown to be correlated with the NK receptor haplotype KIR2DS2 [158]. Intravenous administration of living donor perfusate of NK cells could reduce the HCV-RNA increase after OLT [159]. As acutely infected hepatitis C patients show self-recovery at a rate of 20–30%, a strong NK cell response might control hepatitis C even under immunosuppressive treatment.

Adaptive immune response in post-OLT HBV remains a problem that should be investigated, as this virus continues to be difficult to be eradicated from the infected liver. However, the anti-HCV treatment protocol is drastically changing because several clinical trials of new DAA with >80% viral eradication might result in these drugs being introduced to the market; therefore, the importance of investigating the immune system in post-OLT HCV will probably consolidate to selected refractory patients in the next 10 years.

5. Conclusion

The adaptive immune response in post-OLT hepatitis B recurrence is hidden under strong antiviral HBIG and NA combination treatment. However, the effectiveness of active immunization is dependent upon adaptive immune responses being effective for patients with non-HBV-related disease who have received anti-HBc antibody-positive donor livers and patients with acute liver failure who are not immune tolerant to HBV. Vaccination is not sufficiently effective for patients with liver cirrhosis; nevertheless, the donor immune memory for HBV and the strength of the immunosuppressant drugs have important roles. Adaptive immune responses, especially of the $CD4^+$ and $CD8^+$ T cells and the Treg, have strong effects in post-OLT hepatitis C viral recurrence and in recurrent hepatitis activities. The regulatory T cells and Tr1 cells affect the clinical course and could be used as prediction markers. As IFN-based treatments have risks after OLT, forecasting the patient's course with such markers could be beneficial.

References

[1] A. Takaki, T. Yagi, and K. Yamamoto, "Safe and cost-effective control of post-transplantation recurrence of hepatitis B," *Hepatology Research*, 2014.

[2] G. Dusheiko, "Treatment of HBeAg positive chronic hepatitis B: interferon or nucleoside analogues," *Liver International*, vol. 33, supplement 1, pp. 137–150, 2013.

[3] M. K. Kathryn, A. Corsa, and Y. Liu, "No detectable resistance to tenofovir disoproxil fumarate after 6 years of therapy in patients with chronic hepatitis B," *Hepatology*, vol. 59, no. 2, pp. 434–442, 2014.

[4] D. J. Tenney, R. E. Rose, C. J. Baldick et al., "Long-term monitoring shows hepatitis B virus resistance to entecavir in nucleoside-naïve patients is rare through 5 years-of therapy," *Hepatology*, vol. 49, no. 5, pp. 1503–1514, 2009.

[5] T. Yasunaka, A. Takaki, T. Yagi et al., "Serum hepatitis B virus DNA before liver transplantation correlates with HBV reinfection rate even under successful low-dose hepatitis B immunoglobulin prophylaxis," *Hepatology International*, vol. 5, no. 4, pp. 918–926, 2011.

[6] A. Takaki, T. Yagi, Y. Iwasaki et al., "Short-term high-dose followed by long-term low-dose hepatitis B immunoglobulin and lamivudine therapy prevented recurrent hepatitis B after liver transplantation," *Transplantation*, vol. 83, no. 2, pp. 231–233, 2007.

[7] S. H. Park and B. Rehermann, "Immune responses to HCV and other hepatitis viruses," *Immunity*, vol. 40, no. 1, pp. 13–24, 2014.

[8] M. Utsumi, A. Takaki, Y. Umeda et al., "Frequency of regulatory T-cell and hepatitis C viral antigen-specific immune response in recurrent hepatitis C after liver transplantation," *Transplant Immunology*, vol. 31, no. 1, pp. 33–41, 2014.

[9] K. E. Sherman, S. L. Flamm, N. H. Afdhal et al., "Response-guided telaprevir combination treatment for hepatitis C virus infection," *The New England Journal of Medicine*, vol. 365, no. 11, pp. 1014–1024, 2011.

[10] T. Kanda, F. Imazeki, and O. Yokosuka, "New antiviral therapies for chronic hepatitis C," *Hepatology International*, vol. 4, no. 3, pp. 548–561, 2010.

[11] G. Yamada, S. Iino, T. Okuno et al., "Virological response in patients with hepatitis C virus genotype 1b and a high viral load: impact of peginterferon-α-2a plus ribavirin dose reductions and host-related factors," *Clinical Drug Investigation*, vol. 28, no. 1, pp. 9–16, 2008.

[12] T. Kanda, S. Nakamoto, S. Wu, and O. Yokosuka, "New treatments for genotype 1 chronic hepatitis C—focus on simeprevir," *Therapeutics and Clinical Risk Management*, vol. 10, pp. 387–394, 2014.

[13] L. M. Hagan and R. F. Schinazi, "Best strategies for global HCV eradication," *Liver International*, vol. 33, supplement 1, pp. 68–79, 2013.

[14] M. Berenguer, F. X. López-Labrador, and T. L. Wright, "Hepatitis C and liver transplantation," *Journal of Hepatology*, vol. 35, no. 5, pp. 666–678, 2001.

[15] T. L. Wright, E. Donegan, H. H. Hsu et al., "Recurrent and acquired hepatitis C viral infection in liver transplant recipients," *Gastroenterology*, vol. 103, no. 1, pp. 317–322, 1992.

[16] M. Berenguer, M. Prieto, J. M. Rayón et al., "Natural history of clinically compensated hepatitis C virus-related graft cirrhosis after liver transplantation," *Hepatology*, vol. 32, no. 4 I, pp. 852–858, 2000.

[17] M. Berenguer, L. Ferrell, J. Watson et al., "HCV-related fibrosis progression following liver transplantation: Increase in recent years," *Journal of Hepatology*, vol. 32, no. 4, pp. 673–684, 2000.

[18] M. Charlton and E. Seaberg, "Impact of immunosuppression and acute rejection on recurrence of hepatitis C: results of the national institute of diabetes and digestive and kidney diseases liver transplantation database," *Liver Transplantation and Surgery*, vol. 5, supplement 1, no. 4, pp. S107–S114, 1999.

[19] M. Berenguer, A. Palau, V. Aguilera, J. M. Rayón, F. S. Juan, and M. Prieto, "Clinical benefits of antiviral therapy in patients with recurrent hepatitis C following liver transplantation," *American Journal of Transplantation*, vol. 8, no. 3, pp. 679–687, 2008.

[20] B. Rehermann, C. Ferrari, C. Pasquinelli, and F. V. Chisari, "The hepatitis B virus persists for decades after patients'recovery from acute viral hepatitis despite active maintenance of a cytotoxic T-lymphocyte response," *Nature Medicine*, vol. 2, no. 10, pp. 1104–1108, 1996.

[21] T. Matsui, J. Kang, M. Nojima et al., "Reactivation of hepatitis B virus in patients with undetectable HBsAg undergoing chemotherapy for malignant lymphoma or multiple myeloma," *Journal of Medical Virology*, vol. 85, no. 11, pp. 1900–1906, 2013.

[22] S. Uemoto, K. Sugiyama, H. Marusawa et al., "Transmission of hepatitis B virus from hepatitis B core antibody- positive donors in living related liver transplants," *Transplantation*, vol. 65, no. 4, pp. 494–499, 1998.

[23] M. Levrero, T. Pollicino, J. Petersen, L. Belloni, G. Raimondo, and M. Dandri, "Control of cccDNA function in hepatitis B virus infection," *Journal of Hepatology*, vol. 51, no. 3, pp. 581–592, 2009.

[24] Y. Chen, H. Wei, B. Gao, Z. Hu, S. Zheng, and Z. Tian, "Activation and function of hepatic NK cells in hepatitis B infection: an underinvestigated innate immune response," *Journal of Viral Hepatitis*, vol. 12, no. 1, pp. 38–45, 2005.

[25] L. G. Guidotti and F. V. Chisari, "Noncytolytic control of viral infections by the innate and adaptive immune response," *Annual Review of Immunology*, vol. 19, pp. 65–91, 2001.

[26] A. Boltjes, D. Movita, A. Boonstra, and A. M. Woltman, "The role of Kupffer cells in hepatitis B and hepatitis C virus infections," *Journal of Hepatology*, 2014.

[27] M. Hösel, M. Quasdorff, K. Wiegmann et al., "Not interferon, but interleukin-6 controls early gene expression in hepatitis B virus infection," *Hepatology*, vol. 50, no. 6, pp. 1773–1782, 2009.

[28] H. Li, H. Zheng, H. Chen et al., "Hepatitis B virus particles preferably induce Kupffer cells to produce TGF-β1 over proinflammatory cytokines," *Digestive and Liver Disease*, vol. 44, no. 4, pp. 328–333, 2012.

[29] G. Nebbia, D. Peppa, A. Schurich et al., "Upregulation of the Tim-3/galectin-9 pathway of T cell exhaustion in chronic hepatitis B virus infection," *PLoS ONE*, vol. 7, no. 10, Article ID e47648, 2012.

[30] K. Wallace, A. D. Burt, and M. C. Wright, "Liver fibrosis," *The Biochemical Journal*, vol. 411, no. 1, pp. 1–18, 2008.

[31] G. Sitia, M. Iannacone, R. Aiolfi et al., "Kupffer cells hasten resolution of liver immunopathology in mouse models of viral hepatitis," *PLoS Pathogens*, vol. 7, no. 6, Article ID e1002061, 2011.

[32] P. Ramachandran, A. Pellicoro, M. A. Vernon et al., "Differential Ly-6C expression identifies the recruited macrophage phenotype, which orchestrates the regression of murine liver fibrosis," *Proceedings of the National Academy of Sciences of the United States of America*, vol. 109, no. 46, pp. E3186–E3195, 2012.

[33] M. K. Maini, C. Boni, G. S. Ogg et al., "Direct ex vivo analysis of hepatitis B virus-specific CD8+ T cells associated with the control of infection," *Gastroenterology*, vol. 117, no. 6, pp. 1386–1396, 1999.

[34] A. Schuch, A. Hoh, and R. Thimme, "The role of natural killer cells and $CD8^+$ T cells in hepatitis B virus infection," *Frontiers in Immunology*, vol. 5, article 258, 2014.

[35] A. Takaki, M. Wiese, G. Maertens et al., "Cellular immune responses persist and humoral responses decrease two decades after recovery from a single-source outbreak of hepatitis C," *Nature Medicine*, vol. 6, no. 5, pp. 578–582, 2000.

[36] K. Nitschke, A. Barriga, J. Schmidt et al., "HLA-B*27 subtype specificity determines targeting and viral evolution of a hepatitis C virus-specific CD8+ T cell epitope," *Journal of Hepatology*, vol. 60, no. 1, pp. 22–29, 2014.

[37] A. T. Tan, P. Sodsai, A. Chia et al., "Immunoprevalence and immunodominance of HLA-Cw∗0801-restricted T cell response targeting the hepatitis B virus envelope transmembrane region," *Journal of Virology*, vol. 88, no. 2, pp. 1332–1341, 2014.

[38] A. R. Lopes, P. Kellam, A. Das et al., "Bim-mediated deletion of antigen-specific $CD8^+$T cells in patients unable to control HBV infection," *Journal of Clinical Investigation*, vol. 118, no. 5, pp. 1835–1845, 2008.

[39] V. Appay, R. A. W. Van Lier, F. Sallusto, and M. Roederer, "Phenotype and function of human T lymphocyte subsets: consensus and issues," *Cytometry A*, vol. 73, no. 11, pp. 975–983, 2008.

[40] C. Boni, P. Fisicaro, C. Valdatta et al., "Characterization of hepatitis B virus (HBV)-specific T-cell dysfunction in chronic HBV infection," *Journal of Virology*, vol. 81, no. 8, pp. 4215–4225, 2007.

[41] A. Schurich, P. Khanna, A. R. Lopes et al., "Role of the coinhibitory receptor cytotoxic T lymphocyte antigen-4 on apoptosis-Prone CD8 T cells in persistent hepatitis B virus infection," *Hepatology*, vol. 53, no. 5, pp. 1494–1503, 2011.

[42] P. Fisicaro, C. Valdatta, M. Massari et al., "Antiviral intrahepatic T-cell responses can be restored by blocking programmed death-1 pathway in chronic hepatitis B," *Gastroenterology*, vol. 138, no. 2, pp. 682–693, 2010.

[43] S. Urbani, B. Amadei, E. Cariani et al., "The impairment of CD8 responses limits the selection of escape mutations in acute hepatitis C virus infection," *The Journal of Immunology*, vol. 175, no. 11, pp. 7519–7529, 2005.

[44] M. C. Jung, U. Spengler, W. Schraut et al., "Hepatitis B virus antigen-specific T-cell activation in patients with acute and chronic hepatitis B," *Journal of Hepatology*, vol. 13, no. 3, pp. 310–317, 1991.

[45] E. Loggi, N. Gamal, F. Bihl, M. Bernardi, and P. Andreone, "Adaptive response in hepatitis B virus infection," *Journal of Viral Hepatitis*, vol. 21, no. 5, pp. 305–313, 2014.

[46] K. Dumaidi and A. Al-Jawabreh, "Prevalence of occult HBV among hemodialysis patients in two districts in the northern part of the West Bank, Palestine," *Journal of Medical Virology*, vol. 86, no. 10, pp. 694–1699, 2014.

[47] B. Rehermann, "Chronic infections with hepatotropic viruses: mechanisms of impairment of cellular immune responses," *Seminars in Liver Disease*, vol. 27, no. 2, pp. 152–160, 2007.

[48] L. B. Dustin, S. B. Cashman, and S. M. Laidlaw, "Immune control and failure in HCV infection—tipping the balance," *Journal of Leukocyte Biology*, 2014.

[49] R. Thimme, D. Oldach, K. Chang, C. Steiger, S. C. Ray, and F. V. Chisari, "Determinants of viral clearance and persistence during acute hepatitis C virus infection," *The Journal of Experimental Medicine*, vol. 194, no. 10, pp. 1395–1406, 2001.

[50] J. T. Gerlach, H. M. Diepolder, M. C. Jung et al., "Recurrence of hepatitis C virus after loss of virus-specific CD4+ T- cell response in acute hepatitis C," *Gastroenterology*, vol. 117, no. 4, pp. 933–941, 1999.

[51] H. Wedemeyer, X. He, M. Nascimbeni et al., "Impaired effector function of hepatitis C virus-specific $CD8^+$ T cells in chronic hepatitis C virus infection," *The Journal of Immunology*, vol. 169, no. 6, pp. 3447–3458, 2002.

[52] G. M. Lauer, E. Barnes, M. Lucas et al., "High resolution analysis of cellular immune responses in resolved and persistent hepatitis C virus infection," *Gastroenterology*, vol. 127, no. 3, pp. 924–936, 2004.

[53] F. Rahman, T. Heller, Y. Sobao et al., "Effects of antiviral therapy on the cellular immune response in acute hepatitis C," *Hepatology*, vol. 40, no. 1, pp. 87–97, 2004.

[54] S. I. Khakoo, C. L. Thio, M. P. Martin et al., "HLA and NK cell inhibitory receptor genes in resolving hepatitis C virus infection," *Science*, vol. 305, no. 5685, pp. 872–874, 2004.

[55] S. Knapp, D. Hegazy, L. Brackenbury et al., "Consistent beneficial effects of killer cell immunoglobulin-like receptor 2dl3 and group 1 human leukocyte antigen-c following exposure to hepatitis c virus," *Hepatology*, vol. 51, no. 4, pp. 1168–1175, 2010.

[56] L. B. Dustin and C. M. Rice, "Flying under the radar: the immunobiology of hepatitis C," *Annual Review of Immunology*, vol. 25, pp. 71–99, 2007.

[57] E. O. Long, H. Sik Kim, D. Liu, M. E. Peterson, and S. Rajagopalan, "Controlling natural killer cell responses: integration of signals for activation and inhibition," *Annual Review of Immunology*, vol. 31, pp. 227–258, 2013.

[58] K. Cheent and S. I. Khakoo, "Natural killer cells and hepatitis C: action and reaction," *Gut*, vol. 60, no. 2, pp. 268–278, 2011.

[59] S. I. Khakoo, P. N. Soni, K. Savage et al., "Lymphocyte and macrophage phenotypes in chronic hepatitis C infection: correlation with disease activity," *The American Journal of Pathology*, vol. 150, no. 3, pp. 963–970, 1997.

[60] A. Dolganiuc, O. Norkina, K. Kodys et al., "Viral and host factors induce macrophage activation and loss of toll-like receptor tolerance in chronic HCV infection," *Gastroenterology*, vol. 133, no. 5, pp. 1627–1636, 2007.

[61] S. Chang, A. Dolganiuc, and G. Szabo, "Toll-like receptors 1 and 6 are involved in TLR2-mediated macrophage activation by hepatitis C virus core and NS3 proteins," *Journal of Leukocyte Biology*, vol. 82, no. 3, pp. 479–487, 2007.

[62] Z. Tu, R. H. Pierce, J. Kurtis, Y. Kuroki, I. N. Crispe, and M. S. Orloff, "Hepatitis C virus core protein subverts the antiviral activities of human Kupffer cells," *Gastroenterology*, vol. 138, no. 1, pp. 305–314, 2010.

[63] T. Tordjmann, A. Soulie, C. Guettier et al., "Perforin and granzyme B lytic protein expression during chronic viral and autoimmune hepatitis," *Liver*, vol. 18, no. 6, pp. 391–397, 1998.

[64] H. Kanzler, V. Soumelis, and M. Gilliet, "Dendritic cell lineage, plasticity and cross-regulation," *Nature Immunology*, vol. 2, no. 7, pp. 585–589, 2001.

[65] I. Itose, T. Kanto, M. Inoue et al., "Involvement of dendritic cell frequency and function in virological relapse in pegylated interferon-α and ribavirin therapy for chronic hepatitis C patients," *Journal of Medical Virology*, vol. 79, no. 5, pp. 511–521, 2007.

[66] T. Kanto, N. Hayashi, T. Takehara et al., "Impaired allostimulatory capacity of peripheral blood dendritic cells recovered from hepatitis C virus-infected individuals," *The Journal of Immunology*, vol. 162, no. 9, pp. 5584–5591, 1999.

[67] T. Kanto, M. Inoue, M. Miyazaki et al., "Impaired function of dendritic cells circulating in patients infected with hepatitis C virus who have persistently normal alanine aminotransferase levels," *Intervirology*, vol. 49, no. 1-2, pp. 58–63, 2006.

[68] A. Dolganiuc, K. Kodys, A. Kopasz et al., "Hepatitis C virus core and nonstructural protein 3 proteins induce pro- and anti-inflammatory cytokines and inhibit dendritic cell differentiation," *Journal of Immunology*, vol. 170, no. 11, pp. 5615–5624, 2003.

[69] R. S. Longman, A. H. Talal, I. M. Jacobson, M. L. Albert, and C. M. Rice, "Presence of functional dendritic cells in patients chronically infected with hepatitis C virus," *Blood*, vol. 103, no. 3, pp. 1026–1029, 2004.

[70] R. S. Longman, A. H. Talal, I. M. Jacobson, C. M. Rice, and M. L. Albert, "Normal functional capacity in circulating myeloid and plasmacytoid dendritic cells in patients with chronic hepatitis C," *Journal of Infectious Diseases*, vol. 192, no. 3, pp. 497–503, 2005.

[71] D. Piccioli, S. Tavarini, S. Nuti et al., "Comparable functions of plasmacytoid and monocyte-derived dendritic cells in chronic hepatitis C patients and healthy donors," *Journal of Hepatology*, vol. 42, no. 1, pp. 61–67, 2005.

[72] M. Larsson, E. Babcock, A. Grakoui et al., "Lack of phenotypic and functional impairment in dendritic cells from chimpanzees chronically infected with hepatitis C virus," *Journal of Virology*, vol. 78, no. 12, pp. 6151–6161, 2004.

[73] E. Barnes, M. Salio, V. Cerundolo et al., "Monocyte derived dendritic cells retain their functional capacity in patients following infection with hepatitis C virus," *Journal of Viral Hepatitis*, vol. 15, no. 3, pp. 219–228, 2008.

[74] A. Dolganiuc, S. Chang, K. Kodys et al., "Hepatitis C Virus (HCV) core protein-induced, monocyte-mediated mechanisms of reduced IFN-α and plasmacytoid dendritic cell loss in chronic HCV infection," *Journal of Immunology*, vol. 177, no. 10, pp. 6758–6768, 2006.

[75] A. Takaki, M. Tatsukawa, Y. Iwasaki et al., "Hepatitis C virus NS4 protein impairs the Th1 polarization of immature dendritic cells," *Journal of Viral Hepatitis*, vol. 17, no. 8, pp. 555–562, 2010.

[76] C. Logvinoff, M. E. Major, D. Oldach et al., "Neutralizing antibody response during acute and chronic hepatitis C virus infection," *Proceedings of the National Academy of Sciences of the United States of America*, vol. 101, no. 27, pp. 10149–10154, 2004.

[77] M. W. Yu, B. Bartosch, P. Zhang et al., "Neutralizing antibodies to hepatitis C virus (HCV) in immune globulins derived from anti-HCV-positive plasma," *Proceedings of the National Academy of Sciences of the United States of America*, vol. 101, no. 20, pp. 7705–7710, 2004.

[78] F. Helle, G. Duverlie, and J. Dubuisson, "The hepatitis C virus glycan shield and evasion of the humoral immune response," *Viruses*, vol. 3, no. 10, pp. 1909–1932, 2011.

[79] Y. Miyanari, K. Atsuzawa, N. Usuda et al., "The lipid droplet is an important organelle for hepatitis C virus production," *Nature Cell Biology*, vol. 9, no. 9, pp. 1089–1097, 2007.

[80] M. S. Abdel-Hakeem, N. Bedard, D. Murphy, J. Bruneau, and N. H. Shoukry, "Signatures of protective memory immune responses during hepatitis C virus reinfection," *Gastroenterology*, 2014.

[81] A. Wahid and J. Dubuisson, "Virus-neutralizing antibodies to hepatitis C virus," *Journal of Viral Hepatitis*, vol. 20, no. 6, pp. 369–376, 2013.

[82] W. Kang, P. S. Sung, S. H. Park et al., "Hepatitis C virus attenuates interferon-induced major histocompatibility complex class I expression and decreases $CD8^+$ T cell effector functions," *Gastroenterology*, vol. 146, no. 5, pp. 1351.e4–1360.e4, 2014.

[83] B. Rehermann and A. Bertoletti, "Immunological aspects of antiviral therapy of chronic hepatitis B virus and hepatitis C virus infections," *Hepatology*, vol. 5, pp. 215–229, 2014.

[84] Y. Y. Wan and R. A. Flavell, "TGF-β and regulatory T cell in immunity and autoimmunity," *Journal of Clinical Immunology*, vol. 28, no. 6, pp. 647–659, 2008.

[85] M. Rahmoun, A. Foussat, H. Groux, J. Pène, H. Yssel, and P. Chanez, "Enhanced frequency of CD18- and CD49b-expressing T cells in peripheral blood of asthmatic patients correlates with disease severity," *International Archives of Allergy and Immunology*, vol. 140, no. 2, pp. 139–149, 2006.

[86] C. Miroux, T. Vausselin, and N. Delhem, "Regulatory T cells in HBV and HCV liver diseases: implication of regulatory T lymphocytes in the control of immune response," *Expert Opinion on Biological Therapy*, vol. 10, no. 11, pp. 1563–1572, 2010.

[87] F. Bolacchi, A. Sinistro, C. Ciaprini et al., "Increased hepatitis C virus (HCV)-specific $CD4^+CD25^+$ regulatory T lymphocytes and reduced HCV-specific $CD4^+$ T cell response in HCV-infected patients with normal versus abnormal alanine aminotransferase levels," *Clinical and Experimental Immunology*, vol. 144, no. 2, pp. 188–196, 2006.

[88] T. Manigold, E. Shin, E. Mizukoshi et al., "Foxp3+CD4+CD25+ T cells control virus-specific memory T cells in chimpanzees that recovered from hepatitis C," *Blood*, vol. 107, no. 11, pp. 4424–4432, 2006.

[89] T. Boettler, H. C. Spangenberg, C. Neumann-Haefelin et al., "T cells with a $CD4^+CD25^+$ regulatory phenotype suppress in vitro proliferation of virus-specific $CD8^+$ T cells during chronic hepatitis C virus infection," *Journal of Virology*, vol. 79, no. 12, pp. 7860–7867, 2005.

[90] R. Cabrera, Z. Tu, Y. Xu et al., "An immunomodulatory role for CD4+CD25+ regulatory T lymphocytes in hepatitis C virus infection," *Hepatology*, vol. 40, no. 5, pp. 1062–1071, 2004.

[91] D. C. Kroy, D. Ciuffreda, J. H. Cooperrider et al., "Liver environment and HCV replication affect human T-cell phenotype and expression of inhibitory receptors," *Gastroenterology*, vol. 146, no. 2, pp. 550–561, 2014.

[92] D. Samuel, R. Muller, G. Alexander et al., "Liver transplantation in European patients with the hepatitis B surface antigen," *The New England Journal of Medicine*, vol. 329, no. 25, pp. 1842–1847, 1993.

[93] J. S. Markowitz, P. Martin, A. J. Conrad et al., "Prophylaxis against hepatitis B recurrence following liver transplantation using combination lamivudine and hepatitis B immune globulin," *Hepatology*, vol. 28, no. 2, pp. 585–589, 1998.

[94] J. Dumortier, P. Chevallier, J. Scoazec, F. Berger, and O. Boillot, "Combined lamivudine and hepatitis B immunoglobulin for the prevention of hepatitis B recurrence after liver transplantation: long-term results," *The American Journal of Transplantation*, vol. 3, no. 8, pp. 999–1002, 2003.

[95] E. J. Gane, P. W. Angus, S. Strasser et al., "Lamivudine plus low-dose hepatitis B immunoglobulin to prevent recurrent hepatitis B following liver transplantation," *Gastroenterology*, vol. 132, no. 3, pp. 931–937, 2007.

[96] J. Rosenau, M. J. Bahr, H. L. Tillmann et al., "Lamivudine and low-dose hepatitis B immune globulin for prophylaxis of hepatitis B reinfection after liver transplantation—possible role of mutations in the YMDD motif prior to transplantation as a risk factor for reinfection," *Journal of Hepatology*, vol. 34, no. 6, pp. 895–902, 2001.

[97] D. Di Paolo, G. Tisone, P. Piccolo, I. Lenci, S. Zazza, and M. Angelico, "Low-dose hepatitis B immunoglobulin given "on demand" in combination with lamivudine: a highly cost-effective approach to prevent recurrent hepatitis B virus infection in the long-term follow-up after liver transplantation," *Transplantation*, vol. 77, no. 8, pp. 1203–1208, 2004.

[98] M. Buti, A. Mas, M. Prieto et al., "A randomized study comparing lamivudine monotherapy after a short course of hepatitis B immune globulin (HBIg) and lamivudine with long-term lamivudine plus HBIg in the prevention of hepatitis B virus recurrence after liver transplantation," *Journal of Hepatology*, vol. 38, no. 6, pp. 811–817, 2003.

[99] D. K. Wong, W. Seto, J. Fung et al., "Reduction of hepatitis B surface antigen and covalently closed circular DNA by nucleos(t)ide analogues of different potency," *Clinical Gastroenterology and Hepatology*, vol. 11, no. 8, pp. 1004–1010, 2013.

[100] R. Schilling, S. Ijaz, M. Davidoff et al., "Endocytosis of hepatitis B immune globulin into hepatocytes inhibits the secretion of hepatitis B virus surface antigen and virions," *Journal of Virology*, vol. 77, no. 16, pp. 8882–8892, 2003.

[101] A. U. Neumann, S. Phillips, I. Levine et al., "Novel mechanism of antibodies to hepatitis B virus in blocking viral particle release from cells," *Hepatology*, vol. 52, no. 3, pp. 875–885, 2010.

[102] D. C. Chao and K. Hu, "Update on rescue therapies in patients with lamivudine-resistant chronic hepatitis B," *Drug Design, Development and Therapy*, vol. 7, pp. 777–788, 2013.

[103] E. J. Gane, S. Patterson, S. I. Strasser, G. W. McCaughan, and P. W. Angus, "Combination of lamivudine and adefovir without hepatitis B immune globulin is safe and effective prophylaxis against hepatitis B virus recurrence in hepatitis B surface antigen-positive liver transplant candidates," *Liver Transplantation*, vol. 19, no. 3, pp. 268–274, 2013.

[104] R. Perrillo, M. Buti, F. Durand et al., "Entecavir and hepatitis B immune globulin in patients undergoing liver transplantation for chronic hepatitis B," *Liver Transplantation*, vol. 19, no. 8, pp. 887–895, 2013.

[105] N. J. Yi, J. Y. Choi, K. S. Suh et al., "Post-transplantation sequential entecavir monotherapy following 1-year combination therapy with hepatitis B immunoglobulin," *Journal of Gastroenterology*, vol. 48, no. 12, pp. 1401–1410, 2013.

[106] E. Cholongitas, T. Vasiliadis, N. Antoniadis, I. Goulis, V. Papanikolaou, and E. Akriviadis, "Hepatitis B prophylaxis post liver transplantation with newer nucleos(t)ide analogues after hepatitis B immunoglobulin discontinuation," *Transplant Infectious Disease*, vol. 14, no. 5, pp. 479–487, 2012.

[107] C. Cai, M. Lu, Y. Chen, H. Zhao, M. Li, and G. Chen, "Clinical study on prevention of HBV re-infection by entecavir after liver transplantation," *Clinical Transplantation*, vol. 26, no. 2, pp. 208–215, 2012.

[108] R. T. Stravitz, M. L. Shiffman, M. Kimmel et al., "Substitution of tenofovir/emtricitabine for Hepatitis B immune globulin prevents recurrence of Hepatitis B after liver transplantation," *Liver International*, vol. 32, no. 7, pp. 1138–1145, 2012.

[109] D. J. W. Wesdorp, M. Knoester, A. E. Braat et al., "Nucleoside plus nucleotide analogs and cessation of hepatitis B immunoglobulin after liver transplantation in chronic hepatitis

B is safe and effective," *Journal of Clinical Virology*, vol. 58, no. 1, pp. 67–73, 2013.

[110] M. Wadhawan, S. Gupta, N. Goyal, S. Taneja, and A. Kumar, "Living related liver transplantation for hepatitis B-related liver disease without hepatitis B immune globulin prophylaxis," *Liver Transplantation*, vol. 19, no. 9, pp. 1030–1035, 2013.

[111] J. Rosenau, N. Hooman, K. Rifai et al., "Hepatitis B virus immunization with an adjuvant containing vaccine after liver transplantation for hepatitis B-related disease: failure of humoral and cellular immune response," *Transplant International*, vol. 19, no. 10, pp. 828–833, 2006.

[112] M. Ishigami, H. Kamei, T. Nakamura et al., "Different effect of HBV vaccine after liver transplantation between chronic HBV carriers and non-HBV patients who received HBcAb-positive grafts," *Journal of Gastroenterology*, vol. 46, no. 3, pp. 367–377, 2011.

[113] A. Sanchez-Fueyo, A. Rimola, L. Grande et al., "Hepatitis B immunoglobulin discontinuation followed by hepatitis B virus vaccination: a new strategy in the prophylaxis of hepatitis B virus recurrence after liver transplantation," *Hepatology*, vol. 31, no. 2, pp. 496–501, 2000.

[114] N. Yamashiki, Y. Sugawara, S. Tamura et al., "Double-dose double-phase use of second generation hepatitis B virus vaccine in patients after living donor liver transplantation: not an effective measure in transplant recipients," *Hepatology Research*, vol. 39, no. 1, pp. 7–13, 2009.

[115] N. K. Weber, L. M. Forman, and J. F. Trotter, "HBIg discontinuation with maintenance oral anti-viral therapy and HBV vaccination in liver transplant recipients," *Digestive Diseases and Sciences*, vol. 55, no. 2, pp. 505–509, 2010.

[116] J. Zhang, L. Zhou, and S. S. Zheng, "Clinical management of hepatitis B virus infection correlated with liver transplantation," *Hepatobiliary and Pancreatic Diseases International*, vol. 9, no. 1, pp. 15–21, 2010.

[117] A. Takaki, T. Yagi, T. Yasunaka et al., "Which patients respond best to hepatitis B vaccination after a hepatitis B virus-related liver transplantation?" *Journal of Gastroenterology*, vol. 48, no. 12, pp. 1373–1383, 2013.

[118] H. Tahara, Y. Tanaka, K. Ishiyama et al., "Successful hepatitis B vaccination in liver transplant recipients with donor-specific hyporesponsiveness," *Transplant International*, vol. 22, no. 8, pp. 805–813, 2009.

[119] P. Stärkel, M. Stoffel, J. Lerut, and Y. Horsmans, "Response to an experimental HBV vaccine permits withdrawal of HBIg prophylaxis in fulminant and selected chronic HBV-infected liver graft recipients," *Liver Transplantation*, vol. 11, no. 10, pp. 1228–1234, 2005.

[120] Y. Soejima, T. Ikegami, A. Taketomi et al., "Hepatitis B vaccination after living donor liver transplantation," *Liver International*, vol. 27, no. 7, pp. 977–982, 2007.

[121] J. B. Park, C. H. Kwon, K.-W. Lee et al., "Hepatitis B virus vaccine switch program for prevention of de novo hepatitis B virus infection in pediatric patients," *Transplant International*, vol. 21, no. 4, pp. 346–352, 2008.

[122] S. Shrivastava, N. Trehanpati, S. Patra et al., "Increased regulatory T cells and impaired functions of circulating CD8 T lymphocytes is associated with viral persistence in Hepatitis B virus-positive newborns," *Journal of Viral Hepatitis*, vol. 20, no. 8, pp. 582–591, 2013.

[123] P. T. F. Kennedy, E. Sandalova, J. Jo et al., "Preserved T-cell function in children and young adults with immune-tolerant chronic hepatitis B," *Gastroenterology*, vol. 143, no. 3, pp. 637–645, 2012.

[124] L. Feng, Y. Niu, H. Chen et al., "Immunogenicity of different hepatitis B virus vaccination schedules in liver transplant recipients," *Hepatology Research*, vol. 43, no. 5, pp. 495–501, 2013.

[125] J. Rosenau, N. Hooman, J. Hadem et al., "Failure of hepatitis B vaccination with conventional HBsAg vaccine in patients with continuous HBIG prophylaxis after liver transplantation," *Liver Transplantation*, vol. 13, no. 3, pp. 367–373, 2007.

[126] K. Wursthorn, H. Wedemeyer, and M. P. Manns, "Managing HBV in patients with impaired immunity," *Gut*, vol. 59, no. 10, pp. 1430–1445, 2010.

[127] A. Schumann, M. Lindemann, C. Valentin-Gamazo et al., "Adoptive immune transfer of hepatitis B virus specific immunity from immunized living liver donors to liver recipients," *Transplantation*, vol. 87, no. 1, pp. 103–111, 2009.

[128] Y. Luo, C. M. Lo, C. K. Cheung, G. K. Lau, S. T. Fan, and J. Wong, "Identification of hepatitis B virus-specific lymphocytes in human liver grafts from HBV-immune donors," *Liver Transplantation*, vol. 13, no. 1, pp. 71–79, 2007.

[129] D. Di Paolo, I. Lenci, C. Cerocchi et al., "One-year vaccination against hepatitis B virus with a MPL-vaccine in liver transplant patients for HBV-related cirrhosis," *Transplant International*, vol. 23, no. 11, pp. 1105–1112, 2010.

[130] I. N. Crispe, "The liver as a lymphoid organ," *Annual Review of Immunology*, vol. 27, pp. 147–163, 2009.

[131] M. E. Wachs, W. J. Amend, N. L. Ascher et al., "The risk of transmission of hepatitis B from HBsAg(-), HBcAb(+), HBIgM(-) organ donors," *Transplantation*, vol. 59, no. 2, pp. 230–234, 1995.

[132] R. C. Dickson, J. E. Everhart, J. R. Lake et al., "Transmission of hepatitis B by transplantation of livers from donors positive for antibody to hepatitis B core antigen," *Gastroenterology*, vol. 113, no. 5, pp. 1668–1674, 1997.

[133] C.-C. Lin, C.-L. Chen, A. Concejero et al., "Active immunization to prevent de novo hepatitis B virus infection in pediatric live donor liver recipients," *American Journal of Transplantation*, vol. 7, no. 1, pp. 195–200, 2007.

[134] C. H. D. Kwon, K. Suh, N. Yi et al., "Long-term protection against hepatitis B in pediatric liver recipients can be achieved effectively with vaccination after transplantation," *Pediatric Transplantation*, vol. 10, no. 4, pp. 479–486, 2006.

[135] X. Forns, M. García-Retortillo, T. Serrano et al., "Antiviral therapy of patients with decompensated cirrhosis to prevent recurrence of hepatitis C after liver transplantation," *Journal of Hepatology*, vol. 39, no. 3, pp. 389–396, 2003.

[136] R. P. Francesca, A. Milani, A. Gasbarrini et al., "Treatment of recurrent genotype 4 Hepatitis C after liver transplantation: early virological response is predictive of sustained virological response. An AISF RECOLT-C group study," *Annals of Hepatology*, vol. 11, no. 3, pp. 338–342, 2012.

[137] T. Fukuhara, A. Taketomi, T. Motomura et al., "Variants in IL28B in liver recipients and donors correlate with response to peg-interferon and ribavirin therapy for recurrent hepatitis C," *Gastroenterology*, vol. 139, no. 5, pp. 1577.e3–1585.e3, 2010.

[138] M. Selzner and P.-A. Clavien, "Fatty liver in liver transplantation and surgery," *Seminars in Liver Disease*, vol. 21, no. 1, pp. 105–113, 2001.

[139] S. A. Waits, E. K. Kim, M. N. Terjimanian et al., "Morphometric age and mortality after liver transplant," *JAMA Surgery*, vol. 149, no. 4, pp. 335–340, 2014.

[140] F. Ge, T. Huang, S. Yuan, Y. Zhou, and W. Gong, "Gender issues in solid organ donation and transplantation," *Annals of Transplantation*, vol. 18, pp. 508–514, 2013.

[141] Y. Tanaka, N. Nishida, M. Sugiyama et al., "Genome-wide association of IL28B with response to pegylated interferon-α and ribavirin therapy for chronic hepatitis C," *Nature Genetics*, vol. 41, no. 10, pp. 1105–1109, 2009.

[142] V. Suppiah, M. Moldovan, G. Ahlenstiel et al., "IL28B is associated with response to chronic hepatitis C interferon-α and ribavirin therapy," *Nature Genetics*, vol. 41, no. 10, pp. 1100–1104, 2009.

[143] D. L. Thomas, C. L. Thio, M. P. Martin et al., "Genetic variation in IL28B and spontaneous clearance of hepatitis C virus," *Nature*, vol. 461, no. 7265, pp. 798–801, 2009.

[144] M. J. Sofia, "Beyond sofosbuvir: what opportunity exists for a better nucleoside/nucleotide to treat hepatitis C?" *Antiviral Research*, vol. 107, pp. 119–124, 2014.

[145] C. M. Perry, "Telaprevir: a review of its use in the management of genotype 1 chronic hepatitis C," *Drugs*, vol. 72, no. 5, pp. 619–641, 2012.

[146] V. Garg, R. van Heeswijk, J. Eun Lee, K. Alves, P. Nadkarni, and X. Luo, "Effect of telaprevir on the pharmacokinetics of cyclosporine and tacrolimus," *Hepatology*, vol. 54, no. 1, pp. 20–27, 2011.

[147] T. Takehara, "Simeprevir for the treatment of chronic hepatitis C genotype 1 infection," *Expert Review of Anti-Infective Therapy*, vol. 12, no. 8, pp. 909–917, 2014.

[148] R. Zeiser, V. H. Nguyen, A. Beilhack et al., "Inhibition of $CD4^{+}CD25^{+}$ regulatory T-cell function by calcineurin-dependent interleukin-2 production," *Blood*, vol. 108, no. 1, pp. 390–399, 2006.

[149] A. Bharat, F. Barros, K. Narayanan et al., "Characterization of virus-specific T-cell immunity in liver allograft recipients with HCV-induced cirrhosis," *The American Journal of Transplantation*, vol. 8, no. 6, pp. 1214–1220, 2008.

[150] H. I. Basha, V. Subramanian, A. Seetharam et al., "Characterization of HCV-specific CD4+Th17 immunity in recurrent hepatitis C-induced liver allograft fibrosis," *American Journal of Transplantation*, vol. 11, no. 4, pp. 775–785, 2011.

[151] M. M. Velásquez-Lopera, V. L. Eaton, N. M. Lerret et al., "Induction of transplantation tolerance by allogeneic donor-derived CD4+CD25+Foxp3+ regulatory T cells," *Transplant Immunology*, vol. 19, no. 2, pp. 127–135, 2008.

[152] O. Joffre, T. Santolaria, D. Calise et al., "Prevention of acute and chronic allograft rejection with CD4 +CD25+Foxp3+ regulatory T lymphocytes," *Nature Medicine*, vol. 14, no. 1, pp. 88–92, 2008.

[153] A. Carpentier, F. Conti, F. Stenard et al., "Increased expression of regulatory Tr1 cells in recurrent hepatitis C after liver transplantation," *American Journal of Transplantation*, vol. 9, no. 9, pp. 2102–2112, 2009.

[154] A. Satake, A. M. Schmidt, S. Nomura, and T. Kambayashi, " Inhibition of calcineurin abrogates while inhibition of mTOR promotes regulatory T cell expansion and graft-versus-host disease protection by IL-2 in allogeneic bone marrow transplantation," *PloS One*, vol. 9, no. 3, p. e92888, 2014.

[155] A. S. Gaweco, R. H. Wiesner, M. Porayko et al., "Intragraft localization of activated nuclear factor κB in recurrent hepatitis C virus disease following liver transplantation," *Hepatology*, vol. 31, no. 5, pp. 1183–1191, 2000.

[156] E. Schvoerer, C. Thumann, S. Spohrer et al., "Early decrease in circulating dendritic cells number after liver transplantation could favor hepatitis C virus recurrence," *Journal of Medical Virology*, vol. 78, no. 8, pp. 1070–1075, 2006.

[157] A. Nellore and J. A. Fishman, "NK cells, innate immunity and hepatitis C infection after liver transplantation," *Clinical Infectious Diseases*, vol. 52, no. 3, pp. 369–377, 2011.

[158] M. Askar, R. Avery, R. Corey et al., "Lack of killer immunoglobulin-like receptor 2DS2 (KIR2DS2) and KIR2DL2 is associated with poor responses to therapy of recurrent hepatitis C virus in liver transplant recipients," *Liver Transplantation*, vol. 15, no. 11, pp. 1557–1563, 2009.

[159] M. Ohira, K. Ishiyama, Y. Tanaka et al., "Adoptive immunotherapy with liver allograft-derived lymphocytes induces anti-HCV activity after liver transplantation in humans and humanized mice," *The Journal of Clinical Investigation*, vol. 119, no. 11, pp. 3226–3235, 2009.

9

The Effect of Periodontitis on Expression of Interleukin-21

Archana Mootha, Sankari Malaiappan, N. D. Jayakumar, Sheeja S. Varghese, and Julie Toby Thomas

Department of Periodontics, Saveetha Dental College and Hospitals, No. 162, Poonamallee High Road, Velappanchavadi, Chennai 600077, India

Correspondence should be addressed to Archana Mootha; archanamootha@gmail.com

Academic Editor: Alexander J. Steven

Purpose. Inflammation and tissue breakdown are led by an array of inflammatory destructive mediators associated with initiation and progression of inflammatory diseases like periodontitis. Current evidence shows that these inflammatory mediators have a definitive role in the pathogenesis of various systemic diseases with an inflammatory component. Interleukin-21 (IL-21) has been associated with systemic diseases like rheumatoid arthritis and Crohn's disease that follow a chronic inflammatory cascade. Similarly recent studies have associated Interleukin-21 levels with periodontitis. This systematic review was aimed to assess the levels of IL-21 in subjects with periodontitis. *Methods.* A complete literature search was done in PubMed, Medline, Science Direct, and Cochrane databases and Google Scholar based on the inclusion/exclusion criteria. Six relevant articles were procured. Full text was read individually by two reviewers and data extraction was done based on STROBE statement. *Results.* After data extraction five observational and one interventional study were obtained. All the studies showed an increased expression of IL-21 in periodontitis and the interventional study showed reduction in IL-21 levels after nonsurgical periodontal therapy (NSP). *Conclusion.* Interleukin-21 levels are higher in periodontitis than controls. With this limited evidence further longitudinal studies are required to consider this as a definitive inflammatory marker.

1. Introduction

Periodontitis is a chronic inflammatory condition which was initiated by gram-negative organisms present in the tooth supporting structures [1]. Disease progression occurs as a result of host-immune response to bacteria, leading to destruction of connective tissue and alveolar bone [2]. The pathogens present in the subgingival flora produce various endotoxins which are a prerequisite for periodontal disease [3]. These endotoxins in turn activate a host-immune response to the bacterial challenge by stimulating immune cells like polymorphonuclear neutrophils (PMNs), monocytes, B cells, T cells, and fibroblasts [2] to produce various inflammatory mediators such as cytokines [4, 5], acute phase proteins [6], and proteolytic enzymes [7, 8] that mediate tissue destruction. Progression of the periodontal disease can further trigger the adaptive immune mechanism for release of inflammatory mediators resulting in further periodontal breakdown.

Cytokines are important in expression of the characteristics of the immune response to bacterial endotoxins [9]. Interleukins comprise a large group of cytokines that are naturally occurring glycoproteins produced by the body [10]. They help in recruitment of neutrophils and macrophages to participate and amplify the inflammatory immune reaction [11].

The role of IL-1, IL-6, IL-8, and IL-12 has previously been established in periodontitis [12–15] proving their definitive role in periodontal destruction. Interleukin-21 (IL-21) is an inflammatory cytokine [16] mainly expressed by activated Th1 and Th17 cells which are distinct proinflammatory lineages, and not by Th2 cells in humans pointing out it to be a proinflammatory cytokine [17]. It functions via the receptor IL-21R which is a type I cytokine receptor. Recently

IL-21 has gained importance as it has been associated with the pathogenesis of inflammatory breakdown in various systemic diseases like rheumatoid arthritis [18], colitis [19], and inflammatory bowel disease [20]. On account of the fact that IL-21 plays a paramount role in inflammation [21], its over production leads to amplification of local inflammation, intensifying tissue damage and destruction [22]. Evidences prove that its regulation in vivo has clinical potential in inflammatory diseases like rheumatoid arthritis [23] and is an area for active research. Since periodontitis and rheumatoid arthritis were previously associated with one another [24] this systematic review was aimed to evaluate the expression of IL-21 in periodontitis.

2. Materials and Methods

Based on the aim the following structured questions were formulated:

(a) Is there an increase in Interleukin-21 levels in periodontitis?

(b) Are IL-21 levels associated with severity of periodontitis?

(c) Is there a difference in the IL-21 levels between types of periodontitis?

2.1. Search Strategy. The Cochrane, Medline/PubMed, and Science Direct databases and Google Scholar were searched to identify the relevant studies published through June 2015. A detailed search based on MeSH terms and key words was done. A hand search was carried out in the Journal of Periodontology, Journal of Periodontal Research, Journal of Clinical Periodontology, Journal of Periodontal and Implant Science, and International Journal of Periodontics and Restorative Dentistry to check for relevant additional studies. To locate additional studies, the references of the selected articles were hand-searched. No time limits and language restrictions were applied to include all the potentially relevant articles in the review. Selected studies were screened on the basis of the title and abstract. Full text was then procured for the relevant articles which fulfilled the inclusion criteria. The complete search strategy is mentioned in Table 1 and the flowchart is shown in Figure 1.

2.2. Inclusion and Exclusion Criteria. Studies estimating IL-21 levels in serum, saliva, gingival tissue, or GCF of subjects with chronic periodontitis or aggressive periodontitis, regardless of the methodology followed, were included. All animal studies were excluded. Studies estimating IL-21 levels in other oral lesions in subjects without periodontitis were also excluded.

2.3. Screening Methods and Data Extraction. The excluded and included studies are shown in Tables 2 and 3. Each study's methodological quality was assessed based on the STROBE statement by two reviewers (Archana Mootha and Sankari Malaiappan). The studies included in this review were read independently to extract the descriptive and quantitative information including citation author, year of publication, study design, study sample, number of participants in control and test groups, method of evaluation of IL-21, levels of IL-21, correlation of IL-21 levels with clinical parameters, and results.

TABLE 1: Search methodology.

[[[[[[[[[[[[[[[[[[[[[[[[[[[[aggressive periodontitis [MeSH Terms]] OR chronic periodontitis [MeSH Terms]] OR periapical periodontitis [MeSH Terms]] OR gingivitis [MeSH Terms]]] OR periodontitis] OR periodontal disease]]] AND [[[[[IL21] OR interleukin 21] OR IL-21] OR IL21 protein, human] OR Interleukin 21 protein, human]]]*	10

*Pubmed MESH search.

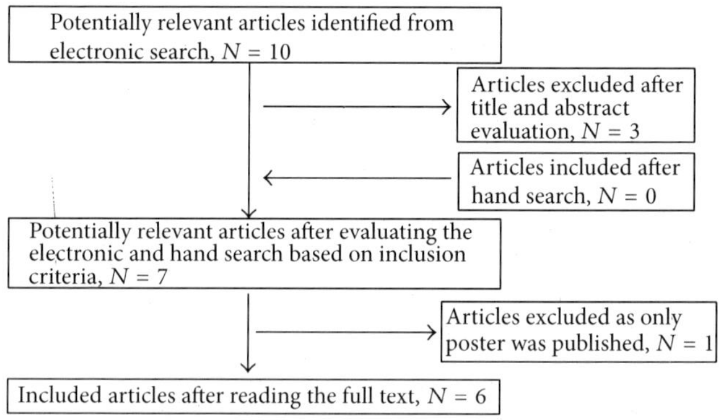

FIGURE 1: Flowchart for selection of articles.

TABLE 2: Excluded studies.

S. number	Citation	Reason for exclusion
1	Ebersole et al. [4]	Animal study
2	Araujo-Pires et al. [25]	IL-21 was estimated in periapical granuloma in subjects without periodontitis
3	Li et al. [26]	Animal study
4	Wang et al. [27]	No abstract/full text available

3. Results

The electronic databases and hand search yielded a total of ten articles (Figure 1). Four articles [4, 25–27] were excluded and the reasons for exclusion are given in Table 2. Full texts for six articles were then procured and data extraction was done. A description of each study is given in Table 3.

The final six studies included five cross-sectional [28, 29, 31–33] and one interventional study [30]. All cross-sectional studies showed increased expression of IL-21 in periodontitis.

The first study estimated salivary IL-21 using ELISA and reported that IL-21 was expressed in all the groups (mild/moderate/no OSAS) with a significant positive correlation with CAL ($p = 0.02$) [28].

TABLE 3: Data summation table.

(a)

Sl. number	Author and journal	Study design	Groups	Parameters	Sample and Methodology	Statistical Analysis	Results
1	Dutzan et al. [29] Journal of Periodontology, 2011 "Levels of Interleukin-21 in Patients with Untreated Chronic Periodontitis"	Case control study	*Group 1*: controls, $n = 19$ *Group 2*: CP, $n = 15$	PI, PD, CAL, PI, BOP, and presence of IL-21	*Gingival and GCF* IL-21 (healthy-extraction site, CP- periodontal lesions) were analysed by IHC and Western blot (for presence of IL-21) and quantification was done by ELISA	Unpaired t-test and Mann-Whitney U test Chi square test	Gingival IL-21 levels were significantly higher in CP group (3.35 pg/mg) than in controls (0.98 pg/mg) ($p < 0.05$) Frequency of GCF IL-21 was greater in CP patients (8/10) than in controls (2/10) ($p = 0.007$) The Western blot and IHC staining confirmed the presence of IL-21 in periodontal tissues and GCF

(b)

Sl. number	Author and journal	Study design	Groups	Parameters	Methodology	Statistical analysis	Results
2	Zhao et al. [30] Journal of Clinical Periodontology, 2011 "Effect of Non-Surgical Periodontal Therapy on the Levels of Th17/Th1/Th2 Cytokines and Their Transcription Factors in Chinese Chronic Periodontitis Patients"	Interventi-onal study	30 participants with CP, $n = 30$	IL-21	*GCF* (before and after treatment) IL-21 was analysed by ELISA	Linear correlation Paired t-test	Downregulation of IL-21 (80.3360 ± 39.4188 versus 31.7741 ± 13.2558 pg/mL) ($p < 0.05$) The quantity of Th17 cells in peripheral blood was decreased especially in IL-17 IFN-γ1 subgroup ($p < 0.05$)

(c)

Sl. number	Author and journal	Study design	Groups	Parameters	Methodology	Statistical analysis	Results
3	Napimoga et al. [32] Scandinavian Journal of Immunology 2011 "Possible Involvement of IL-21 and IL-10 on Salivary IgA Levels in Chronic Periodontitis Subjects"	Case control study	*Group 1*: healthy controls, $n = 15$ *Group2*: CP, $n = 15$	IL-21	*Gingival* IL-21 (healthy-gingivoplasty sites, CP-extraction sites due to advanced periodontitis) using RT-PCR	Student's t-test	The mRNA levels for IL-21 was higher in the CP (1.5-fold) when compared to the healthy group (0.4-fold) ($p < 0.05$)

(d)

Sl. number	Author and journal	Study design	Groups	Parameters	Methodology	Statistical analysis	Results
4	Dutzan et al. [31] Journal of Periodontology, 2012 "Interleukin-21 Expression and Its Association with Proinflammatory Cytokines in Untreated Chronic Periodontitis subjects"	Case control study	*Group 1*: controls, $n = 8$ *Group 2*: CP, $n = 10$	IL-21 mRNA level	*Gingival* IL-21 (healthy-extraction site, CP- periodontal lesions) was analysed using RT-PCR	The RQ expressed as fold change for each studied cytokine Spearman rank correlation test	A significant overexpression of IL-21 in CP affected tissues compared to healthy gingival tissues (120-fold) Significant positive correlations of IL-21 with PD (0.71) ($p = 0.002$) and CAL (0.60) ($p = 0.01$)

(e)

Sl. number	Author and journal	Study design	Groups	Parameters	Methodology	Statistical analysis	Results
5	Isaza-Guzmán et al., 2015 [33] Journal of Archives of Oral Biology "Association Study between Salivary Levels of Interferon (IFN)-Gamma, Interleukin (IL)-17, IL-21, and IL-22 with Chronic Periodontitis"	Cross-sectional study	*Group 1*: CP, $n = 105$ *Group 2*: healthy controls, $n = 44$	IL-21 and IL-21R	*Salivary* IL-21 and levels were analysed using RT-PCR	Pearson's chi square test	In healthy controls IL-21 (0.00–4.54) than CP (0.00 pg/mL) ($p = 0.470$) Low detection frequency of Th17 cytokines in saliva No significant domination in periodontitis

(f)

Sl. number	Author and journal	Study design	Groups	Parameters	Sample and methodology	Statistical analysis	Results
6	Nizam et al. [28] Journal of Periodontology, 2014 "Salivary Cytokines and the Association between Obstructive Sleep Apnea Syndrome and Periodontal Disease"	Case-control study	*Group 1*: controls (non-OSAS), $n = 13$ *Group 2*: mild/moderate OSAS, $n = 17$ *Group 3*: severe OSAS, $n = 22$	PI, PD, CAL, BOP, and *salivary* IL-21	Salivary IL-21 was assessed by ELISA	Spearman r rank correlation analysis	Significant correlation was between CAL and IL-21 ($r = -0.347$) ($p = 0.02$) Borderline significance between PI and IL-21 ($r = -0.287$) ($p = 0.05$) IL-21 levels in healthy controls, moderate OSAS, and severe OSAS (90 pg/mL, 85 pg/mL, and 75 pg/mL)

IL: interleukin, OSAS: obstructive sleep apnea syndrome, GCF: gingival crevicular fluid, GI: Gingival Index, PPD: probing pocket depth, PD: probing depth, CAL: clinical attachment level, BOP: bleeding on probing, PCR: polymerase chain reaction, RT-PCR: real time polymerase chain reaction, IHC: immunohistochemistry, and ELISA: enzyme linked immunosorbant assay.

Next study [29] performed qualitative analysis of gingival tissue samples IL-21 using immunohistochemistry and quantitative analysis of salivary and gingival tissue IL-21 using western blot. Gingival tissue IL-21 (3.35 pg/mL) and GCF IL-21 (8/10) were higher in CP (chronic periodontitis) compared to controls.

Another study showed increased expression of IL-21 in gingival tissue samples using PCR, which were 1.5 times more in CP than controls (0.3) [32]. Another study [31] compared IL-21 levels in gingival tissue between CP and healthy controls using RT-PCR. CP group showed 120-fold increase of IL-21 level and showed a direct positive correlation with probing depth ($p = 0.02$) and CAL ($p = 0.02$).

One study showed reduced expression of salivary IL-21 in periodontitis using ELISA [33]. Salivary estimation of IL-21 using ELISA in CP (smokers were included) showed no significant domination of this cytokine (0.00–4.5 pg/mL) and it was concluded that the detection of IL-21 has no predictive value in health/disease.

In the interventional study, the GCF IL-21 levels were increased in CP group and there was a reduction in IL-21 levels after nonsurgical periodontal therapy when estimated using ELISA [30].

Due to variations in the study population, sample source and the methodology of estimation of IL-21 the data obtained were heterogeneous. One study was conducted in Brazilian [32], one study in Turkish [28], and one study in Chinese population [30], whereas three studies were conducted in the American [29, 31, 33] population. Varied sources were used for analysis of IL-21. Two studies used GCF [29, 30], two studies used gingival tissue [29, 31, 32], and two studies used saliva [28, 33]. All the samples showed increased IL-21 levels in periodontitis, among which GCF [30] showed maximum detection of IL-21 (80.336 pg/mL). Several methodologies were used for qualitative and quantitative analysis of IL-21. Three studies detected IL-21 using RT-PCR [31, 32], one study used western blot and immunohistochemistry [29], and three studies used ELISA [28–30, 33] for analysis of IL-21. All methodologies showed increased IL-21 levels in periodontitis, among which ELISA showed maximum detection of IL-21 [30]. Due to the heterogeneity of the data it was not feasible to pool the data to perform a meta-analysis. Only two studies showed significant correlation of IL-21 level with periodontal disease severity [31, 32]. They found a significant correlation of IL-21 with clinical attachment loss (CAL) and borderline significance between plaque index and IL-21. As CAL is the most reliable indicator of periodontal tissue destruction, this correlation indicates better that IL-21 levels increase with the severity of periodontitis.

4. Discussion

Periodontitis is a chronic inflammatory disease that affects the supporting structures of the teeth and is considered as one of the most common reasons for tooth loss [34]. It is one of the most common pathologies of bone and an important modifying factor of several chronic inflammatory systemic diseases like cardiovascular disease and obesity [35]. Evidence shows association of IL-21 with various systemic conditions such as coronary artery disease [36], rheumatoid arthritis [18], and inflammatory bowel disease [19]. Much about IL-21 has been studied in rheumatoid arthritis (RA), and researchers have reported elevated serum and synovial tissues levels of this cytokine in RA as the disease severity increased [37].

Periodontitis is a chronic inflammatory condition which shows increased local and systemic levels of inflammatory mediators and markers of inflammation like IL-21, and a direct link has been established between periodontitis and rheumatoid arthritis. In this regard, this systematic review aimed to evaluate the expression of IL-21 in periodontitis.

Clinically, periodontal disease is characterized by increase in probing depth and a decrease in clinical attachment level. The ultimate determinant of disease progression and clinical outcome is the immune response of host, which involves the generation of cytokines, activation of osteoclasts, and the recruitment of inflammatory cells like lymphocytes, PMNs, and antigen presenting cells to the site [2]. The recruitment and activation of these host cells lead to overproduction of proinflammatory cytokines like IL-1, IL-6, IL-12, and IL-21 along with other host-destructive mediators that enhance host destruction and activate resident cells to produce proteases which further amplify the host mediated periodontal destruction.

A limited number of eligible studies were identified in this systematic review including five observational [23, 24, 28, 29, 31–33] and one interventional studies [30]. The results of this systematic review show that five [23, 24, 28, 29, 31–33] out of six studies show an increase in IL-21 levels in chronic periodontitis subjects and one study [33] showed no increase in periodontitis. The interventional study [30] showed a reduction in IL-21 levels following nonsurgical therapy.

Nizam et al. [28] hypothesized that OSAS may predispose patients to periodontal disease and associated the salivary cytokines with OSAS severity. He found that salivary IL-6 and IL-33 were similar in OSAS groups but significantly higher than control groups, whereas IL-1β, IL-21, and PTX were similar in all groups with strong and weak positive correlation of IL-21 with CAL and PI, respectively. The authors concluded, it is likely that elevated IL-6 reflects the degree of subclinical inflammation in periodontal tissues, which can be a link between periodontal disease and OSAS, and the presence or severity of OSAS does not affect the level of IL-1β and IL-21 in either plasma or saliva.

Dutzan et al. [31] showed an increase in IL-21 levels in chronic periodontitis, a positive correlation of IL-21 with PD, CAL, IL-1β, IL-6, and Th17 cytokines like IL-17 and IL-23, and a negative correlation with anti-inflammatory cytokines like IL-10 and TGF-β1 [31].

IL-21 influences the actions of various immune cells like Natural Killer (NK) cells, PMNs, and macrophages. NK cells are a part of the innate immune response and serve as a first line of defence against invading pathogens. The development and activation of NK cells are intrinsically dependent on the activity of class I cytokine receptors, and cells treated with IL-21 displayed enhanced effector functions with greater cytolytic activity. IL-21 increased PMN migration to the local inflammatory site and caused greater PMN mediated tissue injury. IL-21 also complemented the phagocytic ability of macrophages. In addition to its action in the innate immune response, it also parades the action of the adaptive immune response. IL-21 drives terminal differentiation of B cells into plasma cells, favours the effector functions of T cell, and accelerates memory cell formation for rapid action on encounter of a pathogen for the second time. Furthermore, IL-6 and IL-21 can stimulate Th17 cells itself to produce increased IL-21. Altogether, IL-21 exaggerates the host-immune response and intensifies the local inflammatory actions, and these data support an important role of IL-21 in the pathogenesis of periodontal disease.

Salivary levels of IgA were increased in periodontitis subjects along with gingival levels of IL-21. As it was previously discussed, IL-21 not only controls Th17 activity, but also controls B cell proliferation and maturation into plasma cells; the elevated IgA levels in periodontitis may be explained, as IgA is predominantly produced by B cells and both IgA and IL-21 are increased in periodontitis compared to healthy controls. IgA is the most predominant Ig secreted by oral mucosal sites and is considered as the most important protein against microbial defence. This indicated the role of IL-21 in Ig-isotype switching in chronic periodontitis and its influence on the adaptive immune response and the immunomodulation of oral mucosa under the challenge of periodontal pathogens [32]. In contrast to these findings, Isaza et al. detected low frequency of Th17 cytokines in saliva samples and concluded that its determination is useless for the detection of disease presence and/or its severity.

After nonsurgical periodontal therapy, Zhao et al. found that Th17 cells might participate in the development of periodontitis by upregulating the expression of cytokines IL-17 and IL-21; meanwhile, Th1 cells increased the expression of IFN-γ, but Th2 cells inhibited the expression of IL-4. He concluded that nonsurgical treatment might decrease the expression of Th17-related cytokines, IL-17 and IL-21, and Th1-related cytokine IFN-g, while increasing the expression of Th2 related cytokine IL-4, thus contributing to the relief of periodontal inflammation [30].

While all the cross-sectional studies showed elevated IL-21 levels in periodontitis, one recent study [33] showed contradictory results by reporting no significant domination of Th17 cytokines in chronic periodontitis. An interesting finding is that there is no positive correlation of smokers with IL-21 levels. No scientific rationale explaining the results is mentioned in the article.

In addition, studies conducted in nonperiodontal oral lesions and animal studies also showed an increase in IL-21 levels in disease state compared to controls. On estimation of IL-21 levels in periapical granulomas, it was demonstrated that IL-21 along with IL-17A, TNF-α (tumour necrosis factor-α), and IFN-γ were higher in active periapical granulomas, while IL-4, IL-9, IL-10, and IL-22 were higher in inactive periapical granulomas. In the secondary lymphoid organs CD4+ T cell subset found in the B cell follicles was described as a major contributor to B cell-mediated antibody responses and an important source of IL-21. Since B cells are predominant in chronic lesions like periapical granulomas, it would be possible to speculate that IL-21 contributes to a Tfh-B cell response axis in periapical areas, similar to that of tertiary lymphoid tissues associated with chronic infection sites. In view of B cells being potential sources of RANKL, Tfh-B cell axis can directly drive the activity of the lesion via RANKL production [34].

Animal study conducted in rhesus monkeys by Ebersole et al. [4] reported that disease initiation/progression was characterized by overexpression of Th17/Treg cytokine genes (IL-1β, IL-6, TGFβ, and IL-21) and downregulation of Th1/Th2 cytokine genes (IL-18 and IL-25). They found that several Th17/Treg cytokine genes positively correlated with tissue destruction genes (TDGs), whereas most Th1/Th2 genes exhibited a negative correlation. Overall their observations were consistent with a cytokine profile driving a Th17 type of response early in the initiation process of periodontitis, followed by a persistence with disease progression.

Isaza-Guzmán et al. [33] showed that rats fed with *Actinobacillus actinomycetemcomitans* containing mash were compared to control; both B and T cells were increased and activated with enhanced IgG switched Ig in 2 weeks. Bone resorption was evident at 12 weeks with early increase in the levels of IL-21 along with IL-2, macrophage-inhibiting factor, IL-19, TNF-α, and CD40 ligand, CD70, while IL-16, TNF-α, lymphotoxin-β, IFN-α1, and IL-1RN were increased from T cells indicating that adaptive immunity appears crucial for bone resorption.

The results of this review conclude that (1) IL-21 was elevated in subjects with chronic periodontitis compared to controls, (2) their levels were correlated with clinical severity of periodontitis (only in 2 studies, and values were given only in one study), and (3) nonsurgical periodontal therapy downregulated IL-21 levels. There are no studies based on comparison of IL-21 levels among types of periodontitis. The present review considers only published data for the interpretation of results and the raw data was not procured form the authors of unpublished studies.

This systematic review included cross-sectional studies (level III) [38] and thus indicates a low level of evidence to prove the definitive role of IL-21 in periodontitis. Future longitudinal studies are required to prove the definitive role of IL-21 in periodontitis and compare IL-21 levels among types of periodontitis. Further research in the field of Interleukin-21 could throw light on a better understanding of its role in the pathogenesis of tissue destruction in periodontitis.

References

[1] H. Loe, "The role of bacteria in periodontal diseases," *Bulletin of the World Health Organization*, vol. 59, no. 6, pp. 821–825, 1981.

[2] G. J. Seymour, "Importance of the host response in the periodontium," *Journal of Clinical Periodontology*, vol. 18, no. 6, pp. 421–426, 1991.

[3] L. Kesic, J. Milasin, M. Igic, and R. Obradovic, "Microbial etiology of periodontal disease," *Facta Universitatis Series: Medicine and Biology*, vol. 15, no. 1, pp. 1–6, 2008.

[4] J. L. Ebersole, S. Kirakodu, M. J. Novak et al., "Cytokine gene expression profiles during initiation, progression and resolution of periodontitis," *Journal of Clinical Periodontology*, vol. 41, no. 9, pp. 853–861, 2014.

[5] D. T. Graves, "The potential role of chemokines and inflammatory cytokines in periodontal disease progression," *Clinical Infectious Diseases*, vol. 28, no. 3, pp. 482–490, 1999.

[6] R. C. Page, "The role of inflammatory mediators in the pathogenesis of periodontal disease," *Journal of Periodontal Research*, vol. 26, no. 3, pp. 230–242, 1991.

[7] F. Trindade, F. G. Oppenheim, E. J. Helmerhorst, F. Amado, P. S. Gomes, and R. Vitorino, "Uncovering the molecular networks in periodontitis," *Proteomics—Clinical Applications*, vol. 8, no. 9-10, pp. 748–761, 2014.

[8] H. M. Fullmer, "Collagenase and periodontal diseases: a review," *Journal of Dental Research*, vol. 50, no. 2, pp. 288–291, 1971.

[9] S. Stenger and M. Röllinghoff, "Role of cytokines in the innate immune response to intracellular pathogens," *Annals of the Rheumatic Diseases*, vol. 60, no. 3, pp. iii43–iii46, 2001.

[10] R. E. Elmslie, S. W. Dow, and G. K. Ogilvie, "Interleukins: biological properties and therapeutic potential," *Journal of Veterinary Internal Medicine*, vol. 5, no. 5, pp. 283–293, 1991.

[11] M. Akdis, S. Burgler, R. Crameri et al., "Interleukins, from 1 to 37, and interferon-γ: receptors, functions, and roles in diseases," *The Journal of Allergy and Clinical Immunology*, vol. 127, no. 3, pp. 701.e70–721.e70, 2011.

[12] S. P. Engebretson, J. T. Grbic, R. Singer, and I. B. Lamster, "GCF IL-1β profiles in periodontal disease," *Journal of Clinical Periodontology*, vol. 29, no. 1, pp. 48–53, 2002.

[13] C. R. Irwin and T. T. Myrillas, "The role of IL-6 in the pathogenesis of periodontal disease," *Oral Diseases*, vol. 4, no. 1, pp. 43–47, 1998.

[14] A. Harada, N. Sekido, T. Akahoshi, T. Wada, N. Mukaida, and K. Matsushima, "Essential involvement of interleukin-8 [IL-8] in acute inflammation," *Journal of Leukocyte Biology*, vol. 56, pp. 559–564, 1994.

[15] I.-S. Tsai, C.-C. Tsai, Y.-P. Ho, K.-Y. Ho, Y.-M. Wu, and C.-C. Hung, "Interleukin-12 and interleukin-16 in periodontal disease," *Cytokine*, vol. 31, no. 1, pp. 34–40, 2005.

[16] C. de Rham, S. Ferrari-Lacraz, S. Jendly, G. Schneiter, J.-M. Dayer, and J. Villard, "The proinflammatory cytokines IL-2, IL-15 and IL-21 modulate the repertoire of mature human natural killer cell receptors," *Arthritis Research and Therapy*, vol. 9, no. 6, article R125, 15 pages, 2007.

[17] M. Sarra, F. Pallone, and G. Monteleone, "Interleukin-21 in chronic inflammatory diseases," *BioFactors*, vol. 39, no. 4, pp. 368–373, 2013.

[18] T. K. Rasmussen, T. Andersen, M. Hvid et al., "Increased interleukin 21 (IL-21) and IL-23 are associated with increased disease activity and with radiographic status in patients with early rheumatoid arthritis," *The Journal of Rheumatology*, vol. 37, no. 10, pp. 2014–2020, 2010.

[19] K. Gerlach, C. Daniel, H. A. Lehr et al., "Transcription factor NFATc2 controls the emergence of colon cancer associated with IL-6-dependent colitis," *Cancer Research*, vol. 72, no. 17, pp. 4340–4350, 2012.

[20] C. Abraham and J. Cho, "Interleukin-23/Th17 pathways and inflammatory bowel disease," *Inflammatory Bowel Diseases*, vol. 15, no. 7, pp. 1090–1100, 2009.

[21] R. Nurieva, X. O. Yang, G. Martinez et al., "Essential autocrine regulation by IL-21 in the generation of inflammatory T cells," *Nature*, vol. 448, no. 7152, pp. 480–483, 2007.

[22] T. Onoda, M. Rahman, H. Nara et al., "Human CD4$^+$ central and effector memory T cells produce IL-21: effect on cytokine-driven proliferation of CD4$^+$ T cell subsets," *International Immunology*, vol. 19, no. 10, pp. 1191–1199, 2007.

[23] F.-L. Yuan, W. Hu, W.-G. Lu et al., "Targeting interleukin-21 in rheumatoid arthritis," *Molecular Biology Reports*, vol. 38, no. 3, pp. 1717–1721, 2011.

[24] F. B. Mercado, R. I. Marshall, A. C. Klestov, and P. M. Bartold, "Relationship between rheumatoid arthritis and periodontitis," *Journal of Periodontology*, vol. 15, pp. 1090–1100, 2001.

[25] A. C. Araujo-Pires, C. F. Francisconi, C. C. Biguetti et al., "Simultaneous analysis of t helper subsets (Th1, Th2, Th9, Th17, Th22, Tfh, Tr1 and Tregs) markers expression in periapical lesions reveals multiple cytokine clusters accountable for lesions activity and inactivity status," *Journal of Applied Oral Science*, vol. 22, no. 4, pp. 336–346, 2014.

[26] Y. Li, C. Messina, M. Bendaoud, D. H. Fine, H. Schreiner, and V. K. Tsiagbe, "Adaptive immune response in osteoclastic bone resorption induced by orally administered *Aggregatibacter actinomycetemcomitans* in a rat model of periodontal disease," *Molecular Oral Microbiology*, vol. 25, no. 4, pp. 275–292, 2010.

[27] Z. M. Wang, J. Zhang, B. S. Pang, L. Q. Zhang, and C. Wang, "Detection of serum interleukin-21 associated with chronic periodontitis," in *Proceedings of the 86th General Session & Exhibition of the IADR*, Toronto, Canada, July 2008.

[28] N. Nizam, O. K. Basoglu, M. S. Tasbakan, A. Nalbantsoy, and N. Buduneli, "Salivary cytokines and the association between obstructive sleep apnea syndrome and periodontal disease," *Journal of Periodontology*, vol. 85, no. 7, pp. e251–e258, 2014.

[29] N. Dutzan, C. Rivas, J. García-Sesnich et al., "Levels of interleukin-21 in patients with untreated chronic periodontitis," *Journal of Periodontology*, vol. 82, no. 10, pp. 1483–1489, 2011.

[30] L. Zhao, Y. Zhou, Y. Xu, Y. Sun, L. Li, and W. Chen, "Effect of non-surgical periodontal therapy on the levels of Th17/Th1/Th2 cytokines and their transcription factors in Chinese chronic periodontitis patients," *Journal of Clinical Periodontology*, vol. 38, no. 6, pp. 509–516, 2011.

[31] N. Dutzan, R. Vernal, J. P. Vaque et al., "Interleukin-21 expression and its association with proinflammatory cytokines in untreated chronic periodontitis subjects," *Journal of Periodontology*, vol. 82, pp. 1483–1489, 2012.

[32] M. H. Napimoga, L. H. A. C. Nunes, A. A. B. Maciel et al., "Possible involvement of IL-21 and IL-10 on salivary IgA levels in chronic periodontitis subjects," *Scandinavian Journal of Immunology*, vol. 74, no. 6, pp. 596–602, 2011.

[33] D. M. Isaza-Guzmán, N. Cardona-Vélez, D. E. Gaviria-Correa, M. C. Martínez-Pabón, M. C. Castaño-Granada, and S. I. Tobón-Arroyave, "Association study between salivary levels of interferon (IFN)-gamma, interleukin (IL)-17, IL-21, and IL-22 with chronic periodontitis," *Archives of Oral Biology*, vol. 60, no. 1, pp. 91–99, 2015.

[34] H. Löe, A. Anerud, H. Boysen, and M. Smith, "The natural history of periodontal disease in man: the rate of periodontal destruction before 40 years of age," *Journal of Periodontology*, vol. 49, no. 12, pp. 607–620, 1978.

[35] F. A. Scannapieco and R. J. Genco, "Association of periodontal infections with atherosclerotic and pulmonary diseases," *Journal of Periodontal Research*, vol. 34, no. 7, pp. 340–345, 1999.

[36] R. Ding, W. Gao, Z. He et al., "Effect of serum interleukin 21 on the development of coronary artery disease," *APMIS*, vol. 122, no. 9, pp. 842–847, 2014.

[37] J. Kim, S. Kang, J. Kim, G. Kwon, and S. Koo, "Elevated levels of T helper 17 cells are associated with disease activity in patients with rheumatoid arthritis," *Annals of Laboratory Medicine*, vol. 33, no. 1, pp. 52–59, 2013.

[38] D. L. Sackett, "Rules of evidence and clinical recommendations on the use of antithrombotic agents," *Chest*, vol. 95, no. 2, pp. 2–4, 1989.

10

Smoking Status Effect on Inflammatory Markers in a Randomized Trial of Current and Former Heavy Smokers

Sami Aldaham,[1] Janet A. Foote,[2] H.-H. Sherry Chow,[3] and Iman A. Hakim[2,3]

[1]*College of Medicine, Al-Imam Mohammad Ibn Saud Islamic University (IMSIU), Riyadh 11432, Saudi Arabia*
[2]*Mel & Enid Zuckerman College of Public Health, University of Arizona, Tucson, AZ 85724, USA*
[3]*Arizona Cancer Center, University of Arizona, Tucson, AZ 85724, USA*

Correspondence should be addressed to Janet A. Foote; jfoote@email.arizona.edu

Academic Editor: Andrew S. Day

Background. The level of systemic inflammation as measured by circulating levels of C-reactive protein (CRP) and interleukin-6 (IL-6) is linked to an increased risk for cardiovascular diseases (CVD) and cancer. *Methods.* We recruited 154 current and former smokers between 40 and 80 years of age with 25 or more pack-years of smoking history to study the relationship between inflammatory markers (CRP and IL-6) and smoking status. *Results.* Our results show that male smokers had significantly higher levels of serum IL-6 compared to male former smokers. We did not find any gender specific differences for smoking and CRP levels but the IL-6 levels were slightly lower in females compared to males. Additionally, our results show that CRP is significantly associated with IL-6 regardless of smoking status. Modelling indicates that the significant predictors of CRP levels were biomarkers of the metabolic syndrome while the significant predictors of IL-6 levels were age and plasma triglycerides among former smokers and the numbers of smoked packs of cigarettes per year among smokers. *Conclusions.* In conclusion, our study showed that CRP levels were not associated with markers of smoking intensity. However, IL-6 levels were significantly associated with smoking especially among current smokers.

1. Introduction

Inflammation is associated with a number of chronic conditions, such as cardiovascular disease and cancer. Reducing inflammation may help prevent or treat these conditions. C-reactive protein (CRP) and interleukin-6 (IL-6) are well-studied proinflammatory cytokines [1, 2]. Inflammation is part of our immune reaction and leads to the release of C-reactive protein (CRP) into the bloodstream [3, 4] and IL-6 is a major factor driving the chronic elevation of CRP [5]. Elevated levels of IL-6 are predictive of future adverse health events in both healthy and clinical populations, even after controlling for both lifestyle and other clinical risk factors [6–9].

Smoking is the major risk factor for lung cancer, the most common cancer worldwide. Cigarette smoking has been associated with increases in CRP and previous investigations have demonstrated that increased CRP levels are a secondary effect of cigarette smoking and reflect tissue injury [10, 11]. The potential significance of IL-6 and CRP has been suggested in the growth and progression of many malignancies [12–14]. Many large-scale epidemiological studies among apparently healthy men and women have found CRP to be an independent and strong predictor of future cardiovascular risk [15–17].

There is great interest in studying the relationship between inflammatory markers and smoking in an attempt to provide explanations for smoking-mediated morbidity and mortality. The current study is unique with the inclusion and comparison of verified former smokers with a similar smoking history (pack-years and years of smoking) to the current smokers. The profile of inflammation markers is expected to differ following smoking cessation. Therefore, we are reporting here the associations of CRP and IL-6 with smoking status among community-dwelling men and women.

2. Methods

Current smokers (CS) and former smokers (FS) between 40 and 80 years of age with 25 pack-years or more of smoking history were recruited to a randomized, double-blind, and placebo controlled chemoprevention trial of green tea and black tea. The study protocol received approval by the University of Arizona Institutional Review Board. Once informed consent had been obtained, each participant completed a set of smoking, dietary, and health assessment questionnaires and was evaluated for health and respiratory history. A blood sample was collected for a comprehensive metabolic panel. Two additional fasting morning blood samples were collected from which plasma, serum, buffy coat, and erythrocytes were isolated and stored at −80°C prior to the sample analysis. Body mass index (BMI) for each participant was calculated as weight divided by height^2 (kg/m^2).

2.1. Human C-Reactive Protein (CRP) Immunoassay and Interleukin-6 (IL-6) Immunoassay in Serum. Aliquots were thawed immediately prior to the analysis. Each immunoassay was completed using a commercially available kit from Quantikine (R & D Systems, Minneapolis, MN, USA). Briefly, specified quantities of the specimen or standard are added to microplates with cells precoated with the CRP antibody or the IL-6 antibody, depending on the assay. The antibodies bind the CRP or IL-6 present in the samples and standards. Any unbound substances are washed away and a monoclonal antibody specific for CRP or a polyclonal antibody specific for IL-6 is added. Again, unbound substances are washed away, substrate solution is added, the plate is incubated, and amplifier solution is added. Color develops in proportion to the amount of CRP or IL-6 present in the well and after stopping the color development in the prescribed time, the wells are measured spectrophotometrically for CRP or IL-6 quantification. Both CRP and IL-6 analyses were completed in duplicate for 154 participants. All data entry and values were checked by additional laboratory personnel for quality control.

2.2. Statistical Analysis. Means and standard errors were calculated for descriptive statistics. Because of value skewness, CRP and IL-6 values were log-transformed. Pearson correlations were calculated to describe the unadjusted relationships between the smoking parameters, inflammatory markers, and other relevant variables. Multivariable linear regression models were created to identify independent predictors of log (CRP) and log (IL-6), using variables that had significant correlations ($p < 0.10$) with these inflammatory markers. A basic model was created for each inflammatory marker that included age, sex, BMI, caloric intake, triglycerides, high-density lipoprotein cholesterol, years of smoking, and cigarette pack-years (cigarettes smoked daily ÷ 20 cigarettes per pack × years of smoking).

3. Results

3.1. Population Characteristics. One hundred and fifty-four current and former smokers (83 women and 71 men) with a mean age of 60.3 ± 0.7 years (mean ± SE) were included in the study. Characteristics of the study population by gender and smoking status are presented in Table 1. There were no significant differences between males and females except in reported pack-years among current smokers. Male smokers reported significantly greater pack-years of smoking compared to females ($p = 0.004$). While the cumulative exposure smoking index of pack-years was not significantly different between current and former smokers among males or females, former smokers reported significantly fewer years of smoking compared to current smokers in both genders ($p \leq 0.001$).

3.2. Inflammation Biomarkers. The differences in the levels of the biomarkers of inflammation and blood lipids between smokers and former smokers are presented in Table 2 for both men and women separately. Male current smokers had significantly higher levels of serum IL-6 compared to male former smokers. Women (smokers and former smokers) had significantly higher levels of HDL compared to men.

Given the fact that there were no significant differences by gender, the correlations among CRP, IL-6, smoking intensity parameters, and other variables are presented by smoking status in Table 3. Log (CRP) and log (IL-6) were significantly correlated regardless of smoking status ($p < 0.001$). Log (CRP) was not associated with any marker of smoking intensity. Among former smokers, log (CRP) was significantly associated with BMI ($r = 0.280$, $p = 0.007$) and low HDL levels ($r = -0.273$, $p = 0.011$). Among smokers, log (IL-6) was significantly associated with age ($r = 0.466$, $p < 0.001$), years of smoking ($r = 0.242$, $p = 0.047$), pack/years ($r = 0.256$, $p = 0.033$), plasma triglycerides ($r = 0.268$, $p = 0.028$), and low HDL levels ($r = -0.029$, $p = 0.017$). The log (CRP) was only associated with age ($r = 0.270$, $p = 0.026$).

3.3. Models of CRP and IL-6 by Smoking Status. The multivariate predictors of inflammatory markers by smoking status are presented in Table 4. The best multivariable model for log (CRP) among former smokers included triglycerides ($p = 0.009$) and the interaction between CRP and IL-6 ($p < 0.001$) and the best multivariable model for log (CRP) among current smokers included HDL ($p = 0.010$), BMI ($p = 0.05$), and the interaction between CRP and IL-6 ($p < 0.001$). The best multivariable model for log (IL-6) among former smokers included triglycerides ($p = 0.002$), age ($p = 0.007$), and the interaction between CRP and IL-6 ($p < 0.001$) and the best multivariable model for log (IL-6) among current smokers included pack/year ($p = 0.005$) and the interaction between CRP and IL-6 ($p < 0.001$).

4. Discussion

In the current study among participants with more than 30 pack-years of smoking exposure, we did not find any significant difference in CRP levels between smokers and former smokers. However, the serum levels of IL-6 were significantly higher among male smokers compared to former smokers ($p = 0.04$). Exposure to cigarette smoke increases oxidative

TABLE 1: Characteristics of the study population by gender and smoking status ($n = 154$).

	Males $n = 71$ mean ± SE	Females $n = 83$ mean ± SE	p value* (males versus females)
Age (years)	60.8 ± 1.0	59.9 ± 1.0	0.54
Former smokers	62.4 ± 1.5	60.9 ± 1.4	0.45
Current smokers	59.5 ± 1.3	59.2 ± 1.4	0.89
p value (former versus current)*	0.14	0.40	
Pack-year	45.6 ± 2.6	40.7 ± 1.9	0.12
Former smokers	41.1 ± 3.4	44.6 ± 3.5	0.49
Current smokers	49.2 ± 3.7	37.7 ± 1.9	0.004
p value (former versus current)*	0.12	0.07	
Years of smoking	34.4 ± 1.1	32.6 ± 1.2	0.28
Former smokers	29.5 ± 1.5	27.6 ± 1.6	0.39
Current smokers	38.4 ± 1.3	36.4 ± 1.5	0.33
p value (former versus current)*	<0.001	0.001	

*χ^2 test.

TABLE 2: Biomarkers of inflammation and lipid profile by gender and smoking status ($n = 154$).

	Males $n = 71$ mean ± SE	Females $n = 83$ mean ± SE	p value (males versus females)
Serum C-reactive protein*	7.4 ± 0.13	7.4 ± 0.11	0.66
Former smokers	7.2 ± 0.20	7.3 ± 0.16	0.58
Current smokers	7.6 ± 0.17	7.4 ± 0.16	0.27
p value (former versus current)	0.10	0.87	
Serum interleukin-6*	0.67 ± 0.10	0.43 ± 0.10	0.09
Former smokers	0.44 ± 0.14	0.33 ± 0.13	0.57
Current smokers	0.86 ± 0.13	0.50 ± 0.14	0.08
p value (former versus current)	0.04	0.40	
Total cholesterol (mg/dL)	193.2 ± 5.1	206.2 ± 4.0	0.04
Former smokers	189.5 ± 6.7	204.6 ± 5.5	0.08
Current smokers	196.1 ± 7.6	207.3 ± 5.7	0.23
p value (former versus current)	0.52	0.74	
High density lipoproteins (mg/dL)	47.0 ± 1.5	61.5 ± 1.6	<0.001
Former smokers	47.1 ± 2.3	59.0 ± 2.7	0.002
Current smokers	47.0 ± 1.9	63.4 ± 1.9	<0.001
p value (former versus current)	0.99	0.17	
Low density lipoproteins (mg/dL)	114.0 ± 4.2	119.7 ± 3.6	0.30
Former smokers	111.8 ± 5.3	118.9 ± 4.6	0.32
Current smokers	116.8 ± 1.9	120.4 ± 5.3	0.67
p value (former versus current)	0.99	0.83	
Total triglycerides (mg/dL)	175.0 ± 18.5	139.5 ± 7.1	0.06
Former smokers	165.4 ± 18.6	142.5 ± 11.2	0.28
Current smokers	182.9 ± 30.3	137.3 ± 9.2	0.12
p value (former versus current)	0.64	0.71	

*Log transformed data for C-reactive protein and interleukin-6.

TABLE 3: Pearson's correlation of CRP* and IL-6* with each parameter by smoking status ($n = 154$).

Variables	CRP		IL-6	
	r	p	r	p
Interleukin-6 (pg/mL)				
Former smoker	0.387	0.000	1.000	
Current smoker	0.589	0.000	1.000	
Age (years)				
Former smoker	0.161	0.140	0.198	0.067
Current smoker	0.270	0.026‡	0.446	0.000‡
Years of smoking				
Former smoker	0.081	0.461	0.202	0.062
Current smoker	0.017	0.889	0.242	0.047‡
Pack/year				
Former smoker	0.136	0.212	0.313	0.003‡
Current smoker	0.028	0.823	0.256	0.033‡
Caloric intake/day				
Former smoker	0.206	0.065	0.014	0.904
Current smoker	0.092	0.474	0.054	0.677
Total fat intake (g/day)				
Former smoker	0.173	0.126	0.007	0.951
Current smoker	0.090	0.488	0.124	0.338
Total cholesterol (mg/dL)				
Former smoker	0.024	0.825	0.024	0.829
Current smoker	0.134	0.275	0.086	0.484
HDL-C (mg/dL)				
Former smoker	−0.273	0.011‡	−0.207	0.056
Current smoker	−0.131	0.287	−0.290	0.017‡
LDL-C (mg/dL)				
Former smoker	0.028	0.799	0.072	0.517
Current smoker	0.182	0.141	0.061	0.623
Total triglycerides (mg/dL)				
Former smoker	0.168	0.123	0.134	0.220
Current smoker	0.196	0.110	0.268	0.028‡
BMI (kg/m^2)				
Former smoker	0.287	0.007‡	0.129	0.236
Current smoker	0.203	0.100	0.130	0.299

CRP: C-reactive protein; HDL-C = high density lipoproteins; LDL-C: low density lipoproteins; BMI: body mass index.
*Log transformed data for CRP (ng/mL) and IL-6 (pg/mL).
‡Significant correlation.

TABLE 4: Stepwise regression analysis for CRP and IL-6 by smoking status.

Subjects	Explanatory variable	β	p	Adjusted R^2
CRP (mg/L)				
Former smokers	Total triglycerides	0.496	0.009	0.455
	CRP ∗ IL-6	<0.001	0.000	
Smokers	HDL-C (mg/dL)	−0.017	0.010	0.369
	BMI (kg/m^2)	0.028	0.052	
	CRP ∗ IL-6	<0.001	0.000	
IL-6 (pg/mL)				
Former smokers	Total triglycerides	0.442	0.002	0.547
	Age	0.027	0.007	
	CRP ∗ IL-6	<0.001	0.000	
Smokers	Pack/year	0.012	0.005	0.436
	CRP ∗ IL-6	<0.001	0.000	

CRP: C-reactive protein; IL-6: interleukin 6; HDL-C: high density lipoprotein; BMI: body mass index, and CRP ∗ IL-6: interaction between CRP and IL-6.
Variables included in the model are gender, age, BMI, total triglycerides, HDL-C, years of smoking, pack/year, caloric intake/day, and interaction between CRP and IL-6.

stress which may lead to vascular inflammation. Because of the possible link between smoking and the initiation of inflammatory pathways, a large number of studies in which serum CRP concentrations have been measured in parallel to smoking status have been published in recent years [2–4, 10, 16]. However, some of these studies provided conflicting results [18]. The complexity of cytokine-mediated inflammation is described in a study showing that although smoking status was associated with a significant elevation in IL-6 levels, the increase in CRP levels observed in smokers was not statistically significant [19]. Another study indicated that mean CRP levels were significantly lower in never-smokers ($p < 0.0001$) compared to current smokers [20]. One study conducted in people of Japanese ethnicity did not find any significant relationship between serum CRP levels and the number of cigarettes smoked per day [4].

The MONICA study from Germany examined gender specific differences for smoking and CRP levels, finding that serum CRP concentrations were significantly higher in male regular smokers than male never-smokers but no significant differences were observed in women [21]. In our study we did not find any gender specific differences for smoking and CRP levels but the IL-6 levels were slightly lower in females compared to males. Also, women had significantly higher levels of HDL compared to men. In addition, our results showed that among smokers, CRP was associated with age while IL-6 was significantly associated with age, smoking variables as measured by years of smoking and number of pack-years, and dyslipidemia as measured by low HDL and high triglycerides levels.

There is strong evidence that IL-6 serum concentration increases with age [22, 23] and it is associated with an increased risk of cardiovascular disease (CVD) mortality, independent of CRP level [24]. Our data showed that the significant predictors of IL-6 levels among former smokers were age and plasma triglycerides. Among smokers, the smoking intensity as measured by the number of smoked packs of cigarettes across the number of years smoked was the main predictor of IL-6 high levels.

Smoking cessation lowers risk for lung and other cancer types along with reducing the risk of coronary heart disease, stroke, and peripheral vascular disease [25]. Inflammation is a key pathological component in these disease processes. Yet in this study among heavy smokers (mean of almost 43 packs per year for 33 years), CRP levels did not differ between former and current smokers. Additionally, former smoker IL-6 levels were significantly lower than the level among current smokers only among the males. These results suggest that CRP levels and IL-6 levels may not be the primary modulators of health improvements following cessation. Alternatively, intense smoking (high frequency over multiple decades) may have more longstanding effects on some types of inflammation. Our CRP results are consistent with results of Asthana et al. among smokers with a similar three-decade history of smoking but with half the pack-years [26].

Numerous studies have now confirmed that CRP levels are elevated in patients with the metabolic syndrome. CRP levels were shown to be strongly associated with BMI, low HDL, triglycerides, and levels of the proinflammatory cytokine, IL-6 [6, 27, 28]. Our results that showed that CRP levels were significantly influenced by HDL, triglycerides, and IL-6 levels support a potential relationship between CRP levels and the metabolic syndrome.

In conclusion, our data supports previous studies that showed that serum CRP is associated with biomarkers of the metabolic syndrome but not with smoking. However, serum IL-6 levels are mainly affected not only by the metabolic syndrome but also by age and smoking status.

Highlights

(i) We conducted a cross-sectional study on a sample of 154 current and former smokers.

(ii) We investigated the relationship between inflammatory biomarkers and smoking status.

(iii) CRP levels were significantly associated with IL-6 levels regardless of smoking status.

(iv) The significant predictors of CRP levels were biomarkers of the metabolic syndrome.

(v) IL-6 levels were significantly associated with smoking especially among current smokers.

Acknowledgment

This work was partially supported by a grant (DOD PR 023104) from the Department of Defense.

References

[1] M. Y. Abeywardena, W. R. Leifert, K. E. Warnes, J. N. Varghese, and R. J. Head, "Cardiovascular biology of interleukin-6," *Current Pharmaceutical Design*, vol. 15, no. 15, pp. 1809–1821, 2009.

[2] V. Pasceri, J. T. Willerson, and E. T. H. Yeh, "Direct proinflammatory effect of C-reactive protein on human endothelial cells," *Circulation*, vol. 102, no. 18, pp. 2165–2168, 2000.

[3] B. G. Nordestgaard and J. Zacho, "Lipids, atherosclerosis and CVD risk: is CRP an innocent bystander?" *Nutrition, Metabolism and Cardiovascular Diseases*, vol. 19, no. 8, pp. 521–524, 2009.

[4] M. Ohsawa, A. Okayama, M. Nakamura et al., "CRP levels are elevated in smokers but unrelated to the number of cigarettes and are decreased by long-term smoking cessation in male smokers," *Preventive Medicine*, vol. 41, no. 2, pp. 651–656, 2005.

[5] R. Roubenoff, T. B. Harris, L. W. Abad, P. W. E. Wilson, G. E. Dallal, and C. A. Dinarello, "Monocyte cytokine production in an elderly population: effect of age and inflammation," *Journals of Gerontology—Series A Biological Sciences and Medical Sciences*, vol. 53, no. 1, pp. M20–M26, 1998.

[6] S. Cheng, A. Lyass, J. M. Massaro, G. T. O'Connor, J. F. Keaney Jr., and R. S. Vasan, "Exhaled carbon monoxide and risk of metabolic syndrome and cardiovascular disease in the community," *Circulation*, vol. 122, no. 15, pp. 1470–1477, 2010.

[7] W. B. Ershler and E. T. Keller, "Age-associated increased interleukin-6 gene expression, late-life diseases, and frailty," *Annual Review of Medicine*, vol. 51, pp. 245–270, 2000.

[8] J. A. Nettleton, L. M. Steffen, E. J. Mayer-Davis et al., "Dietary patterns are associated with biochemical markers of inflammation and endothelial activation in the Multi-Ethnic Study of Atherosclerosis (MESA)," *American Journal of Clinical Nutrition*, vol. 83, no. 6, pp. 1369–1379, 2006.

[9] P. M. Ridker, N. Rifai, M. J. Stampfer, and C. H. Hennekens, "Plasma concentration of interleukin-6 and the risk of future myocardial infarction among apparently healthy men," *Circulation*, vol. 101, no. 15, pp. 1767–1772, 2000.

[10] J. Danesh, R. Collins, P. Appleby, and R. Peto, "Association of fibrinogen, C-reactive protein, albumin, or leukocyte count with coronary heart disease: meta-analyses of prospective studies," *Journal of the American Medical Association*, vol. 279, no. 18, pp. 1477–1482, 1998.

[11] M. Miller, M. Zhan, and S. Havas, "High attributable risk of elevated C-reactive protein level to conventional coronary heart disease risk factors: the third National Health and Nutrition Examination Survey," *Archives of Internal Medicine*, vol. 165, no. 18, pp. 2063–2068, 2005.

[12] M. Groblewska, B. Mroczko, U. Wereszczyńska-Siemiątkowska et al., "Serum interleukin 6 (IL-6) and C-reactive protein (CRP) levels in colorectal adenoma and cancer patients," *Clinical Chemistry and Laboratory Medicine*, vol. 46, no. 10, pp. 1423–1428, 2008.

[13] M. Hara, Y. Matsuzaki, T. Shimuzu et al., "Preoperative serum C-reactive protein level in non-small cell lung cancer," *Anticancer Research*, vol. 27, no. 4, pp. 3001–3004, 2008.

[14] D.-K. Kim, S. Y. Oh, H.-C. Kwon et al., "Clinical significances of preoperative serum interleukin-6 and C-reactive protein level in operable gastric cancer," *BMC Cancer*, vol. 9, article 155, 2009.

[15] J. Danesh, P. Whincup, M. Walker et al., "Low grade inflammation and coronary heart disease: prospective study and updated meta-analyses," *British Medical Journal*, vol. 321, no. 7255, pp. 199–204, 2000.

[16] M. A. Mendall, D. P. Strachan, B. K. Butland et al., "C-reactive protein: relation to total mortality, cardiovascular mortality and cardiovascular risk factors in men," *European Heart Journal*, vol. 21, no. 19, pp. 1584–1590, 2000.

[17] M. Roivainen, M. Viik-Kajander, T. Palosuo et al., "Infections, inflammation, and the risk of coronary heart disease," *Circulation*, vol. 101, no. 3, pp. 252–257, 2000.

[18] D. G. Yanbaeva, M. A. Dentener, E. C. Creutzberg, G. Wesseling, and E. F. M. Wouters, "Systemic effects of smoking," *Chest*, vol. 131, no. 5, pp. 1557–1566, 2007.

[19] J. Helmersson, A. Larsson, B. Vessby, and S. Basu, "Active smoking and a history of smoking are associated with enhanced prostaglandin F2α, interleukin-6 and F2-isoprostane formation in elderly men," *Atherosclerosis*, vol. 181, no. 1, pp. 201–207, 2005.

[20] S. G. Wannamethee, G. D. O. Lowe, A. G. Shaper, A. Rumley, L. Lennon, and P. H. Whincup, "Associations between cigarette smoking, pipe/cigar smoking, and smoking cessation, and haemostatic and inflammatory markers for cardiovascular disease," *European Heart Journal*, vol. 26, no. 17, pp. 1765–1773, 2005.

[21] M. Fröhlich, M. Sund, H. Löwel, A. Imhof, A. Hoffmeister, and W. Koenig, "Independent association of various smoking characteristics with markers of systemic inflammation in men: results from a representative sample of the general population (MONICA Augsburg survey 1994/95)," *European Heart Journal*, vol. 24, no. 14, pp. 1365–1372, 2003.

[22] L. Ferrucci, A. Corsi, F. Lauretani et al., "The origins of age-related proinflammatory state," *Blood*, vol. 105, no. 6, pp. 2294–2299, 2005.

[23] T. B. Harris, L. Ferrucci, R. P. Tracy et al., "Associations of elevated interleukin-6 and C-reactive protein levels with mortality in the elderly," *American Journal of Medicine*, vol. 106, no. 5, pp. 506–512, 1999.

[24] J. K. Lee, R. Bettencourt, D. Brenner, T.-A. Le, E. Barrett-Connor, and R. Loomba, "Association between serum interleukin-6 concentrations and mortality in older adults: the Rancho Bernardo Study," *PLoS ONE*, vol. 7, no. 4, Article ID e34218, 2012.

[25] US Department of Health and Human Services, *How Tobacco Smoke Causes Disease: The Biology and Behavioral Basis for Smoking-Attributable Disease: A Report of the Surgeon General*, US Department of Health and Human Services, Centers for Disease Control and Prevention, National Center for Chronic Disease Prevention and Health Promotion, Office on Smoking and Health, Atlanta, Ga, USA, 2010.

[26] A. Asthana, H. M. Johnson, M. E. Piper, M. C. Fiore, T. B. Baker, and J. H. Stein, "Effects of smoking intensity and cessation on inflammatory markers in a large cohort of active smokers," *American Heart Journal*, vol. 160, no. 3, pp. 458–463, 2010.

[27] A. Festa, R. D'Agostino Jr., G. Howard, L. Mykkänen, R. P. Tracy, and S. M. Haffner, "Chronic subclinical inflammation as part of the insulin resistance syndrome: the insulin resistance atherosclerosis study (IRAS)," *Circulation*, vol. 102, no. 1, pp. 42–47, 2000.

[28] P. M. Ridker, C. H. Hennekens, J. E. Buring, and N. Rifai, "C-reactive protein and other markers of inflammation in the prediction of cardiovascular disease in women," *The New England Journal of Medicine*, vol. 342, no. 12, pp. 836–843, 2000.

11

Anti-Inflammatory Effect of *Emblica officinalis* in Rodent Models of Acute and Chronic Inflammation: Involvement of Possible Mechanisms

Mahaveer Golechha,[1,2] Vikas Sarangal,[1] Shreesh Ojha,[3] Jagriti Bhatia,[1] and Dharmveer S. Arya[1]

[1] *Department of Pharmacology, All India Institute of Medical Sciences, New Delhi 110029, India*
[2] *Public Health Foundation of India, New Delhi 110070, India*
[3] *Department of Pharmacology and Therapeutics, Faculty of Medicine & Health Sciences, UAE University, P.O. Box 17666, Al Ain, UAE*

Correspondence should be addressed to Dharmveer S. Arya; dsarya16@hotmail.com

Academic Editor: Andrew S. Day

Emblica officinalis, commonly known as amla in Ayurveda, is unarguably the most important medicinal plant for prevention and treatment of various ailments. The present study investigated the anti-inflammatory activity of hydroalcoholic extract of *Emblica officinalis* (HAEEO). Acute inflammation in rats was induced by the subplantar injection of carrageenan, histamine, serotonin, and prostaglandin E_2 and chronic inflammation was induced by the cotton pellet granuloma. Intraperitoneal (i.p.) administration of HAEEO at all the tested doses (300, 500, and 700 mg/kg) significantly ($P < 0.001$) inhibited rat paw edema against all phlogistic agents and also reduced granuloma formation. However, at the dose of 700 mg/kg, HAEEO exhibited maximum anti-inflammatory activity in all experimental models, and the effects were comparable to that of the standard anti-inflammatory drugs. Additionally, in paw tissue the antioxidant activity of HAEEO was also measured and it was found that HAEEO significantly ($P < 0.001$) increased glutathione, superoxide dismutase, and catalase activity and subsequently reduced lipid peroxidation evidenced by reduced malondialdehyde. Taken all together, the results indicated that HAEEO possessed potent anti-inflammatory activity and it may hold therapeutic promise in the management of acute and chronic inflammatory conditions.

1. Introduction

Inflammation plays a major role in rheumatoid arthritis and osteoarthritis [1]. In clinics, the nonsteroidal anti-inflammatory drugs (NSAIDs) are commonly prescribed for pain relief in arthritic conditions. However, their continual use is associated with serious adverse effects like gastric mucosal damage, occult blood loss and elevation of serum hepatic transaminases, salt and water retention, and also exacerbation of asthma [2]. In order to circumvent these adverse effects associated with conventional NSAIDs, novel selective COX-2 inhibitors are in progress. However, the development of serious adverse reactions, like cardiovascular events with rofecoxib and Stevens-Johnson syndrome with valdecoxib, has compelled their withdrawal from use [3]. Additionally, the clinical uses of the remaining drugs in this class have been prescribed with caution and have consequently decreased [4].

In milieu of these observations patients as well as health care providers prefer to use alternative therapeutic agents as they are considered to be safe and effective in alleviating inflammation associated with arthritis. Several Indian medicinal plants were reported as an important source of new chemical moieties with potential therapeutic effects [5]. The studies on plants with substantiated folkloric use as anti-inflammatory agents are viewed as a productive and logical research strategy in the search for new anti-inflammatory drugs

Emblica officinalis Gaertn. (*Euphorbiaceae*) commonly known as amla grow in the tropical areas of South-East

Asia. The fruit of the plant is one of the most important medicinal ingredients used in Ayurveda, Siddha, Unani, Arabic, Tibetan, and various other folk systems for the management of myriad chronic ailments [6]. Experimental studies have shown potent antioxidant, analgesic, antipyretic, adaptogenic, immunomodulatory, and antiulcerogenic activities of the fruit of *Emblica officinalis* [6–8].

The fruits are reported to contain thermostable vitamin C, minerals, amino acids, tannins, flavonoids, and other important phytochemicals which are believed to possess diverse pharmacological and biological effects [9]. Earlier studies have shown that the leaf extract possesses anti-inflammatory activities in the carrageenan and dextran-induced rat hind paw edema [10]. However, studies on the fruit extract which is the most used part of amla have never been performed. Therefore, the present study was carried out to evaluate the anti-inflammatory activity of the hydroalcoholic extract of the fruit of *Emblica officinalis* (HAEEO) in both acute and chronic models of inflammation in rats. Further, in order to understand the possible underlying mechanism, the effect of extract on the oxidative stress produced by carrageenan was also studied in the rat paw.

2. Methodology

2.1. Plant Extract. The standardized lyophilized hydroalcoholic extract of the fruit of *Emblica officinalis* (HAEEO) was procured from Sanat Products Limited, India (A WHO-GMP and ISO 9001 Accredited Herbal Extract Manufacturer Company). The voucher specimen of lyophilized extract of the fruits of *Emblica officinalis* (number EO 0114) was deposited at Department of Pharmacology, All India Institute of Medical Sciences, New Delhi, India. The phytochemical analysis was done by using HPLC (Waters, Milford Massachusetts, USA). The extract obtained was of the highest purity with 28.26% w/w of hydrolysable tannins emblicanin A and emblicanin B on dried weight basis.

2.2. Drugs and Chemicals. Carrageenan, histamine, 5-hydroxytryptamine (serotonin), chlorpheniramine, cyproheptadine, prostaglandin E_2 (PGE_2), and bovine serum albumin were purchased from Sigma Chemicals, St. Louis, MO, USA. Indomethacin was procured from Cipla, India. All other chemicals and reagents were of analytical grade.

2.3. Experimental Animals. All experimental procedures described were reviewed and approved by the Institutional Animal Ethics Committee and care of animals was taken as per guidelines of CPCSEA, Ministry of Environment and Forest, Government of India. Wistar albino rats of either sex weighing 180–200 g were used for the study. The animals were procured from the central animal facility in All India Institute of Medical Sciences, New Delhi. The rats were group-housed in polypropylene cages with no more than four animals per cage. They were maintained under standard laboratory conditions with natural dark-light cycle and were allowed free access to standard pellet diet (Golden Feeds, India) and tap water *ad libitum*. All the experiments were carried out using five groups, each containing 6 animals (Groups I–V) except carrageenan-induced paw edema where Groups I–VI were used.

2.4. Determination of Anti-Inflammatory Activity of HAEEO on Acute Inflammation

2.4.1. Carrageenan-Induced Hind Paw Edema in Rats. Acute inflammation was produced by injecting 0.1 mL of carrageenan (1% in saline) locally into the plantar aponeurosis of the right hind paw of the rats [11, 12]. Group I served as normal control, where no inflammation was induced. This group was used for evaluation of biochemical parameters. Groups II and III received vehicle (saline 1 mL/kg, i.p.) and standard drug indomethacin (10 mg/kg, p.o.), respectively, and served as vehicle and positive controls. HAEEO (300, 500, and 700 mg/kg, i.p.) was administered to Groups IV, V, and VI, respectively. The HAEEO or vehicle was administered 30 min prior to injection of carrageenan and indomethacin was orally administered 1 h prior to the injection of carrageenan. The pedal volume up to the ankle joint was measured using a digital plethysmometer (Ugo Basile, 7140 Comerio, Varese, Italy) at 0 h (just before carrageenan injection) and then at 3 h. The different timing was chosen because of the different route of drug administration. The % inhibition of edema volume between treated and control groups was calculated as follows: % Inhibition = $V_c - V_t \times 100/V_c$, where V_c and V_t represent the mean increase in paw volume in control and treated groups, respectively.

2.4.2. Autacoids-Induced Hind Paw Edema in Rats. This experiment was conducted according to the method described by Singh and Pandey [13]. The autacoids serotonin (1 mg/mL), histamine (1 mg/mL), and prostaglandin E_2 (1 μg/mL) were employed as phlogistic agents. The effect of HAEEO (300, 500, and 700 mg/kg, i.p.) and vehicle was tested individually against each autacoid. The anti-inflammatory effect of HAEEO was compared with that of standard drugs against each autacoid: phenylbutazone (PBZ, 100 mg/kg, p.o.) against prostaglandin E_2, chlorpheniramine (CPM, 3 mg/kg, p.o.) against histamine, and cyproheptadine (CPH, 3 mg/kg, p.o.) against serotonin. Right hind paw edema was induced by the subplantar injection of 0.1 mL of different phlogistic agents in the respective groups. HAEEO was administered i.p. 30 min prior to inflammatory insult and standard reference drugs were administered p.o. 1 h prior to the inflammatory insult. The pedal volume was measured just before (0 h) and then at 3 h after the phlogistic challenge.

2.5. Determination of Anti-Inflammatory Activity of HAEEO on Chronic Inflammation

2.5.1. Cotton Pellet-Induced Granuloma in Rats. The cotton pellet-induced granuloma in rats was studied according to the method of D'Arcy et al. [14]. The animals were divided into five groups with six animals in each group. The rats were anaesthetized and sterile cotton pellets weighing 10 ± 1 mg were implanted subcutaneously into both sides of the groin

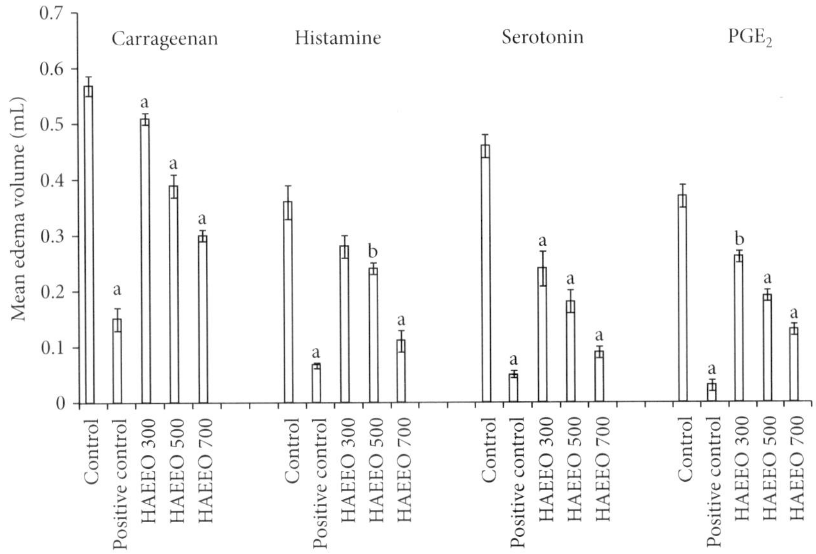

FIGURE 1: Effect of HAEEO on carrageenan- and autacoids-induced hind paw edema in rats. Each value represents the mean ± S.E.M. ($n = 6$). $^{a}P < 0.001$ and $^{b}P < 0.01$ compared to control. Positive control carrageenan (indomethacin 10 mg/kg), histamine (chlorpheniramine 3 mg/kg), serotonin (cyproheptadine 3 mg/kg), and PGE_2 (phenylbutazone 100 mg/kg). HAEEO: hydroalcoholic extract of *Emblica officinalis*.

region of each rat. Group I served as control and received the vehicle. HAEEO in the doses of 300, 500, and 700 mg/kg, i.p. was administered to animals in groups II, III, and IV for seven consecutive days from the day of cotton pellet implantation. Group V received indomethacin (10 mg/kg, p.o.) for the same period. On day 8, the animals were anaesthetized and the pellets together with the attached granuloma tissue were carefully removed and freed from extraneous tissues. The wet pellets were weighed and then dried in an oven at 60°C for 24 h to a constant weight; after that the dried pellets were weighed again. Increment in the dry weight of the pellets was taken as a measure of granuloma formation.

2.6. Determination of Levels of Oxidative Stress Parameters. The biochemical markers of oxidative stress were determined in the carrageenan-induced rat paw edema model. Animals were euthanized 3 h after measurement of paw volume and the inflamed paw tissue was removed and processed for the estimation of oxidative stress. Paw tissue samples were thawed and homogenized with 10 times (w/v) ice-cold 0.1 M phosphate buffer (pH 7.4). Aliquots of homogenates from paw tissue were used to determine the malondialdehyde (MDA) [15] and glutathione [16]. The remaining homogenates were centrifuged at 7000 rpm for 30 min at 4°C temperature and the supernatant was used for estimation of superoxide dismutase (SOD) [17], catalase [18], and protein [19].

2.7. Statistical Analysis. Data were expressed as mean ± S.E.M. Statistical differences between the treatment and the respective control groups were evaluated by one-way ANOVA followed by Tukey-Kramer post hoc test. $P < 0.05$ was considered to be statistically significant.

3. Results

3.1. Carrageenan-Induced Hind Paw Edema in Rats. The mean increase in paw edema volume was 1.0 ± 0.02 mL in the vehicle-treated control rats. All the three doses of HAEEO (300, 500, and 700 mg/kg, i.p.) produced a dose-dependent significant ($P < 0.001$) reduction in the mean paw edema volume (Figure 1). The percentage inhibition in paw edema volume as compared to the vehicle treated group was 48.9, 60.2, and 70.0% for HAEEO, respectively. The standard drug, indomethacin (10 mg/kg, p.o.), exhibited maximum anti-inflammatory activity with 84.27% inhibition.

3.2. Effect of HAEEO on Changes in Tissue Levels of MDA, GSH, SOD, and Catalase. Carrageenan injection into the subplantar tissue of the rat paw decreased the tissue GSH, catalase, and SOD levels (Table 1). Both HAEEO and indomethacin produced a significant increase in the endogenous antioxidants in a dose dependent manner to maintain oxidative homeostasis. Carrageenan injection produced significant lipid peroxidation, as evidenced by a marked increase in the levels of MDA. Both HAEEO and indomethacin produced a significant decrease in the levels of MDA. HAEEO at 700 mg/kg dose most effectively stabilized the oxidative stress parameters.

3.3. Autacoid-Induced Hind Paw Edema in Rats. A dose-dependent effect of HAEEO on hind paw edema was observed. The 700 mg/kg dose of HAEEO was the most effective (Figure 1). It significantly ($P < 0.001$) inhibited hind paw edema induced by histamine (68.47%), serotonin (79.26%), and PGE_2 (64.00%). Phenylbutazone (100 mg/kg, p.o.), chlorpheniramine (3 mg/kg, p.o.), and cyproheptadine

TABLE 1: Effect of HAEEO on oxidative stress parameters in carrageenan-induced paw edema in rats.

Treatment	GSH (μg g^{-1} tissue)	MDA (nmol g^{-1} tissue)	SOD (U mg^{-1} protein)	Catalase (U mg^{-1} protein)
Normal control	32.91 ± 2.13	27.14 ± 2.96	40.54 ± 2.23	57.19 ± 2.48
Carrageenan control (vehicle treated)	13.33 ± 1.39^a	88.45 ± 4.79^a	15.19 ± 1.21^a	14.48 ± 0.75^a
Indomethacin (10 mg kg^{-1})	26.66 ± 1.66^b	28.54 ± 6.85^b	31.96 ± 1.08^b	49.30 ± 1.86^b
HAEEO (300 mg kg^{-1})	19.16 ± 1.53	63.18 ± 4.51^d	21.18 ± 1.80	27.44 ± 1.66^b
HAEEO (500 mg kg^{-1})	22.29 ± 2.80^d	49.14 ± 5.83^b	24.87 ± 0.98^d	36.1 ± 0.83^b
HAEEO (700 mg kg^{-1})	26.25 ± 2.18^c	35.10 ± 2.78^b	29 ± 1.66^b	41.82 ± 1.41^b

Values given are mean ± S.E.M. ($n = 6$). $^aP < 0.001$ compared to normal control and $^bP < 0.001$, $^cP < 0.01$, and $^dP < 0.05$ compared to carrageenan control. HAEEO: hydroalcoholic extract of *Emblica officinalis*; GSH: glutathione; MDA: malondialdehyde; SOD: superoxide dismutase.

TABLE 2: Effect of HAEEO on cotton pellet-induced granuloma in rats.

Group	Weight of cotton pellet granuloma (mg)	Protection percentage
Control (vehicle treated)	53.81 ± 1.94	—
Positive control (indomethacin 10 mg kg^{-1})	18.96 ± 2.18^a	64.76
HAEEO (300 mg kg^{-1})	35.23 ± 1.48^a	34.52
HAEEO (500 mg kg^{-1})	30.30 ± 0.94^a	43.69
HAEEO (700 mg kg^{-1})	25.63 ± 1.29^a	52.36

Each value represents the mean ± S.E.M. ($n = 6$). $^aP < 0.001$ compared to control. HAEEO: hydroalcoholic extract of *Emblica officinalis*.

(3 mg/kg, p.o.) also significantly ($P < 0.001$) inhibited hind paw edema induced by PGE_2 (92.00%), histamine (82.06%), and serotonin (89.56%), respectively (Figure 1).

3.4. Cotton Pellet-Induced Granuloma. The study of HAEEO on proliferative phase of inflammation indicated that HAEEO (300, 500, and 700 mg/kg, i.p.) significantly ($P < 0.001$) and dose-dependently reduced the granuloma formation (Table 2). Indomethacin (10 mg/kg, p.o.) exhibited significant ($P < 0.001$) and maximum inhibition on granuloma formation.

4. Discussion and Conclusion

In the present study, it was observed that *Emblica officinalis* possessed potent anti-inflammatory activity both in acute and chronic rat models of inflammation. Inflammation is part of the host defense system and is triggered by a variety of noxious stimuli. It involves a complex interplay between cell-cell, cell-mediator, and tissue interactions [20]. Carrageenan-induced rat paw edema model is a well-established model for evaluating anti-inflammatory drugs [21]. The edema and inflammation induced by carrageenan are a biphasic event. In the initial 1 h after carrageenan administration, the edema and inflammation are mediated by histamine and serotonin. Later, the increased vascular permeability is maintained by the release of kinins up to about 2.30 h. Thereafter from 2.30 h to 6 h, inflammation is mediated by prostaglandins and is also associated with migration of leucocytes into the inflamed site [22].

Carrageenan-induced paw edema model in rats is known to be sensitive to cyclooxygenase (COX) inhibitors and has been used to investigate the effect of nonsteroidal anti-inflammatory agents [23]. The result of the present study indicated that HAEEO afforded protection against the carrageenan-induced acute inflammation in dose dependent manner. HAEEO at a dose of 700 mg/kg exhibited significant anti-inflammatory activity with 70.0% inhibition of paw edema and was comparable to the indomethacin group. In autacoid-induced models of inflammations (against serotonin, histamine, and PGE_2), HAEEO produced significant inhibitory activity. The present study exhibited HAEEO's anti-inflammatory action by means of inhibiting the synthesis, release, or action of inflammatory mediators like histamine, serotonin, and prostaglandins that are involved in inflammation. In earlier study on the anti-inflammatory activity of leaf extracts of *Emblica officinalis* in carrageenan- and dextran-induced rat paw edema models, it was reported that the extracts did not inhibit the synthesis of the lipid mediators LTB_4, TXB_2, or PAF [24]. Therefore, it is quite possible that a composite effect may have been responsible for the observed protection against autacoids-induced inflammation.

The role of excess generation of nitric oxide (NO) in inflammatory response is well studied. Inflammation or tissue damage leads to induction of iNOS (inducible nitric oxide synthase); consequently large amounts of NO are generated at the site of inflammation [25]. NO reacts with superoxide anion to form peroxynitrite, an oxidizing molecule capable of eliciting lipid peroxidation. In lipid peroxidation there is oxidative deterioration of polyunsaturated lipids to form radical intermediates that causes cellular damage [26]. MDA is a major end product of this reaction and an index of lipid peroxidation that is measurable by estimating as thiobarbituric acid reactive substance (TBARS) [27]. The present study showed that both HAEEO (500 and 700 mg/kg) and indomethacin (10 mg/kg) decreased the levels of MDA.

The infiltrating inflammatory cells also generate reactive oxygen species (ROS) and free radicals. The most common

ROS include the superoxide anion, hydroxyl radical, singlet oxygen, and hydrogen peroxide. The enzyme superoxide dismutase catalyzes the dismutation of superoxide into oxygen and hydrogen peroxide. The activity of SOD reduces during severe inflammation as well as in the presence of oxidative stress [28]. The large quantities of hydrogen peroxide generated are then taken care of by catalase and glutathione peroxidase (GPx) to water. Excessive production of lipid hydroperoxide may also lead to reduced activity of GPx in inflammatory conditions [29]. Besides the enzymatic antioxidants, the level of glutathione, a nonenzymatic reducing agent that traps free radicals and prevents oxidative damage, is also diminished in inflammatory conditions [30]. Both HAEEO (700 mg/kg) and indomethacin (10 mg/kg) maintained the oxidative homeostasis, and the levels of reduced glutathione and activities of catalase and SOD were comparable to the control animals.

Experimental studies have shown the potent antioxidant property of the fruit of *Emblica officinalis* [31]. Various phytochemical constituents of the plant such as emblicanins A and B, gallic acid, and ellagic acids have been identified as powerful free radical scavengers [9]. Moreover, other phytochemicals with NO scavenging properties like Geraniin, Corilagin, and Furosin have been reported in the *Emblica officinalis* fruit extract [32]. Recently, it has also been reported that the superoxide scavenging properties of *Emblica officinalis* extract approximate those of L-ascorbic acid, a well-established antioxidant [33].

In order to assess the efficacy of HAEEO against chronic inflammation, the cotton pellet granuloma model in rats was employed. HAEEO at all doses tested significantly ($P < 0.001$) reduced the granuloma formation. The maximum effect was observed at the dose of 700 mg/kg with 52.36% inhibition in granuloma formation as compared to the control group. Although the exact mechanism of anti-inflammatory activity of HAEEO on proliferative phase of inflammation in this model is not known, it may be hypothesized that both the antioxidant and the immunomodulatory properties of the plant may have been responsible for the protective action of the extract. *Emblica officinalis* extract has been reported to inhibit NF-κB activation, a key transcription factor involved in chronic inflammatory response and ageing [34]. The inhibition of NF-κB leads to reduction in the iNOS and COX-2 enzyme levels.

The main adverse effect of nonsteroidal anti-inflammatory drugs is their ability to produce gastric lesions [35]. Furthermore, Sairam et al. [36] demonstrated the ulcer protective potential of *Emblica officinalis* in different acute gastric ulcer models in rats induced by aspirin, ethanol, cold restraint stress, and pyloric ligation and healing effect in chronic gastric ulcers induced by acetic acid in rats. The antiulcerogenic activity of *Emblica officinalis* is definitely complementary to the good anti-inflammatory and antioxidant activity observed in the present study. Further, it has been shown that *Emblica officinalis* was well tolerated in mice even at the dose of 2.5 g/kg [37].

In conclusion, the present study clearly demonstrated that HAEEO possessed potent anti-inflammatory activity and also scientifically validated the traditional use of this plant for treating inflammatory disorders in the folk medicine. The advantages of HAEEO, namely, better and safer anti-inflammatory profile with potent antiulcerogenic activity, deserve further studies to establish the therapeutic value and elucidate the mechanism of action in the treatment of different inflammatory diseases.

References

[1] K. D. Moudgil and B. M. Berman, "Traditional Chinese medicine: potential for clinical treatment of rheumatoid arthritis," *Expert Review of Clinical Immunology*, vol. 10, no. 7, pp. 819–822, 2014.

[2] Z. Varga, M. Kriška, V. Kristová, and M. Petrová, "Analysis of non-steroidal anti-inflammatory drug use in hospitalized patients and perception of their risk," *Interdisciplinary Toxicology*, vol. 6, no. 3, pp. 141–144, 2013.

[3] E. Z. Dajani and K. Islam, "Cardiovascular and gastrointestinal toxicity of selective cyclo-oxygenase-2 inhibitors in man," *Journal of Physiology and Pharmacology*, vol. 59, no. 2, pp. 117–133, 2008.

[4] T. Santiago and J. A. P. da Silva, "Safety of low- to medium-dose glucocorticoid treatment in rheumatoid arthritis: myths and reality over the years," *Annals of the New York Academy of Sciences*, pp. 41–49, 2014.

[5] Galib, B. Patgiri, and P. Prajapati, "Pharmacological attributes of Indian medicinal plants with special reference to their anti-inflammatory activity," *Ancient Science of Life*, vol. 28, no. 3, pp. 36–39, 2009.

[6] K. R. Thilakchand, R. T. Mathai, P. Simon, R. T. Ravi, M. P. Baliga-Rao, and M. S. Baliga, "Hepatoprotective properties of the Indian gooseberry (*Emblica officinalis* Gaertn): a review," *Food & Function*, vol. 4, no. 10, pp. 1431–1441, 2013.

[7] M. S. Baliga and J. J. Dsouza, "Amla (*Emblica officinalis* Gaertn), a wonder berry in the treatment and prevention of cancer," *European Journal of Cancer Prevention*, vol. 20, no. 3, pp. 225–239, 2011.

[8] M. S. Baliga, S. Meera, B. Mathai, M. P. Rai, V. Pawar, and P. L. Palatty, "Scientific validation of the ethnomedicinal properties of the Ayurvedic drug Triphala: a review," *Chinese Journal of Integrative Medicine*, vol. 18, no. 12, pp. 946–954, 2012.

[9] M. J. Feeney, "Fruits and the prevention of lifestyle-related diseases," *Clinical and Experimental Pharmacology and Physiology*, vol. 31, supplement 2, pp. S11–S13, 2004.

[10] M. Z. Asmawi, H. Kankaanranta, E. Moilanen, and H. Vapaatalo, "Anti-inflammatory activities of *Emblica officinalis* Gaertn leaf extracts," *Journal of Pharmacy and Pharmacology*, vol. 45, no. 6, pp. 581–584, 1993.

[11] G. Amresh, G. D. Reddy, C. V. Rao, and P. N. Singh, "Evaluation of anti-inflammatory activity of *Cissampelos pareira* root in rats," *Journal of Ethnopharmacology*, vol. 110, no. 3, pp. 526–531, 2007.

[12] C. A. Winter, E. A. Risley, and G. W. Nuss, "Carrageenin-induced edema in hind paw of the rat as an assay for anti-iflammatory drugs," *Proceedings of the Society for Experimental Biology and Medicine*, vol. 111, pp. 544–547, 1962.

[13] R. K. Singh and B. L. Pandey, "Anti-inflammatory activity of seed extracts of *Pongamia pinnata* in rat," *Indian Journal of Physiology and Pharmacology*, vol. 40, no. 4, pp. 355–358, 1996.

[14] P. F. D'Arcy, E. M. Howard, P. W. Muggleton, and S. B. Townsend, "The anti-inflammatory action of griseofulvin in experimental

animals," *Journal of Pharmacology and Pharmacotherapeutics*, vol. 12, no. 1, pp. 659–565, 1960.

[15] H. Ohkawa, N. Ohishi, and K. Yagi, "Assay for lipid peroxides in animal tissues by thiobarbituric acid reaction," *Analytical Biochemistry*, vol. 95, no. 2, pp. 351–358, 1979.

[16] G. L. Ellman, "Tissue sulfhydryl groups," *Archives of Biochemistry and Biophysics*, vol. 82, no. 1, pp. 70–77, 1959.

[17] S. Marklund and G. Marklund, "Involvement of the superoxide anion radical in the autoxidation of pyrogallol and a convenient assay for superoxide dismutase," *European Journal of Biochemistry*, vol. 47, no. 3, pp. 469–474, 1974.

[18] H. Aebi, "[13] Catalase *in vitro*," *Methods in Enzymology*, vol. 105, pp. 121–126, 1984.

[19] M. M. Bradford, "A rapid and sensitive method for the quantitation of microgram quantities of protein utilizing the principle of protein dye binding," *Analytical Biochemistry*, vol. 72, no. 1-2, pp. 248–254, 1976.

[20] A. Geremia, P. Biancheri, P. Allan, G. R. Corazza, and A. di Sabatino, "Innate and adaptive immunity in inflammatory bowel disease," *Autoimmunity Reviews*, vol. 13, no. 1, pp. 3–10, 2014.

[21] C. J. Morris, "Carrageenan-induced paw edema in the rat and mouse," *Methods in Molecular Biology*, vol. 225, pp. 115–121, 2003.

[22] R. F. Queiroz, A. K. Jordão, A. C. Cunha et al., "Nitroxides attenuate carrageenan-induced inflammation in rat paws by reducing neutrophil infiltration and the resulting myeloperoxidase-mediated damage," *Free Radical Biology and Medicine*, vol. 53, no. 10, pp. 1942–1953, 2012.

[23] S. Bansal, M. Bala, S. K. Suthar et al., "Design and synthesis of novel 2-phenyl-5-(1,3-diphenyl-1H-pyrazol-4-yl)-1,3,4-oxadiazoles as selective COX-2 inhibitors with potent anti-inflammatory activity," *European Journal of Medicinal Chemistry*, vol. 80C, pp. 167–174, 2014.

[24] A. Ihantola-Vormisto, J. Summanen, H. Kankaanranta, H. Vuorela, Z. M. Asmawi, and E. Moilanen, "Anti-inflammatory activity of extracts from leaves of *Phyllanthus emblica*," *Planta Medica*, vol. 63, no. 6, pp. 518–524, 1997.

[25] C. Ziskoven, M. Jäger, J. Kircher et al., "Physiology and pathophysiology of nitrosative and oxidative stress in osteoarthritic joint destruction," *Canadian Journal of Physiology and Pharmacology*, vol. 89, no. 7, pp. 455–466, 2011.

[26] S. Saeidnia and M. Abdollahi, "Toxicological and pharmacological concerns on oxidative stress and related diseases," *Toxicology and Applied Pharmacology*, vol. 273, no. 3, pp. 442–455, 2013.

[27] E. Ho, K. K. Galougahi, C.-C. Liu, R. Bhindi, and G. A. Figtree, "Biological markers of oxidative stress: applications to cardiovascular research and practice," *Redox Biology*, vol. 1, no. 1, pp. 483–491, 2013.

[28] G.-J. Huang, S. S. Huang, and J.-S. Deng, "Anti-inflammatory activities of inotilone from *Phellinus linteus* through the inhibition of MMP-9, NF-κB, and MAPK activation *in vitro* and *in vivo*," *PLoS ONE*, vol. 7, no. 5, Article ID e35922, 2012.

[29] S. Mohsin, G. M. Kurup, and R. Mahadevan, "Effect of ascophyllan from brown algae *Padina tetrastromatica* on inflammation and oxidative stress in carrageenan-induced rats," *Inflammation*, vol. 36, no. 6, pp. 1268–1278, 2013.

[30] A. Bishayee and M. Chatterjee, "Time course effects of vanadium supplement on cytosolic reduced glutathione level and glutathione S-transferase activity," *Biological Trace Element Research*, vol. 48, no. 3, pp. 275–285, 1995.

[31] B. Hazra, R. Sarkar, S. Biswas, and N. Mandal, "Comparative study of the antioxidant and reactive oxygen species scavenging properties in the extracts of the fruits of *Terminalia chebula*, *Terminalia belerica* and *Emblica officinalis*," *BMC Complementary and Alternative Medicine*, vol. 10, article 20, 15 pages, 2010.

[32] S. K. Jain and D. S. Khurdiya, "Vitamin C enrichment of fruit juice based ready-to-serve beverages through blending of Indian gooseberry (*Emblica officinalis* Gaertn.) juice," *Plant Foods for Human Nutrition*, vol. 59, no. 2, pp. 63–66, 2004.

[33] A. Muthuraman, S. Sood, and S. K. Singla, "The antiinflammatory potential of phenolic compounds from *Emblica officinalis* L. in rat," *Inflammopharmacology*, vol. 19, no. 6, pp. 327–334, 2011.

[34] T. Yokozawa, H. Y. Kim, H. J. Kim, T. Okubo, D.-C. Chu, and L. R. Juneja, "Amla (*Emblica officinalis* Gaertn.)prevents dyslipidaemia and oxidative stress in the ageing process," *British Journal of Nutrition*, vol. 97, no. 6, pp. 1187–1195, 2007.

[35] M. Pairet, L. Churchill, G. Trummlitz, and G. Engelhardt, "Differential inhibition of cyclooxygenase-1 (COX-1) and -2 (COX-2) by NSAIDs: consequences on anti-inflammatory activity versus gastric and renal safety," *Inflammopharmacology*, vol. 4, no. 1, pp. 61–70, 1996.

[36] K. Sairam, C. V. Rao, M. D. Babu, K. V. Kumar, V. K. Agrawal, and R. K. Goel, "Antiulcerogenic effect of methanolic extract of *Emblica officinalis*: an experimental study," *Journal of Ethnopharmacology*, vol. 82, no. 1, pp. 1–9, 2002.

[37] K. B. Hari Kumar, M. C. Sabu, P. S. Lima, and R. Kuttan, "Modulation of haematopoetic system and antioxidant enzymes by *Emblica officinalis* Gaertn and its protective role against γ-radiation induced damages in mice," *Journal of Radiation Research*, vol. 45, no. 4, pp. 549–555, 2004.

Intravenous Immunoglobulins: Mode of Action and Indications in Autoimmune and Inflammatory Dermatoses

Lyubomir A. Dourmishev, Dimitrina V. Guleva, and Ljubka G. Miteva

Department of Dermatology and Venereology, Medical University-Sofia, Bulgaria

Correspondence should be addressed to Lyubomir A. Dourmishev; l_dourmishev@yahoo.com

Academic Editor: David A. Hart

Intravenous immunoglobulins (IVIGs), a mixture of variable amounts of proteins (albumin, IgG, IgM, IgA, and IgE antibodies), as well as salt, sugar, solvents, and detergents, are successfully used to treat a variety of dermatological disorders. For decades, IVIGs have been administered for treatment of infectious diseases and immune deficiencies, since they contain natural antibodies that represent a first-line defense against pathogens. Today their indication has expanded, including the off-label therapy for a variety of autoimmune and inflammatory diseases. In dermatology, IVIGs are administered for treatment of different disorders at different therapeutic regimens, mostly with higher doses then those administered for treatment of infectious diseases. The aim of this prospective review is to highlight the indications, effectiveness, side effects, and perspectives of the systemic treatment with IVIGs for patients with severe, life-threatening, and resistant to conventional therapies autoimmune or inflammatory dermatoses.

1. Introduction

Intravenous immunoglobulins (IVIGs) have been initially used to treat primary and secondary immune deficiencies, since they contain natural antibodies (Ab) that are first-line defense against pathogens. However over the past decades their indications have expanded tremendously, including the off-label therapy for a variety of autoimmune and inflammatory diseases in dermatology.

IVIG consists of mainly IgG (IgG_3, IgG_4) antibodies as well as variable amounts of proteins; IgA, IgE, and IgM Ab; albumin; salt and sugar content; solvents and detergents, depending of the methods of commercial preparation. There are different preparations of IVIG in the market for intravenous administration in two forms—lyophilized and liquid. The first form has to be diluted with water, saline, or 5% glucose while the liquid form (0.5% or 10% solution) is ready to use.

The mechanism of action of IVIG in most autoimmune diseases remains unclear [1]; however various mechanisms have been proposed. IVIGs have an immunomodulatory activity based on biological processes that are implicated in innate or acquired immune response (Table 1).

2. Material and Methods

We reviewed prospective clinical studies on the effectiveness of IVIG for treatment of various allergic, autoimmune, inflammatory, and drug induced dermatoses. A standardized literature search was performed using MEDLINE database and the criteria were limited to case reports, clinical studies, and abstracts. Several indications are still controversial due to the lack of controlled clinical research results.

3. Results and Discussion

Although in second line, IVIGs have shown promising results in treatment of various autoimmune and inflammatory dermatoses.

4. Adverse Drug Reactions

The most significant and potentially life-threatening disorders from the adverse drug reactions group are *Stevens-Johnson syndrome (SJS)* and *toxic epidermal necrolysis (TEN)*. SJS/TEN are adverse skin drug reactions that typically involve

Table 1: Mechanism of action of IVIG in inflammatory and autoimmune dermatoses.

Biologic target	Mode of action	Reference
T-lymphocytes	Inhibition of T cell derived IL-2, IL-10, TNF-β, and IFN-γ Antibodies against CD4 cells, HLA class I and II molecules, and T cell receptor β chain	[2–4]
B-lymphocytes	Antibody neutralization and inhibition of Ab production due B-lymphocytes binding Inhibition of IL-6 and TNF-α production Induction of B-cell apoptosis	[5–7]
Monocyte/macrophage system	Suppressing the phagocytosis of antibody-coated cells by Fc blockade Anti-inflammatory activity of IVIG through the surface expression of inhibitory Fc γRIIB receptor IVIG increasing the synthesis of IL-8 in cultures of monocytes	[8] [9] [2, 10]
Dendritic cells	Suppression of the dendritic cells differentiation maturation and capacity to secrete IL-12 on activation	[11, 12]
Keratinocytes	Blockage of Fas-mediated keratinocyte death by binding to the CD95 (death receptor)	[13, 14]
Complement system	IVIG having immediate and long-lasting attenuating effect on complement amplification *in vivo* by stimulating inactivation of C3 convertase precursors	[15] [16]

the skin and the mucous membranes representing the same disease at different levels of severity. These diseases are characterized by the rapid onset of keratinocyte cell death resulting in the separation of the epidermis from the dermis. The difference between SJS and TEN relates to the body surface affected. SJS consists of less than 10% of the body surface detachment; between 10% and 30% is SJS/TEN overlap syndrome, and if more than 30% of the body surface is affected, the diagnosis is TEN [16]. Moreover it was found that IVIG perfusions bring a significant increase in IgG concentration in the serum, blister fluid, and epidermis of both TEN-involved and clinically uninvolved skin. This highlights the direct effect of infused IgG in the local areas in addition to being present in general circulation, since IgA and IgM remain unchanged [17]. There is still no consensus about the treatment of both disorders, since SJS tend to be distinguished from TEN not only in clinical affection, but in therapeutic responses to corticosteroids and IVIG [18]. Numerous case reports have analyzed the therapeutic effect of IVIG in TEN using total doses greater than 2 g/kg over 3-4 days [13, 19–21], suggesting that total doses of 2 g/kg or less are more likely insufficient to obtain optimal therapeutic effect [22]. In contrast, even low doses IVIG (0.4 g/kg per day) administrated for 5 consecutive days are found highly effective in 87.5% of SJS patients [23]. Hence IVIG together with the systemic steroids should be considered as an important treatment modality for patients with refractory SJS/TEN [23].

5. Autoimmune Bullous Diseases

Pemphigus is a group of autoimmune bullous diseases caused by circulating Ab against adhesion molecules located on the keratinocyte surface. In *pemphigus vulgaris*, the Ab are directed against desmoglein-3 and/or desmoglein-1 while in *pemphigus foliaceus* they are directed only against desmoglein-1. High doses of corticosteroids and immunosuppressive drugs are used as first-line therapy in autoimmune bullous dermatoses. In some cases patients do not respond or tolerate high doses of these drugs or the tapering of the steroids can cause new disease flare-ups or in other cases the therapy could lead to side effects. IVIG is an alternative treatment. It is suggested that IVIG decreases serum level of pemphigus Ab by increased catabolism or by manipulating the idiotypic network [24]. Another suggestion is that IVIG can inhibit the binding of antidesmoglein-3 Ab to recombinant desmoglein-3 in a dose dependent manner in vivo and in vitro. In 2002 Bystryn et al. [25] and in 2006 Baum et al. [26] reported 6 and 12 cases of therapy-resistant patients with pemphigus vulgaris which have been treated with IVIGs with a rapid improvement of the diseases activity. The therapy scheme protocol proposed 2 g/kg over 3–5 days (1 cycle) every month with minor side effects. The treatment with IVIGs in *pemphigus foliaceus* has shown also very good response with long remission after the discontinuation of the study drug [27].

Bullous pemphigoid, a subepidermal blistering disease, is characterized by the presence of IgG Ab against hemidesmosomal antigens BP230 (BPAg1) and BP180 (BPAg2). There are reported cases with a positive response of BP to IVIG with dose of 2 g/kg per month cycle over 3 months or initially as an adjunctive therapy [28, 29].

Pemphigoid gestationis (PG), an autoimmune blistering disease in pregnancy, is characterized by the Ab against BP antigens in the basement membrane zone (BMZ). Although a second-line treatment, IVIG (2 g/kg/cycle, every two weeks antepartum and every three weeks for three months postpartum) was successfully used in a case with clinical and immunological cure, healthy neonate, and lack of adverse events [30].

Cicatricial pemphigoid is a form of pemphigoid, affecting the mucous membranes. IVIGs have been given at 2 g/kg/cycle initially every 2-3 weeks as an alternative option to suppress the disease progression [31, 32].

Epidermolysis bullosa acquisita (EBA), an autoimmune subepidermal blistering disease of the skin and mucus membranes, is characterized by the presence of IgG Ab (in most patients) targeting the noncollagenous (NC1) domain of type

VII collagen, the major component of anchoring fibrils that connect the basement membrane to dermal structures. The disease is often difficult to treat. There are various cases of a possible benefit of IVIG usually in association with previously introduced immunosuppressive therapy [33, 34].

Linear IgA dermatosis is an autoimmune subepidermal vesiculobullous disease characterized by the linear deposition of IgA at the BMZ. It is suggested the IVIGs may be useful in not responding to the conventional therapy patients [35, 36].

6. Connective Tissue Diseases

Dermatomyositis is an autoimmune disease that affects the skin and muscle as a consequence of a complement mediated microangiopathy and T cell mediated muscle destruction. The first-line treatment is high doses of systemic steroids as a monotherapy or combined with immunosuppressive drugs (azathioprine, methotrexate, and cyclosporine) but the side effects are common. It is believed that IVIG could limit the migration of activated T cells from capillaries towards the muscle fibers. Dalakas et al. [37] have conducted a controlled trial of high doses of IVIGs. They found that IVIG at a dose of 2 mg/kg per month was proven to be highly effective in improving both skin and muscle involvement. Other regimens include IVIG 0.1 g/kg/day for 5 days/week for 2 weeks [38] or 0.4 g/kg/day for 5 consecutive days [39]. The response is observed within 3 to 4 months in about 80% of the treated patients. Those patients who do not respond to the first-line therapy should receive IVIG in association with corticosteroids. Similar results, showing an improvement of both muscle and skin disease, have been reported in various forms of inflammatory myopathies as *polymyositis, juvenile dermatomyositis* [40], or *necrotizing myopathy* [41]. Moreover IVIG treatment affects well the dermatomyositis complications as ulcerative skin lesions and *calcinosis cutis* [42].

Although first results were not encouraging, IVIGs now present excellent efficacy in steroid resistant cases of *subacute cutaneous lupus erythematosus* and *systemic lupus erythematosus* in a regimen of two-day course (1 g/kg/24 h) every 4 weeks [43]. Other regimens include IVIG 1 g/kg/24 h on 2 consecutive days, followed by 0.4 mg/kg per month for 6 months, or 0.5 g/kg/24 h on 4 consecutive days (2 g/kg/month) for 3 months [44].

Systemic sclerosis (SSc), other connective tissue disease, is characterized with cutaneous fibrosis and internal organ affection. IVIG administered at 2 g/kg over 5 days monthly for 6 months was found to reduce the disease activity in an open label study [45]. Other case reports also show improvements in skin scores suggesting that IVIG could be of benefit to treating SSc's skin involvement. Same results have been reported for treatment of *mixed connective tissue disease* with or without myositis overlap [46].

7. Allergic Diseases

Atopic dermatitis, a chronic inflammatory skin diseases characterized by a dysregulation of the immune response, usually starts in early infancy but an adult-onset variant is also recognized. Data in literature showed significant children improvement by monotherapy IVIG, given as 2 g/kg [47], but in adults it does not appear to have the same efficacy [48].

Chronic urticaria is a skin disorder characterized by recurrent transitory itchy wheals affecting patients for 6 weeks or longer. In the largest study in chronic urticaria, 2 g/kg IVIG has been used over 5 days. Most patients responded clinically with complete and prolonged remission [49].

8. Vasculitis and Vasculopathies

Idiopathic thrombocytopenic purpura (ITP) is an isolated thrombocytopenia with normal bone marrow and in the absence of other causes of thrombocytopenia presents clinically with petechiae or purpura on skin and signs of mucosal bleeding (gastrointestinal, menometrorrhagia, and haematuria). Therapeutic regimens depend on the patient age (childhood or adults) and clinical course (early diagnosed or chronic) as well as the economical concerns. The standard scheme in childhood ITP is IVIG at a total dose of 0.8–1.0 g/kg given on 1 or 2 consecutive days [50]; however excellent results with very low doses of IVIG (0.1–0.2 g/kg) have also been reported [51]. In adults with ITP, the leukopenia or the serum anti-GPIb-IX Ab are signs for poor IVIG treatment response [52].

Kawasaki disease (KD) is an acute febrile vasculitic syndrome of early childhood, affecting predominantly medium-sized blood vessels and particularly the coronary arteries. Skin and mucous membrane lesions include maculopapular or target-like exanthema, followed by desquamation, pharyngitis, and conjunctivitis. In a trial of 549 children with KD, Newburger et al. [53] have shown that a single dose IVIG 2 g/kg in addition to acetylsalicylate is more effective than the conventional regimen of acetylsalicylate and 4 days of IVIG 0.4 g/kg/day.

Pyoderma gangrenosum (PG) is uncommon, ulcerative cutaneous disorder of uncertain etiology, claimed by some authors to be as Wegener's arteritis—a type of segmental ulcerative vasculitis [54]. It is associated with systemic diseases in at least 50% of patients [55]. Immunosuppressors are the first line of treatment but the therapeutic effects are variable. Significant improvement, long-lasting remissions, or complete healing is reported in all observed patients with PG treated with 2 g/kg/cycle IVIG [56–58]. Thus IVIG is an important therapeutic option in pyoderma gangrenosum refractory to standard immunomodulatory treatment.

9. Other Noninfectious Cutaneous Disorders

Scleromyxoedema is a rare skin disorder characterized by fibroblast proliferation and mucin deposition in the dermis of unclear etiology. Lesions can be localized on the skin of the head, neck, and dorsum of the hands but in some cases there is extracutaneous manifestation in heart, lung, joints, and oesophagus. The treatment is difficult and often ineffective. Many therapeutic approaches have been tried. Improvement in skin and systemic involvement of the disease was observed in patients treated with 2 g/kg IVIG over 5 days [59, 60].

Pretibial myxoedema (PTM) is characterized by localized lesions of the skin resulting from the deposition of hyaluronic acid, usually as a component of thyroid disease. Although the condition is most often confined to the pretibial area, it may occur anywhere on the skin and it is typically associated with Grave's disease. All patients with localized myxoedema have high serum concentrations of thyroid-stimulating hormone receptor Ab, indicating the severity of the autoimmune condition. Current treatment modalities are at the most cases palliative. There are two studies' data of the use of IVIG published in literature. The largest one [61] showed clinical improvement of the skin lesions, ophthalmopathy, and decreasing of Ab levels with a dose of 2 g/kg in 3 weekly cycles for a total of 7–15 cycles of IVIG compared with a group of patients treated with systemic steroids as monotherapy without improvement. Terheyden et al. [62] reported a group of patients with an elephantiasic form of PTM with no response to 2 g/kg IVIG after 6 monthly cycles but there is a reduction in anti-TSH receptor antibody levels.

10. Interactions, Contraindications, and Adverse Effects

Before the initiation of IVIG infusion, it is important to test liver and renal function and complete blood cell count, as well as to perform viral hepatitis screening. Vital signs should be monitored before the infusion, every 15 minutes for the first hour of infusion, and every 30 minutes for the rest of the infusion. The infusion should be at a slow rate and then increasing every 15 minutes. There are no known drug interactions; however IVIG should not be applied at the time of attenuated live vaccinations or within the 3-month period after vaccine.

The therapeutic usage of IVIGs is associated in most cases with a low incidence of side effects according to WHO criteria. IVIGs are basically considered as a safe and efficacious therapeutic option but it is still associated with some adverse effects. They are divided into two groups—minor and severe side effects [63]. Side effects in the first group are transient and often appear during the infusion or up to 72 h following the infusion. It is characterized by headache, nausea, fever, vomiting, cough, malaise, muscle, join and abdominal pain, flushing, urticarial lesions, and variations in heart rate and blood pressure. These reactions are probably due to aggregated immunoglobulin molecules that cause the complement system activation, antigen-antibody, contaminants, or stabilizers reactions [64]. Premedication with systemic steroids, antihistamines (diphenhydramine 50 mg), and nonsteroidal anti-inflammatory drugs (acetaminophen 650 mg) can minimize or prevent them [63]. Leukopenia, neutropenia, and monocytopenia are also seen in IVIGs therapy; however in most of cases those side effects appear to be self-limited and do not lead to increased susceptibility to infection.

Adverse effects in the second group are rare but severe. Most of them appear during or after the first infusion; hence it is important to have a complete medical history before the administration of IVIG. Some of these group side effects are aseptic meningitis, acute renal failure, stroke, exacerbation of the preexisting congestive heart failure, infections, hemolysis, deep venous thrombosis, pulmonary embolism, and anaphylactic shock [26, 63, 64]. Skin adverse effects include severe dermatitis resembling pompholyx initially localized to the palms or soles that then extends to the rest of the body [65], suggesting that a rapid increase in serum IgG levels may be involved in the development of skin lesions [66].

11. Conclusion

The number of first-line or high- or medium-priority indications for IVIG treatment in hematology, neurology, rheumatology, intensive care, and dermatology continues to extend. At present,the use of IVIGs is an important step in the treatment of autoimmune dermatoses. As was already stated, they are safe, well-tolerated, and well-accepted therapeutic modality. Reports in literature about the benefits of IVIG are increasing although we still need evidence-based data to improve the safety and efficacy of the drug, however, and supporting data in many indications.

Acknowledgments

The author thanks a number of colleagues from the Department of Dermatology and Venereology, Medical University-Sofia, who have discussed the issues highlighted in the paper.

References

[1] M. D. Kazatchkine and S. V. Kaveri, "Immunomodulation of autoimmune and inflammatory diseases with intravenous immune globulin," *The New England Journal of Medicine*, vol. 345, no. 10, pp. 747–755, 2001.

[2] J. Andersson, U. Skansen-Saphir, E. Sparrelid, and U. Andersson, "Intravenous immune globulin affects cytokine production in T lymphocytes and monocytes/macrophages," *Clinical & Experimental Immunology*, vol. 104, pp. 10–21, 1996.

[3] V. Hurez, S. V. Kaveri, A. Mouhoub et al., "Anti-CD4 activity of normal human immunoglobulin G for therapeutic use. (Intravenous immunoglobulin, IVIg)," *Therapeutic Immunology*, vol. 1, no. 5, pp. 269–277, 1994.

[4] J. J. Marchalonis, H. Kaymaz, F. Dedeoglu, S. F. Schluter, D. E. Yocum, and A. B. Edmundson, "Human autoantibodies reactive with synthetic autoantigens from T-cell receptor β chain," *Proceedings of the National Academy of Sciences of the United States of America*, vol. 89, no. 8, pp. 3325–3329, 1992.

[5] T. Tha-In, J. Bayry, H. J. Metselaar, S. V. Kaveri, and J. Kwekkeboom, "Modulation of the cellular immune system by intravenous immunoglobulin," *Trends in Immunology*, vol. 29, no. 12, pp. 608–615, 2008.

[6] M. Toyoda, A. Pao, A. Petrosian, and S. C. Jordan, "Pooled human gammaglobulin modulates surface molecule expression and induces apoptosis in human B cells," *American Journal of Transplantation*, vol. 3, no. 2, pp. 156–166, 2003.

[7] M. D. Kazatchkine, G. Dietrich, V. Hurez et al., "V region-mediated selection of autoreactive repertoires by intravenous immunoglobulin (i.v.Ig)," *Immunological Reviews*, vol. 139, no. 1, pp. 79–107, 1994.

[8] J. M. Dwyer, "Manipulating the immune system with immune-globulin," *The New England Journal of Medicine*, vol. 326, pp. 107–116, 1992.

[9] A. Samuelsson, T. L. Towers, and J. V. Ravetch, "Anti-inflammatory activity of IVIG mediated through the inhibitory Fc receptor," *Science*, vol. 291, no. 5503, pp. 484–486, 2001.

[10] V. Ruiz de Souza, M.-P. Carreno, S. V. Kaveri et al., "Selective induction of interleukin-1 receptor antagonist and interleukin-8 in human monocytes by normal polyspecific IgG (intravenous immunoglobulin)," *European Journal of Immunology*, vol. 25, no. 5, pp. 1267–1273, 1995.

[11] J. Bayry, S. Lacroix-Desmazes, C. Carbonneil et al., "Inhibition of maturation and function of dendritic cells by intravenous immunoglobulin," *Blood*, vol. 101, no. 2, pp. 758–765, 2003.

[12] J. Bayry, S. Lacroix-Desmazes, S. Delignat et al., "Intravenous immunoglobulin abrogates dendritic cell differentiation induced by interferon-α present in serum from patients with systemic lupus erythematosus," *Arthritis & Rheumatism*, vol. 48, no. 12, pp. 3497–3502, 2003.

[13] I. Viard, P. Wehrli, R. Bullani et al., "Inhibition of toxic epidermal necrolysis by blockade of CD95 with human intravenous immunoglobulin," *Science*, vol. 282, no. 5388, pp. 490–493, 1998.

[14] N. K. A. Prasad, G. Papoff, A. Zeuner et al., "Therapeutic preparations of normal polyspecific IgG (IVIg) induce apoptosis in human lymphocytes and monocytes: a novel mechanism of action of IVIg involving the Fas apoptotic pathway," *Journal of Immunology*, vol. 161, no. 7, pp. 3781–3790, 1998.

[15] M. Basta, L. F. Fries, and M. M. Frank, "High doses of intravenous Ig inhibit in vitro uptake of C4 fragments onto sensitized erythrocytes," *Blood*, vol. 77, no. 2, pp. 376–380, 1991.

[16] H. U. Lutz, P. Stammler, V. Bianchi et al., "Intravenously applied IgG stimulates complement attenuation in a complement-dependent autoimmune disease at the amplifying C3 convertase level," *Blood*, vol. 103, no. 2, pp. 465–472, 2004.

[17] P. Paquet, S. Kaveri, E. Jacob, J. Pirson, P. Quatresooz, and G. E. Piérard, "Skin immunoglobulin deposition following intravenous immunoglobulin therapy in toxic epidermal necrolysis," *Experimental Dermatology*, vol. 15, no. 5, pp. 381–386, 2006.

[18] R. A. Schwartz, P. H. McDonough, and B. W. Lee, "Toxic epidermal necrolysis: part I. Introduction, history, classification, clinical features, systemic manifestations, etiology, and immunopathogenesis," *Journal of the American Academy of Dermatology*, vol. 69, no. 2, pp. 173.e1–173.e13, 2013.

[19] J. T. Trent, R. S. Kirsner, P. Romanelli, and F. A. Kerdel, "Analysis of intravenous immunoglobulin for the treatment of toxic epidermal necrolysis using SCORTEN: the university of Miami experience," *Archives of Dermatology*, vol. 139, no. 1, pp. 39–43, 2003.

[20] A. W. Tan, B. Y. Thong, L. W. Yip, H. H. Chng, and S. K. Ng, "High-dose intravenous immunoglobulins in the treatment of toxic epidermal necrolysis: an Asian series," *Journal of Dermatology*, vol. 32, no. 1, pp. 1–6, 2005.

[21] S.-K. Tan and Y.-K. Tay, "Profile and pattern of Stevens-Johnson syndrome and toxic epidermal necrolysis in a general hospital in Singapore: treatment outcomes," *Acta Dermato-Venereologica*, vol. 92, no. 1, pp. 62–66, 2012.

[22] J. Trent, M. Halem, L. E. French, and F. Kerdel, "Toxic epidermal necrolysis and intravenous immunoglobulin: a review," *Seminars in Cutaneous Medicine and Surgery*, vol. 25, no. 2, pp. 91–93, 2006.

[23] M. Aihara, Y. Kano, H. Fujita et al., "Efficacy of additional i.v. immunoglobulin to steroid therapy in Stevens-Johnson syndrome and toxic epidermal necrolysis," *The Journal of Dermatology*, vol. 42, no. 8, pp. 768–777, 2015.

[24] Y. Shoenfeld, "The idiotypic network in autoimmunity: antibodies that bind antibodies that bind antibodies," *Nature Medicine*, vol. 10, no. 1, pp. 17–18, 2004.

[25] J.-C. Bystryn, D. Jiao, and S. Natow, "Treatment of pemphigus with intravenous immunoglobulin," *Journal of the American Academy of Dermatology*, vol. 47, no. 3, pp. 358–363, 2002.

[26] S. Baum, A. Scope, A. Barzilai, E. Azizi, and H. Trau, "The role of IVIg treatment in severe pemphigus vulgaris," *Journal of the European Academy of Dermatology and Venereology*, vol. 20, no. 5, pp. 548–552, 2006.

[27] A. R. Ahmed and N. Sami, "Intravenous immunoglobulin therapy for patients with pemphigus foliaceus unresponsive to conventional therapy," *Journal of the American Academy of Dermatology*, vol. 46, no. 1, pp. 42–49, 2002.

[28] R. C. Y. Beckers, A. Brand, B. J. Vermeer, and B. W. Boom, "Adjuvant high-dose intravenous gammaglobulin in the treatment of pemphigus and bullous pemphigoid: experience in six patients," *British Journal of Dermatology*, vol. 133, no. 2, pp. 289–293, 1995.

[29] A. R. Ahmed, "Intravenous immunoglobulin therapy for patients with bullous pemphigoid unresponsive to conventional immunosuppressive treatment," *Journal of the American Academy of Dermatology*, vol. 45, no. 6, pp. 825–835, 2001.

[30] T. Nguyen, E. Alraqum, and A. Razzaque Ahmed, "Positive clinical outcome with IVIg as monotherapy in recurrent pemphigoid gestationis," *International Immunopharmacology*, vol. 26, no. 1, pp. 1–3, 2015.

[31] M. L. Urcelay, A. McQueen, and W. S. Douglas, "Cicatricial pemphigoid treated with intravenous immunoglobulin," *British Journal of Dermatology*, vol. 137, no. 3, pp. 477–478, 1997.

[32] N. Sami, K. C. Bhol, and A. Razzaque Ahmed, "Intravenous immunoglobulin therapy in patients with multiple mucosal involvement in mucous membrane pemphigoid," *Clinical Immunology*, vol. 102, no. 1, pp. 59–67, 2002.

[33] F. Meier, K. Sonnichsen, G. Schaumburg-Lever, R. Dopfer, and G. Rassner, "Epidermolysis bullosa acquisita: efficacy of high-dose intravenous immunoglobulins," *Journal of the American Academy of Dermatology*, vol. 29, no. 2, pp. 334–337, 1993.

[34] K. Gourgiotou, D. Exadaktylou, K. Aroni et al., "Epidermolysis bullosa acquisita: treatment with intravenous immunoglobulins," *Journal of the European Academy of Dermatology and Venereology*, vol. 16, no. 1, pp. 77–80, 2002.

[35] I. U. Khan, K. C. Bhol, and A. R. Ahmed, "Linear IgA bullous dermatosis in a patient with chronic renal failure: response to intravenous immunoglobulin therapy," *Journal of the American Academy of Dermatology*, vol. 40, no. 3, pp. 485–488, 1999.

[36] M. Goebeler, C. Seitz, C. Rose et al., "Successful treatment of linear IgA disease with salazosulphapyridine and intravenous immunoglobulins," *British Journal of Dermatology*, vol. 149, pp. 912–914, 2003.

[37] M. C. Dalakas, I. Illa, J. M. Dambrosia et al., "A controlled trial of high-dose intravenous immune globulin infusions as treatment for dermatomyositis," *The New England Journal of Medicine*, vol. 329, no. 27, pp. 1993–2000, 1993.

[38] T. Sadayama, S. Miyagawa, and T. Shirai, "Low-dose intravenous immunoglobulin therapy for intractable dermatomyositis skin lesions," *Journal of Dermatology*, vol. 26, no. 7, pp. 457–459, 1999.

[39] E. Saito, T. Koike, H. Hashimoto et al., "Efficacy of high-dose intravenous immunoglobulin therapy in Japanese patients with steroid-resistant polymyositis and dermatomyositis," *Modern Rheumatology*, vol. 18, no. 1, pp. 34–44, 2008.

[40] G. Imataka and O. Arisaka, "Long-term, high-dose intravenous immunoglobulin therapy in a patient with banker-type juvenile dermatomyositis," *Cell Biochemistry and Biophysics*, vol. 69, no. 3, pp. 747–748, 2014.

[41] A. K. B. Patil, A. T. Prabhakar, A. Sivadasan, M. Alexander, and G. Chacko, "An unusual case of inflammatory necrotizing myopathy and neuropathy with pipestem capillaries," *Neurology India*, vol. 63, no. 1, pp. 72–76, 2015.

[42] M. G. Danieli, S. Gambini, L. Pettinari, F. Logullo, G. Veronesi, and A. Gabrielli, "Impact of treatment on survival in polymyositis and dermatomyositis. A single-centre long-term follow-up study," *Autoimmunity Reviews*, vol. 13, no. 10, pp. 1048–1054, 2014.

[43] C. E. Lampropoulos, G. R. V. Hughes, and D. P. D'Cruz, "Intravenous immunoglobulin in the treatment of resistant subacute cutaneous lupus erythematosus: a possible alternative," *Clinical Rheumatology*, vol. 26, no. 6, pp. 981–983, 2007.

[44] C. Ky, B. Swasdibutra, S. Khademi, S. Desai, V. Laquer, and S. A. Grando, "Efficacy of intravenous immunoglobulin monotherapy in patients with cutaneous lupus erythematosus: results of proof-of-concept study," *Dermatology Reports*, vol. 7, no. 1, article 5804, 2015.

[45] Y. Levy, H. Amital, P. Langevitz et al., "Intravenous immunoglobulin modulates cutaneous involvement and reduces skin fibrosis in systemic sclerosis: an open-label study," *Arthritis & Rheumatism*, vol. 50, no. 3, pp. 1005–1007, 2004.

[46] M. Matsuda, J. Miki, K. Oguchi, K. Tabata, and S.-I. Ikeda, "Fasciitis in mixed connective tissue disease successfully treated with high-dose intravenous immunoglobulin," *Internal Medicine*, vol. 42, no. 9, pp. 910–911, 2003.

[47] M. Wakim, M. Alazard, A. Yajima, D. Speights, A. Saxon, and E. R. Stiehm, "High dose intravenous immunoglobulin in atopic dermatitis and hyper-IgE syndrome," *Annals of Allergy, Asthma and Immunology*, vol. 81, no. 2, pp. 153–158, 1998.

[48] C. Paul, M. Lahfa, H. Bachelez, S. Chevret, and L. Dubertret, "A randomized controlled evaluator-blinded trial of intravenous immunoglobulin in adults with severe atopic dermatitis," *British Journal of Dermatology*, vol. 147, no. 3, pp. 518–522, 2002.

[49] B. F. O'Donnell, R. M. Barr, A. Kobza Black et al., "Intravenous immunoglobulin in autoimmune chronic urticaria," *British Journal of Dermatology*, vol. 138, no. 1, pp. 101–106, 1998.

[50] E. Parodi, P. Giordano, E. Rivetti et al., "Efficacy of combined intravenous immunoglobulins and steroids in children with primary immune thrombocytopenia and persistent bleeding symptoms," *Blood Transfusion*, vol. 12, no. 3, pp. 340–345, 2014.

[51] J. H. Lee and K. S. Lee, "Efficacy of very low-dose (200 mg/kg/d) with short-term intravenous immunoglobulin G therapy according to individual response of acute immune thrombocytopenic purpura in childhood," *Clinical Pediatric Hematology-Oncology*, vol. 13, no. 2, pp. 143–149, 2006.

[52] J. Peng, S.-H. Ma, J. Liu et al., "Association of autoantibody specificity and response to intravenous immunoglobulin G therapy in immune thrombocytopenia: a multicenter cohort study," *Journal of Thrombosis and Haemostasis*, vol. 12, no. 4, pp. 497–504, 2014.

[53] J. W. Newburger, M. Takahashi, A. S. Beiser et al., "A single intravenous infusion of gamma globulin as compared with four infusions in the treatment of acute Kawasaki syndrome," *The New England Journal of Medicine*, vol. 324, no. 23, pp. 1633–1639, 1991.

[54] A. L. Dourmishev, D. K. Serafimova, S. G. Vassileva, L. A. Dourmishev, and R. A. Schwartz, "Segmental ulcerative vasculitis: a cutaneous manifestation of Takayasu's arteritis," *International Wound Journal*, vol. 2, no. 4, pp. 332–345, 2005.

[55] E. M. DeFilippis, S. R. Feldman, and W. W. Huang, "The genetics of pyoderma gangrenosum and implications for treatment: a systematic review," *British Journal of Dermatology*, vol. 172, no. 6, pp. 1487–1497, 2014.

[56] A. K. Gupta, N. H. Shear, and D. N. Sauder, "Efficacy of human intravenous immune globulin in pyoderma gangrenosum," *Journal of the American Academy of Dermatology*, vol. 32, no. 1, pp. 140–142, 1995.

[57] C. M. Dobson, R. A. Parslew, and S. Evans, "Superficial granulomatous pyoderma treated with intravenous immunoglobulin," *Journal of the American Academy of Dermatology*, vol. 48, no. 3, pp. 456–460, 2003.

[58] J. Cafardi and N. Sami, "Intravenous immunoglobulin as salvage therapy in refractory pyoderma gangrenosum: report of a case and review of the literature," *Case Reports in Dermatology*, vol. 6, no. 3, pp. 239–244, 2014.

[59] R. K. Lister, S. Jolles, S. Whittaker et al., "Scleromyxedema: response to high-dose intravenous immunoglobulin (hdIVIg)," *Journal of the American Academy of Dermatology*, vol. 43, no. 2, pp. 403–408, 2000.

[60] N. Kumar and M. Rodriguez, "Scleromyxedema in a patient with multiple sclerosis and monoclonal gammopathy on interferon beta-1a," *Multiple Sclerosis*, vol. 10, no. 1, pp. 85–86, 2004.

[61] A. Antonelli, A. Navarranne, R. Palla et al., "Pretibial myxedema and high-dose intravenous immunoglobulin treatment," *Thyroid*, vol. 4, no. 4, pp. 399–408, 1994.

[62] P. Terheyden, G. J. Kahaly, D. Zillikens, and E.-B. Bröcker, "Lack of response of elephantiasic pretibial myxoedema to treatment with high-dose intravenous immunoglobulins," *Clinical and Experimental Dermatology*, vol. 28, no. 2, pp. 224–226, 2003.

[63] C. Prins, E. W. Gelfand, and L. E. French, "Intravenous immunoglobulin: properties, mode of action and practical use in dermatology," *Acta Dermato-Venereologica*, vol. 87, no. 3, pp. 206–218, 2007.

[64] F. R. Palabrica, S. L. Kwong, and F. R. Padua, "Adverse events of intravenous immunoglobulin infusions: a ten-year retrospective study," *Asia Pacific Allergy*, vol. 3, no. 4, pp. 249–256, 2013.

[65] G. Vecchietti, K. Kerl, C. Prins, G. Kaya, J.-H. Saurat, and L. E. French, "Severe eczematous skin reaction after high-dose intravenous immunoglobulin infusion: report of 4 cases and review of the literature," *Archives of Dermatology*, vol. 142, no. 2, pp. 213–217, 2006.

[66] M. Kurata, C. Horie, Y. Kano, and T. Shiohara, "Pompholyx as a clinical manifestation suggesting increased serum IgG levels in a patient with drug-induced hypersensitivity syndrome/drug reaction with eosinophilia and systemic symptoms," *British Journal of Dermatology*, 2015.

13

Macrophage Derived Platelet Activating Factor Implicated in the Resolution Phase of Gouty Inflammation

Darshna Yagnik

Department of Natural Sciences, School of Science and Technology, Middlesex University, The Burroughs, London NW4 4BT, UK

Correspondence should be addressed to Darshna Yagnik; d.yagnik@mdx.ac.uk

Academic Editor: B. L. Slomiany

Human blood derived *in vitro* differentiated monocytes or macrophages are a population of cells which have been investigated over the years to determine the role these cells play in the resolution phase of gout. Macrophages are able to phagocytose monosodium urate monohydrate (MSU) crystals without releasing inflammatory factors. This study analysed macrophage platelet activating factor secretion and its possible role in the pathway of gout resolution. Analysis of sunatants from *in vitro* differentiated macrophages stimulated with MSU crystals revealed the secretion of platelet activating factor (PAF) 1.54 ± 0.10 mean ± SEM; ng/mL per 10^6 cells. This secretion was absent in immature monocytes treated similarly. When these monocytes were pretreated with recombinant human PAF-acetylhydrolase (rhuPAF-AH) and MSU crystals resulted in TNFα suppression. Addition of WEB2086, a platelet activating factor (PAF) antagonist, to differentiated macrophages with MSU crystals unmasked TNFα secretion 0.7 ± 0.06 mean ± SEM; ng/mL per 10^6 cells. This study identifies a role for PAF and the PAF receptor antagonist in the pathway by which macrophages ingest MSU crystals and resolve the concomitant inflammation.

1. Introduction

An acute attack of gouty arthritis includes clinical features such as joint inflammation, erythema, fever, and extreme, unbearable pain resulting in reduced mobility of the afflicted joint [1]. Prophylactic therapy is recommended to control gouty arthritis flares [2, 3]. The symptoms are caused by monosodium urate monohydrate (MSU) crystal deposition into the intra-articular joint spaces. Crystal precipitation provokes mass polymorphonuclear (PMN) leukocyte infiltration into the joints where these cells release inflammatory cytokines which mediate joint damage [4, 5]. However, in the absence of clinical intervention, gout is self-limiting in nature and is able to spontaneously resolve over a period of a week [6–9]. The exact theory behind the resolution phase of gout remains an enigma although macrophages and their cofactors have been implicated in the mechanism [10–12].

Platelet activating factor (PAF, 1-0-alkyl-2-acetyl-sn-glycero-3-phosphocholine) was discovered in 1972, it is known as one of the most potent phospholipids, involved in platelet aggregation and anaphylaxis [13]. It is produced by a variety of immune cells including monocytes/macrophages, neutrophils, eosinophils, basophils, and platelets [14, 15]. There are two main pathways which lead to cellular synthesis of PAF, the de nova pathway and remodelling pathway. Inflammatory or immune stimuli induce PAF primarily via the remodelling pathway whereby membrane bound PAF-acetylhydrolase (PAF-AH) which is an extracellular phospholipase A2 catalyses the transfer of an acetyl residue from acetyl-CoA to 1-alkyl-sn-glycero-3-phosphocholine (lyso-PAF). This is produced by the action of phospholipase A2 on phosphatidylcholine [16–18].

However, the full mechanisms and the exact role of various enzymes on PAF degradation have not been fully elucidated to date.

To exert its effect, PAF binds directly to a specific G protein coupled receptor and is an important mediator of juxtacrine and paracrine signals between cells [19]. PAF is well regarded as a potent mediator of inflammatory pathologies such as acute pancreatitis [20], diabetes [21], and renal failure [22]. However, recent studies suggest PAF could also play a crucial role in regulating immune responses. Studies have highlighted the necessity of PAF receptor activation in deactivation of ultraviolet B (UVB) induced suppression of hypersensitivity responses [23]. In addition, PAF administration to equine alveolar macrophages increased phagocytic capacity and superoxide anion production [24]. Moreover, during immunological defence, PAF can play an immunomodulatory role including monocyte or macrophage degranulation, cytokine release, phagocytosis, and cell adhesion [25, 26].

2. Materials and Methods

2.1. Reagents and Antibodies. WEB2086 was purchased from Tocris Bioscience (UK). Human TNFα ELISA kit was purchased from R and D systems Europe. PAF ELISA kit was purchased from Blue Gene Biotech, China. LPS, antimonoclonal anti-human CD62, anti-mouse IgG FITC, and mouse IgG1 were purchased from Sigma-Aldrich (Poole, UK). MSU crystals were purchased from Enzo Life Sciences, Germany. HUVEC cells were purchased from ATCC cell lines, UK. Recombinant human PAF-acetylhydrolase was purchased from Sigma-Aldrich, USA.

2.2. Monocyte Isolation Procedure. Leucocyte rich cones were obtained from volunteer donors collected from NHS Cord Blood and Transplant Bank at Colindale, London. Briefly, the cones were washed with PBS to harvest leucocytes. The leucocyte rich cells were then spun on Histopaque at 1200 RPM for 20 mins. The mononuclear portion was obtained and washed in HANKS balanced solution. Cells were counted and cultured into 24 wells at 4×10^6/mL. Cells were allowed to adhere for an hour after which nonadherent cells were washed and full media replenished with Dulbecco's media containing AB serum. Differentiated macrophages were determined by light microscopy and flow cytometry phenotypic analysis of differentiation markers. Cells were washed and fed at days 1, 3, 5, and 7 of culture and stimulated with LPS (10 μg/mL) or MSU crystals (0.5 mg/mL) with or without pretreatment with WEB2086 for 16–24 hours after which supernatants were collected and stored in aliquots at −70°C prior to analysis. Pretreatment with rhuPAF-AH at concentrations of 2.5–20 μg/mL was carried out for half an hour prior to addition of MSU crystals to monocyte cells. Supernatants were collected and analysed for TNFα after 16 hours.

2.3. Enzyme Linked Immunosorbant Assays (ELISA). PAF and TNFα levels in cultured supernatants were determined by ELISA (purchased from Blue Gene Biotech, China, and R and D Systems Europe, resp.) using manufacturer's recommendations. For PAF determination, culture supernatants were pretreated with balance solution provided in the ELISA kit, mixed, and then processed according to manufacturer's instructions. The antibodies to PAF formed solid phase ELISA. All samples were measured in duplicate, with results expressed as the mean ± SEM cytokine concentration (ng/mL) from at least 4 experiments.

2.4. Flow Cytometric Analysis. Indirect flow cytometric analysis was performed as previously described (12), using primary antibodies at 10 μg/mL and secondary antibodies at 1:64 dilution. Endothelial cells were detached by trypsin/EDTA and the trypsin activity was quenched in excess growth medium supplemented with serum. Monocyte/macrophage cultures were detached by 15-minute incubation in ice-cold phosphate buffered saline (PBS) containing 2.5 mM of EDTA, followed by scraping and washing in growth medium containing serum. Data analysis was performed using a flow cytometer analyser purchased from Beckton Dickinson (BD), UK. Results were analysed using BD Cell Quest Pro software.

HUVEC E-Selectin expression was calculated by dividing the staining intensity (mean fluorescent intensity (MFI)) of E-Selectin by the staining intensity of class-matched control antibody, thus resulting in a relative fluorescent intensity (RFI) of expression (where an RFI of 1.00 is equivalent to no antigen expression). Results were expressed as the mean ± SD RFI from at least 3 separate experiments.

2.5. Statistical Analysis. Analysis of inhibition by WEB2086 on TNFα secretion and endothelial cell E-Selectin expression was carried out using 1-way analysis of variance (ANOVA) with Dunnett's correction.

3. Results and Discussion

Figure 1 shows that monocytes secrete detectable PAF when incubated with MSU crystals. This detection of PAF occurs at day 5 and peaks at day 7 of monocyte differentiation. The phenotype of monocytes as they differentiate into macrophages has been well characterised and it has previously been postulated that they can acquire an anti-inflammatory phenotype. A similar model showed that at days 5–7 of monocyte culture, upon stimulation with MSU crystals, an anti-inflammatory phenotypic response was enabled [11]. This was corroborated by the detection of TGFβ1 secretion by human *in vitro* differentiated macrophages in response to MSU crystal challenge. Coincubation of day 7 *in vitro* differentiated macrophages with the PAF receptor antagonist (WEB2086) and MSU crystals resulted in a decrease in PAF secretion (Figure 2). To investigate whether PAF production was autocrine suppressive, MSU crystal stimulated macrophages were incubated in the presence of increasing concentrations of the PAF receptor antagonist and this time TNFα production was analysed. Inclusion of WEB2086 at concentrations of 25–100 μM in these cultures resulted in peak TNFα production (Figure 3(b)). In fact, this TNFα production was comparable to that released by day 1 monocytes after MSU crystal stimulation which had been determined in a previous study [11].

Prior investigations have reported that macrophage cell lines and human *in vitro* differentiated macrophages can ingest MSU crystals without releasing inflammatory cytokines (TNFα, IL-1β, and IL-6) [11, 12]; indeed, it was identified that instead macrophages produced anti-inflammatory TGFβ1. In addition, it was observed that TGFβ1 was able to

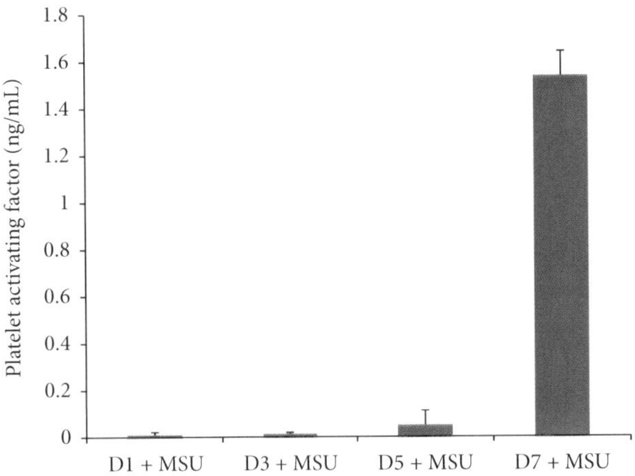

FIGURE 1: Monocyte differentiation and time course of platelet activating factor (PAF) production after challenge with MSU crystals. Isolated monocytes were differentiated over 7 days *in vitro* and incubated with MSU crystals for 17 hours at day 1 (D1), day 3 (D3), day 5 (D5), and day 7 (D7) of culture. Collected supernatants were analysed for PAF secretion by ELISA. Results are mean and SEM of 4 experiments.

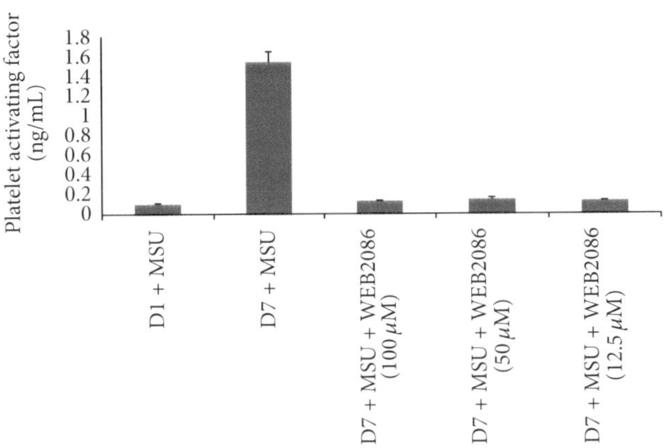

FIGURE 2: Platelet activating factor (PAF) production by D7 *in vitro* differentiated macrophages incubated with MSU crystals and with or without WEB2086 (WEB). Monocytes were cultured for 1 and 7 days and stimulated with MSU crystals and collected supernatants were analysed for PAF by ELISA. Results are mean and SEM of 4 experiments. D7 = supernatants from day 7 macrophages, D1 = supernatants from day 1 Monocytes, and WEB = WEB2086. Macrophages also secreted PAF when incubated with LPS (1.48 ± 0.10 mean ± SEM; ng/mL per 10^6 cells), data not shown.

inhibit endothelial cell activation and E-Selectin expression [12]. Essentially in this study coincubation of endothelial cells with anti-TGFβ1 and a mixture of day 1 and day 7 MSU crystal stimulated supernatants unmasked only a partial degree of endothelial E-Selectin reexpression even with using maximum concentrations of neutralising antibody against TGFβ1. This suggested that other anti-inflammatory factors could also be released by macrophages upon phagocytosis of MSU crystals. Figures 1 and 2 identify macrophage derived PAF in this mechanism. Another anti-inflammatory model whereby macrophages play an active role in regulating inflammation and resulting in PAF mediated activity by macrophages is the phagocytosis of apoptotic neutrophils. Indeed, this mechanism also results in a lack of proinflammatory cytokine release and associated inflammation [27–29]. Pretreatment of freshly isolated monocytes with rhuPAF-AH and MSU crystals resulted in partial suppression of TNFα release. Full suppression of TNFα was not expected as manufacturers reference data indicated that rhuPAF-AH cleaved the PAF analogue by approximately 50% at 10 μg/mL, which was observed in Figure 3(a).

It is likely that PAF exerts an immunomodulatory effect on MSU crystal stimulated macrophages as coincubation in the presence of WEB2086 unmasked TNFα production, implicating that PAF may be involved in autocrine and paracrine suppression of macrophages.

There are studies that highlight PAF's role in endocrine, autocrine, and intercrine signalling [28]. Endothelial activation precedes the inflammatory response by MSU crystals which has been observed *in vitro* and *in vivo* [27]. An antagonist of PAF was able to reduce E-Selectin mediated endothelial activation (Figure 4). Although PAF is well regarded as a potent mediator of inflammation, emerging research suggests that PAF can mediate inflammation control [30–32]. Impaired anaphylactic responses were reported in mice lacking the PAF receptor [23, 26]. Another study showed that mice stimulated with LPS were protected from endotoxin shock when injected with PAF systemically. In these mice, a reduction in proinflammatory cytokine secretion, namely, interferon gamma, IL-1, and TNFα, was also observed [32]. Researchers have highlighted the role of PAF mediated interference in microbial associated damage as well. PAF was pivotal in the extent of pathological consequences due to *H. pylori* infection and gastric mucin synthesis [33]. Another report implicated PAF in *Porphyromonas gingivalis*, LPS mediated interference with salivary mucin [34]. Moreover, prophylactic administration of PAF antagonist to rats with gastric injury exerted an anti-inflammatory effect reducing mucosal apoptosis, TNFα, and nitric oxide synthase 2 activity and resulted in rapid gastric ulcer healing [35].

In fact, PAF has been identified as a molecular sensor recognising cellular damage and exerting effects on cytokines and COX-2 transcription which resulted in systemic immune suppression [36]. Deposition of MSU crystals into intra-articular joints causes joint swelling and joint damage as well as oxidative stress [2, 3, 5, 37]. Hence, it is feasible that a similar sensory mechanism of cell damage detection by PAF and PAF receptor signalling could be underpinning gouty arthritis.

4. Conclusion

This study identifies macrophage derived PAF and PAF related molecules in the noninflammatory phagocytosis of MSU crystals by human blood derived differentiated macrophages. In this model, the PAF receptor antagonist was able to have a number of effects; it was able to inhibit endothelial cell activation measured by E-Selectin

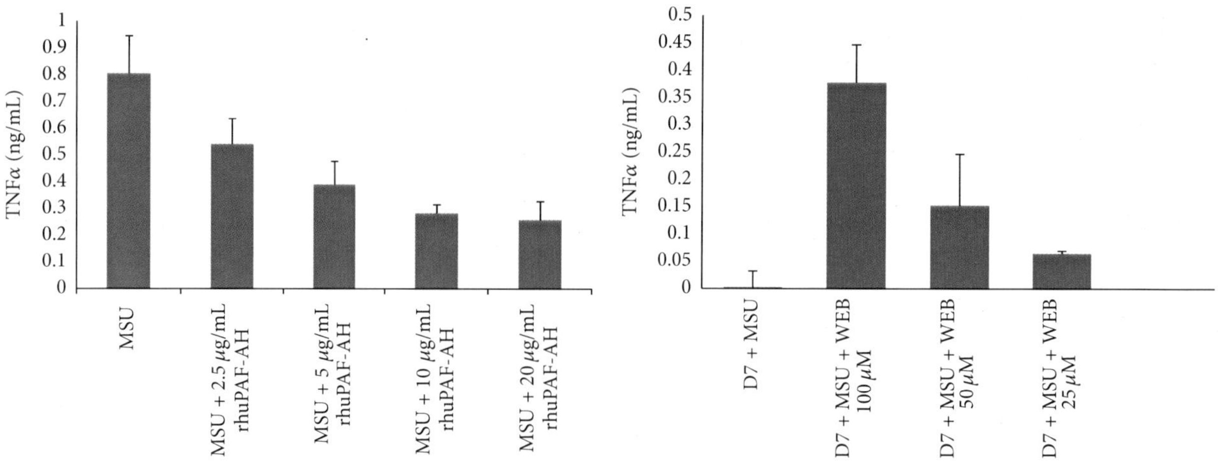

FIGURE 3: (a) Effect of recombinant human platelet activating factor acetylhydrolase (rhuPAF-AH) on TNFα release from monocytes. Freshly isolated monocytes were cultured overnight and treated with rhuPAF-AH at concentrations of 2.5, 5, 10, and 20 μg/mL, respectively, for 45 minutes prior to addition of MSU crystals for 24 hours. Afterwards, collected supernatants were analysed for TNFα by ELISA. Results are mean and SEM of 3 experiments. (b). TNFα production unmasked by costimulation of *in vitro* differentiated macrophages with MSU crystals and WEB2086. Monocytes were cultured *in vitro* for 7 days and stimulated with MSU crystals for 24 hours with or without the PAF antagonist (WEB2086). At 100 μM, coincubation with WEB2086 and urate crystals caused the release of TNFα with $P = 0.002$ (Student's paired t-test). Conditioned supernatants were analysed for TNFα production by ELISA. Differentiated macrophages were also coincubated with WEB2086 at 100 μM which reduced the amount of TNFα unmasked. Values are mean and SEM of 4 experiments. D7 = supernatants from day 7 macrophages, D1 = supernatants from day 1 monocytes, and WEB = WEB2086 (PAF antagonist).

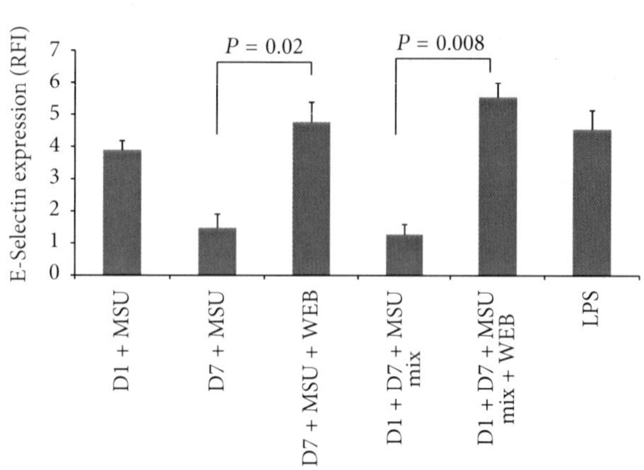

FIGURE 4: Inhibition of endothelial cell activation by platelet activating factor derived from supernatants from MSU crystal stimulated macrophages. Monocytes or macrophages were cultured for 1 and 7 days, respectively, and stimulated with MSU crystals. Collected supernatants were cocultured with human umbilical vein endothelial cells (HUVEC) for 4 hours at a 1:2 dilution or 1:1 mix, either alone or in the presence of WEB2086 (a PAF receptor antagonist). HUVEC expression of E-Selectin was measured by flow cytometry. WEB2086 was added to supernatant mixtures in culture at 100 μM which relieved the suppression of E-Selectin seen in the 1:1 mix condition ($P = 0.008$ by Student's paired t-test). Relief of E-Selectin suppression by supernatants from day 7 macrophages stimulated with MSU crystals was also observed ($P = 0.02$ by Student's paired t-test). Results are the mean and SD of 3 experiments. RFI = relative fluorescence intensity. D7 = supernatants from day 7 macrophages, D1 = supernatants from day 1 monocytes, and WEB = WEB2086.

upregulation and was also implicated in downregulating TNFα secretion by MSU crystal stimulated monocyte cells. Essentially, the immune response to MSU crystals is clearly multifaceted in nature involving a complex interplay by inflammatory and noninflammatory mechanisms involving various leukocyte derived factors which act in coordination during the resolution phase of gouty arthritis. Noticeably, little is known about the role that PAF-acetylhydrolases play in PAF activation and degradation or how PAF exerts its effects through its receptors. These pathways remain to be defined. The model of monocyte, macrophage, and MSU crystal induced inflammation could be used to further examine these molecular mechanisms and unravel the associated PAF signalling and receptor pathways. In conclusion, this study suggests a role for PAF and related molecules in the anti-inflammatory pathway by which macrophages phagocytose MSU crystals.

Acknowledgment

This work was funded by research grants from Middlesex University.

References

[1] M. P. Keith and W. R. Gilliland, "Updates in the management of Gout," *The American Journal of Medicine*, vol. 120, no. 3, pp. 221–224, 2007.

[2] R. A. Terkeltaub, "Gout," *The New England Journal of Medicine*, vol. 349, no. 17, pp. 1647–1655, 2003.

[3] Z.-H. Fang and H. Waizy, "Current concepts in the treatment of gouty arthritis," *Orthopaedic Surgery*, vol. 5, no. 1, pp. 6–12, 2013.

[4] P. A. Dieppe, P. R. Crocker, C. F. Corker, D. V. Doyle, E. C. Huskisson, and D. A. Willoughby, "Synovial fluid crystals," *Quarterly Journal of Medicine*, vol. 48, no. 192, pp. 533–553, 1979.

[5] R. Terkeltaub, C. Zachariae, D. Santoro, J. Martin, P. Peveri, and K. Matsushima, "Monocyte-derived neutrophil chemotactic factor/interleukin-8 is a potential mediator of crystal-induced inflammation," *Arthritis & Rheumatism*, vol. 34, no. 7, pp. 894–903, 1991.

[6] E. Pascual, E. Batlle-Gualda, A. Martínez, J. Rosas, and P. Vela, "Synovial fluid analysis for diagnosis of intercritical gout," *Annals of Internal Medicine*, vol. 131, no. 10, pp. 756–759, 1999.

[7] W. Louthrenoo, M. Sieck, G. Clayburne, S. Rothfuss, and H. R. Schumacher Jr., "Supravital staining of cells in noninflammatory synovial fluids: analysis of the effect of crystals on cell populations," *The Journal of Rheumatology*, vol. 18, no. 3, pp. 409–413, 1991.

[8] E. Pascual and V. Jovani, "A quantitative study of the phagocytosis of urate crystals in the synovial fluid of asymptomatic joints of patients with gout," *British Journal of Rheumatology*, vol. 34, no. 8, pp. 724–726, 1995.

[9] H. R. Schmacher, M. G. Stineman, S. Magge, A. Huppert, and M. Rahman, "The association between synovial fluid and treatment response in osteoarthritis," *Internal Medicine Journal*, vol. 4, pp. 25–34, 1996.

[10] D. R. Yagnik, P. Hillyer, D. Marshall et al., "Noninflammatory phagocytosis of monosodium urate monohydrate crystals by mouse macrophages. Implications for the control of joint inflammation in gout," *Arthritis and Rheumatism*, vol. 43, no. 8, pp. 1779–1789, 2000.

[11] R. C. Landis, D. R. Yagnik, O. Florey et al., "Safe disposal of inflammatory monosodium urate monohydrate crystals by differentiated macrophages," *Arthritis and Rheumatism*, vol. 46, no. 11, pp. 3026–3033, 2002.

[12] D. R. Yagnik, B. J. Evans, O. Florey, J. C. Mason, R. C. Landis, and D. O. Haskard, "Macrophage release of transforming growth factor $\beta 1$ during resolution of monosodium urate monohydrate crystal-induced inflammation," *Arthritis and Rheumatism*, vol. 50, no. 7, pp. 2273–2280, 2004.

[13] J. Benveniste, "Platelet activating factor, a new mediator of anaphylaxis and immune complex deposition from rabbit and human basophils," *Nature*, vol. 249, no. 5457, pp. 581–582, 1974.

[14] P. Braquet and M. Rola-Pleszczynski, "The role of PAF in immunological responses: a review," *Prostaglandins*, vol. 34, no. 2, pp. 143–148, 1987.

[15] G. Camussi, C. Tetta, and C. Baglioni, "The role of platelet-activating factor in inflammation," *Clinical Immunology and Immunopathology*, vol. 57, no. 3, pp. 331–338, 1990.

[16] F. Snyder, "Platelet-activating factor: the biosynthetic and catabolic enzymes," *Biochemical Journal*, vol. 305, no. 3, pp. 689–705, 1995.

[17] L. W. Tjoelker, C. Wilder, C. Eberhardt et al., "Anti-inflammatory properties of a platelet-activating factor acetylhydrolase," *Nature*, vol. 374, no. 6522, pp. 549–553, 1995.

[18] L. W. Tjoelker, C. Eberhardt, J. Unger et al., "Plasma platelet-activating factor acetylhydrolase is a secreted phospholipase A2 with a catalytic triad," *Journal of Biological Chemistry*, vol. 270, no. 43, pp. 25481–25487, 1995.

[19] D. E. Lorant, K. D. Patel, T. M. McIntyre, R. P. McEver, S. M. Prescott, and G. A. Zimmerman, "Coexpression of GMP-140 and PAF by endothelium stimulated by histamine or thrombin: a juxtacrine system for adhesion and activation of neutrophils," *Journal of Cell Biology*, vol. 115, no. 1, pp. 223–234, 1991.

[20] C. D. Johnson, "Platelet-activating factor and platelet-activating factor antagonists in acute pancreatitis," *Digestive Surgery*, vol. 16, no. 2, pp. 93–101, 1999.

[21] B. Ersoy, A. Hüseyinov, and Ş. Darcan, "The role of platelet-activating factor in pathogenesis of type 1 diabetes," *Diabetes Care*, vol. 28, no. 4, p. 980, 2005.

[22] D. Schlondorff and R. Neuwirth, "Platelet-activating factor and the kidney," *The American Journal of Physiology*, vol. 251, no. 1, part 2, pp. F1–F11, 1986.

[23] Q. Zhang, Y. Yao, R. L. Konger et al., "UVB radiation-mediated inhibition of contact hypersensitivity reactions is dependent on the platelet-activating factor system," *Journal of Investigative Dermatology*, vol. 128, no. 7, pp. 1780–1787, 2008.

[24] L. A. Muehlmann, P. V. Michelotto, E. A. Nunes, F. C. C. Grando, F. T. D. Silva, and A. Nishiyama, "PAF increases phagocytic capacity and superoxide anion production in equine alveolar macrophages and blood neutrophils," *Research in Veterinary Science*, vol. 93, no. 1, pp. 393–397, 2012.

[25] S. M. Prescott, G. A. Zimmerman, D. M. Stafforini, and T. M. McIntyre, "Platelet-activating factor and related lipid mediators," *Annual Review of Biochemistry*, vol. 69, pp. 419–445, 2000.

[26] S. Ishii, T. Kuwaki, T. Nagase et al., "Impaired anaphylactic responses with intact sensitivity to endotoxin in mice lacking a platelet-activating factor receptor," *Journal of Experimental Medicine*, vol. 187, no. 11, pp. 1779–1788, 1998.

[27] V. A. Fadok, M. L. Warner, D. L. Bratton, and P. M. Henson, "CD36 is required for phagocytosis of apoptotic cells by human macrophages that use either a phosphatidylserine receptor or the vitronectin receptor ($\alpha(V)\beta 3$)," *The Journal of Immunology*, vol. 161, no. 11, pp. 6250–6257, 1998.

[28] L. C. Meagher, J. S. Savill, A. Baker, R. W. Fuller, and C. Haslett, "Phagocytosis of apoptotic neutrophils does not induce macrophage release of thromboxane B2," *Journal of Leukocyte Biology*, vol. 52, no. 3, pp. 269–273, 1992.

[29] J. S. Savill, A. H. Wyllie, J. E. Henson, M. J. Walport, P. M. Henson, and C. Haslett, "Macrophage phagocytosis of aging neutrophils in inflammation. Programmed cell death in the neutrophil leads to its recognition by macrophages," *Journal of Clinical Investigation*, vol. 83, no. 3, pp. 865–875, 1989.

[30] N. G. Bazan, S. P. Squinto, P. Braquet, T. Panetta, and V. L. Marcheselli, "Platelet-activating factor and polyunsaturated fatty acids in cerebral ischemia or convulsions: intracellular PAF-binding sites and activation of a fos/jun/AP-1 transcriptional signaling system," *Lipids*, vol. 26, no. 12, pp. 1236–1242, 1991.

[31] S. Ishii and T. Shimizu, "Platelet-activating factor (PAF) receptor and genetically engineered PAF receptor mutant mice," *Progress in Lipid Research*, vol. 39, no. 1, pp. 41–82, 2000.

[32] Y.-I. Jeong, I. D. Jung, C.-M. Lee et al., "The novel role of platelet-activating factor in protecting mice against lipopolysaccharide-induced endotoxic shock," *PLoS ONE*, vol. 4, no. 8, Article ID e6503, 2009.

[33] B. L. Slomiany and A. Slomiany, "Platelet activating factor mediates helicobacter pylori lipopolysaccharide interference with gastric mucin synthesis," *IUBMB Life*, vol. 56, no. 1, pp. 41–46, 2004.

[34] B. L. Slomiany and A. Slomiany, "Platelet-activating factor mediates Porphyromonas gingivalis lipopolysaccharide interference with salivary mucin synthesis via phosphatidylinositol 3-kinase-dependent constitutive nitric-oxide synthase activation," *Journal of Physiology and Pharmacology*, vol. 55, no. 1, part 1, pp. 85–98, 2004.

[35] B. L. Slomiany and A. Slomiany, "Differential role of platelet-activating factor in gastric mucosal ulcer healing," *Inflammopharmacology*, vol. 11, no. 3, pp. 237–248, 2003.

[36] J. P. Walterscheid, S. E. Ullrich, and D. X. Nghiem, "Platelet-activating factor, a molecular sensor for cellular damage, activates systemic immune suppression," *Journal of Experimental Medicine*, vol. 195, no. 2, pp. 171–179, 2002.

[37] P. Gasse, N. Riteau, S. Charron et al., "Uric acid is a danger signal activating NALP3 inflammasome in lung injury inflammation and fibrosis," *The American Journal of Respiratory and Critical Care Medicine*, vol. 179, no. 10, pp. 903–913, 2009.

14

Curbing Inflammation in Skin Wound Healing

Rodrigo G. Rosique, Marina J. Rosique, and Jayme A. Farina Junior

Division of Plastic Surgery, Department of Surgery and Anatomy, Ribeirão Preto School of Medicine, University of São Paulo, Avenida Bandeirantes 3900, 14048-900 Ribeirão Preto, SP, Brazil

Correspondence should be addressed to Jayme A. Farina Junior; jafarinajr@fmrp.usp.br

Academic Editor: B. L. Slomiany

Wound healing is a complex regulated process that results in skin scar formation in postnatal mammals. Chronic wounds are major medical problems that can confer devastating consequences. Currently, there are no treatments to prevent scarring. In the early fetus wounds heal without scarring and the healing process is characterized by relatively less inflammation compared to adults; therefore, research aimed at reducing the inflammatory process related to wound healing might speed healing and improve the final scar appearance.

1. Introduction

The skin is the largest organ of the body and acts as the first line of defense against pathogens, toxins, and trauma. It also plays a critical role in fluid homeostasis and provides sensory functions and thermal regulation. Damage or loss of skin integrity resulting from an injury or disease can lead to significant morbidity and even death.

Wound healing is a complex, regulated process in which regulated collagen deposition, in response to tissue injury, results in scar formation. Its mechanisms include inflammation, fibroplasia, and scar maturation.

Sometimes cutaneous wounds do not progress to normal healing with formation of a final mature scar formation but to a continuing inflammatory process, which can lead to a more aggressive carcinogenic transformation in long time of evolution (Marjolin's Ulcer). Many chronic wounds are the result of chronic inflammation. In contrast to adult wound healing, the early gestation fetus displays a remarkable ability to heal wounds without scarring. Fetal wounds heal rapidly and are characterized by a relative lack of inflammation [1]. The introduction of inflammation into normally scarless wounds produces scarring [2]. Conversely, reduction of inflammation in postnatal wounds can reduce scarring [3].

In this paper, we review how to curb inflammation in cutaneous wound healing; the following lists the main topics discussed in this paper.

Topics about Curbing Inflammation in Wound Healing

General Topics

(i) Wet environment.

(ii) Primary closure and sutures.

(iii) Drugs or supplement:

- (a) curcumin,
- (b) protein supplementation,
- (c) nutraceuticals,
- (d) neurotensin (NT),
- (e) photodynamic therapy (PDT),
- (f) doxycycline,
- (g) tumour necrosis factor-alpha (TNF-α) antibody.

(iv) Technology:

- (a) transcutaneous electrical nerve stimulation (TENS),
- (b) hyperbaric oxygen,
- (c) silver dressings,
- (d) negative pressure wound therapy (NPWT).

(v) Biomaterials and cellular therapy.

Specific Wounds

(i) Diabetic wounds.

(ii) Vascular wounds.

(iii) Irradiated wounds.

2. Postnatal Wound Healing Process

Repair of the skin consists of three phases: an initial inflammatory phase and then a proliferative/repair phase and it concludes with a remodeling phase, which results in scar formation in postnatal mammals.

In response to tissue injury, inflammatory cells are recruited to wounded tissue. The acute inflammatory response is followed by proliferation of fibroblasts, which are responsible for synthesizing collagen and extracellular matrix. Fibroblasts can differentiate into myofibroblasts, which are responsible for collagen deposition and wound contraction. Ultimately, a scar results from accumulation of extracellular matrix. Despite scar remodeling during maturation, normal architecture is never completely restored [4]; only 70 percent of the tensile strength of normal skin is recovered [5].

The early stage of inflammation is regarded as a critical period of the wound healing process, essential for clearing contaminating bacteria and creating an environment conducive to the succeeding events of tissue repair and regeneration [6]. The injury causes a gap, which is immediately filled by clots in the presence of platelet aggregates. Then, during the inflammatory phase, leukocytes, such as neutrophils, monocytes, and macrophages, infiltrate the site, remove the breakdown products of the injured cells and clots, and release various growth factors and cytokines [7]. In response to growth factors and cytokines, the proliferative phase starts. In this phase, epidermal cells migrate, proliferate to fill the wound gap, and displace remnants of the original clots. Thus, it is generally accepted that leukocyte and macrophage infiltration is essential to wound healing.

Cytokines have been widely studied because they are important to wound healing; they regulate the activity of the cells that produce the healing response to tissue injury [8]. Several cytokines, including interleukin- (IL-) 1β and tumor necrosis factor- (TNF-) α, have been shown to regulate the recruitment and function of neutrophils. In irradiated mice, an investigation of the ability of exogenous IL-1β or transforming growth factor-β to reverse radiation-induced defective wound healing found that IL-1β enhanced wound tensile strength [9]. TNF-α is a major cytokine secreted by macrophages and neutrophils during the inflammation phase of wound healing; it is elevated in early wound healing [10].

In all phases of wound repair, extracellular matrix (ECM) proteins play a key role in directing the fate and activities of progenitor and reparative cells. Immediately after injury, the ECM orchestrates the recruitment of platelets and directs the inflammatory cell response that initiates the hemostatic and the cellular debridement phases [11]. These cells, which migrate into the wound bed of the ECM of the initial hemostatic plug and then migrate into the provisional matrix, respond to individual ECM components and growth factors (which may be bound to this matrix). These cells, in turn, recruit and direct stem/progenitor and reparative cells from both distant and local sites to mediate the proliferative/repair phase of healing. Particularly, in this rebuilding phase of healing, adult stem cells participate critically in replenishing cells that were damaged or lost after injury. In addition to their role after trauma, adult stem cells participate in the maintenance of the skin as well as wound healing [12].

3. General Topics

3.1. Wet Environment. A wet or moist environment in wounds has been shown to promote reepithelialization and result in reduced scar formation more than a dry environment [13]. The inflammatory reaction is reduced in the wet environment, thereby limiting injury progression. Several studies have compared wet, moist, and dry healing. A wet or moist incubator-like microenvironment achieves fastest healing with fewest aberrations and least scar formation.

The modern approach of employing a moist environment for the treatment of wounds was introduced in the early 1960s by Winter [14], who showed in a pig model that the rate of epithelialization after wounding was doubled by using a moist dressing as compared to dry conditions. This was a new concept that opposed the generally accepted idea that a dry environment could best fight wound infection.

Manufacturers responded to Winter's research findings and provided a wide range of moist dressings, such as hydrocolloids that absorb the wound fluid beneath a semiocclusive dressing [15], foams [16, 17], alginates [18], and hydrogels [19, 20]. Using the Cochrane database, Dumville et al. [21–24] performed systematic reviews of the four types of wound dressings to evaluate their contribution to the healing of diabetic ulcers. A systematic review by Wiechula [25] suggests that moist wound healing products have distinct clinical advantages over dry products for the management of split-thickness skin donor sites.

Adult human skin wounds heal with varying degrees of scar formation [26]. Scarring is correlated with the intensity and duration of inflammation during healing [27]. In 2009, Reish et al. [28] published an experimental study of porcine wounds treated either in a moist environment or with gauze: inflammation was compared by evaluating the number of inflammatory cells/high-power field 3 days after wounding. Inflammation was greatly reduced in the wounds treated in the wound chamber, and the number of inflammatory cells on day 3 was very strongly correlated with the amount of scarring at day 28. Compared with dry wounds, wet wounds created under sterile conditions and treated with low concentrations of antibiotics exhibited a significantly smaller macroscopic scar surface area in all experimental wound groups. Wounds with a greater inflammatory cell infiltrate could be predicted to develop more residual scarring.

3.2. Primary Closure and Sutures. Surgical sutures are used universally to achieve proper wound approximation by supporting the strain of closure until sufficient healing has occurred. Approximating the wound wedges with sutures decreases the wound area subjected to the healing process and abbreviates the inflammatory phase, which decreases scarring due to the faster pace of healing. All sutures are foreign bodies; therefore their presence triggers a local immune response. Thereby sutures may, paradoxically, potentiate and extend the inflammatory phase of wound healing, resulting in undesirable outcomes, such as wound breakdown, suture "spitting," hypertrophic scar, or keloid formation. The degree of inflammation induced varies with suture composition, which ranges from relatively inert polypropylene and nylon to highly inflammatory silk and plain gut suture. As a result, numerous investigations have attempted to alter suture composition with the goal of reducing the inflammatory response; however, no specific composition has gained clinical relevance or widespread practice [29].

3.3. Drugs or Supplement

3.3.1. Curcumin. Kant et al. [30] found that curcumin, an anti-inflammatory and antioxidant agent, caused faster and better wound healing in diabetic rats. This effect was attributed to a decreased expression of inflammatory cytokines and enzymes, TNF-α, IL-1β, and MMP-9, and increased levels of the anti-inflammatory cytokine IL-10 and antioxidant enzymes, SOD, catalase, and GPx, at the wound site in diabetic rats. This data allows us to suggest that curcumin could be an additional novel therapeutic agent for the management of impaired wound healing in diabetics and radiated tissues [31, 32].

3.3.2. Protein Supplementation. Abdel-Salam [33] demonstrated that whey (milk serum) protein could contribute to cutaneous wound healing. In this investigation, wound closure was significantly delayed in the diabetic group. Moreover, the results clearly demonstrated that whey protein supplementation of diabetic animals enhanced wound closure and restored proinflammatory (IL-1β, IL-6, and TNF-α) and anti-inflammatory cytokine (IL-4 and IL-10) levels nearly to the levels of control animals. These findings support the hypothesis that delayed wound healing in diabetic animals is caused by deregulation of signaling molecules that are critical mediators of the inflammatory response.

3.3.3. Nutraceuticals. Serra et al. [34] evaluated the effects of a new nutraceutical on both clinical and molecular parameters in patients with chronic vascular ulcers, since bioflavonoids were shown to have provessel activities along with anti-inflammatory, antioxidant, and phlebotonic effects in the treatment of chronic venous disease. They found that it decreases inflammatory cytokine, MMPs and NGAL, levels and both improved symptoms and accelerated wound healing.

3.3.4. Neurotensin (NT). Based on findings that peripheral nerves and cutaneous neurobiology contribute to correct wound healing [35], Moura et al. [36] studied the effect of neurotensin (NT), a neuropeptide that acts as an inflammatory modulator in wound healing. They prepared a collagen-based dressing as vehicle to deliver NT, applied it to diabetic mice, and found that it can effectively support NT's release into diabetic wounds, enhancing the healing process. Nevertheless, compared to treatment with NT alone, a more prominent scar was observed in diabetic wounds treated with the collagen-based dressing.

3.3.5. Photodynamic Therapy (PDT). Reports of animal studies indicate that photodynamic therapy (PDT) improves healing of excisional wounds but the mechanism is uncertain. Mills et al. [37] first reported the effect of PDT on healing of acute excisional wounds in humans. They showed that treatment with methyl aminolevulinate- (MAL-) PDT modulated clinical and microscopic indicators of healing and, ultimately, produced scars with improved dermal matrix architecture. Pivotally, the number of TGF-b3-producing cells was significantly higher in MAL-PDT-treated wounds than in controls after 3 weeks, with an elevated TGF-b3 : b1 ratio. At 9 months, MAL-PDT-treated wounds showed improved deposition and organization of dermal matrix protein at the histological level. Thus, this regimen of PDT of wounds appears to mediate an antiscarring phenotype, with TGF-b3 as a potential key modulator.

3.3.6. Doxycycline. Serra et al. [38] documented that doxycycline improved healing of chronic venous ulcers. In their study, oral low doses of doxycycline 20 mg were administrated for 3 months to a group of patients. The treated patients showed a higher healing rate compared to control group. Doxycycline has anti-inflammatory and immunomodulatory effects, through the inhibition of metalloproteinases, representing a potential solution to support wound healing.

3.3.7. Tumour Necrosis Factor-Alpha (TNF-α) Antibody Infliximab. Therapeutic antibodies such as infliximab can inhibit TNF-α activity. In a case series [39], infliximab was applied topically to eight patients with 14 chronic ulcers of more than 4-month duration, which failed to respond to any previous conventional treatment. Infliximab was applied repeatedly to ulcers either as a 10 mg/mL solution or as a gel formulation (0.45, 1, or 4.5 mg/g). The authors observed, after 8 weeks, that five ulcers completely healed, while another four were reduced by more than 75% in size.

3.4. Technology

3.4.1. Transcutaneous Electrical Nerve Stimulation (TENS). Transcutaneous electrical nerve stimulation (TENS) has been shown to accelerate the healing of chronic wounds in human subjects and induced wounds in animal models [40, 41]. More specifically, it has been shown to significantly increase the rate of wound epithelialization [40] and contraction [42]. Kutlu et al. [43] demonstrated that TENS of incised wounds improves healing by increasing growth factors (epidermal growth factor, platelet-derived growth factor-A, and fibroblast growth factor-2) in the dermis and epidermis. In a later study, Gürgen et al. [44] showed marked decreases in the levels of proinflammatory cytokines in the dermis of the TENS-treated group, which suggests that TENS shortened the healing process by inhibiting the inflammation phase.

3.4.2. Hyperbaric Oxygen. Hyperbaric oxygen therapy (HBOT), an effective tool that helps skin wound healing, is defined as delivery of 100% oxygen at greater than one atmospheric pressure (ATA) into the core of the wound [45]. Delivery of this increased amount of oxygen to the cells of unhealed tissues expedites healing of subacute and chronic cutaneous wounds [46].

Hyperbaric oxygen works by the following four dominant mechanisms:

(1) Augmented hydroxylation: it helps improve collagen synthesis.

(2) Angiogenesis: HBOT creates a large oxygen gradient between the center and periphery of the wound that strongly stimulates angiogenesis, which is seminal for wound healing [47].

(3) Increased bactericidal activity.

(4) Increased collagen deposition.

Kalani et al. showed that when diabetic foot ulcers were treated with HBOT, after 3 years of therapy, they healed completely in 76% of patients, whereas the ulcers of only 48% patients healed completely with conventional treatment [48]. In a randomized study by Kessler et al., either HBOT or standard treatment was given to 28 hospitalized patients with neuropathic ulcers (Wagner grades I to III). After two weeks of treatment, the ulcer area was reduced by half in the HBOT group (41.8 ± 25.5 versus $21.7 \pm 16.9\%$, $P = 0.037$). This improvement, however, disappeared at the two-week follow-up [49].

3.4.3. Silver Dressings. Ionized silver (Ag+) has both anti-inflammatory and antimicrobial properties with a broad spectrum of action [50–52]. Jemec et al. [53] found that treatment with silver dressings during the initial four weeks produced a total cost saving compared with treatment with nonsilver dressings. In addition, the wounds of patients treated with silver dressings closed faster than those treated with nonsilver dressings. Bisson et al. [54] found that silver dressings produced significant anti-inflammatory effects in chronic skin inflammation. It is believed that silver can improve wound healing due to its antimicrobial and anti-inflammatory properties.

Wu et al. [55] found that nanocrystalline silver can also reduce inflammation and promote scald wound healing in animal models. Sibbald et al. [56] concluded that evidence indicates that nanocrystalline silver dressings may reduce bacterial levels, decrease the chronic inflammatory response, and thus promote wound healing. Likewise, healing of chronic venous leg ulcers was associated with less wound bacteria and less neutrophilic inflammation but was associated with persistent or high lymphocyte count; greater numbers of lymphocytes were associated with more reduction in ulcer size.

3.4.4. Negative Pressure Wound Therapy (NPWT). According to prospective and retrospective clinical and experimental studies [57, 58], negative pressure wound therapy (NPWT) has been widely used to facilitate healing of acute and chronic wounds. This therapy has been shown to provide a moist wound healing environment, increase granulation tissue formation, reduce edema, and stimulate angiogenesis and blood flow to the wound margins [59–63]. In a retrospective clinical study, Torbrand et al. [64] attributed these biological effects to the evenly distributed transduction of negative pressure to the wound bed by a vacuum pump.

The impact of NPWT on local expression of proinflammatory cytokines, the number of neutrophils, and the bacterial bioburden living on the wound surface suggest that NPWT of acutely infected soft-tissue wounds leads to increased local IL-1β and IL-8 expression in the early phase of inflammation, which may trigger infiltration of neutrophils and thus accelerate bacterial clearance. Furthermore, the success of NPWT of acute wounds can attenuate the expression of TNF-α, and this effect may partly explain why NPWT does not significantly impair wound healing [65].

NPWT not only enhances the granulation tissue in the more superficial layer of the wound bed but also appears to affect deeper layers, with relief of chronic inflammation and tissue stabilization. It is believed that NPWT removes excess fluid and thereby removes proteolytic enzymes that negatively influence the healing process [66].

Interestingly, studies have shown that the activity of some matrix metalloproteinases (MMPs) is elevated in chronic wounds and the presence of these molecules is related to impairing wound healing. For instance, high concentrations of MMP-9 and high MMP-9 : tissue inhibitors of MMP (TIMP-1) ratio in wound fluid predict poor wound healing in diabetic foot ulcers [67]. In addition, in chronic wound exudates, mainly MMP-1 type collagenase is present [68]. These findings may partially explain the cause of difficult healing in chronic wounds.

On the other hand, data strongly suggest that NPWT influences the microenvironment of the wound by reducing the levels of MMPs and the MMP : TIMP ratio. Mouës et al. [69] found significantly lower levels of pro-MMP-9 and a lower total MMP-9 : TIMP-1 ratio in TNP-treated wounds during 10 days of follow-up. Stechmiller et al. showed that NPWT-treated wounds had decreased levels of MMP-3 and MMP-9 and lower MMP-3 : TIMP-1 ratios in wound fluid from pressure ulcers [70]. NPWT may lower collagenase activity and thereby prevent exaggerated degradation of collagen and promote wound healing.

In addition, some studies compared different types of interface material for the application of NPWT with other common dressings. Tuncel et al. [71], who studied dressings applied to rabbit wounds, found NPWT superior to control saline-moistened gauze dressing but found no difference among three different interface materials (polyurethane foam, saline soaked antimicrobial gauze, and loofah sponge) used in association with NPWT (Figure 1).

3.5. Biomaterials and Cellular Therapy. The use of acellular and cell-based tissue-engineered dermal substitutes has become increasingly routine [72]. Dermal matrices and other biomimetic scaffolds for delivery of adult stem cells have been shown to augment the regenerative potential of mesenchymal

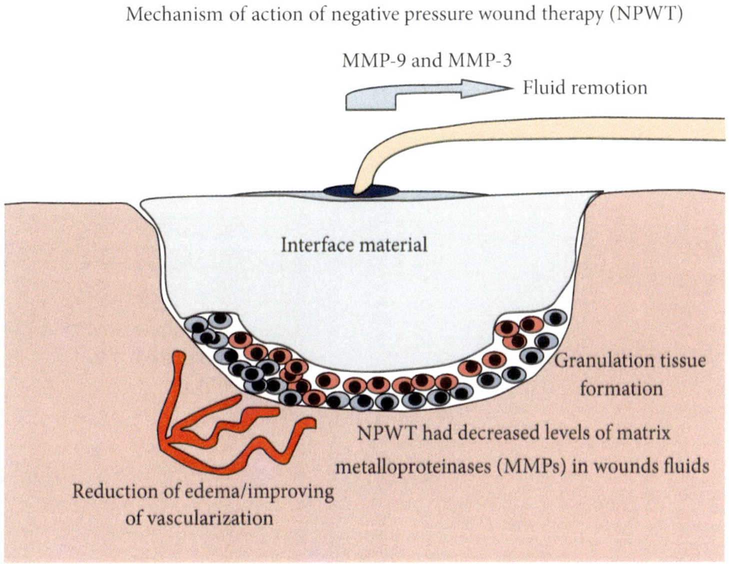

FIGURE 1: Demonstration of the principal mechanisms of action attributed to NPWT.

stem cells (MSCs) and enhance wound healing through their presumptive ability to recreate a regenerative niche [73–75]. Besides their ability to improve the efficiency and quality of cutaneous wound healing, existing products have not yet been able to promote repair that approximates uninjured skin. The continuous evolution of superior biomaterials will depend upon a greater understanding of the role that individual components play in the regenerative niches of uninjured and injured skin, particularly the ECM constituents. Further, the development of successful biomimetic and bioresponsive substrates should incorporate the knowledge of not only how cells interact with these substrates but also how these cells then respond by remodelling and depositing their own ECM.

Of note, tissue engineering and regenerative medicine have shown significant promise in treatment of problematic wounds. Initial proof-of-principle studies that investigated the use of exogenously applied adult stem cells for the treatment of chronic wounds provided support for their vulnerary effects [76, 77]. MSCs have been shown to improve wound healing through their ability to directly contribute cells and ECM components to the repair process, as well as their ability to direct other cells participating in the repair process through their production of paracrine mediators (Figure 2) [78]. Human MSCs appear to have potent immune regulatory actions that make them attractive for use in human diseases that involve tissue injury and/or inflammation. Although initial attempts with injection of cells alone showed improved healing, it is clear that delivery strategies that reproduce complex stem cell niches will be required to maximize their potential. Given the ability of the ECM to influence many key aspects of that niche, such as signaling events, regulation of growth factor bioavailability, and mechanosensation, the identification of specific ECM components that most accurately recreate a functional stem cell niche for incorporation into therapeutic biomaterials remains a focus of intense investigation.

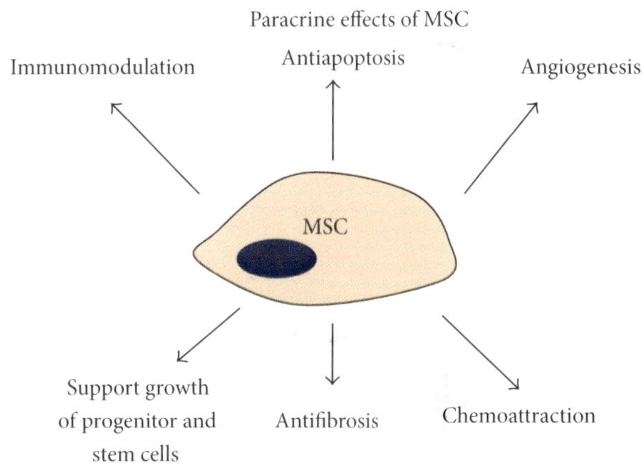

FIGURE 2: Paracrine effects of cultured mesenchymal stem cells (MSCs). It is now believed that the secretion of a wide variety of bioactive molecules may be the major mechanism by which CMMs achieve their therapeutic effect. This mechanism can be categorized into these six major actions: immunomodulatory, antiapoptosis, angiogenesis, support of the growth and differentiation of stem cells and progenitor sites, scarring modulation, and chemotaxis [78].

4. Specific Wounds

4.1. Diabetic Wound. Diabetes is a multisystem disorder, and its complications induce physiological changes in tissues and cells that impair the normal healing process. However, the pathophysiologic relationship between diabetes and impaired healing is complex. Diabetic wounds become halted in the inflammatory phase, which is characterized by a continuing influx of neutrophils that release cytotoxic enzymes, free radicals, and inflammatory mediators that cause extensive collateral damage to surrounding tissue. These destructive processes counteract the healing process in such wounds, and the overproduction of free radicals, which induce oxidative stress, results in detrimental cytotoxic effects that delay wound healing [79, 80].

Increased oxidative stress is one of the most common reasons for the delayed wound healing in the diabetic population [81]. Therefore, reduction/termination of the persistent inflammation and elimination of free radicals by the introduction of anti-inflammatory agents and antioxidants into the treatment of wounds could be an important strategy to improve healing of diabetic wounds [80].

4.2. Vascular Wound. Chronic venous, lower limb ulceration (VLU) affects 1–3% of the adult population worldwide, [82] and some patients suffer repeated cycles of ulceration, healing, and recurrence. The underlying pathogenesis of these hard-to-heal VLUs is complicated by excessive and prolonged inflammation that is often related to critical microbial colonization and early localized infection [83, 84]. A heavy bioburden of colonizing microorganisms in the wound may be one of the most important barriers to wound closure [85].

Pathophysiological events involved in the onset of chronic venous ulceration are inflammation, activation of polymorphonucleates (PMNs), and secretion of proteases such as MMPs, which degrade the ECM that supports the vascular and tissue walls. MMPs, neutrophil gelatinase-associated lipocalin (NGAL), and inflammatory cytokines are overexpressed in VLUs, and they could play a central role in pathophysiological mechanisms of skin lesions and delayed wound healing.

4.3. Irradiated Wound. Approximately 50% of cancer patients receive radiation as an adjuvant therapy. Although radiation therapy technology has progressed substantially in the last decades, patients still suffer from various degrees of nonspecific radiation damage to noncancerous tissues. Radiation ulcers have posed an enormous challenge to reconstructive surgeons; also, they cause great distress to patients, impair their quality of life, and consume high amounts of medical resources. These kinds of chronic wounds can last for several years, and some may even lead to amputations. Strategies for treating these and other chronic wounds may include the use of various growth factors [86–88], hyperbaric oxygen [89], and stem cells [90].

5. Conclusion

Over the last fifty years, the complex wound healing process became clearer allowing the development of strategies, devices, and medications that help achieve a better final scar, mainly through strategies to curb the wound-related inflammation. Nonetheless, we are still far from definitely solving the chronic wounds or the pathologic scarring issue and, even more, achieving the goal of rapid and scarless healing similar to fetal one.

References

[1] K. Moore, R. McCallion, R. J. Searle, M. C. Stacey, and K. G. Harding, "Prediction and monitoring the therapeutic response of chronic dermal wounds," *International Wound Journal*, vol. 3, no. 2, pp. 89–96, 2006.

[2] F. W. Frantz, D. A. Bettinger, J. H. Haynes et al., "Biology of fetal repair: the presence of bacteria in fetal wounds induces an adult-like healing response," *Journal of Pediatric Surgery*, vol. 28, no. 3, pp. 428–434, 1993.

[3] G. S. Ashcroft, X. Yang, A. B. Glick et al., "Mice lacking Smad3 show accelerated wound healing and an impaired local inflammatory response," *Nature Cell Biology*, vol. 1, no. 5, pp. 260–266, 1999.

[4] A. S. Colwell, T.-T. Phan, W. Kong, M. T. Longaker, and P. H. Lorenz, "Hypertrophic scar fibroblasts have increased connective tissue growth factor expression after transforming growth factor-β stimulation," *Plastic and Reconstructive Surgery*, vol. 116, no. 5, pp. 1387–1390, 2005.

[5] J. W. Madden and E. E. Peacock Jr., "Studies on the biology of collagen during wound healing. 3. Dynamic metabolism of scar collagen and remodeling of dermal wounds," *Annals of Surgery*, vol. 174, no. 3, pp. 511–520, 1971.

[6] A. M. Mercado, N. Quan, D. A. Padgett, J. F. Sheridan, and P. T. Marucha, "Restraint stress alters the expression of interleukin-1 and keratinocyte growth factor at the wound site: an in situ hybridization study," *Journal of Neuroimmunology*, vol. 129, no. 1-2, pp. 74–83, 2002.

[7] A. J. Singer and R. A. F. Clark, "Cutaneous wound healing," *The New England Journal of Medicine*, vol. 341, no. 10, pp. 738–746, 1999.

[8] T. Molloy, Y. Wang, and G. A. C. Murrell, "The roles of growth factors in tendon and ligament healing," *Sports Medicine*, vol. 33, no. 5, pp. 381–394, 2003.

[9] V. Vegesna, W. H. McBride, J. M. G. Taylor, and H. R. Withers, "The effect of interleukin-1 beta or transforming growth factor-beta on radiation-impaired murine skin wound healing," *Journal of Surgical Research*, vol. 59, no. 6, pp. 699–704, 1995.

[10] A. Goel, S. Kumar, D. K. Singh, and A. K. Bhatia, "Wound healing potential of *Ocimum sanctum* linn. with induction of tumor necrosis factor-α," *Indian Journal of Experimental Biology*, vol. 48, no. 4, pp. 402–406, 2010.

[11] G. S. Schultz, J. M. Davidson, R. S. Kirsner, P. Bornstein, and I. M. Herman, "Dynamic reciprocity in the wound microenvironment," *Wound Repair and Regeneration*, vol. 19, no. 2, pp. 134–148, 2011.

[12] S. W. Volk, S. A. Iqbal, and A. Bayat, "Interactions of the extracellular matrix and progenitor cells in cutaneous wound healing," *Advances in Wound Care*, vol. 2, no. 6, pp. 261–272, 2013.

[13] J. P. Junker, R. A. Kamel, E. J. Caterson, and E. Eriksson, "Clinical impact upon wound healing and inflammation in moist, wet, and dry environments," *Advances in Wound Care*, vol. 2, no. 7, pp. 348–356, 2013.

[14] G. D. Winter, "Formation of the scab and the rate of epithelization of superficial wounds in the skin of the young domestic pig," *Nature*, vol. 193, no. 4812, pp. 293–294, 1962.

[15] A. Singh, S. Halder, G. R. Menon et al., "Meta-analysis of randomized controlled trials on hydrocolloid occlusive dressing versus conventional gauze dressing in the healing of chronic wounds," *Asian Journal of Surgery*, vol. 27, no. 4, pp. 326–332, 2004.

[16] K. Carter, "Hydropolymer dressings in the management of wound exudate," *British Journal of Community Nursing*, vol. 8, no. 9, supplement, pp. S10–S16, 2003.

[17] J. Fletcher, "The application of foam dressings," *Nursing Times*, vol. 99, no. 31, p. 59, 2003.

[18] D. Piacquadio and D. B. Nelson, "Alginates: a 'new' dressing alternative," *Journal of Dermatologic Surgery and Oncology*, vol. 18, no. 11, pp. 992–995, 1992.

[19] D. Eisenbud, H. Hunter, L. Kessler et al., "Hydrogel wound dressings: where do we stand in 2003?" *Ostomy Wound Manage*, vol. 49, no. 10, pp. 52–57, 2003.

[20] B. Kickhöfen, H. Wokalek, D. Scheel, and H. Ruh, "Chemical and physical properties of a hydrogel wound dressing," *Biomaterials*, vol. 7, no. 1, pp. 67–72, 1986.

[21] J. C. Dumville, S. Deshpande, S. O'Meara, and K. Speak, "Hydrocolloid dressings for healing diabetic foot ulcers," *Cochrane Database of Systematic Reviews*, vol. 2, Article ID CD009099, 2012.

[22] J. C. Dumville, S. Deshpande, S. O'Meara, and K. Speak, "Foam dressings for healing diabetic foot ulcers," *Cochrane Database of Systematic Reviews*, vol. 9, Article ID CD009111, 2011.

[23] J. C. Dumville, S. O'Meara, S. Deshpande, and K. Speak, "Alginate dressings for healing diabetic foot ulcers," *Cochrane Database of Systematic Reviews*, vol. 2, Article ID CD009110, 2012.

[24] J. C. Dumville, S. O'Meara, S. Deshpande, and K. Speak, "Hydrogel dressings for healing diabetic foot ulcers," *Cochrane Database of Systematic Reviews*, no. 9, Article ID CD009101, 2011.

[25] R. Wiechula, "The use of moist wound-healing dressings in the management of split-thickness skin graft donor sites: a systematic review," *International Journal of Nursing Practice*, vol. 9, no. 2, pp. S9–S17, 2003.

[26] B. S. Atiyeh, C. A. Amm, and K. A. El Musa, "Improved scar quality following primary and secondary healing of cutaneous wounds," *Aesthetic Plastic Surgery*, vol. 27, no. 5, pp. 411–417, 2003.

[27] M. C. Robson and A. Barbul, "Guidelines for the best care of chronic wounds," *Wound Repair and Regeneration*, vol. 14, no. 6, pp. 647–648, 2006.

[28] R. G. Reish, B. Zuhaili, J. Bergmann et al., "Modulation of scarring in a liquid environment in the Yorkshire pig," *Wound Repair and Regeneration*, vol. 17, no. 6, pp. 806–816, 2009.

[29] T. Georgiev-Hristov, M. García-Arranz, I. García-Gómez et al., "Sutures enriched with adipose-derived stem cells decrease the local acute inflammation after tracheal anastomosis in a murine model," *European Journal of Cardio-Thoracic Surgery*, vol. 42, no. 3, pp. e40–e47, 2012.

[30] V. Kant, A. Gopal, N. N. Pathak, P. Kumar, S. K. Tandan, and D. Kumar, "Antioxidant and anti-inflammatory potential of curcumin accelerated the cutaneous wound healing in streptozotocin-induced diabetic rats," *International Immunopharmacology*, vol. 20, no. 2, pp. 322–330, 2014.

[31] G. S. Sidhu, H. Mani, J. P. Gaddipati et al., "Curcumin enhances wound healing in streptozotocin induced diabetic rats and genetically diabetic mice," *Wound Repair and Regeneration*, vol. 7, no. 5, pp. 362–374, 1999.

[32] G. C. Jagetia and G. K. Rajanikant, "Acceleration of wound repair by curcumin in the excision wound of mice exposed to different doses of fractionated gamma radiation," *International Wound Journal*, vol. 9, no. 1, pp. 76–92, 2012.

[33] B. K. A.-H. Abdel-Salam, "Modulatory effect of whey proteins in some cytokines involved in wound healing in male diabetic albino rats ," *Inflammation*, vol. 37, no. 5, pp. 1616–1622, 2014.

[34] R. Serra, R. Grande, L. Butrico et al., "Effects of a new nutraceutical substance on clinical and molecular parameters in patients with chronic venous ulceration," *International Wound Journal*, 2014.

[35] L. Pradhan, C. Nabzdyk, N. D. Andersen, F. W. LoGerfo, and A. Veves, "Inflammation and neuropeptides: the connection in diabetic wound healing," *Expert Reviews in Molecular Medicine*, vol. 11, article e2, 2009.

[36] L. I. F. Moura, A. M. A. Dias, E. Suesca et al., "Neurotensin-loaded collagen dressings reduce inflammation and improve wound healing in diabetic mice," *Biochimica et Biophysica Acta—Molecular Basis of Disease*, vol. 1842, no. 1, pp. 32–43, 2014.

[37] S. J. Mills, M. D. Farrar, G. S. Ashcroft, C. E. M. Griffiths, M. J. Hardman, and L. E. Rhodes, "Topical photodynamic therapy following excisional wounding of human skin increases production of transforming growth factor-$\beta 3$ and matrix metalloproteinases 1 and 9, with associated improvement in dermal matrix organization," *British Journal of Dermatology*, vol. 171, no. 1, pp. 55–62, 2014.

[38] R. Serra, L. Gallelli, G. Buffone et al., "Doxycycline speeds up healing of chronic venous ulcers," *International Wound Journal*, vol. 12, no. 2, pp. 179–184, 2015.

[39] M. Streit, Z. Beleznay, and L. R. Braathen, "Topical application of the tumour necrosis factor-α antibody infliximab improves healing of chronic wounds," *International Wound Journal*, vol. 3, no. 3, pp. 171–191, 2006.

[40] O. M. Alvarez, P. M. Mertz, R. V. Smerbeck, and W. H. Eaglstein, "The healing of superficial skin wounds is stimulated by external electrical current," *Journal of Investigative Dermatology*, vol. 81, no. 2, pp. 144–148, 1983.

[41] M. Brown, M. K. McDonnell, and D. N. Menton, "Polarity effects on wound healing using electric stimulation in rabbits," *Archives of Physical Medicine and Rehabilitation*, vol. 70, no. 8, pp. 624–627, 1989.

[42] B. V. Stromberg, "Effects of electrical currents on wound contraction," *Annals of Plastic Surgery*, vol. 21, no. 2, pp. 121–123, 1988.

[43] A. K. Kutlu, D. Çeçen, S. G. Gürgen, O. Sayn, and F. Çetin, "A comparison study of growth factor expression following treatment with transcutaneous electrical nerve stimulation, saline solution, povidone-iodine, and lavender oil in wounds healing," *Evidence-Based Complementary and Alternative Medicine*, vol. 2013, Article ID 361832, 9 pages, 2013.

[44] S. G. Gürgen, O. Sayin, F. Çetin, and A. Tuç Yücel, "Transcutaneous electrical nerve stimulation (TENS) accelerates cutaneous wound healing and inhibits pro-inflammatory cytokines," *Inflammation*, vol. 37, no. 3, pp. 775–784, 2014.

[45] C. E. Fife, C. Buyukcakir, G. Otto, P. Sheffield, T. Love, and R. Warriner III, "Factors influencing the outcome of lower-extremity diabetic ulcers treated with hyperbaric oxygen therapy," *Wound Repair and Regeneration*, vol. 15, no. 3, pp. 322–331, 2007.

[46] A. M. Eskes, D. T. Ubbink, M. J. Lubbers, C. Lucas, and H. Vermeulen, "Hyperbaric oxygen therapy: solution for difficult to heal acute wounds? Systematic review," *World Journal of Surgery*, vol. 35, no. 3, pp. 535–542, 2011.

[47] S. Bhutani and G. Vishwanath, "Hyperbaric oxygen and wound healing," *Indian Journal of Plastic Surgery*, vol. 45, no. 2, pp. 316–324, 2012.

[48] M. Kalani, G. Jörneskog, N. Naderi, F. Lind, and K. Brismar, "Hyperbaric oxygen (HBO) therapy in treatment of diabetic foot ulcers: long-term follow-up," *Journal of Diabetes and its Complications*, vol. 16, no. 2, pp. 153–158, 2002.

[49] L. Kessler, P. Bilbault, F. Ortéga et al., "Hyperbaric oxygenation accelerates the healing rate of nonischemic chronic diabetic foot ulcers a prospective randomized study," *Diabetes Care*, vol. 26, no. 8, pp. 2378–2382, 2003.

[50] M. H. Hermans, "Silver-containing dressings and the need for evidence," *Advances in Skin & Wound Care*, vol. 20, no. 3, pp. 166–165, 2007.

[51] A. B. Lansdown, "Silver. I: its antibacterial properties and mechanism of action," *Journal of Wound Care*, vol. 11, no. 4, pp. 125–130, 2002.

[52] D. J. Leaper, "Silver dressings: their role in wound management," *International Wound Journal*, vol. 3, no. 4, pp. 282–311, 2006.

[53] G. B. E. Jemec, J. C. Kerihuel, K. Ousey, S. L. Lauemløler, and D. J. Leaper, "Cost-effective use of silver dressings for the treatment of hard-to-heal chronic venous leg ulcers," *PLoS ONE*, vol. 9, no. 6, Article ID e100582, 2014.

[54] J.-F. Bisson, S. Hidalgo-Lucas, M. Bouschbacher, and L. Thomassin, "Effects of TLC-Ag dressings on skin inflammation," *Journal of Dermatology*, vol. 40, no. 6, pp. 463–470, 2013.

[55] J. Wu, Y. Zheng, X. Wen, Q. Lin, X. Chen, and Z. Wu, "Silver nanoparticle/bacterial cellulose gel membranes for antibacterial wound dressing: investigation *in vitro* and *in vivo*," *Biomedical Materials*, vol. 9, no. 3, Article ID 035005, 2014.

[56] R. G. Sibbald, J. Contreras-Ruiz, P. Coutts, M. Fierheller, A. Rothman, and K. Woo, "Bacteriology, inflammation, and healing: a study of nanocrystalline silver dressings in chronic venous leg ulcers," *Advances in Skin & Wound Care*, vol. 20, no. 10, pp. 549–558, 2007.

[57] M. J. Morykwas, J. Simpson, K. Punger, A. Argenta, L. Kremers, and J. Argenta, "Vacuum-assisted closure: state of basic research and physiologic foundation," *Plastic and Reconstructive Surgery*, vol. 117, no. 7, supplement, pp. 121S–126S, 2006.

[58] P. E. Banwell and L. Téot, "Topical negative pressure (TNP): the evolution of a novel wound therapy," *Journal of Wound Care*, vol. 12, no. 1, pp. 22–28, 2003.

[59] S. Steingrimsson, M. Gottfredsson, I. Gudmundsdottir, J. Sjögren, and T. Gudbjartsson, "Negative-pressure wound therapy for deep sternal wound infections reduces the rate of surgical interventions for early re-infections," *Interactive Cardiovascular and Thoracic Surgery*, vol. 15, no. 3, pp. 406–410, 2012.

[60] P. E. Banwell, "Topical negative pressure therapy in wound care," *Journal of Wound Care*, vol. 8, no. 2, pp. 79–84, 1999.

[61] M. J. Morykwas, L. C. Argenta, E. I. Shelton-Brown, and W. McGuirt, "Vacuum-assisted closure: a new method for wound control and treatment: animal studies and basic foundation," *Annals of Plastic Surgery*, vol. 38, no. 6, pp. 553–562, 1997.

[62] S.-Z. Chen, J. Li, X.-Y. Li, and L.-S. Xu, "Effects of vacuum-assisted closure on wound microcirculation: an experimental study," *Asian Journal of Surgery*, vol. 28, no. 3, pp. 211–217, 2005.

[63] A. K. Greene, M. Puder, R. Roy et al., "Microdeformational wound therapy: effects on angiogenesis and matrix metalloproteinases in chronic wounds of 3 debilitated patients," *Annals of Plastic Surgery*, vol. 56, no. 4, pp. 418–422, 2006.

[64] C. Torbrand, R. Ingemansson, L. Gustafsson, P. Paulsson, and M. Malmsjö, "Pressure transduction to the thoracic cavity during topical negative pressure therapy of a sternotomy wound," *International Wound Journal*, vol. 5, no. 4, pp. 579–584, 2008.

[65] D. Liu, L. Zhang, T. Li et al., "Negative-pressure wound therapy enhances local inflammatory responses in acute infected soft-tissue wound," *Cell Biochemistry and Biophysics*, vol. 70, no. 1, pp. 539–547, 2014.

[66] F. Bassetto, L. Lancerotto, R. Salmaso et al., "Histological evolution of chronic wounds under negative pressure therapy," *Journal of Plastic, Reconstructive and Aesthetic Surgery*, vol. 65, no. 1, pp. 91–99, 2012.

[67] Y. Liu, D. Min, T. Bolton et al., "Increased matrix metalloproteinase-9 predicts poor wound healing in diabetic foot ulcers," *Diabetes Care*, vol. 32, no. 1, pp. 117–119, 2009.

[68] B. Shi, P. Zhang, W.-Z. Li, S.-Z. Chen, and J.-Q. Li, "Effect of vacuum assisted closure on collagenase activity in human chronic wound," *Zhonghua Zheng Xing Wai Ke Za Zhi*, vol. 22, no. 6, pp. 465–467, 2006.

[69] C. M. Mouës, A. W. Van Toorenenbergen, F. Heule, W. C. Hop, and S. E. R. Hovius, "The role of topical negative pressure in wound repair: expression of biochemical markers in wound fluid during wound healing," *Wound Repair and Regeneration*, vol. 16, no. 4, pp. 488–494, 2008.

[70] J. K. Stechmiller, D. V. Kilpadi, B. Childress, and G. S. Schultz, "Effect of Vacuum-Assisted Closure Therapy on the expression of cytokines and proteases in wound fluid of adults with pressure ulcers," *Wound Repair and Regeneration*, vol. 14, no. 3, pp. 371–374, 2006.

[71] U. Tuncel, A. Turan, F. Markoc, U. Erkorkmaz, C. Elmas, and N. Kostakoglu, "Loofah sponge as an interface dressing material in negative pressure wound therapy: results of an in vivo study," *Ostomy Wound Management*, vol. 60, no. 3, pp. 37–45, 2014.

[72] T. Hodgkinson and A. Bayat, "Dermal substitute-assisted healing: enhancing stem cell therapy with novel biomaterial design," *Archives of Dermatological Research*, vol. 303, no. 5, pp. 301–315, 2011.

[73] K. C. Rustad, V. W. Wong, M. Sorkin et al., "Enhancement of mesenchymal stem cell angiogenic capacity and stemness by a biomimetic hydrogel scaffold," *Biomaterials*, vol. 33, no. 1, pp. 80–90, 2012.

[74] Y. Zhou, Z. Yan, H. Zhang et al., "Expansion and delivery of adipose-derived mesenchymal stem cells on three microcarriers for soft tissue regeneration," *Tissue Engineering—Part A*, vol. 17, no. 23-24, pp. 2981–2997, 2011.

[75] A. M. Altman, N. Matthias, Y. Yan et al., "Dermal matrix as a carrier for in vivo delivery of human adipose-derived stem cells," *Biomaterials*, vol. 29, no. 10, pp. 1431–1442, 2008.

[76] S. W. Volk, A. Radu, L. Zhang, and K. W. Liechty, "Stromal progenitor cell therapy corrects the wound-healing defect in the ischemic rabbit ear model of chronic wound repair," *Wound Repair and Regeneration*, vol. 15, no. 5, pp. 736–747, 2007.

[77] A. T. Badillo, R. A. Redden, L. Zhang, E. J. Doolin, and K. W. Liechty, "Treatment of diabetic wounds with fetal murine mesenchymal stromal cells enhances wound closure," *Cell and Tissue Research*, vol. 329, no. 2, pp. 301–311, 2007.

[78] N. G. Singer and A. I. Caplan, "Mesenchymal stem cells: mechanisms of inflammation," *Annual Review of Pathology*, vol. 6, pp. 457–478, 2011.

[79] V. Falanga, "Classifications for wound bed preparation and stimulation of chronic wounds," *Wound Repair and Regeneration*, vol. 8, no. 5, pp. 347–352, 2000.

[80] J. Dissemond, M. Goos, and S. N. Wagner, "The role of oxidative stress in the pathogenesis and therapy of chronic wounds," *Hautarzt*, vol. 53, no. 11, pp. 718–723, 2002.

[81] A. Soneja, M. Drews, and T. Malinski, "Role of nitric oxide, nitroxidative and oxidative stress in wound healing," *Pharmacological Reports*, vol. 57, supplement, pp. 108–119, 2005.

[82] D. J. Margolis, W. Bilker, J. Santanna, and M. Baumgarten, "Venous leg ulcer: incidence and prevalence in the elderly," *Journal of the American Academy of Dermatology*, vol. 46, no. 3, pp. 381–386, 2002.

[83] C. E. Davies, K. E. Hill, R. G. Newcombe et al., "A prospective study of the microbiology of chronic venous leg ulcers to reevaluate the clinical predictive value of tissue biopsies and swabs," *Wound Repair and Regeneration*, vol. 15, no. 1, pp. 17–22, 2007.

[84] N. J. Trengove, H. Bielefeldt-Ohmann, and M. C. Stacey, "Mitogenic activity and cytokine levels in non-healing and healing chronic leg ulcers," *Wound Repair and Regeneration*, vol. 8, no. 1, pp. 13–25, 2000.

[85] R. J. White and K. F. Cutting, "Critical colonizationg—the concept under scrutiny," *Ostomy Wound Management*, vol. 52, no. 11, pp. 50–56, 2006.

[86] R. Goldman, "Growth factors and chronic wound healing: past, present, and future," *Advances in Skin & Wound Care*, vol. 17, no. 1, pp. 24–35, 2004.

[87] P. A. Efron and L. L. Moldawer, "Cytokines and wound healing: the role of cytokine and anticytokine therapy in the repair response," *Journal of Burn Care and Rehabilitation*, vol. 25, no. 2, pp. 149–160, 2004.

[88] A. E. Brissett and D. B. Hom, "The effects of tissue sealants, platelet gels, and growth factors on wound healing," *Current Opinion in Otolaryngology & Head and Neck Surgery*, vol. 11, no. 4, pp. 245–250, 2003.

[89] P. Kranke, M. Bennett, I. Roeckl-Wiedmann, and S. Debus, "Hyperbaric oxygen therapy for chronic wounds," *Cochrane Database of Systematic Reviews*, no. 2, Article ID CD004123, 2004.

[90] J. Cha and V. Falanga, "Stem cells in cutaneous wound healing," *Clinics in Dermatology*, vol. 25, no. 1, pp. 73–78, 2007.

15

HMGB1 and Histones Play a Significant Role in Inducing Systemic Inflammation and Multiple Organ Dysfunctions in Severe Acute Pancreatitis

Runkuan Yang,[1,2,3] **Jyrki Tenhunen,**[1,4] **and Tor Inge Tonnessen**[3,5]

[1]*Department of Intensive Care Medicine, Tampere University Hospital, University of Tampere, 10 Biokatu, 33014 Tampere, Finland*
[2]*Department of Critical Care Medicine, University of Pittsburgh Medical School, 3550 Terrace Street, Pittsburgh, PA 15261, USA*
[3]*Department of Emergencies and Critical Care, Oslo University Hospital, 4950 Nydalen, 0424 Oslo, Norway*
[4]*Department of Surgical Science, Anesthesiology and Intensive Care Medicine, Uppsala University, 751 85 Uppsala, Sweden*
[5]*Institute of Clinical Medicine, University of Oslo, Blindern, 0316 Oslo, Norway*

Correspondence should be addressed to Runkuan Yang; runkuanyang@gmail.com

Academic Editor: Jean-Marc Cavaillon

Severe acute pancreatitis (SAP) starts as a local inflammation of pancreatic tissue that induces the development of multiple extrapancreatic organs dysfunction; however, the underlying mechanisms are still not clear. Ischemia-reperfusion, circulating inflammatory cytokines, and possible bile cytokines significantly contribute to gut mucosal injury and intestinal bacterial translocation (BT) during SAP. Circulating HMGB1 level is significantly increased in SAP patients and HMGB1 is an important factor that mediates (at least partly) gut BT during SAP. Gut BT plays a critical role in triggering/inducing systemic inflammation/sepsis in critical illness, and profound systemic inflammatory response syndrome (SIRS) can lead to multiple organ dysfunction syndrome (MODS) during SAP, and systemic inflammation with multiorgan dysfunction is the cause of death in experimental SAP. Therefore, HMGB1 is an important factor that links gut BT and systemic inflammation. Furthermore, HMGB1 significantly contributes to multiple organ injuries. The SAP patients also have significantly increased circulating histones and cell-free DNAs levels, which can reflect the disease severity and contribute to multiple organ injuries in SAP. Hepatic Kupffer cells (KCs) are the predominant source of circulating inflammatory cytokines in SAP, and new evidence indicates that hepatocyte is another important source of circulating HMGB1 in SAP; therefore, treating the liver injury is important in SAP.

1. Introduction

Acute pancreatitis (AP) is a relatively common disease, its severe form is potentially fatal, and SAP is associated with high mortality, ranging from 15 to 40% [1–8]. AP starts as a local inflammation of pancreatic tissue that induces the development of multiple extrapancreatic organs dysfunction including acute lung injury [8–10], general endothelial barrier dysfunction, liver injury, and gut barrier dysfunction [2, 6, 8]; systemic inflammation is thought to be the key link to multiple organ dysfunction (MOD) in SAP [11, 12] and gut BT plays a critical role in triggering/inducing systemic inflammation [13, 14]; however, the underlying mechanism of BT in SAP is still poorly understood. The inflammatory cytokines play a crucial role in the pathogenesis of SAP [6, 7, 15, 16] and the late proinflammatory cytokine HMGB1 is particularly important in SAP [17, 18], because the circulating HMGB1 levels can reflect the disease severity and are potent in augmenting systemic inflammation [17, 18], and emerging evidence shows that HMGB1 is also an important factor that mediates 85% of the gut BT in acetaminophen hepatotoxicity [19]; therefore, it is possible that HMGB1 also mediates BT in SAP. Except HMGB1, new investigations show that extracellular histones and DNAs might also significantly contribute to multiple organ injury during SAP [20–23]. Because hepatic KCs are the predominant source of circulating inflammatory cytokines (including HMGB1) in SAP [8], and new evidence indicates that hepatocyte is another important source of circulating HMGB1 in SAP [15, 16]; therefore, the inflamed liver is an important contributor to the circulating HMGB1 and the liver is a promising therapeutic target to prevent BT and systemic inflammation during SAP. This manuscript focuses on the new development in gut BT and provides evidences to show that HMGB1, histones, and DNAs might significantly contribute to systemic inflammation and multiple organ injury during SAP.

1.1. Ischemia-Reperfusion, Circulating Inflammatory Cytokines, and Possible Bile Cytokines Contribute to Gut Barrier Dysfunction in SAP. Gut barrier dysfunction is frequently seen in SAP [6, 11, 24, 25] and clarifying the underlying mechanisms is important because the intestine is the biggest reservoir of bacteria in the body and leakage of bacteria or microbial products, notably LPS, from the intestinal lumen into the systemic circulation, leads to initiation or amplification of a systemic inflammation and MOD [26].

Intestinal ischemia-reperfusion significantly contributes to small intestinal injury during SAP [27, 28] by inducing gut mucosal injury and affecting gut muscular layer to impair gut motility, which is frequently seen in SAP [14], and the reduced intestinal motility significantly contributes to disrupted intestinal microflora and BT [14].

The circulating inflammatory cytokines including TNF-α, IL-6, and HMGB1 also contribute to gut mucosal injury [29–32], among these inflammatory cytokines, extracellular HMGB1 triggers and sustains the inflammatory response by inducing cytokine release and by recruiting leucocytes [33]. However, HMGB1 undergoes extensive posttranslational modifications, in particular acetylation and oxidation, which significantly modulate the functions of HMGB1 [33, 34]. High levels of serum HMGB1, in particular of the hyperacetylated and disulfide isoforms, are sensitive disease biomarkers [33], and SAP patients have significantly increased serum HMGB1 levels [35, 36], which can reflect the severity of gut barrier injury [35]. The circulating HMGB1 contributes to gut mucosal hyperpermeability and induces evident BT during hemorrhagic shock and reperfusion [37], and exogenous HMGB1 injection is able to induce gut hyperpermeability and BT in normal mice [29].

Except from the circulating HMGB1, bile HMGB1 might also significantly contribute to intestinal mucosa injury and induces evident BT in SAP because SAP patients have significantly increased circulating LPS levels [38], and LPS injection reduces 40% of bile flow in normal rats [31]; adequate bile is important to maintain gut epithelial tight junction and intestinal bacterial homeostasis [31] and decreased gut luminal bile volume not only impairs intestinal tight junction, but also changes intestinal bacterial homeostasis to facilitate BT [31]. In addition, LPS injection (to normal animals) markedly increases bile TNF-α and HMGB1 levels, and the endotoxemic bile can induce gut mucosal hyperpermeability and evident BT in normal mice [31], and neutralization of bile HMGB1 can reverse endotoxemic bile induced intestinal mucosal hyperpermeability and BT in normal mice [31], suggesting that bile HMGB1 is able to cause gut mucosal injury and intestinal BT.

1.2. HMGB1 Plays a Significant Role in Mediating BT in SAP. SAP induces significant small intestinal injury [27, 28], and the failure of gut barrier is associated with BT [27], which is evident in SAP [6, 24, 25]. SAP patients have significantly increased serum LPS level, which is likely derived from the gut lumen or from translocated intestinal bacteria [38]. 68.8% of the SAP patients have bacteraemia and these bacteria have been tested as gut-derived opportunistic pathogens [24], which likely derive from small bowel rather than from the colon [25]. Therefore, it is important to identify the key factor that mediates intestinal BT in SAP. Gut bacteria can adhere to the injured intestinal mucosa that is necessary but not sufficient to induce gut BT in which HMGB1 and other unknown factors are also needed, because evidence shows that exogenous HMGB1 injection can induce gut mucosal injury and evident BT in normal mice [29], and HMGB1 also contributes to gut barrier dysfunction in rats with SAP [32]; blockade of HMGB1 reduces 85% of BT but does not significantly improve gut mucosal injury during acetaminophen hepatotoxicity [19]; similarly, ethyl pyruvate (EP), which is a HMGB1 inhibitor [39], reduces 80% of the gut BT but did not significantly decrease intestinal mucosal hyperpermeability in a lethal SAP animal model [6]; this BT-inhibition effect is associated with EP inhibiting 80% of the hepatic tissue HMGB1 release [15]. These evidences indicate that HMGB1 might mediate gut BT in SAP, and this hypothesis is confirmed by the following experiment: neutralization of HMGB1 decreased 70% of the gut BT (4252 $\pm$ 205 CFU/g for the sham antibody group versus 1235 $\pm$ 41 CFU/g for the anti-HMGB1 group, results are mean $\pm$ SEM, $n = 6$ for each group, unpublished data) but did not reduce gut mucosal hyperpermeability in another commonly used murine SAP model (7 hourly 50 μg/kg intraperitoneal injections of cerulean and a single intraperitoneal injection of 4 mg/kg *Escherichia coli* lipopolysaccharide). These data indicate that intestinal mucosal injury is essential but not sufficient for gut BT during SAP; HMGB1 plays a significant role in mediating (at least partly) gut BT in experimental SAP and BT is likely an active "transcellular" procedure.

1.3. Gut BT Induces/Triggers Systemic Inflammation and Sepsis. Gut BT not only contributes to pancreatic infection [14, 25], but also induces/triggers systemic inflammation/sepsis in critical illness [13, 14], and the profound systemic inflammation can lead to MOD and mortality in SAP [9, 14, 27, 40]. This is one of the important underlying mechanisms that SAP frequently affects extrapancreatic organs [3, 6], and the incidence of MOD in SAP is not available but certainly higher than the 20–30% of mortality rate in SAP [3]. Systemic inflammation with multiorgan dysfunction is the cause of death in a murine ligation-induced SAP, and systemic inflammation and MOD can lead to the preponderance of mortality (75%) in this lethal SAP model [11] while bile duct ligation does not have mortality [11]. Therefore, the gut is thought to act as the starter of SIRS [27] and HMGB1 is an important factor that links gut barrier dysfunction and MOD during SAP.

1.4. The Liver Itself Plays an Important Role in BT in SAP. AP frequently affects the liver [6, 15] that plays an important role in BT during SAP by virtue of its unique structure and immune surveillance function [14, 41]. The liver is the largest organ in the body, hepatocytes account for 70–80% of the hepatic cytoplasmic mass and nonparenchymal cells make up 20–30% of the hepatic cytoplasmic mass [41]. Among the nonparenchymal cells, KCs, sinusoidal endothelial cells, and the natural killer (NK) lymphocytes exert cellular defence functions for the whole body but also for the liver itself [41]. The liver has a large number of immune cells that can be rapidly expanded in response to infection or injury by recruiting leukocytes from the circulations [42]. SAP frequently injures the liver [6, 15, 16, 40] and impairs the phagocytic function [14, 40]; the impaired host defence fails to clear regional lymph nodes and resultantly facilitates BT [14, 40].

1.5. HMGB1, Extracellular Histones, and DNAs Contribute to Multiple Organ Injuries. About 20–30% of acute pancreatitis patients develop SAP in clinical practice; the mortality rate in SAP is 20–30% [3]; however, most of the SAP related mortality is not due to pancreatic injury itself; systemic inflammation with multiorgan dysfunction is the cause of death [11]. Early inflammatory cytokines are certainly involved in the pathogenesis of SAP; however, due to the narrow window time of the early cytokines in clinic, the clinical significance of the early inflammatory cytokines is limited. Attention should be focused on the late inflammatory cytokines such as HMGB1 and the newly recognized histones because these damage associated molecular patterns (DAMPs) have much wider window time to treat the patients and these DAMPs also significantly contribute to multiple organ injuries. The circulating HMGB1 level is significantly higher in SAP patients than in patients with mild pancreatitis [43]; the serum HMGB1 levels are higher in SAP patients with organ dysfunction and infection than in patients without organ dysfunction or infection [36]; the serum HMGB1 levels in nonsurvivors are higher than those in survivors [36]; serum HMGB1 levels are positively correlated with disease severity scores [36]. Pancreatic tissue HMGB1 levels are significantly increased in experimental SAP [44]; HMGB1 promotes the pathogenesis of pancreatitis [39, 45], and inhibiting HMGB1 therapy ameliorates the pancreatic injury [46]. HMGB1 contributes to liver injury in ischemia-reperfusion [47]. Exogenous HMGB1 injection is able to induce liver injury in normal mice [29]. HMGB1 impairs hepatocyte regeneration during acetaminophen hepatotoxicity and blockade of HMGB1 improves hepatocyte regeneration in acetaminophen overdose-induced fatal liver injury [48]. Anti-HMGB1 treatment protects against APAP hepatotoxicity in rats [49]. HMGB1 also contributes to renal ischemia-reperfusion injury [50], sepsis-induced kidney injury [51], and severe acute pancreatitis related kidney injury [52]. HMGB1 is also found to significantly contribute to hemorrhagic shock related acute lung injury (ALI) [53], hypoxia-induced ALI [54], and severe acute pancreatitis related ALI [55].

The extracellular histones are another group of important DAMPs molecules [56], which are toxic to host cells and elicit immunostimulatory effect that results in tissue damage and inflammation [56, 57]. The necrotic tissue/the dying cells release HMGB1 and histones as DAMPs [57]; therefore, circulating histones are significantly increased in both SAP patients and experimental animals with SAP [20–23] and the circulating histones levels reflect the disease severity in experimental AP [21].

The on-admission circulating nucleosome (containing DNA and histones) levels can predict organ dysfunction during the hospitalization of AP patients [20], suggesting that extracellular histones might contribute to multiple organ dysfunctions in SAP. Reduced pancreatic injury is associated with decreased histones 3 and histone 4 levels in the pancreas in response to taurocholate challenge [23], suggesting that histones are associated with pancreatic injury during SAP. The extracellular histones kill endothelial cells and are one of the major mediators of death in sepsis [58]. Extracellular histones contribute to two different acute fatal liver injury models [57]; TLR2 and TLR4 are the major receptors for extracellular histone mediated sterile inflammation, tissue injury, and organ failure in acute liver failure (ALF) [57]; neutralization of histones can ameliorate these two different fatal liver injury models in mice [57]. Extracellular histones can induce microvascular endothelial injury and the TLR2/4-mediated inflammation can lead to acute tubular necrosis in acute kidney injury (AKI) [59, 60]. Extracellular histones injure endothelial cells causing microvascular thrombosis and hemorrhage in acute lung injury (ALI) [61]. Histones also contribute to stroke in acute brain injury, and blockade of histones can reduce infarct size [62]. Histone H4 and increased circulating neutrophil extracellular traps (NETs) activate platelets, which trigger platelet aggregation and clotting that result in microvascular thrombosis and vascular and parenchymal injury in sepsis [57, 58, 60]. Therefore, extracellular histones contribute to the microvascular complications of sepsis, small vessel vasculitis, acute fatal liver injury, acute kidney, and acute lung injuries [58, 60].

Cell-free plasma DNA is significantly increased in SAP patients [20, 22] and in experimental animal with SAP [22]. Damaged cells from SAP can release nucleosomes, which contain DNA and histones, into the circulation to promote inflammation, and the circulating nucleosomes levels can predict AP patients who present no clinical signs of organ dysfunction on admission and are bound to develop organ dysfunction during hospitalization [20], suggesting that DNA/or histones likely play a significant role in the development of organ dysfunction during SAP. Neutrophils play an active role in the development of AP [22]. Except the secretion of antimicrobial compounds, activated neutrophils eliminate invading microorganisms by expelling nuclear DNA and histones to form extracellular web-like structures called neutrophil extracellular traps (NETs) [22]. NETs form in the pancreas in a murine SAP model; addition of NETs and histones to the acinar cells induces trypsin formation and activates the signal transducer and transcription [22]. NETs are able to activate platelets leading to thrombosis and the major contributor to this process is histone 4 [52]. NETs contribute to organ dysfunction in patients with infectious diseases and regulate organ inflammation and injury in mice with AP [22]. SAP patients have increased plasma levels of NETs [22]. Administration of DNase 1 (to deplete DNA and NETs) decreases circulating HMGB1 level and reduces neutrophil infiltration and tissue damage in the inflamed pancreas and lung [22], suggesting that DNA also significantly contributes to the development of SAP.

1.6. The Inflamed Liver Is an Important Source of Circulating HMGB1 and Has an Impaired Capacity to Clear Histones in SAP. Proinflammatory mediators are thought to play a crucial role in the pathogenesis of SAP [6, 8, 15, 16, 63, 64]. The amount of cytokines released from the liver represents about 50% of the total cytokine content in the body [64], suggesting that the liver is the major contributor of the circulating cytokines. KCs are the largest number of tissue resident macrophages in the body and a predominant source of circulating inflammatory cytokines in SAP [8], and KCs play a major role in amplifying systemic inflammation during AP [11, 12, 64–68]. Except KCs, emerging evidence is showing that hepatocyte is another important source of circulating HMGB1 in two different experimental SAP models [15, 16]: especially in this triple-hit lethal SAP model, the inflamed liver releases nearly 90% of the hepatic tissue HMGB1 (detected by liver tissue whole cell lysis) [15]. EP is a potent HMGB1 inhibitor that ameliorates SAP via the reduced serum HMGB1 level [17], which is potent in augmenting SIRS in SAP [17, 18]. EP is also found to ameliorate intestinal barrier dysfunction by reducing the ileal mucosal HMGB1 expression [32]. EP not only inhibits LPS-stimulated macrophages to release TNF-α and HMGB1 [69], but also inhibits the inflamed liver to release both early (TNF-α, IL-6) and late (HMGB1) inflammatory mediators during SAP [15, 16] and resultantly ameliorates the SAP related multiple distant organs injuries (including the liver injury) [6, 15–18]. These evidences indicate that both KCs and the hepatocytes are an important source of circulating HMGB1 in SAP, and the inflamed liver might play a critical role in the translation of pancreatic injury into systemic inflammation and MOD. In addition, the liver is an important organ to rapidly clear extracellular histones [21]; however, SAP can induce severe liver injury and impair its capacity of clearing histones, and this can lead to the increased circulating histones levels, which can significantly contribute multiple organ injury as described above. Therefore, the liver could be a promising therapeutic target to treat SAP.

2. Conclusions

Increased circulating HMGB1, histones, and cell-free DNAs levels in SAP patients might play a significant role in contributing to systemic inflammation and multiple organ injury during SAP. HMGB1 is an important factor that might link gut BT and systemic inflammation in SAP. The inflamed liver is an important source of circulating HMGB1 and treating the liver injury is important in SAP.

Competing Interests

The authors declare that they have no competing interests.

Acknowledgments

This investigation was supported by South-Eastern Norway Regional Health Authority, Grant no. 2013121.

References

[1] M. Yousaf, K. McCallion, and T. Diamond, "Management of severe acute pancreatitis," *British Journal of Surgery*, vol. 90, no. 4, pp. 407–420, 2003.

[2] R. Hegazi, A. Raina, T. Graham et al., "Early jejunal feeding initiation and clinical outcomes in patients with severe acute pancreatitis," *Journal of Parenteral and Enteral Nutrition*, vol. 35, no. 1, pp. 91–96, 2011.

[3] Z.-W. Yang, X.-X. Meng, and P. Xu, "Central role of neutrophil in the pathogenesis of severe acute pancreatitis," *Journal of Cellular and Molecular Medicine*, vol. 19, no. 11, pp. 2513–2520, 2015.

[4] S. Isaji, T. Takada, Y. Kawarada et al., "JPN Guidelines for the management of acute pancreatitis: surgical management," *Journal of Hepato-Biliary-Pancreatic Surgery*, vol. 13, no. 1, pp. 48–55, 2006.

[5] S. L. Triester and K. V. Kowdley, "Prognostic factors in acute pancreatitis," *Journal of Clinical Gastroenterology*, vol. 34, no. 2, pp. 167–176, 2002.

[6] R. Yang, T. Uchiyama, S. M. Alber et al., "Ethyl pyruvate ameliorates distant organ injury in a murine model of acute necrotizing pancreatitis," *Critical Care Medicine*, vol. 32, no. 7, pp. 1453–1459, 2004.

[7] J. Escobar, J. Pereda, A. Arduini et al., "Role of redox signaling, protein phosphatases and histone acetylation in the inflammatory cascade in acute pancreatitis: therapeutic implications," *Inflammation and Allergy—Drug Targets*, vol. 9, no. 2, pp. 97–108, 2010.

[8] H. Akbarshahi, A. H. Rosendahl, G. Westergren-Thorsson, and R. Andersson, "Acute lung injury in acute pancreatitis—a waiting the big leap," *Respiratory Medicine*, vol. 106, no. 9, pp. 1199–1210, 2012.

[9] D. Closa, L. Sabater, L. Fernández-Cruz, N. Prats, E. Gelpí, and J. Roselló-Catafau, "Activation of alveolar macrophages in lung injury associated with experimental acute pancreatitis is mediated by the liver," *Annals of Surgery*, vol. 229, no. 2, pp. 230–236, 1999.

[10] D. Closa, M. Bardaji, G. Hotter et al., "Hepatic involvement in pancreatitis-induced lung damage," *American Journal of Physiology—Gastrointestinal and Liver Physiology*, vol. 270, no. 1, pp. G6–G13, 1996.

[11] Z. Yuan, D. K. Meyerholz, E. C. Twait, D. Kempuraj, D. E. Williard, and I. Samuel, "Systemic inflammation with multiorgan dysfunction is the cause of death in murine ligation-induced acute pancreatitis," *Journal of Gastrointestinal Surgery*, vol. 15, no. 10, pp. 1670–1678, 2011.

[12] E. Puy-Folch, "Importance of the liver in systemic complications associated with acute pancreatitis: the role of Kupffer cells," *Journal of Pathology*, vol. 211, no. 4, pp. 383–388, 2007.

[13] M. Y. Z. Fanous, A. J. Phillips, and J. A. Windsor, "Mesenteric lymph: the bridge to future management of critical illness," *Journal of the Pancreas*, vol. 8, no. 4, pp. 374–399, 2007.

[14] N. Runkel, "Bacterial translocation in acute pancreatitis," *Digestive Surgery*, vol. 13, no. 4-5, pp. 269–272, 1996.

[15] R. Yang, A. L. Shaufl, M. E. Killeen, and M. P. Fink, "Ethyl pyruvate ameliorates liver injury secondary to severe acute pancreatitis," *Journal of Surgical Research*, vol. 153, no. 2, pp. 302–309, 2009.

[16] Z.-G. Luan, H. Zhang, X.-C. Ma, C. Zhang, and R.-X. Guo, "Therapeutic treatment with ethyl pyruvate attenuates the severity of liver injury in rats with severe acute pancreatitis," *Pancreas*, vol. 41, no. 5, pp. 729–737, 2012.

[17] Z.-Y. Yang, Y. Ling, T. Yin et al., "Delayed ethyl pyruvate therapy attenuates experimental severe acute pancreatitis via reduced serum high mobility group box 1 levels in rats," *World Journal of Gastroenterology*, vol. 14, no. 28, pp. 4546–4550, 2008.

[18] B.-Q. Cheng, C.-T. Liu, W.-J. Li et al., "Ethyl pyruvate improves survival and ameliorates distant organ injury in rats with severe acute pancreatitis," *Pancreas*, vol. 35, no. 3, pp. 256–261, 2007.

[19] R. Yang, X. Zou, J. Tenhunen et al., "HMGB1 neutralization is associated with bacterial translocation during acetaminophen hepatotoxicity," *BMC Gastroenterology*, vol. 14, no. 1, article 66, 2014.

[20] A. K. Penttilä, A. Rouhiainen, L. Kylänpää et al., "Circulating nucleosomes as predictive markers of severe acute pancreatitis," *Journal of Intensive Care*, vol. 4, article 14, 2016.

[21] X. Ou, Z. Cheng, T. Liu et al., "Circulating histone levels reflect disease severity in animal models of acute pancreatitis," *Pancreas*, vol. 44, no. 7, pp. 1089–1095, 2015.

[22] M. Merza, H. Hartman, M. Rahman et al., "Neutrophil extracellular traps induce trypsin activation, inflammation, and tissue damage in mice with severe acute pancreatitis," *Gastroenterology*, vol. 149, no. 7, pp. 1920–1931e8, 2015.

[23] M. Merza, M. Rahman, S. Zhang et al., "Human thrombin-derived host defense peptides inhibit neutrophil recruitment and tissue injury in severe acute pancreatitis," *American Journal of Physiology—Gastrointestinal and Liver Physiology*, vol. 307, no. 9, pp. G914–G921, 2014.

[24] Q. Li, C. Wang, C. Tang, Q. He, N. Li, and J. Li, "Bacteremia in patients with acute pancreatitis as revealed by 16S ribosomal RNA gene-based techniques," *Critical Care Medicine*, vol. 41, no. 8, pp. 1938–1950, 2013.

[25] S. Fritz, T. Hackert, W. Hartwig et al., "Bacterial translocation and infected pancreatic necrosis in acute necrotizing pancreatitis derives from small bowel rather than from colon," *American Journal of Surgery*, vol. 200, no. 1, pp. 111–117, 2010.

[26] M. P. Fink, "Leaky gut hypothesis: a historical perspective," *Critical Care Medicine*, vol. 18, no. 5, pp. 579–580, 1990.

[27] G. Capurso, G. Zerboni, M. Signoretti et al., "Role of the gut barrier in acute pancreatitis," *Journal of Clinical Gastroenterology*, vol. 46, pp. S46–S51, 2012.

[28] Z.-Z. Guo, P. Wang, Z.-H. Yi, Z.-Y. Huang, and C.-W. Tang, "The crosstalk between gut inflammation and gastrointestinal disorders during acute pancreatitis," *Current Pharmaceutical Design*, vol. 20, no. 7, pp. 1051–1062, 2014.

[29] P. L. Sappington, R. Yang, H. Yang, K. J. Tracey, R. L. Delude, and M. P. Fink, "HMGB1 B box increases the permeability of Caco-2 enterocytic monolayers and impairs intestinal barrier function in mice," *Gastroenterology*, vol. 123, no. 3, pp. 790–802, 2002.

[30] P. L. Sappington, X. Han, R. Yang, R. L. Delude, and M. P. Fink, "Ethyl pyruvate ameliorates intestinal epithelial barrier dysfunction in endotoxemic mice and immunostimulated caco-2 enterocytic monolayers," *Journal of Pharmacology and Experimental Therapeutics*, vol. 304, no. 1, pp. 464–476, 2003.

[31] R. Yang, K. Miki, N. Oksala et al., "Bile high-mobility group box 1 contributes to gut barrier dysfunction in experimental endotoxemia," *American Journal of Physiology—Regulatory Integrative and Comparative Physiology*, vol. 297, no. 2, pp. R362–R369, 2009.

[32] Z.-G. Luan, H. Zhang, X.-C. Ma, C. Zhang, and R.-X. Guo, "Role of high-mobility group box 1 protein in the pathogenesis of intestinal barrier injury in rats with severe acute pancreatitis," *Pancreas*, vol. 39, no. 2, pp. 216–223, 2010.

[33] E. Venereau, F. De Leo, R. Mezzapelle, G. Careccia, G. Musco, and M. E. Bianchi, "HMGB1 as biomarker and drug target," *Pharmacological Research*, vol. 111, pp. 534–544, 2016.

[34] U. Andersson, D. J. Antoine, and K. J. Tracey, "The functions of HMGB1 depend on molecular localization and post-translational modifications," *Journal of Internal Medicine*, vol. 276, no. 5, pp. 420–424, 2014.

[35] G.-F. Xu, M. Guo, Z.-Q. Tian, G.-Z. Wu, X.-P. Zou, and W.-J. Zhang, "Increased of serum high-mobility group box chromosomal protein 1 correlated with intestinal mucosal barrier injury in patients with severe acute pancreatitis," *World Journal of Emergency Surgery*, vol. 9, article 61, 2014.

[36] T. Yasuda, T. Ueda, Y. Takeyama et al., "Significant increase of serum high-mobility group box chromosomal protein 1 levels in patients with severe acute pancreatitis," *Pancreas*, vol. 33, no. 4, pp. 359–363, 2006.

[37] R. Yang, T. Harada, K. P. Mollen et al., "Anti-HMGB1 neutralizing antibody ameliorates gut barrier dysfunction and improves survival after hemorrhagic shock," *Molecular Medicine*, vol. 12, no. 4–6, pp. 105–114, 2006.

[38] H. Chen, F. Li, J.-G. Jia, Y.-P. Diao, Z.-X. Li, and J.-B. Sun, "Effects of traditional chinese medicine on intestinal mucosal permeability in early phase of severe acute pancreatitis," *Chinese Medical Journal*, vol. 123, no. 12, pp. 1537–1542, 2010.

[39] X. Shen and W.-Q. Li, "High-mobility group box 1 protein and its role in severe acute pancreatitis," *World Journal of Gastroenterology*, vol. 21, no. 5, pp. 1424–1435, 2015.

[40] X. Wang, R. Andersson, V. Soltesz, P. Leveau, and I. Ihse, "Gut origin sepsis, macrophage function, and oxygen extraction associated with acute pancreatitis in the rat," *World Journal of Surgery*, vol. 20, no. 3, pp. 299–308, 1996.

[41] G. Ramadori, F. Moriconi, I. Malik, and J. Dudas, "Physiology and pathophysiology of liver inflammation, damage and repair," *Journal of Physiology and Pharmacology*, vol. 59, no. 1, pp. 107–117, 2008.

[42] P. F. Lalor and D. H. Adams, "The liver: a model of organ-specific lymphocyte recruitment," *Expert reviews in molecular medicine*, vol. 4, no. 2, pp. 1–16, 2002.

[43] Á. K. Kocsis, A. Szabolcs, P. Hofner et al., "Plasma concentrations of high-mobility group box protein 1, soluble receptor for advanced glycation end-products and circulating DNA in patients with acute pancreatitis," *Pancreatology*, vol. 9, no. 4, pp. 383–391, 2009.

[44] L. Schneider, B. Jabrailova, O. Strobel, T. Hackert, and J. Werner, "Inflammatory profiling of early experimental necrotizing pancreatitis," *Life Sciences*, vol. 126, Article ID 14285, pp. 76–80, 2015.

[45] G. Li, X. Wu, L. Yang et al., "TLR4-mediated NF-κB signaling pathway mediates HMGB1-induced pancreatic injury in mice with severe acute pancreatitis," *International Journal of Molecular Medicine*, vol. 37, no. 1, pp. 99–107, 2016.

[46] T. Zhang, M. Xia, Q. Zhan, Q. Zhou, G. Lu, and F. An, "Sodium butyrate reduces organ injuries in mice with severe acute

pancreatitis through inhibiting HMGB1 expression," *Digestive Diseases and Sciences*, vol. 60, no. 7, pp. 1991–1999, 2015.

[47] A. Tsung, R. Sahai, H. Tanaka et al., "The nuclear factor HMGB1 mediates hepatic injury after murine liver ischemia-reperfusion," *Journal of Experimental Medicine*, vol. 201, no. 7, pp. 1135–1143, 2005.

[48] R. Yang, S. Zhang, A. Cotoia, N. Oksala, S. Zhu, and J. Tenhunen, "High mobility group B1 impairs hepatocyte regeneration in acetaminophen hepatotoxicity," *BMC Gastroenterology*, vol. 12, article 45, 2012.

[49] D. J. Antoine, D. P. Williams, A. Kipar, H. Laverty, and B. Kevin Park, "Diet restriction inhibits apoptosis and HMGB1 oxidation and promotes inflammatory cell recruitment during acetaminophen hepatotoxicity," *Molecular Medicine*, vol. 16, no. 11-12, pp. 479–490, 2010.

[50] A. Lau, S. Wang, W. Liu, A. Haig, Z.-X. Zhang, and A. M. Jevnikar, "Glycyrrhizic acid ameliorates HMGB1-mediated cell death and inflammation after renal ischemia reperfusion injury," *American Journal of Nephrology*, vol. 40, no. 1, pp. 84–95, 2014.

[51] Y.-M. Hu, M.-H. Pai, C.-L. Yeh, Y.-C. Hou, and S.-L. Yeh, "Glutamine administration ameliorates sepsis-induced kidney injury by downregulating the high-mobility group box protein-1-mediated pathway in mice," *American Journal of Physiology—Renal Physiology*, vol. 302, no. 1, pp. F150–F158, 2012.

[52] H. Sawa, T. Ueda, Y. Takeyama et al., "Blockade of high mobility group box-1 protein attenuates experimental severe acute pancreatitis," *World Journal of Gastroenterology*, vol. 12, no. 47, pp. 7666–7670, 2006.

[53] R. L. C. Kao, X. Xu, A. Xenocostas et al., "Induction of acute lung inflammation in mice with hemorrhagic shock and resuscitation: role of HMGB1," *Journal of Inflammation*, vol. 11, no. 1, pp. 30–37, 2014.

[54] M. Entezari, M. Javdan, D. J. Antoine et al., "Inhibition of extracellular HMGB1 attenuates hyperoxia-induced inflammatory acute lung injury," *Redox Biology*, vol. 2, no. 1, pp. 314–322, 2014.

[55] Z.-G. Luan, X.-J. Zhang, X.-H. Yin et al., "Downregulation of HMGB1 protects against the development of acute lung injury after severe acute pancreatitis," *Immunobiology*, vol. 218, no. 10, pp. 1261–1270, 2013.

[56] R. Allam, S. V. R. Kumar, M. N. Darisipudi, and H.-J. Anders, "Extracellular histones in tissue injury and inflammation," *Journal of Molecular Medicine*, vol. 92, no. 5, pp. 465–472, 2014.

[57] J. Xu, X. Zhang, M. Monestier, N. L. Esmon, and C. T. Esmon, "Extracellular histones are mediators of death through TLR2 and TLR4 in mouse fatal liver injury," *Journal of Immunology*, vol. 187, no. 5, pp. 2626–2631, 2011.

[58] J. Xu, X. Zhang, R. Pelayo et al., "Extracellular histones are major mediators of death in sepsis," *Nature Medicine*, vol. 15, no. 11, pp. 1318–1321, 2009.

[59] R. Allam, C. R. Scherbaum, M. N. Darisipudi et al., "Histones from dying renal cells aggravate kidney injury via TLR2 and TLR4," *Journal of the American Society of Nephrology*, vol. 23, no. 8, pp. 1375–1388, 2012.

[60] D. L. Rosin and M. D. Okusa, "Dying cells and extracellular histones in AKI: beyond a NET effect?" *Journal of the American Society of Nephrology*, vol. 23, no. 8, pp. 1275–1277, 2012.

[61] M. Bosmann, J. J. Grailer, R. Ruemmler et al., "Extracellular histones are essential effectors of C5aR- and C5L2-mediated tissue damage and inflammation in acute lung injury," *FASEB Journal*, vol. 27, no. 12, pp. 5010–5021, 2013.

[62] S. F. De Meyer, G. L. Suidan, T. A. Fuchs, M. Monestier, and D. D. Wagner, "Extracellular chromatin is an important mediator of ischemic stroke in mice," *Arteriosclerosis, Thrombosis, and Vascular Biology*, vol. 32, no. 8, pp. 1884–1891, 2012.

[63] S. Hoyos, S. Granell, N. Heredia, O. Bulbena, D. Closa, and L. Fernández-Cruz, "Influence of portal blood on the development of systemic inflammation associated with experimental acute pancreatitis," *Surgery*, vol. 137, no. 2, pp. 186–191, 2005.

[64] B. Gloor, T. A. Blinman, D. A. Rigberg et al., "Kupffer cell blockade reduces hepatic and systemic cytokine levels and lung injury in hemorrhagic pancreatitis in rats," *Pancreas*, vol. 21, no. 4, pp. 414–420, 2000.

[65] H.-B. Liu, N.-Q. Cui, D.-H. Li, and C. Chen, "Role of Kupffer cells in acute hemorrhagic necrotizing pancreatitis-associated lung injury of rats," *World Journal of Gastroenterology*, vol. 12, no. 3, pp. 403–407, 2006.

[66] C. M. Pastor, A. Vonlaufen, F. Georgi, A. Hadengue, P. Morel, and J.-L. Frossard, "Neutrophil depletion-but not prevention of Kupffer cell activation-decreases the severity of cerulein-induced acute pancreatitis," *World Journal of Gastroenterology*, vol. 12, no. 8, pp. 1219–1224, 2006.

[67] Y. Sailai, X. Yu, P. Baiheti, H. Tang, Y. Li, and M. Xu, "Influence of nuclear factor κb activation on inflammatory mediators of alveolar macrophages in rats with acute necrotizing pancreatitis," *Journal of Investigative Medicine*, vol. 58, no. 1, pp. 38–42, 2010.

[68] L. Schneider, T. Hackert, T. Longerich et al., "Effects of gadolinium chloride and glycine on hepatic and pancreatic tissue damage in alcoholic pancreatitis," *Pancreas*, vol. 39, no. 4, pp. 502–509, 2010.

[69] L. Ulloa, M. Ochani, H. Yang et al., "Ethyl pyruvate prevents lethality in mice with established lethal sepsis and systemic inflammation," *Proceedings of the National Academy of Sciences of the United States of America*, vol. 99, no. 19, pp. 12351–12356, 2002.

16

Serum Levels of Proinflammatory Cytokines in Painful Knee Osteoarthritis and Sensitization

Marta Imamura,[1] Fernando Ezquerro,[2] Fábio Marcon Alfieri,[1,3] Lucy Vilas Boas,[4] Tania Regina Tozetto-Mendoza,[4] Janini Chen,[5] Levent Özçakar,[6] Lars Arendt-Nielsen,[7] and Linamara Rizzo Battistella[1]

[1] *Clinical Research Center, Institute of Physical Medicine and Rehabilitation, University of São Paulo School of Medicine, Rua Jandiatuba, 580 Vila Andrade, 05716-150 São Paulo, SP, Brazil*

[2] *University of São Paulo School of Medicine, Avenida Dr. Arnaldo, 455 Cerqueira César, 01246903 São Paulo, SP, Brazil*

[3] *São Paulo Adventist University Center, Estrada de Itapecerica, 5859 Jardim IAE, 05858-001 São Paulo, SP, Brazil*

[4] *Tropical Hematology Laboratory, Institute of Tropical Medicine of São Paulo and Medical Research Laboratory, LIM 52, University of São Paulo, Avenida Dr. Arnaldo, 455 Cerqueira César, 01246903 São Paulo, SP, Brazil*

[5] *Institute of Physical Medicine and Rehabilitation, University of São Paulo School of Medicine, Rua Domingo de Soto 100, Vila Mariana, 04116-030 São Paulo, SP, Brazil*

[6] *Department of Physical Medicine and Rehabilitation, Hacettepe University Medical School, Hacettepe University Faculty of Medicine, Sıhhiye, 06100 Ankara, Turkey*

[7] *Center for Sensory-Motor Interaction, School of Medicine, Aalborg University, Fredrik Bajers Vej 7, Building D3, 9220 Aalborg E, Denmark*

Correspondence should be addressed to Fábio Marcon Alfieri; fabiomarcon@bol.com.br

Academic Editor: David A. Hart

Osteoarthritis (OA) is the most common joint disorder in the world. Among the mechanisms involved in osteoarthritis, biomarkers (cytokines profile) may be related to pain and pain intensity, functional capacity, and pressure pain thresholds (PPT). Thus, the study of these relationships may offer useful information about pathophysiology and associated mechanisms involved in osteoarthritis. Therefore, the objective of this study was to investigate the seric concentration of pro (IL-6, IL-8, and TNF-α) and anti-inflammatory (IL-10) cytokines in patients with painful knee osteoarthritis and to correlate the levels of these biomarkers with the patients' functional capacity and pressure pain threshold (PPT) values.

1. Introduction

Osteoarthritis (OA) is the most common joint disorder in the world [1]. In the United States, the symptomatic knee OA occurs in 10% of the male and 13% of the female population with 60 years of age or more, with an estimated financial burden of US$ 47.8 billion annually [2, 3]. In Brazil, this disease is estimated to affect 6% to 12% of the adults with more than one third of those aged 65 years or over [4]. Due to the current trend of population aging and the increasing prevalence of obesity, it is estimated that the number of people suffering from knee OA will probably increase in the coming years [5] with substantial reduction in quality of life for the individual and massive costs for societies.

Different mechanisms may underlie the heterogeneous and multifactorial presentation of OA and inflammation is considered as one of the factors involved at some stages in the OA progression. The inflammatory process may be associated with alterations in the cytokines profile (e.g., interleukin-6) [6]. In addition, specific cytokines may provoke damage of the extracellular matrix of the joint tissue [7]. Some cytokines may act as biochemical markers of OA severity and pain [8]. Recent studies have indicated that specific pain mechanisms in OA may relate to biomarkers associated with cartilage and bone degradation [9]. Yet articular cartilage and subchondral bone damage are key factors in OA and can be assessed by a variety of new biomarkers [10] such as C-telopeptide of Type I collagen (CTX-I), CTX-II, Type III collagen N-propeptide, and matrix metalloproteinase (MMP) mediated degradation fragments of connective tissue turnover (C1M and C2M) and synovium (C3M) connective tissue turnover [11]. Ishijima et al. [12] showed that pain and Type II collagen degradation (sC2C and uCTX-II) and formation (sCPII), bone resorption (uNTx), and hence, for example, synovitis may contribute to joint pain. Another novel biomarker specific of MMP cleavage is the CRPM that reflects local inflammation, whereas circulating, uncleaved C-reactive protein (CRP) reflects systemic inflammation [13]. It is therefore of relevance to investigate how joint damage, measured by these novel disease related biomarkers, is related to pain mechanisms. Further, many authors have reported on the effects of different variables, such as functional performance [14], obesity [15], clinical aspects [16], and radiological severity of OA [6], on the serum or intra-articular levels of cytokines. In obesity, more and more studies have shown hypersensitivity to pain and that those individuals are more vulnerable to developing pain possibly due to the low inflammatory processes initiated by cytokine release from adipose tissue [17]. It has been already shown that pain in knee OA patients may be associated with generalized pain sensitization rather than peripheral inflammation and injury [18–21]. It is well known that joint damage in the individual OA patient is not strongly associated with pain [22, 23], suggesting many other factors are involved in driving the clinical manifestations in OA.

To further address this issue, the current study (1) investigated serum concentrations of proinflammatory cytokines (IL-6, IL-8, and TNF-α) and an anti-inflammatory cytokine (IL-10) in OA patients (with painful knee osteoarthritis) and healthy controls and (2) correlated these serum levels with pain intensity, functional capacity, and pressure pain thresholds (PPTs).

2. Method

This study was approved by the Ethics Committee for Analysis of Research Projects (CAPPesq), Hospital of Clinics of University of São Paulo Medical School, São Paulo, Brazil, research protocol CAPPesq 0131/10. All participants were informed about the study procedure and they all signed an informed consent. The procedures that followed were in accordance with the ethical standards of the responsible committee on human experimentation (institutional and national) and with the Helsinki Declaration of 1975, as revised in 2000.

2.1. Study Population. The recruitment of 101 subjects was done through referrals from various departments of the Hospital of Clinics and via contact with friends or family members who volunteered to participate.

Knee OA subjects ($N = 53$) were enrolled if they had the following: age ≥ 60 years, diagnosis of knee OA according to the American College of Rheumatology criteria and Kellgren/Lawrence scale grades of 2–4 [24, 25], and moderate to severe pain (visual analogue scale (VAS) > 4), as general averaged level of pain experienced during the day for the past month, lasting ≥ 3 months.

Healthy volunteers without any pain ($N = 48$) participated as controls. Those who had any rheumatic disease, fibromyalgia and other chronic painful condition, a history of malignancy, psychiatric disorder, or previous knee surgery were not included in the study.

2.2. Assessment of Function and Pain. Participants answered the Western Ontario and McMaster Universities Arthritis Index (WOMAC) questionnaire for the assessment of pain and function during daily activities [26].

Pain intensity was assessed using the 10 cm VAS ruler graded from zero (no pain) to ten (average pain intensity during the past 48 hours, during daily activities).

The pressure pain threshold (PTT) was measured by a pressure algometer (Pain Diagnostics, Great Neck, NY, USA) having a hard rubber 1 cm^2 at the end of the apparatus. The pressure was applied perpendicular to the skin at a constant speed (1 Kg/s) and the patients indicated when they felt pain. The reading is expressed in kg/cm^2.

Pressure pain thresholds were assessed over vastus medialis, adductor longus, rectus femoris, vastus lateralis, tibialis anterior, peroneus longus, iliacus, sartorius, gracilis, quadratus lumborum, and popliteus as previously described [18]. For this evaluation, the subject remained supine and prone and in the lateral position for better evaluation. We have not performed measures over the knee joints. In addition, PPT values were assessed over the ligaments located over the supraspinous ligaments (L) between L1-L2, L2-L3, L3-L4, L4-L5, and L5-S1 and sacral (S) areas S1-S2. During this assessment, the volunteer lied in the lateral decubitus position with hip flexion and the evaluator applied the pressure directly over the region. The pinch and roll maneuver at the L1, L2, L3, L4, L5, S1, and S2 dermatomes was done to evaluate subcutaneous hyperalgesia [27]. Except for the supraspinous ligaments and the L5–S1 and S1–S2 sacral areas (6 sites), all measurements were done bilaterally [28].

2.3. Blood Samples. Serum concentrations of proinflammatory cytokines (IL-6, IL-8, and TNF-α) and an anti-inflammatory cytokine (IL-10) were collected by blood samples (5 mL), taken from the antecubital vein between 8:00 am and 11:00 am. A Vacutainer tube, without the addition of anticoagulants, was used in order to obtain serum after the centrifugation process at 500 g, 4°C. Samples of sera were separated in 100 uL aliquots in Eppendorf cryotube and stored at −80°C until processing. Data was obtained by measuring the fluorescence intensity. Human Inflammatory Cytokines Kit (BDTM Bioscience CBA Cytometric Bead Array, San Jose, CA) was used to quantitatively measure serum concentrations of interleukin-6 (IL-6), interleukin-8 (IL-8), and tumor necrosis factor (TNF-α) according to the manufacturer's instructions. Individual cytokine concentrations (pg/mL) were computed using the standard reference curve of CELLQUEST and CBA software. The reading of the serum samples was performed by the cytometer FACS Calibur (BD Biosciences, USA) from the Laboratory of Medical Investigation (LIM 56), University of São Paulo School of Medicine. The serum measurements of proinflammatory cytokines (IL-6, IL-8, and TNF-α) and an anti-inflammatory cytokine (IL-10) were performed by an independent investigator blinded to the patients' status (knee osteoarthritis or healthy volunteers).

2.4. Statistics. Kolmogorov-Smirnov test and the observation of the morphology of the histogram were used to test for a normal distribution for all studied variables.

Quantitative characteristics with use of summary measures (median, interquartile interval) were compared between groups using Mann-Whitney U test. Correlations between age, pain duration, VAS, WOMAC scores, and the PPT values were evaluated using scatter plots and Spearman's rank correlation coefficients. Stepwise multiple linear regression models analyzed the relationships of VAS, WOMAC subscales, and the PPT measures. Napierian logarithm transformation was used to stabilize variability of serum cytokine values. Analyses were performed using SPSS software, version 15 (SPSS, Chicago, IL). P values less than 0.05 (2-tailed) were considered significant.

3. Results

Mean age values of symptomatic patients (71.23 ± 7.62 years, n = 53 (women)) and controls (68.21 ± 7.17 years, n = 48, 2 men and 46 women) were not significantly different (Table 1). All patients reported pain duration of at least 24 months (median, 96 months; range 36–150). About the use of drugs in the group of OA knee individuals, 36 were taking drugs, 22 with several medications such as antidepressants and antihypertensive, among other items, and 14 were using mediation analgesic. In the control group, 41 were taking several medications such as antidepressants and antihypertensive, among others.

3.1. Function and Pain. Mean WOMAC (pain, stiffness, and function) scores in the OA patients were 10.90 ± 2.35, 4.20 ± 2.35, and 42.53 ± 14.59, respectively. Mean pain intensity in the OA patients was 7.6 cm ± 1.59.

Knee OA patients showed lower PPTs compared to the matched controls ($P < 0.05$) in all 24 muscular, ligamentous, and subcutaneous points tested, both at the knees and at distant sites (Table 2).

3.2. Blood Samples. Serum levels of IL-8 and TNF-α were similar between patients and controls (Table 2). IL-6 (P = 0.031) and IL-10 (P = 0.030) levels were significantly elevated in patients (Table 3).

3.3. Correlation Analysis. Correlation analyses of variables are given in Table 4. Both IL-6 and IL-10 correlated positively with VAS and WOMAC scores for rigidity. Only IL-6 correlated positively with WOMAC scores for pain. IL-6 and IL-10 did not correlate with any PPT measurements.

PPTs from muscular, ligamentous, or subcutaneous sources showed the most consistent positive associations with TNF-α (Table 4).

For the pinch and roll cutaneous assessment, consistent positive associations were found with TNF-α (Table 4).

TABLE 1: Comparison of age and BMI (body mass index) between the knee osteoarthritis (OA) and healthy control groups.

	Knee OA	Control	P
N	53	48	
Age (years)	71.23 ± 7.62	68.21 ± 7.17	0.066
BMI (kg/cm^2)	28.33 ± 5.95	27.42 ± 4.86	0.55

Note: values are presented as mean and standard deviation (SD). Kg: kilogram. Cm: centimeter. BMI: body mass index.

3.4. Regression Analysis. Stepwise analysis revealed that a combination of three variables added gain to the equation. Besides VAS, combined PPT values over pes anserinus and supraspinous ligaments at L1-L2 were the best predictors (R^2 = 0.244) for serum TNF-α (Tables 4 and 5). For serum IL-6, we found that WOMAC rigidity and VAS could be added to the equation (R^2 = 0.186) (Tables 4 and 5).

We could not find any predictors for serum IL-8 or IL-10 (Tables 4 and 5).

4. Discussion

4.1. Main Findings. The present cross sectional observational study (i) explored the serum concentration of proinflammatory cytokines (IL-6, IL-8, and TNF-α) and anti-inflammatory cytokines (IL-10) in patients with knee OA and healthy controls and (ii) associated those with clinical pain manifestations and pain hyperalgesia as assessed by PPTs and function. OA patients presented spreading sensitization as assessed by pressure pain hyperalgesia from all the structures investigated. IL-6 and IL-10 were higher in the knee OA patients compared with matched controls. As an exploratory study, we have not corrected for multiple analyses, and therefore, for 30 comparisons, two positive results can be by chance.

4.2. Cytokines Profile. Cytokines are glycoproteins of light molecular weight, responsible for the communication among cells of the immune system [29]. Several authors identified the correlation of higher levels of serum cytokines and knee OA, such as IL-6, TNF-α, and TNF-α soluble receptors sTNFR1 and sTNFR2, and C-reactive protein (CRP) [15, 30]. Classically, increased levels of proinflammatory cytokines are related to development and progression of OA due to upregulation of metalloproteinase gene expression, stimulation of reactive oxygen species production, alteration of chondrocyte metabolism, and increased osteoclastic bone reabsorption [15, 30–33].

TABLE 2: Pressure pain threshold (PPT) values from the assessed structures.

Variable	Group						Mean difference	CI (95%)		P	Cohen's d
	Healthy control			Knee OA							
	Mean	SD	N	Mean	SD	N		Lower	Upper		
Vastus M	6.00	2.08	48	3.30	1.81	53	2.70	1.93	3.47	**<0.001**	1.38
Adductor L	4.97	2.20	48	2.73	1.44	53	2.24	1.51	2.97	**<0.001**	1.21
Rectus fem	7.44	2.29	48	4.19	2.18	53	3.25	2.37	4.13	**<0.001**	1.45
Vastus L	6.13	2.09	48	3.47	2.10	53	2.66	1.83	3.49	**<0.001**	1.27
Tibialis ant	7.43	2.53	48	4.04	2.10	53	3.39	2.48	4.31	**<0.001**	1.46
Peroneus	7.40	2.33	48	4.21	2.96	53	3.19	2.13	4.25	**<0.001**	1.20
Gracilis	5.97	2.47	48	2.82	1.89	53	3.15	2.28	4.01	**<0.001**	1.43
Iliopsoas	6.45	3.36	48	3.50	1.34	53	2.95	1.96	3.95	**<0.001**	1.15
Quadratus L	6.86	2.04	48	4.10	1.86	53	2.77	2.00	3.54	**<0.001**	1.42
Pes anserinus	5.40	2.49	48	2.75	2.01	53	2.65	1.76	3.55	**<0.001**	1.17
Popliteus	7.05	2.36	48	3.87	2.20	53	3.18	2.28	4.08	**<0.001**	1.39
Lig L1-L2	7.98	3.12	48	4.46	2.07	53	3.52	2.48	4.55	**<0.001**	1.33
Lig L2-L3	8.38	3.11	48	4.37	2.21	53	4.01	2.95	5.06	**<0.001**	1.49
Lig L3-L4	8.09	3.10	48	4.58	2.31	53	3.51	2.44	4.58	**<0.001**	1.29
Lig L4-L5	8.29	2.89	48	4.64	2.10	53	3.65	2.66	4.64	**<0.001**	1.44
Lig L5-S1	8.70	2.98	48	4.42	2.27	53	4.28	3.24	5.32	**<0.001**	1.62
Lig S1-S2	8.72	3.21	48	4.90	2.81	53	3.82	2.63	5.01	**<0.001**	1.27
PRL1	3.79	2.11	48	2.39	3.45	53	1.40	0.25	2.54	**<0.001**	0.40
PRL2	3.67	1.83	48	1.77	1.33	53	1.90	1.27	2.53	**<0.001**	1.19
PRL3	4.26	1.74	48	2.01	1.34	53	2.25	1.64	2.86	**<0.001**	1.45
PRL4	5.58	2.17	48	2.95	1.77	53	2.63	1.85	3.41	**<0.001**	1.33
PRL5	5.09	1.98	48	2.47	1.58	53	2.62	1.92	3.33	**<0.001**	1.46
PR S1	5.51	1.59	48	3.02	1.59	53	2.50	1.87	3.12	**<0.001**	1.57
PR S2	4.80	1.92	48	2.77	1.49	53	2.03	1.35	2.70	**<0.001**	1.18

OA: osteoarthritis; Vastus M: vastus medialis; Adductor L: adductor longus; Rectus fem: rectus femoris; Vastus L: vastus lateralis; Tibialis ant: tibialis anterior. PR: pinch and roll maneuver; Lig: supraspinous ligaments; Quad L: quadratus lumborum; L: lumbar; S: sacral.
SD: standard deviation; CI: confidence interval; N: number; P: probability of significance.

TABLE 3: Comparison of cytokine concentrations between groups.

Variable	Group	Mean	SD	Median	Quartile 1	Quartile 3	N	P
TNFα (pg/mL)	Healthy	1.40	1.02	1.29	0.0	2.8	48	0.457
	Knee OA	2.20	4.52	1.30	1.1	1.5	53	
	All	1.82	3.36	1.26	0.0	24.2	101	
IL-10 (pg/mL)	Healthy	0.89	0.87	1.30	0.0	2.3	48	**0.030**
	Knee OA	1.58	2.36	1.17	0.0	1.2	53	
	All	1.25	1.84	1.09	0.0	15.7	101	
IL-6 (pg/mL)	Healthy	2.55	1.06	2.9	2.3	4.0	48	**0.031**
	Knee OA	4.38	4.61	2.4	1.7	3.1	53	
	All	3.48	3.53	2.50	1.2	19.3	101	
IL-8 (pg/mL)	Healthy	9.72	5.28	8.80	5.4	16.0	48	0.984
	Knee OA	10.56	8.51	9.00	6.2	12.7	53	
	All	10.16	7.14	8.83	0.0	53.5	101	

OA: osteoarthritis; Healthy: healthy control; IL: interleukin; TNF: tumor necrosis factor; SD: standard deviation; N: number of subjects; P: probability.

Several authors have described the association of disability, measured by the WOMAC scores, with higher levels of proinflammatory cytokines [14, 15, 18, 34]. TNF has been compared to other proinflammatory cytokines and shown to be elevated in elderly patients with knee osteoarthritis [6, 35, 36]. Regarding knee OA, the most commonly measured cytokines in the literature are IL-6 and TNF-α [6, 37, 38]. Similar to previous reports [6, 35, 39], we observed that serum levels of IL-6 had a twofold increase in patients when compared to controls, comparable to a study that

TABLE 4: Correlation among cytokines, age, pain duration, VAS, WOMAC scores, and PPT values over 24 anatomical structures.

Variables		TNF-α	IL-10	IL-6	IL-8
Age	Spearman*	−0.154	−0.019	0.016	−0.006
	P	0.123	0.854	0.873	0.954
	N	101	101	101	101
Pain duration (months)	Spearman*	−0.039	0.185	0.166	−0.001
	P	0.706	0.070	0.105	0.993
	N	97	97	97	97
VAS	Spearman*	−0.029	0.203	0.238	0.020
	P	0.774	0.042	0.017	0.842
	N	101	101	101	101
WOMAC pain	Spearman*	−0.145	0.177	0.251	0.019
	P	0.151	0.078	0.012	0.850
	N	100	100	100	100
WOMAC rigidity	Spearman*	−0.050	0.271	0.303	0.059
	P	0.626	0.007	0.002	0.562
	N	99	99	99	99
WOMAC difficulties	Spearman*	−0.134	0.166	0.192	0.013
	P	0.182	0.097	0.055	0.896
	N	101	101	101	101
Vastus M	Spearman*	0.283	0.075	−0.070	0.113
	P	0.004	0.453	0.488	0.259
	N	101	101	101	101
Adductor L	Spearman*	0.337	0.054	−0.076	0.097
	P	0.001	0.589	0.449	0.335
	N	101	101	101	101
Rectus A	Spearman*	0.229	0.034	−0.056	0.133
	P	0.021	0.737	0.580	0.185
	N	101	101	101	101
Vastus L	Spearman*	0.252	−0.006	0.015	0.154
	P	0.011	0.955	0.880	0.124
	N	101	101	101	101
Tibialis ant	Spearman*	0.236	−0.067	−0.065	0.096
	P	0.017	0.507	0.519	0.338
	N	101	101	101	101
Peroneal	Spearman*	0.322	0.001	−0.075	0.067
	P	0.001	0.992	0.456	0.503
	N	101	101	101	101
Pes anserinus	Spearman*	0.339	0.113	0.009	0.099
	P	0.001	0.259	0.932	0.326
	N	101	101	101	101
Gracilis	Spearman*	0.322	0.050	−0.031	0.101
	P	0.001	0.623	0.761	0.316
	N	101	101	101	101
Iliopsoas	Spearman*	0.136	−0.098	−0.060	−0.058
	P	0.175	0.330	0.554	0.564
	N	101	101	101	101
Quad L	Spearman*	0.228	−0.080	−0.087	−0.030
	P	0.022	0.424	0.384	0.764
	N	101	101	101	101
Lig L1-L2	Spearman*	0.204	−0.122	−0.032	0.084
	P	0.041	0.223	0.750	0.406
	N	101	101	101	101

TABLE 4: Continued.

Variables		TNF-α	IL-10	IL-6	IL-8
Lig L2-L3	Spearman*	0.192	−0.100	−0.031	0.034
	P	0.055	0.322	0.762	0.733
	N	101	101	101	101
Lig L3-L4	Spearman*	0.139	−0.117	−0.068	0.037
	P	0.165	0.243	0.496	0.711
	N	101	101	101	101
Lig L4-L5	Spearman*	0.187	−0.091	−0.034	0.098
	P	0.061	0.367	0.737	0.330
	N	101	101	101	101
L5-S1	Spearman*	0.188	−0.045	−0.048	0.102
	P	0.060	0.656	0.635	0.312
	N	101	101	101	101
Lig S1-S2	Spearman*	0.171	−0.100	−0.067	0.081
	P	0.087	0.318	0.504	0.420
	N	101	101	101	101
Popliteus	Spearman*	0.266	−0.102	−0.067	0.056
	P	0.007	0.308	0.503	0.581
	N	101	101	101	101
PRL1	Spearman*	0.328	0.089	−0.077	0.057
	P	0.001	0.377	0.445	0.574
	N	101	101	101	101
PRL2	Spearman*	0.323	0.052	−0.063	0.123
	P	0.001	0.607	0.529	0.221
	N	101	101	101	101
PRL3	Spearman*	0.313	0.017	−0.046	0.059
	P	0.001	0.870	0.645	0.559
	N	101	101	101	101
PRL4	Spearman*	0.253	−0.061	−0.094	0.138
	P	0.011	0.547	0.349	0.169
	N	101	101	101	101
PRL5	Spearman*	0.278	−0.049	−0.013	0.073
	P	0.005	0.627	0.896	0.470
	N	101	101	101	101
PR S1	Spearman*	0.275	−0.104	−0.151	−0.026
	P	0.005	0.303	0.132	0.798
	N	101	101	101	101
PR S2	Spearman*	0.221	0.000	−0.068	−0.008
	P	0.026	0.998	0.497	0.938
	N	101	101	101	101

*Spearman's rank correlation coefficients.
Vastus M: vastus medialis; Adductor L: adductor longus; Rectus A: rectus femoris; Vastus L: vastus lateralis; Tibialis ant: tibialis anterior; PR: pinch and roll maneuver; Lig: supraspinous ligaments; Quad L: quadratus lumborum; L: lumbar; S: sacral; IL: interleukin; TNF: tumor necrosis factor; WOMAC: Western Ontario and McMaster Universities Arthritis Index; *r*: Spearman correlation; *P*: probability.

showed increased IL-6 in patients with more severe disease as measured by radiologic knee OA findings [6]. On the other hand, serum concentrations of the other cytokines are very heterogeneous to draw any conclusions. We also demonstrated that symptomatic patients presented less resistance to algometer-induced PPT than did the healthy controls in all 24 muscular, ligamentous, and subcutaneous points

TABLE 5: Stepwise multiple linear regression models for IL-6 and TNF-α and age, VAS, WOMAC pain subscale, WOMAC rigidity subscale, WOMAC physical activity subscale, and pressure pain threshold values (in kg/cm^2) in 24 studies structures.

IL-6 (pg/mL)	R^2	0.186	P
Independent variables	Estimated parameter	Standard error	
(Constant)	0.961	0.125	<0.000
WOMAC rigidity	0.157	0.034	<0.000
VAS L	0.050	0.019	0.012
TNF-α (pg/mL)	R^2	0.244	P
Independent variables	Estimated parameter	Standard error	
(Constant)	0.356	0.189	0.062
Pes anserinus	0.167	0.033	0.000
VAS	0.049	0.018	0.007
Ligaments L1-L2	−0.059	0.027	0.032

L: left.

tested, not only at the knees. Both IL-6 and IL-10 correlated positively with VAS and WOMAC scores for rigidity. Only IL-6 correlated positively with WOMAC pain scores.

In fact, many have investigated the effect of different presentations of OA on the serum or intra-articular levels of cytokines [6, 14–16]. However, to the best of our knowledge, this is the first report regarding the association between serum proinflammatory cytokines and PPTs that are located further beyond the painful area at the involved joint. This indicates a sclerotome-wide phenomenon that can be explained only neurologically. On the other hand, the lack of relation between this particular cytokine and pain duration, WOMAC scores, or VAS remains to be clarified. Additionally, since cytokine IL-10 was not detectable in the cerebrospinal fluid of patients with knee OA, the concept of central sensitization as an important mechanism in the causal chain of disability would be noteworthy [40]. Several authors have already demonstrated that proinflammatory mediators as interleukins are increased in fibromyalgia patients [41, 42]. It seems that chronic pain, hyperalgesia, and fatigue are associated with increased levels of IL-6 and IL-8 in these patients [18, 41]. Similarly, tissue lesion may, in most cases, not be the major issue determining loss of function and quality of life in OA.

Interestingly, muscle tender points and lower tolerance to pressure areas have higher levels of TNF-α when compared to healthy individuals without spontaneous pain or asymptomatic subjects [43–45]. In subjects with spontaneous pain, areas distant from the site of pain also showed a significant increase of these chemical mediators [45]. Cytokine production has also been demonstrated in nonimmune tissue under special conditions such as acute inflammation. Production of proinflammatory cytokines such as IL-1-β, IL-6, and TNF-α has recently been found in skeletal muscle tissue during special conditions such as endotoxemia [46]. However, the influence of hyperalgesia found in muscle tissues of patients with OA on serum cytokines has not been determined, although leaking from local microenvironment could be a possible mechanism.

Still, we must remember that the process called inflammaging indicating a regulation of the inflammatory response that occurs with aging can result in the production of inflammatory cytokines, which generates a low level of chronic and systemic proinflammatory state [47, 48]. This may occur due to the presence of chronic diseases associated with aging such as OA, as well as other conditions such as obesity and physical inactivity [47].

A possible source of local cytokine production, different from the inflammatory cells, may be the adipose tissue. It is known that adipose tissue produces and secretes several proinflammatory cytokines, including IL-6 and TNF-α [49]. Despite the lack of correlations between IL-6 and the PPT values over any of the assessed tissues, we observed that PPT value over supraspinous ligament L1-L2 combined with pes anserinus and VAS can predict serum levels of TNF-α. Yet increased production and secretion of proinflammatory cytokines (biomarkers) by adipose cells have been hypothesized as the role played by obesity as a risk factor for OA [50]. According to Livshits et al. [6], when inflammation occurs, cytokine profile changes and seems to be influenced by obesity and aging [15, 16]. In fact, we have recently demonstrated that aging may play a role in cytokine profile, a finding not so extensively addressed in the literature and that should be further investigated [51]. In the elderly population, body metabolism and composition, as well as the response to acute inflammation, may be altered and influenced in a different pattern by cytokines than in the acute-phase response, all of which are altered with increasing age [52]. TNF-α seems to act as a biomarker of physiologic status and a major predictor of strength and functional status in the elderly [6]. IL-1α, IL-1β, and TNF-α seem to induce production of IL-6 [52]. To the best of our knowledge, the contribution of inflammatory factors such as IL-6 and TNF-α to the involvement of structures outside the knee joint has not been adequately explored yet, in particular, the correlation of structures that are innervated by the same spinal nerve constituting the metameres.

Our study had some limitations. First, we did not measure other cytokines such as IL-1 or IL-Ra, due to the budget of the study. Another item is the lack of radiographic evaluation of the control subjects. But it is noteworthy that, in the clinical evaluation of these patients, absence of pain was observed and evaluated. However, further studies with radiographic classification of healthy volunteers, with other cytokines, are needed to confirm our findings and to explore the local production of cytokines by skeletal muscle (myocytes), adipose cells, and the surrounding connective tissue.

5. Conclusion

This study showed that serum levels of IL-6 and IL-10 were higher in knee OA than in healthy controls. A positive association between IL-10 and IL-6 with VAS and WOMAC for pain and rigidity scores was found. These findings align with a physiopathological understanding of pain and functionality that surpasses the one which currently provides basis for therapeutics in OA.

Acknowledgment

For this study, there was no sponsorship. The study was conducted with the authors' own resources.

References

[1] B. M. Alkan, F. Fidan, A. Tosun, and Ö. Ardiçoğlu, "Quality of life and self-reported disability in patients with knee osteoarthritis," *Modern Rheumatology*, vol. 24, no. 1, pp. 166–171, 2014.

[2] H. Kotlarz, C. L. Gunnarsson, H. Fang, and J. A. Rizzo, "Insurer and out-of-pocket costs of osteoarthritis in the US: evidence from national survey data," *Arthritis and Rheumatism*, vol. 60, no. 12, pp. 3546–3553, 2009.

[3] D. C. Ang, G. James, and T. E. Stump, "Clinical appropriateness and not race predicted referral for joint arthroplasty," *Arthritis Care and Research*, vol. 61, no. 12, pp. 1677–1685, 2009.

[4] A. J. Fellet, A. F. Afonso, and L. F. Barbosa, "Osteoarthrosis: uma revisão," *Revista Brasileira de Medicina*, vol. 64, no. 11, pp. 55–61, 2007.

[5] W. Zhang, G. Nuki, R. W. Moskowitz et al., "OARSI recommendations for the management of hip and knee osteoarthritis. Part III: changes in evidence following systematic cumulative update of research published through January 2009," *Osteoarthritis and Cartilage*, vol. 18, no. 4, pp. 476–499, 2010.

[6] G. Livshits, G. Zhai, D. J. Hart et al., "Interleukin-6 is a significant predictor of radiographic knee osteoarthritis: the Chingford Study," *Arthritis and Rheumatism*, vol. 60, no. 7, pp. 2037–2045, 2009.

[7] M. B. Goldring, M. Otero, D. A. Plumb et al., "Roles of inflammatory and anabolic cytokines in cartilage metabolism: signals and multiple effectors converge upon MMP-13 regulation in osteoarthritis," *European Cells and Materials*, vol. 21, pp. 202–220, 2011.

[8] N. Saetan, S. Honsawek, A. Tanavalee, S. Tantavisut, P. Yuktanandana, and V. Parkpian, "Association of plasma and synovial fluid interferon-γ inducible protein-10 with radiographic severity in knee osteoarthritis," *Clinical Biochemistry*, vol. 44, no. 14-15, pp. 1218–1222, 2011.

[9] J. Kumm, A. Tamm, M. Lintrop, and A. Tamm, "The value of cartilage biomarkers in progressive knee osteoarthritis: cross-sectional and 6-year follow-up study in middle-aged subjects," *Rheumatology International*, vol. 33, no. 4, pp. 903–911, 2013.

[10] E. B. Dam, I. Byrjalsen, L. Arendt-Nielsen, C. Christiansen, and M. A. Karsdal, "Relationships between knee pain and osteoarthritis biomarkers based on systemic fluids and magnetic resonance imaging," *Journal of Musculoskeletal Pain*, vol. 19, no. 3, pp. 144–153, 2011.

[11] P. Garnero, "Biochemical markers of bone remodeling," *Annales de Biologie Clinique*, vol. 59, article 298, 2001.

[12] M. Ishijima, T. Watari, K. Naito et al., "Relationships between biomarkers of cartilage, bone, synovial metabolism and knee pain provide insights into the origins of pain in early knee osteoarthritis," *Arthritis Research & Therapy*, vol. 13, article R22, 2011.

[13] D. M. Vigushin, M. B. Pepys, and P. N. Hawkins, "Metabolic and scintigraphic studies of radioiodinated human C-reactive protein in health and disease," *Journal of Clinical Investigation*, vol. 91, no. 4, pp. 1351–1357, 1993.

[14] L. Ferrucci, B. W. J. H. Penninx, S. Volpato et al., "Change in muscle strength explains accelerated decline of physical function in older women with high interleukin-6 serum levels," *Journal of the American Geriatrics Society*, vol. 50, no. 12, pp. 1947–1954, 2002.

[15] G. D. Miller, B. J. Nicklas, and R. F. Loeser, "Inflammatory biomarkers and physical function in older, obese adults with knee pain and self-reported osteoarthritis after intensive weight-loss therapy," *Journal of the American Geriatrics Society*, vol. 56, no. 4, pp. 644–651, 2008.

[16] B. W. J. H. Penninx, H. Abbas, W. Ambrosius et al., "Inflammatory markers and physical function among older adults with knee osteoarthritis," *Journal of Rheumatology*, vol. 31, no. 10, pp. 2027–2031, 2004.

[17] K. C. Deere, J. Clinch, K. Holliday et al., "Obesity is a risk factor for musculoskeletal pain in adolescents: findings from a population-based cohort," *Pain*, vol. 153, no. 9, pp. 1932–1938, 2012.

[18] M. Imamura, S. T. Imamura, H. H. S. Kaziyama et al., "Impact of nervous system hyperalgesia on pain, disability, and quality of life in patients with knee osteoarthritis: a controlled analysis," *Arthritis Care and Research*, vol. 59, no. 10, pp. 1424–1431, 2008.

[19] L. Arendt-Nielsen, H. Nie, M. B. Laursen et al., "Sensitization in patients with painful knee osteoarthritis," *Pain*, vol. 149, no. 3, pp. 573–581, 2010.

[20] T. Graven-Nielsen, T. Wodehouse, R. M. Langford, L. Arendt-Nielsen, and B. L. Kidd, "Normalization of widespread hyperesthesia and facilitated spatial summation of deep-tissue pain in knee osteoarthritis patients after knee replacement," *Arthritis and Rheumatism*, vol. 64, no. 9, pp. 2907–2916, 2012.

[21] A. K. Suokas, D. A. Walsh, D. F. McWilliams et al., "Quantitative sensory testing in painful osteoarthritis: a systematic review and meta-analysis," *Osteoarthritis and Cartilage*, vol. 20, no. 10, pp. 1075–1085, 2012.

[22] D. T. Felson, "The sources of pain in knee osteoarthritis," *Current Opinion in Rheumatology*, vol. 17, no. 5, pp. 624–628, 2005.

[23] P. H. Finan, L. F. Buenaver, S. C. Bounds et al., "Discordance between pain and radiographic severity in knee osteoarthritis: findings from quantitative sensory testing of central sensitization," *Arthritis and Rheumatism*, vol. 65, no. 2, pp. 363–372, 2013.

[24] R. Altman, E. Asch, and D. Bloch, "Development of criteria for the classification and reporting of osteoarthritis. Classification of osteoarthritis of the knee. Diagnostic and Therapeutic Criteria Committee of the American Rheumatism Association," *Arthritis and Rheumatism*, vol. 29, no. 8, pp. 1039–1049, 1986.

[25] P. Ravaud, G.-R. Auleley, C. Chastang et al., "Knee joint space width measurement: an experimental study of the influence of radiographic procedure and joint positioning," *British Journal of Rheumatology*, vol. 35, no. 8, pp. 761–766, 1996.

[26] N. Bellamy, W. W. Buchanan, C. H. Goldsmith, J. Campbell, and L. W. Stitt, "Validation study of WOMAC: a health status instrument for measuring clinically important patient relevant outcomes to antirheumatic drug therapy in patients with

osteoarthritis of the hip or knee," *Journal of Rheumatology*, vol. 15, no. 12, pp. 1833–1840, 1988.

[27] J. Keegan and F. D. Garrett, "The segmental distribution of the cutaneous nerves in the limbs of man," *The Anatomical Record*, vol. 102, no. 4, pp. 409–437, 1948.

[28] A. D. Farasyn, R. Meeusen, and J. Nijs, "Validity of cross-friction algometry procedure in referred muscle pain syndromes: preliminary results of a new referred pain provocation technique with the aid of a Fischer pressure algometer in patients with nonspecific low back pain," *Clinical Journal of Pain*, vol. 24, no. 5, pp. 456–462, 2008.

[29] J. Curfs, J. Meis, and J. Hoogkamp-Korstanje, "A primer on cytokines: sources, receptors, effects, and inducers," *Clinical Microbiology Reviews*, vol. 10, no. 4, pp. 742–780, 1997.

[30] J.-P. Pelletier, J. Martel-Pelletier, and S. B. Abramson, "Osteoarthritis, an inflammatory disease: potential implication for the selection of new therapeutic targets," *Arthritis & Rheumatism*, vol. 44, no. 6, pp. 1237–1247, 2001.

[31] F. A. J. van de Loo, S. Veenbergen, B. van den Brand et al., "Enhanced suppressor of cytokine signaling 3 in arthritic cartilage dysregulates human chondrocyte function," *Arthritis and Rheumatism*, vol. 64, no. 10, pp. 3313–3323, 2012.

[32] T. Saxne, M. Lindell, B. Månsson, I. F. Petersson, and D. Heinegård, "Inflammation is a feature of the disease process in early knee joint osteoarthritis," *Rheumatology*, vol. 42, no. 7, pp. 903–904, 2003.

[33] T. D. Spector, D. J. Hart, D. Nandra et al., "Low-level increases in serum C-reactive protein are present in early osteoarthritis of the knee and predict progressive disease," *Arthritis and Rheumatism*, vol. 40, no. 4, pp. 723–727, 1997.

[34] K. F. Ferraro and T. L. Booth, "Age, body mass index, and functional illness," *Journals of Gerontology—Series B Psychological Sciences and Social Sciences*, vol. 54, no. 6, pp. S339–S348, 1999.

[35] O. Stannus, G. Jones, F. Cicuttini et al., "Circulating levels of IL-6 and TNF-α are associated with knee radiographic osteoarthritis and knee cartilage loss in older adults," *Osteoarthritis and Cartilage*, vol. 18, no. 11, pp. 1441–1447, 2010.

[36] C. Ding, F. Cicuttini, V. Parameswaran, O. Stannus, J. Burgess, and G. Jones, "045 serum levels of inflammatory markers, knee radiographic osteoarthritis, and knee cartilage loss in older adults," *Osteoarthritis and Cartilage*, vol. 17, p. S33, 2009.

[37] C. R. Scanzello, E. Umoh, F. Pessler et al., "Local cytokine profiles in knee osteoarthritis: elevated synovial fluid interleukin-15 differentiates early from end-stage disease," *Osteoarthritis and Cartilage*, vol. 17, no. 8, pp. 1040–1048, 2009.

[38] A. D. Pearle, C. R. Scanzello, S. George et al., "Elevated high-sensitivity C-reactive protein levels are associated with local inflammatory findings in patients with osteoarthritis," *Osteoarthritis and Cartilage*, vol. 15, no. 5, pp. 516–523, 2007.

[39] M. L. A. S. Santos, W. F. Gomes, D. S. Pereira et al., "Muscle strength, muscle balance, physical function and plasma interleukin-6 (IL-6) levels in elderly women with knee osteoarthritis (OA)," *Archives of Gerontology and Geriatrics*, vol. 52, no. 3, pp. 322–326, 2011.

[40] C. Lundborg, M. Hahn-Zoric, B. Biber, and E. Hansson, "Glial cell line-derived neurotrophic factor is increased in cerebrospinal fluid but decreased in blood during long-term pain," *Journal of Neuroimmunology*, vol. 220, no. 1-2, pp. 108–113, 2010.

[41] D. J. Wallace, M. Linker-Israeli, D. Hallegua, S. Silverman, D. Silver, and M. H. Weisman, "Cytokines play an aetiopathogenetic role in fibromyalgia: a hypothesis and pilot study," *Rheumatology*, vol. 40, no. 7, pp. 743–749, 2001.

[42] A. Gur, M. Karakoc, S. Erdogan, K. Nas, R. Cevik, and A. J. Sarac, "Regional cerebral blood flow and cytokines in young females with fibromyalgia," *Clinical and Experimental Rheumatology*, vol. 20, no. 6, pp. 753–760, 2002.

[43] J. P. Shah, T. M. Phillips, J. V. Danoff, and L. H. Gerber, "An in vivo microanalytical technique for measuring the local biochemical milieu of human skeletal muscle," *Journal of Applied Physiology*, vol. 99, no. 5, pp. 1977–1984, 2005.

[44] J. P. Shah and E. A. Gilliams, "Uncovering the biochemical milieu of myofascial trigger points using in vivo microdialysis: an application of muscle pain concepts to myofascial pain syndrome," *Journal of Bodywork and Movement Therapies*, vol. 12, no. 4, pp. 371–384, 2008.

[45] J. P. Shah, J. V. Danoff, M. J. Desai et al., "Biochemicals associated with pain and inflammation are elevated in sites near to and remote from active myofascial trigger points," *Archives of Physical Medicine and Rehabilitation*, vol. 89, no. 1, pp. 16–23, 2008.

[46] B. Å. S. Borge, K.-H. Kalland, S. Olsen, A. Bletsa, E. Berggreen, and H. Wiig, "Cytokines are produced locally by myocytes in rat skeletal muscle during endotoxemia," *The American Journal of Physiology—Heart and Circulatory Physiology*, vol. 296, no. 3, pp. H735–H744, 2009.

[47] D. Baylis, D. B. Bartlett, H. P. Patel, and H. C. Roberts, "Understanding how we age: insights into inflammaging," *Longevity & Healthspan*, vol. 2, no. 1, article 8, 2013.

[48] J. A. Woods, K. R. Wilund, A. S. Martin, and B. M. Kistler, "Exercise, inflammation and aging," *Aging and Disease*, vol. 3, no. 1, pp. 130–140, 2012.

[49] V. Mohamed-Ali, S. Goodrick, A. Rawesh et al., "Subcutaneous adipose tissue releases interleukin-6, but not tumor necrosis factor-alpha, in vivo," *Journal of Clinical Endocrinology and Metabolism*, vol. 82, no. 12, pp. 4196–4200, 1997.

[50] M. Bulló, P. García-Lorda, I. Megias, and J. Salas-Salvadó, "Systemic inflammation, adipose tissue tumor necrosis factor, and leptin expression," *Obesity Research*, vol. 11, no. 4, pp. 525–531, 2003.

[51] M. Imamura, R. A. Targino, W. T. Hsing et al., "Concentration of cytokines in patients with osteoarthritis of the knee and fibromyalgia," *Clinical Interventions in Aging*, vol. 9, pp. 939–944, 2014.

[52] K. J. Tracey and A. Cerami, "Tumor necrosis factor, other cytokines and disease," *Annual Review of Cell Biology*, vol. 9, pp. 317–343, 1993.

17

Inflammatory Serum Protein Profiling of Patients with Lumbar Radicular Pain One Year after Disc Herniation

Aurora Moen,[1,2] Anne-Li Lind,[3] Måns Thulin,[4] Masood Kamali-Moghaddam,[5] Cecilie Røe,[2,6] Johannes Gjerstad,[1,2,7] and Torsten Gordh[3]

[1]*National Institute of Occupational Health, 0033 Oslo, Norway*
[2]*Department of Physical Medicine and Rehabilitation, Oslo University Hospital, 0424 Oslo, Norway*
[3]*Department of Surgical Sciences, Uppsala University, 751 85 Uppsala, Sweden*
[4]*Department of Statistics, Uppsala University, 751 20 Uppsala, Sweden*
[5]*Department of Immunology, Genetics and Pathology, Science for Life Laboratory, Uppsala University, 751 85 Uppsala, Sweden*
[6]*Faculty of Medicine, University of Oslo, 0316 Oslo, Norway*
[7]*Department of Molecular Biosciences, University of Oslo, 0371 Oslo, Norway*

Correspondence should be addressed to Johannes Gjerstad; johannes.gjerstad@stami.no

Academic Editor: Sarah Howie

Earlier studies suggest that lumbar radicular pain following disc herniation may be associated with a local or systemic inflammatory process. In the present study, we investigated the serum inflammatory protein profile of such patients. All 45 patients were recruited from Oslo University Hospital, Ullevål, Norway, during the period 2007–2009. The new multiplex proximity extension assay (PEA) technology was used to analyze the levels of 92 proteins. Interestingly, the present data showed that patients with radicular pain 12 months after disc herniation may be different from other patients with regard to many measurable serum cytokines. Given a false discovery rate (FDR) of 0.10 and 0.05, we identified 41 and 13 proteins, respectively, which were significantly upregulated in the patients with severe pain one year after disc herniation. On the top of the list ranked by estimated increase we found C-X-C motif chemokine 5 (CXCM5; 217% increase), epidermal growth factor (EGF; 142% increase), and monocyte chemotactic protein 4 (MCP-4; 70% increase). Moreover, a clear overall difference in the serum cytokine profile between the chronic and the recovered patients was demonstrated. Thus, the present results may be important for future protein serum profiling of lumbar radicular pain patients with regard to prognosis and choice of treatment. We conclude that serum proteins may be measurable molecular markers of persistent pain after disc herniation.

1. Introduction

Lumbar radicular pain, also referred to as "sciatica," is characterized by radiating pain that typically follows the dermatome of the affected nerve-root. When strict criteria are used, the prevalence rate is approximately 2% [1, 2]. Roughly 90% of the lumbar radicular pain cases are caused by intervertebral disc herniation with nerve-root compression [3]. Although a spontaneous recovery is seen in most of these patients, only 30% are completely pain-free one year after onset [4]. At present, there are no measurable molecular markers for patient prognosis, choice of treatment, or development of new compounds for persistent pain after disc herniation.

Earlier studies suggest that leakage of nucleus pulposus into the spinal canal after disc herniation may initiate immunological and inflammatory responses close to the nerve-roots [5, 6] that increase the activity in nociceptive pathways [7–11]. This inflammatory influence has been attributed to an upregulation of interleukins (ILs), tumor necrosis factor (TNF), matrix metalloproteinases (MMPs), nitric oxide (NO), and prostaglandins (PGs) in or around the herniated disc [12–14].

In addition, recent data point to increased levels of circulating cytokines in patients with chronic pain. For example, higher systemic IL-2 and TNF levels have been observed in patients with painful neuropathies compared to painless neuropathies [15]. Moreover, IL-6 and IL-8 appear to be elevated in serum of patients with radicular pain due to disc herniation [16, 17]. Thus, earlier observations suggest that disc herniation may be associated with an upregulation of several inflammatory molecules. In these previous studies, however, the methodological hindrance has limited the number of markers to a few proteins.

In the present study, in contrast, we take advantage of the new multiplex proximity extension assay (PEA) technology to simultaneously analyze the levels of 92 inflammatory proteins [18]. To adjust for multiplicity, we used the false discovery rate (FDR) approach in the statistical analysis of the data [19]. The aim of the present study was to investigate if it is possible to define an inflammatory fingerprint in the serum of patients with persistent lumbar radicular pain after disc herniation. Our results indicate that the PEA technology may be important for future protein serum profiling of lumbar radicular pain patients with regard to prognosis and choice of treatment.

2. Materials and Methods

2.1. Patients. Patients with lumbar radicular pain were recruited from the outpatient clinic at Oslo University Hospital, Ullevål, Norway, during the period 2007–2009. The inclusion criteria were age between 18 and 60 years, lumbar disc herniation confirmed by magnetic resonance imaging (MRI) with corresponding radicular pain, and positive Straight Leg Raising (SLR). The exclusion criteria were lumbar spinal stenosis, previous surgery for herniated disc at the same level or fusion at any level in lumbar spine, generalized musculoskeletal pain, inflammatory rheumatic disease, diabetic polyneuropathy, cardiovascular disease (NYHA III and IV), cancer, psychiatric disease, cauda equine syndrome, alcohol or drug abuse, recent surgery (within one month), pregnancy, poor Norwegian language, or non-European-Caucasian ethnicity. In total, 122 patients (82%) of the 148 patients who met the eligibility requirement were included in the intended follow-up assessment.

Surgical treatment was given to patients with persistent radicular pain lasting for more than 8 weeks, neurological deficits (sensory changes, muscle weakness, and depressed or absent deep tendon reflexes), and corresponding magnetic resonance imaging findings in the anticipated location. Patients who did not clearly fulfill these criteria were managed conservatively by a treatment comprised of a brief cognitive intervention, activity guidance during the acute phase of disc herniation, and, for the majority of patients, physiotherapy.

At inclusion, at 6 weeks and at 12-month follow-up, the patients were asked to rate their pain intensity in activity during the last week on a 10 cm visual analog scale (VAS) with endpoints "no pain" and "worst possible pain." Hopkins symptom checklist (HSCL), a 25-item questionnaire, was used to register psychological distress, that is, anxiety and depression. The drop-out rate was 8% and ultimately, 112 patients were assessed at 12-month follow-up.

Among these 112 patients, patients with VAS > 6 at 12-month follow-up were defined as a high pain group ($n = 23$). Moreover, a gender and age matched sample from the same 112 patients with VAS < 1 at 12-month follow-up was defined as a low pain group ($n = 22$). The serum levels in inflammatory-related proteins in the high pain group versus the low pain group were analyzed. All participants received written information and signed an informed consent form. The study was approved by the Norwegian Regional Committee for Medical Research Ethics and the Norwegian Social Science Data Services.

2.2. Blood Sampling. At 12-month follow-up, venous blood was collected and kept on ice for 45 minutes. After centrifugation at 2,000 g for 10 min at 4°C, the supernatant serum was collected and stored in aliquots at −80°C until further analysis. Serum was used to analyze the biomarkers for the levels of 92 inflammatory proteins.

2.3. Proximal Extension Assay. In the present study we took advantage of the multiplex proximity extension assay (PEA) technology in which a panel of 92 proteins (see Supplementary Table 1 in Supplementary Material available online at http://dx.doi.org/10.1155/2016/3874964) is simultaneously analyzed [18]. The serum samples were assessed with Proseek Multiplex Inflammation I (Olink Bioscience, Uppsala, Sweden) using the PEA according to the manufacturer's instructions. Briefly, 3 μL incubation mix containing two PEA probes, that is, antibodies equipped with single strand DNA oligonucleotide, against each protein was mixed with 1 μL serum and the mixture was incubated at 8°C overnight. The mixture was then mixed with 96 μL extension mix containing PEA enzyme and PCR reagents and incubated for 5 min at room temperature before the plate was transferred to a thermal cycler for 17 cycles of DNA amplification. A 96.96 Dynamic Array IFC (Fluidigm, CA, USA) was prepared and primed according to the manufacturer's instructions. 2.8 μL of sample mixture was mixed with 7.2 μL detection mix in a new 96-well plate and 5 μL was loaded into the right side of the primed 96.96 Dynamic Array IFC. The unique primer pairs for each cytokine were loaded into the left side of the 96.96 Dynamic Array IFC, and the protein expression program was run in Fluidigm Biomark reader according to the instructions for Proseek.

2.4. Statistics. For the baseline characteristics, the Kolmogorov-Smirnov test was applied to test for normality. Unpaired Student's t-test was chosen to compare mean values for normally distributed data, whereas for nonnormally distributed data the mean values were compared by a nonparametric two-sided Mann-Whitney U test. Pearson Chi-square test was used to analyze the frequency of baseline categorical variables between the high and low pain group.

In order to identify differentially expressed serum proteins between the two groups of patients, protein-level analyses for each individual biomarker were performed. For a group of patients, the protein expression levels of some proteins were below the laboratory's limit of detection (LoD). Therefore, we used a multiple linear regression model with LoD imputed values in place of below-LoD values to test the differences between the groups.

TABLE 1: Baseline characteristics of patients grouped in the high and low pain group.

	Low pain	High pain	p value
Gender, men/women (%)	11/11/(50/50)	12/11 (52/48)	0.884[a]
Age, mean (SD)	40 (9)	41 (12)	0.697[b]
Current smoker, yes/no (%)	6/16 (27/73)	13/10 (57/43)	0.047[a]
Treatment, surgery/conservative (%)	10/12 (45/55)	8/15 (35/65)	0.465[a]
HSCL total score, mean (SD)	1.53 (0.41)	2.09 (0.56)	0.001[c]

[a]Pearson Chi-square, [b]unpaired Student's t-test, and [c]Mann-Whitney U test. SD: standard deviation, and HSCL: Hopkins symptom checklist.

Because of the difficulties associated with analyzing data with a high proportion of below-LoD values [20–22], only proteins for which the proportion of below-LoD values was less than 20% were included in the analyses. The false discovery rate (FDR) was controlled using the procedure of Benjamini and Hochberg (1995) [19]. The difference in expression levels was estimated by computing the ratio of the group medians on the original non-log scale.

The linear discriminant analysis [23, 24] was performed to visualize the differences between the two groups. Using vector notation and letting $\mathbf{x}_{ij}$ denote the vector of protein measurements of patient j in group i (with $i = 1$ corresponding to high pain and $i = 2$ corresponding to low pain), $\bar{\mathbf{x}}_i$ denote the sample mean vector in group i, and n_i denote the number of patients in group i, the discriminant score for each individual was computed as

$$(\bar{\mathbf{x}}_1 - \bar{\mathbf{x}}_2)' \left(\sum_{i=1}^{2} \sum_{j=1}^{n_i} (\mathbf{x}_{ij} - \bar{\mathbf{x}}_i)(\mathbf{x}_{ij} - \bar{\mathbf{x}}_i)' \right)^{-1} \cdot \left(\mathbf{x}_{ij} - \frac{1}{2}(\bar{\mathbf{x}}_1 + \bar{\mathbf{x}}_2) \right). \quad (1)$$

This resulted in a score, essentially based on a weighted average of the differentially expressed proteins, such that positive values indicated high levels of inflammatory proteins and negative values indicated low levels of inflammatory proteins.

The weighted protein score was visualized in a simple dot plot where each patient was represented by one dot. A positive score indicated a high inflammatory activity, whereas a negative score indicated a low inflammatory activity.

3. Results

The high pain group had more pain when they arrived at the hospital, at 6 weeks and 12-month follow-up, than the low pain group (Figure 1). More smoking and higher HSCL score were also observed in the high pain group (Table 1). Therefore, smoking and HSCL were corrected for in the further analyses, that is, in the multiple linear regression model to test the differences between the high and low pain group.

The analyses of the levels of 92 proteins showed 76 proteins for which at most 20% of the patients had expression levels below the LoD. Among these 76 proteins, we identified 41 with FDR < 0.10 and 13 with FDR < 0.05, which were considered upregulated in the patients with severe pain one year after disc herniation (Table 2). The analyses of the inflammation-related protein levels showed increased expression of many proteins in the high pain group compared to the low pain group.

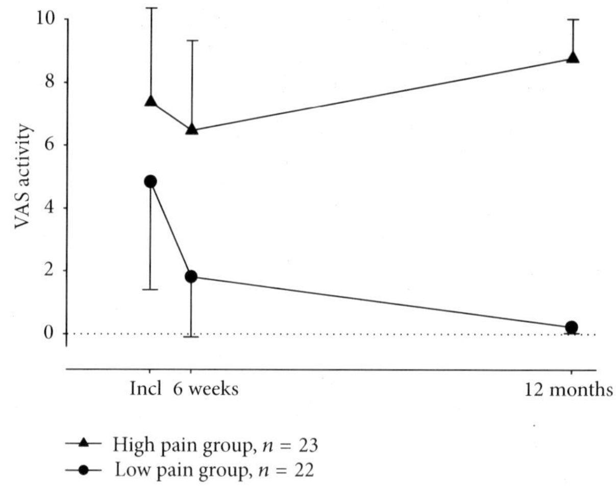

FIGURE 1: Intensity of pain in 45 disc herniation patients recruited from Oslo University Hospital, Ullevål, Norway. The patients were divided into two groups based on their clinical outcome measured by VAS at 12-month follow-up. The data are shown as mean ± SD.

On the top of the list ranked by estimated increase we found C-X-C motif chemokine 5 (CXCM5; 217% increase), epidermal growth factor (EGF; 142% increase), and monocyte chemotactic protein 4 (MCP-4; 70% increase).

For each patient, an inflammation score, that is, weighted average of the 41 protein levels, was also constructed. Notably, the two groups were completely separated; all high pain patients had positive scores, whereas all low pain patients had negative scores (Figure 2). Thus, an inflammatory fingerprint in the serum of the patients with persistent lumbar radicular pain after disc herniation was demonstrated. The data showed a clear increase in cytokine levels in the patients that developed chronic pain (Figure 3).

4. Discussion

In the present study, we examined the serum levels of 92 inflammatory proteins in patients one year after lumbar disc herniation. Among these, 41 proteins with FDR < 0.10, including IL-6 and IL-8, seemed to be upregulated in the chronic pain patients compared to the patients that fully recovered within one year. Hence, in accordance with our earlier ELISA findings from the same cohort where IL-6 and IL-8 in almost all patients were increased the first weeks after disc herniation [17, 25], the present data showed that patients that develop long lasting radicular pain may be different from patients that recover with regard to measurable cytokines in serum. Moreover, a clear overall difference in the serum cytokine profile between the chronic and the recovered patients was demonstrated.

TABLE 2: List of biomarkers which are significantly differentially expressed when the false discovery rate (FDR) is 0.10 and 0.05. The rightmost column shows the estimated increase on the original non-log scale.

Biomarker	p value	FDR adjusted p value	Estimated increase		
MCP-3/CCL7	0.0006	0.047	50.6%	↑	↑
M-CSF/CSF-1	0.001	0.047	20.2%		
VEGF-A	0.0015	0.047	47.6%		
CXCL10/IP10	0.0017	0.047	55.2%		
MCP-2	0.0023	0.047	56.6%		
CXCL5	0.0024	0.047	217.0%		
CCL-4	0.0034	0.047	43.4%		
IL-15-R-alpha	0.0036	0.047	15.2%		
MCP-4	0.004	0.047	69.9%		
TGF-beta-1	0.0041	0.047	52.3%		
CASP-8	0.0051	0.047	14.3%		
EGF	0.0064	0.047	142.0%		
STAMPB	0.0071	0.047	40.4%		FDR < 0.05
IFNg	0.0102	0.0553	25.0%		
IL-6	0.0118	0.0596	68.5%		
TRAIL	0.0119	0.0596	16.6%		
LIGHT-TNFSF14	0.0147	0.0656	35.6%		
CX3CL1	0.0147	0.0656	18.5%		
CXCL6	0.0153	0.0656	82.4%		
CXCL9-MIG	0.0165	0.0656	39.7%		
SIRT2	0.0173	0.0656	44.9%		
IL-10-R-beta	0.0179	0.0656	19.6%		
MCP-1-CCL2	0.0191	0.0656	36.2%		
HGF	0.0195	0.0656	37.9%		
Eotaxin-1	0.0198	0.0656	31.3%		
AXIN1	0.021	0.0656	11.2%		
CCL19	0.0217	0.0656	44.0%		
CDCP1	0.0223	0.0656	26.7%		
CD40	0.0233	0.0656	18.8%		
IL-8	0.0238	0.0656	47.5%		
SULT1A1	0.0256	0.0656	21.0%		
Beta-NGF	0.0286	0.0679	11.8%		
OSM	0.0298	0.0685	78.7%		
CCL20	0.0298	0.0685	43.7%		
TWEAK-TNFSF12	0.0316	0.0687	21.7%		
EIF4EBP1	0.0339	0.0716	59.2%		
MIP-1-alpha-CCL3	0.0384	0.0788	16.1%		
CXCL11	0.0384	0.0788	54.6%		
IL12B	0.0386	0.0788	28.9%		
IL18R1	0.0436	0.0828	20.8%		
CXCL1	0.0459	0.0852	52.8%	FDR < 0.10	

Many of the upregulated proteins with FDR < 0.05 were chemokines and other molecules associated with inflammation, activation of macrophages, and/or immune responses including regulators of glial cells. For example, C-X-C motif chemokine 5 (CXCL5) is a neutrophil chemoattractant which increases the expression of several proinflammatory mediators [26]. Moreover, monocyte chemotactic proteins 2, 3, and 4 (MCP-2, MCP-3/CCL7, and MCP-4) recruit macrophages [27], whereas C-X-C motif chemokine 10 (CXCL10/IP10) activates T-cells [28] and microglia [29]. Macrophages and microglia cells may also be activated by macrophage colony stimulating factor (M-CSF/CSF-1) thought to be upregulated in nucleus pulposus tissue after disc herniation [10, 30].

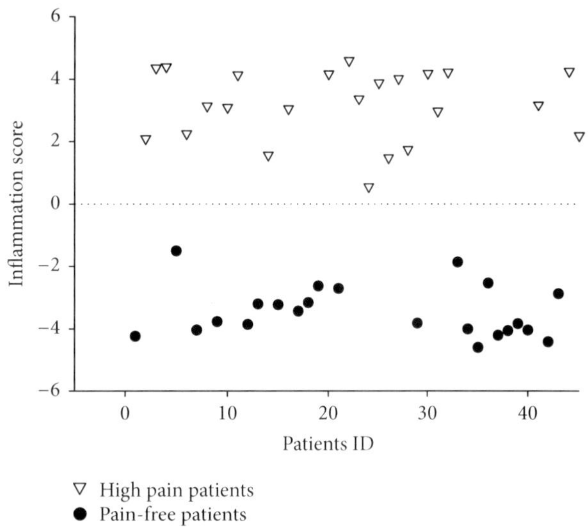

FIGURE 2: Linear discriminant analysis. An inflammation score was computed for each patient as a weighted average of the protein expression levels for the 41 biomarkers (FDR < 0.10). The scores were adjusted so that positive values indicate an ongoing inflammation and negative values indicate lack of inflammation. The scores are plotted for all patients (patient ID 1–45) in the study.

Several of the upregulated proteins with FDR < 0.05 have also previously been linked to healing and tissue regeneration. C-C motif chemokine 4 (CCL4) that reduces the expression of TNF and IL-1β [31] may be involved in nucleus pulposus resorption after disc herniation [32]. Vascular endothelial growth factor A (VEGF-A) supports healing, regeneration, and revascularization [33–35] and facilitates opening of the blood-nerve-barrier [36]. Interleukin-15 receptor-α (IL-15Rα) is expressed in monocytes, NK cells, and T-cells [37].

In addition, some of the upregulated proteins with FDR < 0.05 may induce cell differentiation, apoptosis, and neuronal loss and influence cell cycle regulation. Epidermal growth factor (EGF) stimulates cell growth, proliferation, and differentiation [38]. Moreover, transforming growth factor β (TGFβ) has important immune-regulative role and may reverse inflammation [39], whereas caspase-8 (CASP-8) is involved in FAS mediated apoptosis [40, 41] and cleavage of cytoskeletal proteins. STAM-binding protein (STAMBP) is a zinc metalloprotease involved in cell cycle regulation recently linked to the neuronal loss underlying microcephaly-capillary malformation syndrome [42].

4.1. Methodological Considerations. In PEA, each target molecule is recognized by a pair of affinity binders in which both have to bind the same target molecule prior to signal amplification via qPCR. Similar to other proximity assays [43, 44], the PEA technology also has an increased assay specificity. The specificity of the assay has been validated using a complete pool of PEA probes to analyze either all or submixes of eight antigens, for which significant signal over background was obtained only when the cognate antigen was present [18]. As previously described, the PEA technology has a sensitivity in low pM range [18].

Still, as some of the protein expressions were below the LoD, the actual expression levels of these proteins remain unknown. As high proportions of below-LoD measurements lead to tests with low power, we opted to only analyze the proteins for which the proportion of below-LoD measurements was at most 20%. Moreover, the two groups were balanced in terms of age, sex, and treatment but differed in smoking habits and HSCL scores (Table 1). Our linear regression model was therefore adjusted for smoking and HSCL scores to exclude the possibility that any differences found actually were due to differences in smoking and HSCL.

In the present study, we examined 92 serum proteins. Thus, the analyses of the data include multiple testing, that is, associated with many challenges. Clearly, we cannot control the family wise error rate by Bonferroni correction as such corrections tend to be far too conservative, resulting in statistical procedures with very low power. However, since this is a study where the focus is on evaluation of the methodology (proof of concept), a limited rate of false positives is acceptable. We therefore controlled the false discovery rate using the procedure of Benjamini and Hochberg [19].

Given a FDR of 0.10 and 0.05, up to 1/10 and 1/20 of our findings are likely to be false positives. Importantly, however, almost all inflammatory markers moved in the same direction. Moreover, although a few false positive markers may be present, our study clearly demonstrated that inflammatory profiling can be used to characterize chronic sciatica patients. The present data also showed that the PEA is a reliable and sensitive method to study proteins in serum associated with clinical measures.

Despite the above mentioned challenges, the linear discriminant analysis demonstrated a clear difference between the high pain group and the low pain group. A weighted average of the differentially expressed proteins with FDR < 0.10 was used [24]. This allowed us to summarize our multivariate data in a single objective measure [19]. Notably, the two groups were completely separated; all high pain patients had positive scores, whereas all low pain patients had negative scores. Thus, even though there might be one or two false positive markers, an inflammatory fingerprint in the serum of the patients that developed persistent lumbar radicular pain after disc herniation was defined by the PEA technology.

4.2. Study Limitations. Although the present study had a prospective design when it comes to the pain ratings, the serum protein levels of the patients were only measured at one time point, that is, 12 months after disc herniation. Thus, it is hard to tell whether the observed differences in serum proteins are a trait or a state of the patients that develop chronic pain. Moreover, medication and other life style factors may also influence the serum protein levels. However, the analgesics and anti-inflammatory-drugs taken by the patients were higher in the high pain group than in the low pain group. Therefore, it seems likely that the effect of medication reduces rather than increases the difference in inflammatory serum proteins. Nevertheless, the results demonstrated that it is possible to detect differences between persistent and nonpersistent pain patients. The fact that this

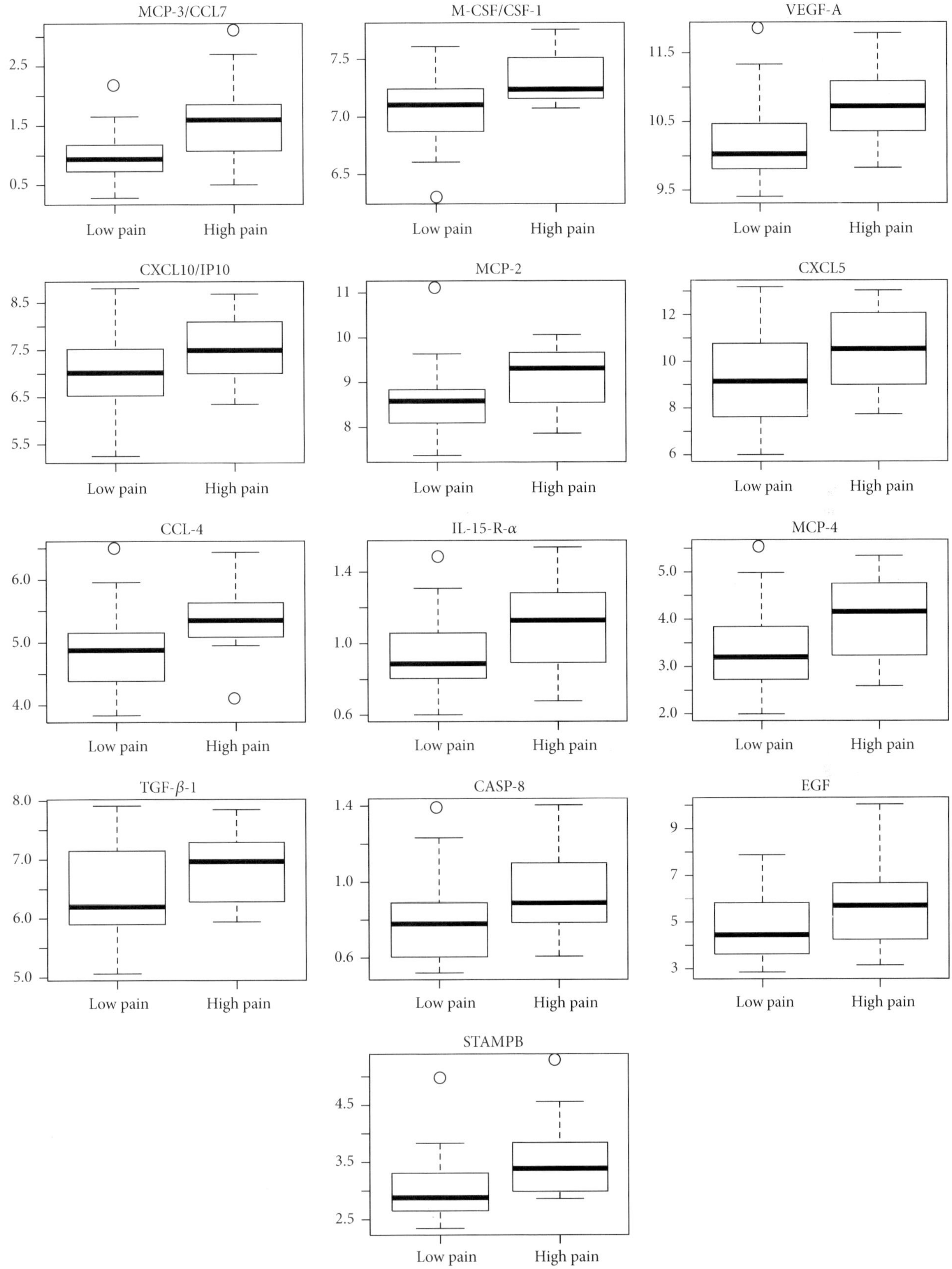

FIGURE 3: The expression of the 13 most significant proteins (FDR < 0.05). All 45 patients were included. The data are shown by box plot; median and IQR ± min/max.

protein pattern can be detected in serum suggests that the PEA technology may have a clinical potential.

5. Conclusion

In summary, the present data demonstrated that sciatica patients with a chronic outcome have increased levels of inflammatory proteins in serum one year after disc herniation. This is to our knowledge the first protein serum profiling study of patients with chronic lumbar radicular pain. An inflammatory PEA-based fingerprint of these persistent pain patients was demonstrated. We conclude that serum proteins may be measurable molecular markers of patients that develop persistent pain after disc herniation. The pathophysiological relevance of these proteins, however, remains to be investigated.

Competing Interests

The authors declare that there are no competing interests regarding the publication of this paper.

Acknowledgments

This research project was supported by Uppsala Berzelii Technology Centre for Neurodiagnostics, with financing from the Swedish Governmental Agency for Innovation Systems (Vinnova) and the Swedish Research Council (Grant no. P29797-1). The present study also received financial support from the South Eastern Norway Regional Health Authority (Grant no. 2013/20589). The authors thank Elina I. Schistad and Anette Storesund for data collection.

References

[1] R. A. Deyo and Y.-J. Tsui-Wu, "Functional disability due to back pain. A population-based study indicating the importance of socioeconomic factors," *Arthritis & Rheumatism*, vol. 30, no. 11, pp. 1247–1253, 1987.

[2] M. Younes, I. Béjia, Z. Aguir et al., "Prevalence and risk factors of disk-related sciatica in an urban population in Tunisia," *Joint Bone Spine*, vol. 73, no. 5, pp. 538–542, 2006.

[3] J.-P. Valat, S. Genevay, M. Marty, S. Rozenberg, and B. Koes, "Sciatica," *Best Practice & Research: Clinical Rheumatology*, vol. 24, no. 2, pp. 241–252, 2010.

[4] F. Balagué, M. Nordin, A. Sheikhzadeh et al., "Recovery of severe sciatica," *Spine*, vol. 24, no. 23, pp. 2516–2524, 1999.

[5] R. F. McCarron, M. W. Wimpee, P. G. Hudkins, and G. S. Laros, "The inflammatory effect of nucleus pulposus: a possible element in the pathogenesis of low-back pain," *Spine*, vol. 12, no. 8, pp. 760–764, 1987.

[6] K. Olmarker, J. Blomquist, J. Strömbarg et al., "Inflammatogenic properties of nucleus pulposus," *Spine*, vol. 20, no. 6, pp. 665–669, 1995.

[7] H. Anzai, M. Hamba, A. Onda, S. Konno, and S. Kikuchi, "Epidural application of nucleus pulposus enhances nociresponses of rat dorsal horn neurons," *Spine*, vol. 27, no. 3, pp. E50–E55, 2002.

[8] H. Brisby and I. Hammar, "Thalamic activation in a disc herniation model," *Spine*, vol. 32, no. 25, pp. 2846–2852, 2007.

[9] J. M. Cuellar, P. X. Montesano, J. F. Antognini, and E. Carstens, "Application of nucleus pulposus to L5 dorsal root ganglion in rats enhances nociceptive dorsal horn neuronal windup," *Journal of Neurophysiology*, vol. 94, no. 1, pp. 35–48, 2005.

[10] N. G. Egeland, A. Moen, L. M. Pedersen, H. Brisby, and J. Gjerstad, "Spinal nociceptive hyperexcitability induced by experimental disc herniation is associated with enhanced local expression of Csf1 and FasL," *Pain*, vol. 154, no. 9, pp. 1743–1748, 2013.

[11] T. Takebayashi, J. M. Cavanaugh, A. Cüneyt Özaktay, S. Kallakuri, and C. Chen, "Effect of nucleus pulposus on the neural activity of dorsal root ganglion," *Spine*, vol. 26, no. 8, pp. 940–944, 2001.

[12] P. Andrade, G. Hoogland, M. A. Garcia, H. W. Steinbusch, M. A. Daemen, and V. Visser-Vandewalle, "Elevated IL-1b and IL-6 levels in lumbar herniated discs in patients with sciatic pain," *European Spine Journal*, vol. 22, no. 4, pp. 714–720, 2013.

[13] J. D. Kang, M. Stefanovic-Racic, L. A. McIntyre, H. I. Georgescu, and C. H. Evans, "Toward a biochemical understanding of human intervertebral disc degeneration and herniation. Contributions of nitric oxide, interleukins, prostaglandin E2, and matrix metalloproteinases," *Spine*, vol. 22, no. 10, pp. 1065–1073, 1997.

[14] H. Takahashi, T. Suguro, Y. Okazima, M. Motegi, Y. Okada, and T. Kakiuchi, "Inflammatory cytokines in the herniated disc of the lumbar spine," *Spine*, vol. 21, no. 2, pp. 218–224, 1996.

[15] N. Üçeyler, J. P. Rogausch, K. V. Toyka, and C. Sommer, "Differential expression of cytokines in painful and painless neuropathies," *Neurology*, vol. 69, no. 1, pp. 42–49, 2007.

[16] A. Geiss, E. Varadi, K. Steinbach, H. W. Bauer, and F. Anton, "Psychoneuroimmunological correlates of persisting sciatic pain in patients who underwent discectomy," *Neuroscience Letters*, vol. 237, no. 2-3, pp. 65–68, 1997.

[17] L. M. Pedersen, E. Schistad, L. M. Jacobsen, C. Røe, and J. Gjerstad, "Serum levels of the pro-inflammatory interleukins 6 (IL-6) and -8 (IL-8) in patients with lumbar radicular pain due to disc herniation: a 12-month prospective study," *Brain, Behavior, and Immunity*, vol. 46, pp. 132–136, 2015.

[18] E. Assarsson, M. Lundberg, G. Holmquist et al., "Homogenous 96-plex PEA immunoassay exhibiting high sensitivity, specificity, and excellent scalability," *PLoS ONE*, vol. 9, no. 4, Article ID e95192, 2014.

[19] Y. Benjamini and Y. Hochberg, "Controlling the false discovery rate: a practical and powerful approach to multiple testing," *Journal of the Royal Statistical Society Series B (Methodological)*, vol. 57, no. 1, pp. 289–300, 1995.

[20] D. R. Helsel, "More than obvious: better methods for interpreting nondetect data," *Environmental Science & Technology*, vol. 39, no. 20, pp. 419A–423A, 2005.

[21] D. R. Helsel, *Statistics for Censored Environmental Data Using Minitab and R*, vol. 77, John Wiley & Sons, New York, NY, USA, 2011.

[22] D. Zhang, C. Fan, J. Zhang, and C.-H. Zhang, "Nonparametric methods for measurements below detection limit," *Statistics in Medicine*, vol. 28, no. 4, pp. 700–715, 2009.

[23] R. A. Fisher, *The Use of Multiple Measurements in Taxonomic Problems*, vol. 7 of *Annals of Eugenics*, 1936.

[24] R. A. Johnson and D. W. Wichern, *Applied Multivariate Statistical Analysis*, Prentice Hall, Englewood Cliffs, NJ, USA, 6th edition, 2007.

[25] E. I. Schistad, A. Espeland, L. M. Pedersen, L. Sandvik, J. Gjerstad, and C. Røe, "Association between baseline IL-6 and 1-year recovery in lumbar radicular pain," *European Journal of Pain*, vol. 18, no. 10, pp. 1394–1401, 2014.

[26] B. Chandrasekar, P. C. Melby, H. M. Sarau et al., "Chemokine-cytokine cross-talk: the ELR$^+$ CXC chemokine LIX (CXCl5) amplifies a proinflammatory cytokine response via a phosphatidylinositol 3-kinase-NF-κB pathway," *The Journal of Biological Chemistry*, vol. 278, no. 7, pp. 4675–4686, 2003.

[27] T. Kimura, S. Kobayashi, F. Hanihara-Tatsuzawa, A. Sayama, T. MaruYama, and T. Muta, "Responses of macrophages to the danger signals released from necrotic cells," *International immunology*, vol. 26, no. 12, pp. 697–704, 2014.

[28] D. D. Taub, A. R. Lloyd, K. Conlon et al., "Recombinant human interferon-inducible protein 10 is a chemoattractant for human monocytes and T lymphocytes and promotes T cell adhesion to endothelial cells," *The Journal of Experimental Medicine*, vol. 177, no. 6, pp. 1809–1814, 1993.

[29] G. Flynn, S. Maru, J. Loughlin, I. A. Romero, and D. Male, "Regulation of chemokine receptor expression in human microglia and astrocytes," *Journal of Neuroimmunology*, vol. 136, no. 1-2, pp. 84–93, 2003.

[30] M. Sawada, A. Suzumura, H. Yamamoto, and T. Marunouchi, "Activation and proliferation of the isolated microglia by colony stimulating factor-1 and possible involvement of protein kinase C," *Brain Research*, vol. 509, no. 1, pp. 119–124, 1990.

[31] F. Saika, N. Kiguchi, Y. Kobayashi, Y. Fukazawa, and S. Kishioka, "CC-chemokine ligand 4/macrophage inflammatory protein-1β participates in the induction of neuropathic pain after peripheral nerve injury," *European Journal of Pain*, vol. 16, no. 9, pp. 1271–1280, 2012.

[32] H. Haro, K. Shinomiya, H. Komori et al., "Upregulated expression of chemokines in herniated nucleus pulposus resorption," *Spine*, vol. 21, no. 14, pp. 1647–1652, 1996.

[33] H. Haro, T. Kato, H. Komori, M. Osada, and K. Shinomiya, "Vascular endothelial growth factor (VEGF)-induced angiogenesis in herniated disc resorption," *Journal of Orthopaedic Research*, vol. 20, no. 3, pp. 409–415, 2002.

[34] S. I. Nikolaev, A. R. Gallyamov, G. V. Mamin, and Y. A. Chelyshev, "Poly(ε-caprolactone) nerve conduit and local delivery of *vegf* and *fgf2* genes stimulate neuroregeneration," *Bulletin of Experimental Biology and Medicine*, vol. 157, no. 1, pp. 155–158, 2014.

[35] F. Zor, M. Deveci, A. Kilic et al., "Effect of vegf gene therapy and hyaluronic acid film sheath on peripheral nerve regeneration," *Microsurgery*, vol. 34, no. 3, pp. 209–216, 2014.

[36] T. K. Y. Lim, X. Q. Shi, H. C. Martin et al., "Blood-nerve barrier dysfunction contributes to the generation of neuropathic pain and allows targeting of injured nerves for pain relief," *Pain*, vol. 155, no. 5, pp. 954–967, 2014.

[37] C. Bergamaschi, J. Bear, M. Rosati et al., "Circulating IL-15 exists as heterodimeric complex with soluble IL-15Rα in human and mouse serum," *Blood*, vol. 120, no. 1, pp. e1–e8, 2012.

[38] Y. Shirakata, T. Komurasaki, H. Toyoda et al., "Epiregulin, a novel member of the epidermal growth factor family, is an autocrine growth factor in normal human keratinocytes," *The Journal of Biological Chemistry*, vol. 275, no. 8, pp. 5748–5753, 2000.

[39] M. O. Li, Y. Y. Wan, S. Sanjabi, A.-K. L. Robertson, and R. A. Flavell, "Transforming growth factor-β regulation of immune responses," *Annual Review of Immunology*, vol. 24, pp. 99–146, 2006.

[40] D. Han, Y. Ding, S.-L. Liu et al., "Double role of Fas ligand in the apoptosis of intervertebral disc cells in vitro," *Acta Biochimica et Biophysica Sinica*, vol. 41, no. 11, pp. 938–947, 2009.

[41] J.-B. Park, H. Chang, and K.-W. Kim, "Expression of Fas ligand and apoptosis of disc cells in herniated lumbar disc tissue," *Spine*, vol. 26, no. 6, pp. 618–621, 2001.

[42] L. M. McDonell, G. M. Mirzaa, D. Alcantara et al., "Mutations in STAMBP, encoding a deubiquitinating enzyme, cause microcephaly-capillary malformation syndrome," *Nature Genetics*, vol. 45, no. 5, pp. 556–562, 2013.

[43] S. Darmanis, R. Y. Nong, M. Hammond et al., "Sensitive plasma protein analysis by microparticle-based proximity ligation assays," *Molecular and Cellular Proteomics*, vol. 9, no. 2, pp. 327–335, 2010.

[44] S. Darmanis, R. Y. Nong, J. Vänelid et al., "ProteinSeq: high-performance proteomic analyses by proximity ligation and next generation sequencing," *PLoS ONE*, vol. 6, no. 9, Article ID e25583, 2011.

18

The Role of Toll-Like Receptors in Autoimmune Diseases through Failure of the Self-Recognition Mechanism

Mark Farrugia and Byron Baron

Centre for Molecular Medicine and Biobanking, Faculty of Medicine and Surgery, University of Malta, Msida MSD 2080, Malta

Correspondence should be addressed to Byron Baron; angenlabs@gmail.com

Academic Editor: B. L. Slomiany

Toll-like receptors (TLRs), part of the innate immune system that recognises molecular signatures, are important in the recognition of pathogenic components. However, when specific cellular contexts develop in which TLRs are inappropriately activated by self-components, this may lead to sterile inflammation and result in the occurrence of autoimmunity. This review analyses the available data regarding TLR biochemistry, the specific mechanisms which are brought about by TLR activation, and the importance of these mechanisms in the light of any existing and potential therapies in the field of autoimmunity.

1. Introduction

The innate immune system relies on a limited number of germline-encoded receptors, known as pattern recognition receptors (PRRs), that have evolved to recognise molecular signatures [1]. Toll-like receptors (TLRs) are just one of several distinct classes of PRRs including Nod-like receptors (NLRs), C-type lectin receptors (CLRs), AIM2-like receptors (ALRs), RIG-I-like receptors (RLRs), and intracellular DNA sensors including cyclic GMP-AMP synthase (cGAS) [2, 3], which recognise structures as diverse as flagellins, nucleic acids, saccharides (mainly mannose and lipopolysaccharide), peptidoglycans (such as lipoteichoic peptidoglycans), and lipoproteins. An adaptive immune response is triggered by the recognition of such antigens, mediated by proinflammatory cytokine production together with antigen-presenting cell (APC) stimulation.

TLRs are a family of type I transmembrane glycoproteins [4] consisting of a single transmembrane helix, which connects an extracellular ligand-binding domain to an intracellular signalling domain [5]. The extracellular domain can bind either directly to the ligand or to coreceptor-ligand complexes, and it then initiates ligand-mediated multimerisation of the receptor. TLRs generally are found as dimers, with most being homodimers, although TLR2 can be found preferentially as heterodimers either with TLR1 or with TLR6, even when a ligand is absent [6]. The intracellular signalling domains of TLRs have significant sequence similarity with the interleukin-1 receptor (IL-1) and are thus termed Toll/IL-1R homology (TIR) domains [4]. TLRs are located either at the cell surface or in the endosomes. TLR1, TLR2, TLR4, TLR5, and TLR6 are expressed on the cell membrane, whereas TLR3, TLR7, TLR8, and TLR9 are localised mainly in the endosomal compartment [7]. TLR expression has been identified in various immune cells, including T-cells, B-cells, different subsets of dendritic cells, and macrophages [8, 9].

The TLR family can recognise a wide variety of bacterial, fungal, protozoan, and viral components, generally referred to as pathogen-associated molecular patterns (PAMPs). These TLR ligands can be grouped into three categories: lipids and lipopeptides (recognised by TLR2/TLR1, TLR2/TLR6, and TLR4), proteins (recognised by TLR5), and nucleic acids (recognised by TLR3, TLR7, TLR8, and TLR9). Different types of nucleic acid have their unique TLR, with viral double-stranded RNA (dsRNA) being recognised by TLR3, single-stranded RNA (ssRNA) being recognised by TLR7 and TLR8, and DNA containing unmethylated CG dinucleotides (whether from bacteria, viruses, or synthetic oligodeoxynucleotides, referred to as ODNs) being recognised by TLR9 [1, 10, 11].

TLRs play an important role in both innate and acquired immune responses [4, 12, 13]. However, the inappropriate

Table 1: TLRs involved in autoimmune disease with the ligands causing the immune reaction. (EDN: eosinophil-derived neurotoxin; Hsp: heat shock protein; HMGB1: high-mobility group box 1 protein.)

TLRs	Potential endogenous ligands
TLR2	HSP60, HSP70, HSP90 fragments, hyaluronic acid, versican, HMGB1, biglycan, EDN
TLR3	mRNA, dsRNA
TLR4	HSP22, HSP60, HSP70, HSP72, HSP90, HMGB1, oxidised phospholipids, heparin sulfate, fibronectin, tenascin-C, β-defensin 2, versican, hyaluronic acid, minimally modified-low-density lipoprotein, fibrinogen, lung surfactant protein A
TLR7	U1snRNP RNA, ssRNA
TLR8	ssRNA
TLR9	Hypomethylated CpG-DNA

TLR activation triggered by self-components brings about sterile inflammation and autoimmunity. Autoimmunity is the result of several mechanisms that are associated with the presence of autoreactive immune cell subsets and loss of immunological tolerance [9]. Organ-specific autoimmune diseases are the culmination of hereditary and environmental factors related to the failure of adaptive immune response regulation to self-antigens [14]. In fact, overexpression of PRRs was identified in the tissues of patients with organ-specific autoimmunity, type 1 diabetes and Crohn's disease [15, 16].

Autoimmunity and infection have been linked together in several studies due to PAMPs being found in tissues after episodes of infection [17]. These are part of a substantial body of experimental data indicating that PRR activation on innate immune cells by either PAMPs or pathogens has the ability to dysregulate self-tolerance and subsequently activate autoreactive T- and B-cells.

However, TLRs are also known to recognise host-derived endogenous ligands which have undergone some form of change from their native state or accumulated excessively in nonphysiologic compartments [18]. Such ligands are referred to as damage associated molecular patterns (DAMPs) and are commonly released from damaged tissues or apoptotic cells such as high mobility group box 1 (HMGB1), saturated fatty acids, and amyloid β and can result in chronic or acute inflammation [19–21]. However, under certain conditions TLRs can bind to such kind of self-molecules and as a result contribute to the development, progression, and resolution of autoimmune diseases [22]. A list of potential endogenous ligands and their respective TLRs can be found in Table 1.

In order to prevent TLR-induced inflammation, TLR-activated DCs cross-talk with and are suppressed by regulatory T-cells (T_{regs}), while the suppressive action of regulatory T-cells is blocked by APCs which have been stimulated through TLRs [23]. TLR stimulation can conversely be inhibited by cytokines such as interleukin- (IL-) 10 secreted by regulatory T-cells [24, 25]. Different subsets of T_{regs} exist and their impairment has been reported in a number of human autoimmune conditions, including oral tolerance [26].

2. TLR Signalling Pathways

The stimulation of TLRs by the respective ligands results in the recruitment of downstream adaptor molecules, such as myeloid differentiation factor 88 (MyD88), myeloid Toll/interleukin- (IL-) 1 receptor- (TIR-) domain-containing adaptor-inducing interferon-β (TRIF a.k.a. TIR-domain-containing molecule 1; TICAM1), TIR-associated protein (TIRAP a.k.a. MyD88 adaptor-like; Mal), TRIF-related adaptor molecule (TRAM), or sterile α- and armadillo-motif containing protein (SARM) [6, 27, 28], which trigger a number of downstream molecules activating signalling cascades converging at the nuclear factor-kB (NF-kB), interferon (IFN) response factors (IRFs), and mitogen-activated protein (MAP) kinases. These transcription factors induce the transcription of various immune response genes, including inflammatory cytokines (such as interleukin- (IL-) 6, IL-12, IL-23, and tumour necrosis factor α (TNF-α)), stimulatory immune cytokines, chemokines, and costimulatory molecules [29, 30] (Figure 1).

TLRs specifically recruit and signal via TRIF, TIRAP, TRAM, or direct MyD88 activation to produce a different response, despite this recruitment being always through heterotypic TIR-TIR interactions. More specifically, except for TLR3, MyD88 is utilised by all TLRs and activates NF-kB and mitogen-activated protein kinases (MAPKs) to induce the genes encoding inflammatory cytokines [31]. TIRAP acts as a sorting adaptor by recruiting MyD88 to TLRs at the cell surface. One study has also shown that TIRAP is involved in endosomal TLR signalling (such as TLR9) by binding to different lipids [32, 33]. The recruitment of TRIF to TLR3 and TLR4 promotes an alternative pathway to that of MyD88 [34]. Interestingly, TRAM has been shown to be recruited specifically to TLR4 but not TLR3 and serves as the link between TRIF and TLR4 [35]. Thus, depending on what adaptor protein is used, one can divide TLR signalling into two pathways: MyD88-dependent and TRIF-dependent pathways.

In the MyD88-dependent pathway, TLR binding leads to MyD88 forming a complex with IRAK kinases [36], such that IRAK4 activates IRAK1 [37, 38]. IRAK1 then associates with TRAF6, a RING-domain E3 ubiquitin ligase, which polyubiquitinates and activates TAK1 [39, 40]. This results in the activation of the NF-kB and MAPK pathways. NF-kB is activated through the IKK complex (composed of the IKKα and IKKβ catalytic subunits and the IKKγ regulatory subunit), which phosphorylates the NF-kB inhibitory protein IkBα, allowing the translocation of NF-kB to the nucleus inducing the expression of proinflammatory genes. The MAPK pathways are induced through ERK1/2, p38, and JNK, which mediate activation of AP-1 and regulate inflammatory responses [2, 41].

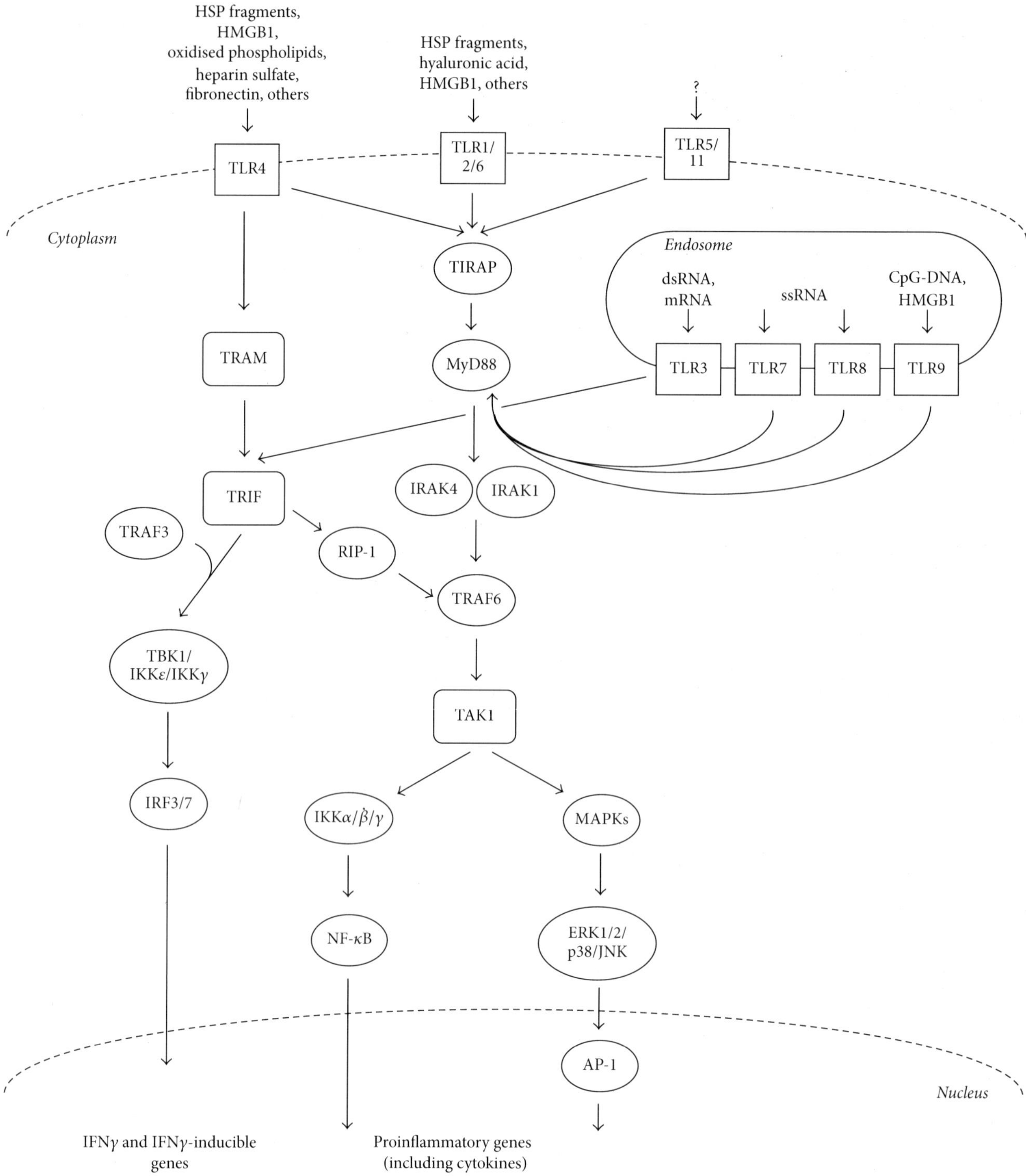

FIGURE 1: TLR signalling pathways. The two main pathways by which TLR signalling occurs upon stimulation by their ligands. These pathways are characterised depending on which of the adaptor molecules MyD88 or TRIF are involved. These signalling cascades result in the activation of NF-kB, IRFs, and MAP kinases, which promote the transcription of various immune response genes, including inflammatory cytokines and IFNγ-related genes. (AP-1, activator protein 1; ERK, extracellular signal-regulated kinase; IKK, inhibitor of kappa light polypeptide gene enhancer in B-cell kinase; IRAK, IL-1 receptor-associated kinase; JNK, c-Jun N-terminal kinase; MKK, MAPK kinase; RIP1, receptor interacting protein 1; TAK, transforming growth factor-activated kinase; TBK1, TANK-binding kinase 1; TRAF, tumour necrosis factor receptor-associated factor.)

In the TRIF-dependent pathway, once TRIF is activated by either TLR3 or TLR4, it binds to TRAF6 via the recruitment of RIP-1 kinase, which leads to the activation of TAK1. This results in the NF-kB and MAPKs induction of inflammatory cytokines as discussed above. Meanwhile, TRIF also activates TRAF3 which recruits IKK-related kinases (TBK1 and IKKε) and IKKγ for IRF3 phosphorylation, which translocates into the nucleus inducing the expression of type I IFN genes [2, 41]. On the other hand, TRAF3 binds to the MyD88 complex causing its degradation and leading to TAK1 activation. This implies that TRAF3 promotes the TRIF-dependent pathway via direct activation, while concurrently inhibiting the MyD88-dependent pathway.

3. Nucleic-Acid-Sensing TLRs in Autoimmune Disease

The nucleic-acid-sensing TLRs are endosomal and consist of TLR3 (which recognises viral dsRNA [42]), TLR7 and TLR8 (which recognise viral ssRNA [43–45]), and TLR9 (which recognises bacterial and viral unmethylated CpG-containing DNA motifs [46]). TLR3 signalling is distinguished from the rest in that it signals via the adaptor TRIF, while TLR7, TLR8, and TLR9 signal through the adaptor molecule MyD88 [47]. TLR3 also binds to self-mRNA [48].

The restricted access to these TLRs is one mechanism by which to prevent them from being aberrantly activated by self-nucleic acids (as those released by apoptotic cells), which could bring about autoimmune diseases. However, the dysregulation of TLR7, TLR8, and TLR9 plays a major role in numerous autoimmune diseases.

Studies show that immune complexes (ICs) composed of DNA and the immunoglobulin G (IgG) that recognises them stimulate pDCs in humans to produce IFNα [11, 20, 49, 50] and the production of autoantibodies in mice via a process which involves TLR7 and/or TLR9 [51, 52]. Such ICs containing self-nucleic acids are recognised via the FcRγIIa receptor expressed on the surface of plasmacytoid dendritic cells (pDCs; innate immune cells) [53]. Once antibodies are captured, the FcR allows ICs to enter pDC and activates the endosomal pathway [54]. In the endosome, the nucleic acid component of the IC is likely released by the low pH. The nucleic acids then trigger TLR7 or TLR9 which brings about the maturation of the pDC and induces IFNα production [50, 54, 55].

The trafficking of nucleic-acid-sensing TLRs from the endoplasmic reticulum to endosomes for ligand recognition as well as their nucleic acid-sensing function is controlled by the multipass transmembrane protein Unc93B1 [56]. This protein is also involved in the localisation regulation of nucleic-acid-sensing TLRs, with studies presenting evidence of competition between TLR7 and TLR9 for Unc93B1-dependent trafficking, where TLR9 predominates due to a higher affinity for Unc93B1 than TLR7 [56–59]. Thus, Unc93B1 regulates excessive TLR7 activation by balancing TLR9 to TLR7 trafficking. The mutation of Unc93B1 by an amino acid substitution (D34A) resulted in a phenotype which presents TLR7-hyperreactivity together with TLR9-hyporeactivity, which was linked to systemic lethal inflammation, known to be TLR7-dependent [59]. It is thus hypothesised that in some autoimmune diseases deficiency of either TLR8 or TLR9 will result in decreased competition of these endosomal TLRs to bind to Unc93B1, making TLR7 more available and resulting in higher TLR7 trafficking and response. This manifests itself as autoimmune phenotypes [60]. Consequently, altering the TLR7 to TLR9 balance can be envisioned as a potential regulatory mechanism in the context of autoimmunity [59].

TLR7 activity regulation appears to be cell type dependent, with the TLR7 response being controlled by TLR8 on dendritic cells and by TLR9 on B-cells. This has been shown using the TLR7 agonist R848 on TLR8$^{-/-}$ and TLR8/9$^{-/-}$ derived from bone marrow (which produced significantly higher amounts of IFNβ mRNA (at 4 h), IL-6, and TNF, compared with WT or TLR9$^{-/-}$ cells) and TLR8/9$^{-/-}$ and TLR9$^{-/-}$ B-cells (which presented significant CD69 and CD86 upregulation, when compared to TLR8$^{-/-}$ or WT B-cells) [60]. Concomitantly, TLR8$^{-/-}$ and TLR8/9$^{-/-}$ B-cells presented a significant increase in TLR7 mRNA levels compared to WT or TLR9$^{-/-}$ cells. Furthermore, TLR8/9$^{-/-}$ mice had a significantly higher percentage of activated and memory CD4 and CD8 T-cells compared to WT or TLR9$^{-/-}$ mice, while in TLR8$^{-/-}$ mice the values were only significantly higher when compared to WT mice [60].

4. Protein-Sensing TLRs in Autoimmune Disease

TLR2 and TLR4, which are both cell surface TLRs, are involved in regulating Th immune responses. In fact, it was shown that, depending on which TLRs are ligated, the Th responses can be skewed towards a Th1 or Th2 cytokine profile [61]. This is in contrast with a previous model in which Th2 differentiation was driven forward without any TLR-mediated signals. Despite the promotion of Th2 responses (and allergic inflammation) in some contexts by low-doses of inhaled LPS [62], generally TLR4 stimulated by LPS brings about the maturation of DCs associated with strong Th1-type responses as a consequence of IL-12 release [63]. Moreover, both TLR2 and TLR4 were found to be involved in regulating $\gamma\delta$ T-cell [64] and CD4+ T-helper 17 (Th17) [65] production of IL-17. More specifically, in vitro studies showed that in $\gamma\delta$ T-cells expansion and IL-17 production are promoted by the activation of TLR4 [65]. TLR2 signalling could also stimulate naïve cells to expand and undergo polarisation towards the Th17 lineage [65] and provide CD4^{+} and CD8^{+} T-cells with a costimulatory signal [66, 67].

TLR2 and TLR4 have been shown to also respond to endogenous heat-shock proteins [68, 69]. Clinical observations confirm that HSPs are involved in the regulation of some autoimmune disease such as autoimmune arthritis, type 1 diabetes, atherosclerosis, multiple sclerosis, and others [70].

5. Role of TLRs in Autoantibody Production

TLRs are known to play a critical role in autoantibody production because genetic mutations which lead to some deficiency in either TLR7, TLR9, or MyD88 most commonly also lead to a reduction in autoantibody production, while an increase in TLR7 production generally leads to a susceptibility towards developing autoimmune diseases [71]. Moreover, the engagement of B-cell receptor by chromatin-IgG complexes and TLR9 signalling were shown to be essential and act synergistically in the activation of autoreactive B-cells in vitro [51].

However, it is difficult to gauge the direct contribution of TLR signalling in B-cells in vivo since the activation of both DCs and plasmacytoid DCs is brought about by the same TLR ligands and play just as important roles in the pathogenesis of autoimmune diseases [20]. Furthermore, TLRs are expressed by a variety of cell types that have the ability to regulate the functions of B-cell through the activation of their TLRs. So far evidence seems to suggest that the intrinsic TLR signalling of B-cells is a requirement for the production of autoantibodies in vivo [72–74].

6. Spectrum of TLR Action in Autoimmune Disease Contexts

The involvement of TLRs in early inflammatory immune responses is responsible for their ability to develop autoreactive B- and T-cells. There is now a well-established link between a variety of infections and autoimmune diseases, both in animal models and in the clinical setting. Such autoimmune responses are thought to be the result of molecular mimicry of the pathogen-derived antigens to self-antigens or a form of nonspecific activation of the innate immune system (through loss of immunological tolerance) that results in the production of T-cells and antibody responses specific to self-antigens, implicating TLRs in numerous autoimmune diseases. Here we would like to point out three disease settings.

6.1. TLRs in Rheumatoid Arthritis. Several of the risk alleles linked to rheumatoid arthritis (RA) are associated with immune regulation such as NF-κB-dependent signalling, T-cell stimulation, activation, and functional differentiation. This suggests that these immunologic pathways are amongst the key modulators of the development of the autoimmune inflammation in RA [75, 76]. Through the use of human synovial membrane cultures from patients with RA it has been shown that expression of TLR2 and TLR4 in conjunction with the release of endogenous ligands to these two TLRs may play a role in inflammation and damage to joints in RA patients [77]. The alarmin heterogeneous nuclear ribonucleoprotein (hnRNP) was also found to play a role in human RA and pristane-induced arthritis in rats. This RNA- and DNA-binding complex binds to most nuclear antigen-specific B and T-cells in systemic autoimmune diseases. Moreover hnRNP was shown to activate APCs causing arthritis mediated by TLR7 and TLR9, which can then activate harmful T-cells [78].

6.2. TLRs in Type 2 Diabetes Mellitus. Innate immune responses leading to Type 2 Diabetes Mellitus (T2DM) can be initiated by adipose tissue inflammation, as has been shown through LPS-treatment of adipocytes which showed significant increase in TLR2, TRAF-6, and NF-κB levels as well as increased secretion of potentially diabetogenic proinflammatory cytokines. Similarly, abdominal subcutaneous adipose tissue isolated from diabetic patients presented increases in the expression of TLR2, MyD88, TRAF6, and NF-κB. It has thus been proposed that obesity may increase proinflammatory cytokines in the host and subsequently increase the risk of T2DM [79]. TLR4 is thought to be an important mediator of obesity and insulin resistance because of its activation by saturated fatty acids and LPS, known to cause insulin resistance in adipose tissue amongst others. Obesity is associated with insulin resistance and is considered to be amongst the major risk factors in the development of T2DM and cardiovascular diseases. Thus, TLR4 is being considered as a potential therapeutic target in the treatment of these metabolic diseases [4].

6.3. TLRs in Other Diseases Not Generally Classified as Autoimmune. Two widespread diseases that are considered to have an autoimmune component are atherosclerosis and cancers. Both have now been shown to display TLR-directed responses. In the case of atherosclerosis a link has been found with TLR-induced IFNα [18, 80, 81], while, in cancer, the cells dying from chemotherapy release endogenous molecules that bring about an innate immune response following TLR-mediated recognition, which has been found to be critical for cancer elimination [82].

7. Therapeutic Application of TLR Regulators

TLR signalling is negatively regulated by a number of molecules, which act through a variety of mechanisms in order to prevent or control excessive immune responses. In autoimmunity and inflammatory diseases these processes could be nonfunctional, dysregulated, or simply not enough to overcome the TLR signalling in place. In an attempt to control aberrant immune responses both natural and synthetic negative regulators targeting each of the key molecules in the TLR signalling pathways have been identified. In fact, blocking the activation signal at the TLR level rather than targeting individual PAMPs or DAMPs is a more preferred and effective therapeutic approach since sterile inflammation contexts tend to be induced by similar signalling pathways and there may be multiple autoimmunity inducing peptides following tissue injury.

Cationic peptides (such as LL-37 or polymyxin), for example, are known to facilitate the uptake of self-DNA by plasmacytoid dendritic cells (pDCs) to activate TLR9 signalling and can lead to preferential localisation in the early endosomes of pDCs [81, 83], leading to significant IFNα production [83, 84]. One context in which this applies is psoriasis, in which the DNA is not transported in the form of an IC but associated with the antimicrobial cationic peptide, LL-37 [81]. Synthetic ligands of TLRs that effectively regulate innate and adaptive immune responses thus have the potential of being a new class of therapeutic molecules [85].

Some of these agents act directly on the TLRs themselves. Vitamin D3 has been shown to downregulate TLR2 and TLR4 expression on monocytes [86]. Endosomal TLRs like TLR7, TLR8, and TLR9 can be inhibited by Chloroquine and related compounds, which act as antagonists that specifically target and inhibit signalling through these TLRs [87–91]. Nucleic acid-binding polymers are another class of endosomal TLR inhibitors which recognise ssRNA, dsRNA, or hypomethylated DNA and bind to them, thus inhibiting nucleic acid-mediated activation of these TLRs [30]. 9-Benzyl-8-hydroxy-2-(2-methoxyethoxy) adenine on the other hand acts as a TLR7 agonist, which induces hyporesponsiveness or tolerance, thus still inhibiting TLR7 activation [92]. Research in such agonists could lead the way to the synthesis of drugs which could inhibit TLR overactivation while still sparing the side-effects related to total inhibition of these pathways.

At the protein level activation of the MyD88-dependent pathway is suppressed by the synthetic inhibitor ST2825, which is a heptapeptide analog specifically designed to inhibit MyD88 dimerisation, thus interfering with the recruitment of IRAK1 and IRAK4 by MyD88 [93]. Compound 4a is also responsible for inhibiting the MyD88 dependent pathway activation by interfering with the interaction between MyD88 and the TIR domains of TLRs [94]. Other inhibitors of MyD88 include Suppressor of Cytokine Signalling 1 (SOCS1) and the E3 Ubiquitin Protein Ligase Cbl-b. Further down the pathway IRAK1 and IRAK4 are targeted by RO0884 which acts as a dual inhibitor of both these protein kinases resulting in the blocking of proinflammatory cytokine production [95]. TRAF6 is targeted by a number of inhibitory molecules such as Tumour Necrosis Factor Inducible Protein A20 (A20), Ubiquitin Specific Peptidase 4 (USP4), Ubiquitin-Specific-Processing Protease CYLD (CYLD), TRAF Family Member Associated NF-κB Activator (TANK), Tripartite Motif Containing Protein 38 (TRIM38), and Small Heterodimer Partner (SHP) [96–98]. TAK1 activation is inhibited by Tripartite Motif Containing 5 (TRIM5; TRIM30a in mouse) and A20 [99]. In addition to these signalling molecules, the transcription factor NF-κB is suppressed by B-Cell Lymphoma 3-Encoded Protein (Bcl-3), NF-κB Inhibitor Delta (IkBNS), Nuclear Receptor Related 1 (Nurr1), Activating Transcription Factor 3 (ATF3), and PDZ and LIM Domain Protein 2 (PDLIM2) [100].

Activation of the TRIF-dependent pathway is suppressed by Sterile Alpha and TIR Motif Containing 1 (SARM) and a splice variant of the adaptor TRAM called TAG [101–103], both acting as direct TRIF inhibitors. TRAF3 activation is negatively regulated by Suppressor of Cytokine Signalling 3 (SOCS3) and Deubiquitinating Enzyme A (DUBA) [104]. SOCS3 is itself upregulated by high molecular weight hyaluronan (HA900), making it also a key molecule in regulating TRAF3 activation [105]. IRF3 activation is negatively regulated by Peptidylprolyl Cis/Trans Isomerase, NIMA-Interacting 1 (PIN1) and Ubiquitin Protein Ligase E3C (UBE3C or RAUL) [100]. (Figure 2).

At the RNA level, micro-RNAs (miRNAs) such as miR-146a, miR-199a, miR-155, miR-126, miR-21, miR-29, miR-148/152, and miR-466l regulate the stability of mRNAs that encode TLR signalling molecules [98]. Furthermore, the stability of mRNAs encoding cytokines are regulated by Regnase-1 and the zinc finger protein Tristetraprolin (TTP) [41, 98]. It was shown that, after being treated with a variety of TLR ligands, Regnase-1-deficient macrophages produce large amounts of cytokines and increased autoantibody production in Regnase-1-deficient mice [106].

One of the more interesting areas of research for therapeutic application of TLR modulators is the development of atypical, nonstimulatory DNA sequences called immune-regulatory DNA sequences (IRS) to regulate immune-stimulatory ligands of TLR7 and TLR9 as well as altogether inhibiting TLR7 and TLR9 stimulation [107]. Ligands of TLR9 include CpG-containing immune-stimulatory sequences (CpG-ISS) of diverse origin, including sequences of viral origin, CpG sequences which have been mutated, or mammalian telomere TTAGGG motif repeats [107–115].

A kind of TLR7 inhibitor (exemplified by IRS 661) acted specifically on mouse splenocytes to reduce their response to the TLR7 agonist R848, while having no effect on the response to a CpG-ISS, which is a TLR9 agonist. It also efficiently blocked antiribonucleoproteins (RNPs) but not anti-DNA-induced IFNα, indicating the role of TLR7 in this process. On the other hand, the TLR9 inhibitor IRS 869 was effective in inhibiting TLR9 activation by CpG-ISS, while having no effect when the TLR7 ligand R848 was used to activate the splenocytes, proving that anti-dsDNA-induced IFNα is TLR9-dependent. A newer type of inhibitor, exemplified by IRS 954 (derived by combining the three $5'$ residues from the TLR7 inhibitor IRS 661 (TGC) with the TLR9 inhibitor IRS 869), could significantly inhibit splenocyte activation by ligands to TLR7 and TLR9 [50]. This IRS 954 was shown to strongly inhibit IFNα production by pDCs in response to ICs containing DNA or RNA. R848, through its mechanism of being a TLR7 agonist, was also found to induce production of IFN-γ in invariant NKT cells, which can alleviate allergic inflammation [116].

TLR modulators and inhibitors offer great promise with high selectivity and effectiveness when tested out in animal model for most autoimmune diseases. However it is important to recall when attempting to test inhibitors targeting TLRs and their signalling pathways for therapeutic applications using disease models in mice that humans and mice have different expression and distribution of TLRs and that any responses produced are just as different; for example, in humans, treatment with a TLR9 ligand produces a response dominated by the IFNα pathway [117–119] (stimulating numerous IFN-regulated genes elevated in lupus [120, 121]), while in mice TLR9 activation leads to the expression of proinflammatory cytokines such as IL-6, IL-12, or TNF-α via macrophage and myeloid DC activation.

8. Conclusion

TLRs have been shown to cover a much greater recognition repertoire than originally thought and a number of autoimmune diseases are either initiated or aggravated by TLR dysregulation. Thus further work in the field will definitely focus on uncovering more pieces to this ever growing signalling puzzle providing researchers and clinicians a clearer

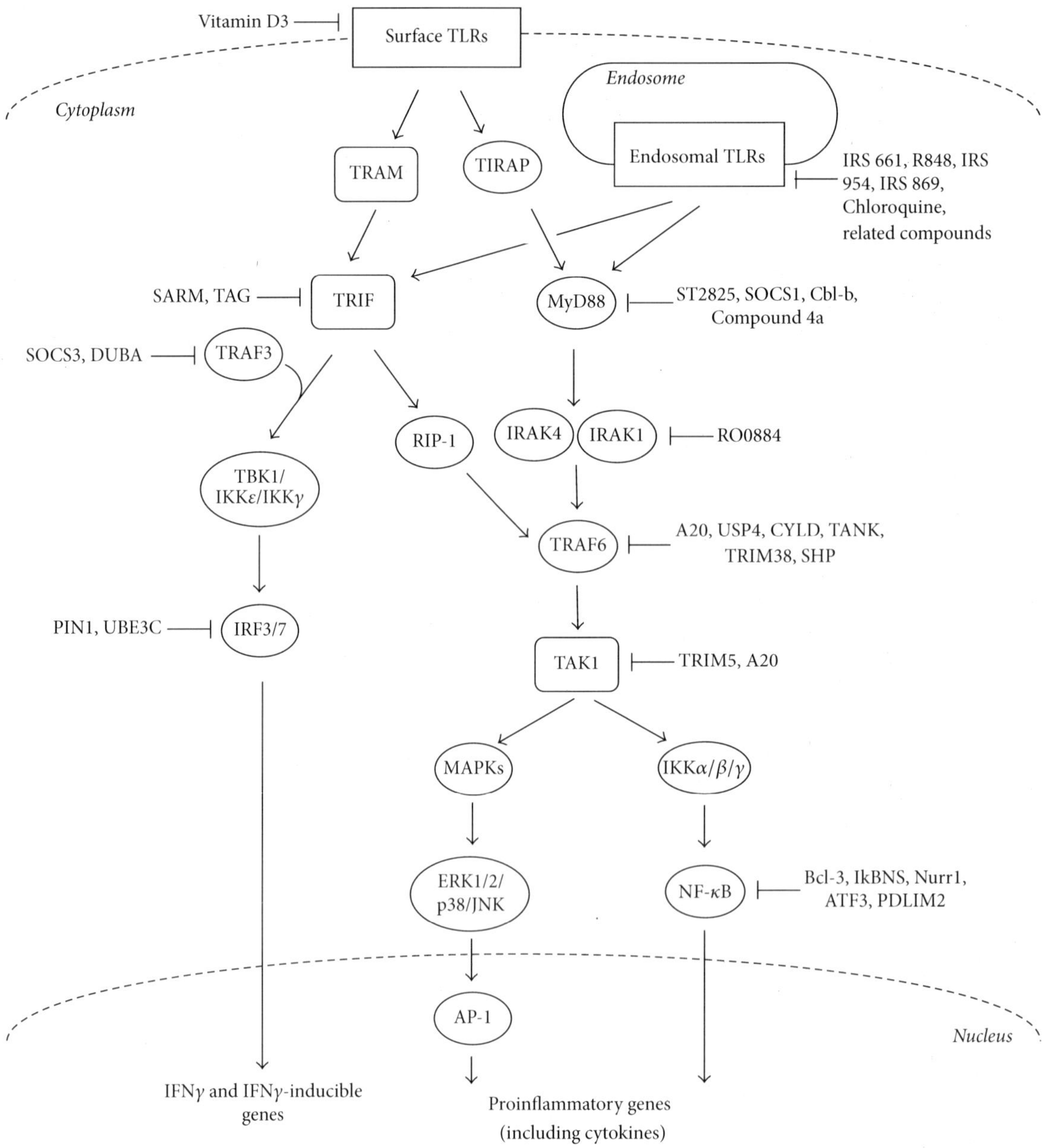

FIGURE 2: TLR signalling inhibitors. The regulation of TLR signalling has been achieved through the application of both natural and synthetic inhibitory molecules, which target each of the key molecules in the TLR signalling pathways, acting through a wide range of mechanisms. (AP-1, activator protein 1; ATF, activating transcription factor; ERK, extracellular signal-regulated kinase; IKK, inhibitor of kappa light polypeptide gene enhancer in B-cell kinase; IRAK, IL-1 receptor-associated kinase; JNK, c-Jun N-terminal kinase; MKK, MAPK kinase; RIP1, receptor interacting protein 1; TAB, transforming growth factor-b-activated kinase 1/MAP3K7-binding protein; TAK, transforming growth factor-activated kinase; TRAF, tumour necrosis factor receptor-associated factor); A20, Tumour Necrosis Factor Inducible Protein A20; ATF3, Activating Transcription Factor 3; Bcl-3, B-Cell Lymphoma 3-Encoded Protein; Cbl-b, E3 Ubiquitin Protein Ligase Cbl-b; CYLD, Ubiquitin-Specific-Processing Protease CYLD; DUBA, Deubiquitinating Enzyme A; HA900, high molecular weight hyaluronan; IkBNS, NF-κB Inhibitor Delta; Nurr1, Nuclear Receptor Related 1; PDLIM2, PDZ and LIM Domain Protein 2; PIN1, Peptidylprolyl Cis/Trans Isomerase, NIMA-Interacting 1; SARM, Sterile Alpha and TIR Motif Containing 1; SHP, Small Heterodimer Partner; SOCS1, Suppressor of Cytokine Signalling 1; SOCS3, Suppressor of Cytokine Signalling 3; TAG, splice variant of the adaptor TRAM; TANK, TRAF Family Member Associated NF-κB Activator; TRIM5, Tripartite Motif Containing 5; TRIM38, Tripartite Motif Containing Protein 38; UBE3C, Ubiquitin Protein Ligase E3C; USP4, Ubiquitin Specific Peptidase 4.

picture of the actual signalling pathways and viable, effective, druggable targets.

In fact a number of clinical trials are currently underway. These include antagonists of TLR4, such as TLR4 targeted monoclonal antibody NI-0101, by Novimmune, which has several potential applications including asthma and rheumatoid arthritis and is the first antibody for TLR4 to pass Phase I clinical trials for safety and tolerability [122]. Antagonists of the endosomal TLRs (specifically TLR7, TLR8, and TLR9) are also being studied, such as IRS954 by Dynavax and IMO3100 by Idera, who have published results from their Phase II trials for this drug [123], amongst others. As indicated by such clinical trials, the inhibition of aberrant TLR signalling induced by endogenous DAMPs or exogenous PAMPs has high potential as a viable therapeutic approach in humans for the treatment of autoimmune diseases.

The insight from such TLR signalling research should also direct the medical field to rethink the classification of some diseases or the way in which they are treated. Over the past decade lots of new components and interactions have been discovered and it is plausible to postulate that there is much more to be discovered. This being said, the position of the classification, development, and treatment of complexes or multifactorial diseases should also be reconsidered to include elements of autoimmunity.

Moreover, we are now starting to gain the ability to modulate specific TLR activity, which should be used to the benefit of patients suffering from such TLR-dependent autoimmune diseases. In order to achieve this goal, more studies on the inhibitors mentioned above and others are required in order to provide alternatives to the current limited therapeutic options, providing a long-term solution, with reduced off-target effects.

References

[1] C. A. Janeway Jr. and R. Medzhitov, "Innate immune recognition," *Annual Review of Immunology*, vol. 20, pp. 197–216, 2002.

[2] S. Akira, S. Uematsu, and O. Takeuchi, "Pathogen recognition and innate immunity," *Cell*, vol. 124, no. 4, pp. 783–801, 2006.

[3] X. Cai, Y.-H. Chiu, and Z. J. Chen, "The cGAS-cGAMP-STING pathway of cytosolic DNA sensing and signaling," *Molecular Cell*, vol. 54, no. 2, pp. 289–296, 2014.

[4] M. Li, Y. Zhou, G. Feng, and S. B. Su, "The critical role of toll-like receptor signaling pathways in the induction and progression of autoimmune disease," *Current Molecular Medicine*, vol. 9, no. 3, pp. 365–374, 2009.

[5] N. J. Gay and M. Gangloff, "Structure and function of toll receptors and their ligands," *Annual Review of Biochemistry*, vol. 76, pp. 141–145, 2007.

[6] S. Akira and K. Takeda, "Toll-like receptor signalling," *Nature Reviews Immunology*, vol. 4, no. 7, pp. 499–511, 2004.

[7] T. Kawai and S. Akira, "TLR signaling," *Seminars in Immunology*, vol. 19, no. 1, pp. 24–32, 2007.

[8] I. Berglová, J. Krejsek, M. Koláčková, and R. Slezák, "B cell toll-like receptors with respect to the pathogenesis of sjögren's syndrome," *Acta Medica (Hradec Kralove, Czech Republic)*, vol. 54, no. 2, pp. 51–57, 2011.

[9] H. J. Anders, D. Zecher, R. D. Pawar, and P. S. Patole, "Molecular mechanisms of autoimmunity triggered by microbial infection," *Arthritis Research Therapy*, vol. 7, no. 5, pp. 215–224, 2005.

[10] S. Akira and H. Hemmi, "Recognition of pathogen-associated molecular patterns by TLR family," *Immunology Letters*, vol. 85, no. 2, pp. 85–95, 2003.

[11] H. Kanzler, F. J. Barrat, E. M. Hessel, and R. L. Coffman, "Therapeutic targeting of innate immunity with Toll-like receptor agonists and antagonists," *Nature Medicine*, vol. 13, no. 5, pp. 552–559, 2007.

[12] J. Booth, H. Wilson, S. Jimbo, and G. Mutwiri, "Modulation of B cell responses by Toll-like receptors," *Cell and Tissue Research*, vol. 343, no. 1, pp. 131–140, 2011.

[13] L. M. Skivka and V. V. Pozur, "Responses with participation of toll-like receptors in protective immunity and in pathologic states," *Ukraïns'kyi Biokhimichnyi Zhurnal*, vol. 80, no. 3, pp. 5–20, 2008.

[14] K. H. G. Mills, "Induction, function and regulation of IL-17-producing T cells," *European Journal of Immunology*, vol. 38, no. 10, pp. 2636–2649, 2008.

[15] Y. Park, S. Park, E. Yoo, D. Kim, and H. Shin, "Association of the polymorphism for toll-like receptor 2 with type 1 diabetes susceptibility," *Annals of the New York Academy of Sciences*, vol. 1037, pp. 170–174, 2004.

[16] J. Hong, E. Leung, A. G. Fraser, T. R. Merriman, P. Vishnu, and G. W. Krissansen, "TLR2, TLR4 and TLR9 polymorphisms and Crohn's disease in a New Zealand Caucasian cohort," *Journal of Gastroenterology and Hepatology*, vol. 22, no. 11, pp. 1760–1766, 2007.

[17] B. Serafini, B. Rosicarelli, D. Franciotta et al., "Dysregulated Epstein-Barr virus infection in the multiple sclerosis brain," *Journal of Experimental Medicine*, vol. 204, no. 12, pp. 2899–2912, 2007.

[18] I. R. Rifkin, E. A. Leadbetter, L. Busconi, G. Viglianti, and A. Marshak-Rothstein, "Toll-like receptors, endogenous ligands, and systemic autoimmune disease," *Immunological Reviews*, vol. 204, pp. 27–42, 2005.

[19] E. Andreakos, B. Foxwell, and M. Feldmann, "Is targeting Toll-like receptors and their signaling pathway a useful therapeutic approach to modulating cytokine-driven inflammation?" *Immunological Reviews*, vol. 202, pp. 250–265, 2004.

[20] A. Marshak-Rothstein, "Toll-like receptors in systemic autoimmune disease," *Nature Reviews Immunology*, vol. 6, no. 11, pp. 823–835, 2006.

[21] K. H. G. Mills, "TLR-dependent T cell activation in autoimmunity," *Nature Reviews Immunology*, vol. 11, no. 12, pp. 807–822, 2011.

[22] F. Y. Liew, D. Xu, E. K. Brint, and L. A. J. O'Neill, "Negative regulation of toll-like receptor-mediated immune responses," *Nature Reviews Immunology*, vol. 5, no. 6, pp. 446–458, 2005.

[23] C. Pasare and R. Medzhitov, "Toll pathway-dependent blockade of $CD4^+CD25^+$ T cell-mediated suppression by dendritic cells," *Science*, vol. 299, no. 5609, pp. 1033–1036, 2003.

[24] K. W. Moore, R. de Waal Malefyt, R. L. Coffman, and A. O'Garra, "Interleukin-10 and the interleukin-10 receptor," *Annual Review of Immunology*, vol. 19, pp. 683–765, 2001.

[25] O. Duramad, K. L. Fearon, J. H. Chan et al., "IL-10 regulates plasmacytoid dendritic cell response to CpG-containing immunostimulatory sequences," *Blood*, vol. 102, no. 13, pp. 4487–4492, 2003.

[26] M. Farrugia and B. Baron, "Role of regulatory t-cells in oral tolerance and immunotherapy," *Biochemistry Physiology: Open Access*, vol. 5, no. 199, 7 pages, 2016.

[27] D. M. Underhill, "Collaboration between the innate immune receptors dectin-1, TLRs, and Nods," *Immunological Reviews*, vol. 219, no. 1, pp. 75–87, 2007.

[28] L. A. J. O'Neill and A. G. Bowie, "The family of five: TIR-domain-containing adaptors in Toll-like receptor signalling," *Nature Reviews Immunology*, vol. 7, no. 5, pp. 353–364, 2007.

[29] K. Honda, H. Yanai, H. Negishi et al., "IRF-7 is the master regulator of type-I interferon-dependent immune responses," *Nature*, vol. 434, no. 7034, pp. 772–777, 2005.

[30] J. Lee, J. W. Sohn, Y. Zhang, K. W. Leong, D. Pisetsky, and B. A. Sullenger, "Nucleic acid-binding polymers as anti-inflammatory agents," *Proceedings of the National Academy of Sciences of the United States of America*, vol. 108, no. 34, pp. 14055–14060, 2011.

[31] O. Adachi, T. Kawai, K. Takeda et al., "Targeted disruption of the MyD88 gene results in loss of IL-1- and IL-18-mediated function," *Immunity*, vol. 9, no. 1, pp. 143–150, 1998.

[32] T. Horng, G. M. Barton, R. A. Flavell, and R. Medzhitov, "The adaptor molecule TIRAP provides signalling specificity for Toll-like receptors," *Nature*, vol. 420, no. 6913, pp. 329–333, 2002.

[33] J. C. Kagan and R. Medzhitov, "Phosphoinositide-mediated adaptor recruitment controls Toll-like receptor signaling," *Cell*, vol. 125, no. 5, pp. 943–955, 2006.

[34] L. Sun, L. Deng, C.-K. Ea, Z.-P. Xia, and Z. J. Chen, "The TRAF6 ubiquitin ligase and TAK1 kinase mediate IKK activation by BCL10 and MALT1 in T lymphocytes," *Molecular Cell*, vol. 14, no. 3, pp. 289–301, 2004.

[35] M. Yamamoto, S. Sato, H. Hemmi et al., "TRAM is specifically involved in the Toll-like receptor 4-mediated MyD88-independent signaling pathway," *Nature Immunology*, vol. 4, no. 11, pp. 1144–1150, 2003.

[36] S.-C. Lin, Y.-C. Lo, and H. Wu, "Helical assembly in the MyD88-IRAK4-IRAK2 complex in TLR/IL-1R signalling," *Nature*, vol. 465, no. 7300, pp. 885–890, 2010.

[37] Z. Jiang, J. Ninomiya-Tsuji, Y. Qian, K. Matsumoto, and X. Li, "Interleukin-1 (IL-1) receptor-associated kinase-dependent IL-1-induced signaling complexes phosphorylate TAK1 and TAB2 at the plasma membrane and activate TAK1 in the cytosol," *Molecular and Cellular Biology*, vol. 22, no. 20, pp. 7158–7167, 2002.

[38] C. Kollewe, A.-C. Mackensen, D. Neumann et al., "Sequential autophosphorylation steps in the interleukin-1 receptor-associated kinase-1 regulate its availability as an adapter in interleukin-1 signaling," *The Journal of Biological Chemistry*, vol. 279, no. 7, pp. 5227–5236, 2004.

[39] Z. J. Chen, "Ubiquitination in signaling to and activation of IKK," *Immunological Reviews*, vol. 246, no. 1, pp. 95–106, 2012.

[40] A. A. Ajibade, H. Y. Wang, and R.-F. Wang, "Cell type-specific function of TAK1 in innate immune signaling," *Trends in Immunology*, vol. 34, no. 7, pp. 307–316, 2013.

[41] T. Kawai and S. Akira, "The role of pattern-recognition receptors in innate immunity: update on toll-like receptors," *Nature Immunology*, vol. 11, no. 5, pp. 373–384, 2010.

[42] L. Alexopoulou, A. C. Holt, R. Medzhitov, and R. A. Flavell, "Recognition of double-stranded RNA and activation of NF-κB by toll-like receptor 3," *Nature*, vol. 413, no. 6857, pp. 732–738, 2001.

[43] S. S. Diebold, T. Kaisho, H. Hemmi, S. Akira, and C. Reis E Sousa, "Innate antiviral responses by means of TLR7-mediated recognition of single-stranded RNA," *Science*, vol. 303, no. 5663, pp. 1529–1531, 2004.

[44] F. Heil, H. Hemmi, H. Hochrein et al., "Species-specific recognition of single-stranded RNA via toll-like receptor 7 and 8," *Science*, vol. 303, no. 5663, pp. 1526–1529, 2004.

[45] J. M. Lund, L. Alexopoulou, A. Sato et al., "Recognition of single-stranded RNA viruses by toll-like receptor 7," *Proceedings of the National Academy of Sciences of the United States of America*, vol. 101, no. 15, pp. 5598–5603, 2004.

[46] H. Hemmi, O. Takeuchi, T. Kawai et al., "A Toll-like receptor recognizes bacterial DNA," *Nature*, vol. 408, no. 6813, pp. 740–745, 2000.

[47] T. Kawai and S. Akira, "Toll-like receptor and RIG-1-like receptor signaling," *Annals of the New York Academy of Sciences*, vol. 1143, pp. 1–20, 2008.

[48] K. Karikó, H. Ni, J. Capodici, M. Lamphier, and D. Weissman, "mRNA is an endogenous ligand for toll-like receptor 3," *The Journal of Biological Chemistry*, vol. 279, no. 13, pp. 12542–12550, 2004.

[49] L. Rönnblom and G. V. Alm, "Systemic lupus erythematosus and the type I interferon system," *Arthritis Research Therapy*, vol. 5, pp. 68–75, 2003.

[50] F. J. Barrat, T. Meeker, J. Gregorio et al., "Nucleic acids of mammalian origin can act as endogenous ligands for Toll-like receptors and may promote systemic lupus erythematosus," *Journal of Experimental Medicine*, vol. 202, no. 8, pp. 1131–1139, 2005.

[51] E. A. Leadbetter, I. R. Rifkin, A. M. Hohlbaum, B. C. Beaudette, M. J. Shlomchik, and A. Marshak-Rothstein, "Chromatin-IgG complexes activate B cells by dual engagement of IgM and Toll-like receptors," *Nature*, vol. 416, no. 6881, pp. 603–607, 2002.

[52] C. M. Lau, C. Broughton, A. S. Tabor et al., "RNA-associated autoantigens activate B cells by combined B cell antigen receptor/Toll-like receptor 7 engagement," *Journal of Experimental Medicine*, vol. 202, no. 9, pp. 1171–1177, 2005.

[53] U. Båve, M. Magnusson, M.-L. Eloranta, A. Perers, G. V. Alm, and L. Rönnblom, "FcγRIIa is expressed on natural IFN-α-producing cells (plasmacytoid dendritic cells) and is required for the IFN-α production induced by apoptotic cells combined with lupus IgG," *The Journal of Immunology*, vol. 171, no. 6, pp. 3296–3302, 2003.

[54] T. K. Means, E. Latz, F. Hayashi, M. R. Murali, D. T. Golenbock, and A. D. Luster, "Human lupus autoantibody-DNA complexes activate DCs through cooperation of CD32 and TLR9," *The Journal of Clinical Investigation*, vol. 115, no. 2, pp. 407–417, 2005.

[55] J. Vollmer, S. Tluk, C. Schmitz et al., "Immune stimulation mediated by autoantigen binding sites within small nuclear RNAs involves Toll-like receptors 7 and 8," *The Journal of Experimental Medicine*, vol. 202, no. 11, pp. 1575–1585, 2005.

[56] B. L. Lee, J. E. Moon, J. H. Shu et al., "UNC93B1 mediates differential trafficking of endosomal TLRs," *eLife*, vol. 2, Article ID e00291, 2013.

[57] R. Fukui, S.-I. Saitoh, A. Kanno et al., "Unc93B1 restricts systemic lethal inflammation by orchestrating toll-like receptor 7 and 9 trafficking," *Immunity*, vol. 35, no. 1, pp. 69–81, 2011.

[58] H. Itoh, M. Tatematsu, A. Watanabe et al., "UNC93B1 physically associates with human TLR8 and regulates TLR8-mediated signaling," *PLoS ONE*, vol. 6, no. 12, Article ID e28500, 2011.

[59] R. Fukui, S.-I. Saitoh, F. Matsumoto et al., "Unc93B1 biases Toll-like receptor responses to nucleic acid in dendritic cells toward DNA- but against RNA-sensing," *Journal of Experimental Medicine*, vol. 206, no. 6, pp. 1339–1350, 2009.

[60] B. Desnues, A. B. Macedo, A. Roussel-Queval et al., "TLR8 on dendritic cells and TLR9 on B cells restrain TLR7-mediated spontaneous autoimmunity in C57BL/6 mice," *Proceedings of the National Academy of Sciences of the United States of America*, vol. 111, no. 4, pp. 1497–1502, 2014.

[61] H. Qi, T. L. Denning, and L. Soong, "Differential induction of interleukin-10 and interleukin-12 in dendritic cells by microbial Toll-like receptor activators and skewing of T-cell cytokine profiles," *Infection and Immunity*, vol. 71, no. 6, pp. 3337–3342, 2003.

[62] S. C. Eisenbarth, D. A. Piggott, J. W. Huleatt, I. Visintin, C. A. Herrick, and K. Bottomly, "Lipopolysaccharide-enhanced, toll-like receptor 4-dependent T helper cell type 2 responses to inhaled antigen," *Journal of Experimental Medicine*, vol. 196, no. 12, pp. 1645–1651, 2002.

[63] F. Re and J. L. Strominger, "Toll-like receptor 2 (TLR2) and TLR4 differentially activate human dendritic cells," *The Journal of Biological Chemistry*, vol. 276, no. 40, pp. 37692–37699, 2001.

[64] B. Martin, K. Hirota, D. J. Cua, B. Stockinger, and M. Veldhoen, "Interleukin-17-producing $\gamma\delta$ T cells selectively expand in response to pathogen products and environmental signals," *Immunity*, vol. 31, no. 2, pp. 321–330, 2009.

[65] J. M. Reynolds, B. P. Pappu, J. Peng et al., "Toll-like receptor 2 signaling in $CD4^+$ T lymphocytes promotes T helper 17 responses and regulates the pathogenesis of autoimmune disease," *Immunity*, vol. 32, no. 5, pp. 692–702, 2010.

[66] M. Komai-Koma, L. Jones, G. S. Ogg, D. Xu, and F. Y. Liew, "TLR2 is expressed activated T cells as a costimulatory receptor," *Proceedings of the National Academy of Sciences of the United States of America*, vol. 101, no. 9, pp. 3029–3034, 2004.

[67] B. C. Mercier, A. Cottalorda, C. A. Coupet, J. Marvel, and N. Bonnefoy-Bérard, "TLR2 engagement on CD8 T cells enables generation of functional memory cells in response to a suboptimal TCR signal," *The Journal of Immunology*, vol. 182, no. 4, pp. 1860–1867, 2009.

[68] S. T. Smiley, J. A. King, and W. W. Hancock, "Fibrinogen stimulates macrophage chemokine secretion through toll-like receptor 4," *Journal of Immunology*, vol. 167, no. 5, pp. 2887–2894, 2001.

[69] A. Biragyn, P. A. Ruffini, C. A. Leifer et al., "Toll-like receptor 4-dependent activation of dendritic cells by β-defensin 2," *Science*, vol. 298, no. 5595, pp. 1025–1029, 2002.

[70] M. Raska and E. Weigl, "Heat shock proteins in autoimmune diseases," *Biomedical Papers*, vol. 149, no. 2, pp. 243–249, 2005.

[71] N. M. Green and A. Marshak-Rothstein, "Toll-like receptor driven B cell activation in the induction of systemic autoimmunity," *Seminars in Immunology*, vol. 23, no. 2, pp. 106–112, 2011.

[72] M. Ehlers, H. Fukuyama, T. L. McGaha, A. Aderem, and J. V. Ravetch, "TLR9/MyD88 signaling is required for class switching to pathogenic IgG2a and 2b autoantibodies in SLE," *Journal of Experimental Medicine*, vol. 203, no. 3, pp. 553–561, 2006.

[73] J. R. Groom, C. A. Fletcher, S. N. Walters et al., "BAFF and MyD88 signals promote a lupuslike disease independent of T cells," *Journal of Experimental Medicine*, vol. 204, no. 8, pp. 1959–1971, 2007.

[74] S. Becker-Herman, A. Meyer-Bahlburg, M. A. Schwartz et al., "WASp-deficient B cells play a critical, cell-intrinsic role in triggering autoimmunity," *Journal of Experimental Medicine*, vol. 208, no. 10, pp. 2033–2042, 2011.

[75] A. B. Begovich, V. E. H. Carlton, L. A. Honigberg et al., "A missense single-nucleotide polymorphism in a gene encoding a protein tyrosine phosphatase (PTPN22) is associated with rheumatoid arthritis," *American Journal of Human Genetics*, vol. 75, no. 2, pp. 330–337, 2004.

[76] R. M. Plenge, C. Cotsapas, L. Davies et al., "Two independent alleles at 6q23 associated with risk of rheumatoid arthritis," *Nature Genetics*, vol. 39, no. 12, pp. 1477–1482, 2007.

[77] S. M. Sacre, E. Andreakos, S. Kiriakidis et al., "The toll-like receptor adaptor proteins MyD88 and Mal/TIRAP contribute to the inflammatory and destructive processes in a human model of rheumatoid arthritis," *American Journal of Pathology*, vol. 170, no. 2, pp. 518–525, 2007.

[78] M. H. Hoffmann, K. Skriner, S. Herman et al., "Nucleic acid-stimulated antigen-presenting cells trigger T cells to induce disease in a rat transfer model of inflammatory arthritis," *Journal of Autoimmunity*, vol. 36, no. 3-4, pp. 288–300, 2011.

[79] S. J. Creely, P. G. McTernan, C. M. Kusminski et al., "Lipopolysaccharide activates an innate immune system response in human adipose tissue in obesity and type 2 diabetes," *American Journal of Physiology—Endocrinology and Metabolism*, vol. 292, no. 3, pp. E740–E747, 2007.

[80] M. F. Denny, S. Thacker, H. Mehta et al., "Interferon-α promotes abnormal vasculogenesis in lupus: a potential pathway for premature atherosclerosis," *Blood*, vol. 110, no. 8, pp. 2907–2915, 2007.

[81] R. Lande, J. Gregorio, V. Facchinetti et al., "Plasmacytoid dendritic cells sense self-DNA coupled with antimicrobial peptide," *Nature*, vol. 449, no. 7162, pp. 564–569, 2007.

[82] S. Rakoff-Nahoum and R. Medzhitov, "Toll-like receptors and cancer," *Nature Reviews Cancer*, vol. 9, no. 1, pp. 57–63, 2009.

[83] C. Guiducci, G. Ott, J. H. Chan et al., "Properties regulating the nature of the plasmacytoid dendritic cell response to Toll-like receptor 9 activation," *The Journal of Experimental Medicine*, vol. 203, no. 8, pp. 1999–2008, 2006.

[84] K. Honda, Y. Ohba, H. Yanai et al., "Spatiotemporal regulation of MyD88-IRF-7 signalling for robust type-I interferon induction," *Nature*, vol. 434, no. 7036, pp. 1035–1040, 2005.

[85] S. Fasciano and L. Li, "Intervention of toll-like receptors-mediated human innate immunity and inflammation by synthetic compunds and naturally occurring products," *Current Medicinal Chemistry*, vol. 13, no. 12, pp. 1389–1395, 2006.

[86] T. Du, Z.-G. Zhou, S. You et al., "Modulation of monocyte hyperresponsiveness to TLR ligands by 1,25-dihydroxy-vitamin D3 from LADA and T2DM," *Diabetes Research and Clinical Practice*, vol. 83, no. 2, pp. 208–214, 2009.

[87] S. Sun, N. L. Rao, J. Venable, R. Thurmond, and L. Karlsson, "TLR7/9 antagonists as the rapeutics for immune-mediated inflammatory disorders," *Inflammation Allergy—Drug Targets*, vol. 6, no. 4, pp. 223–235, 2007.

[88] M. Rutz, J. Metzger, T. Gellert et al., "Toll-like receptor 9 binds single-stranded CpG-DNA in a sequence- and pH-dependent manner," *European Journal of Immunology*, vol. 34, no. 9, pp. 2541–2550, 2004.

[89] A. M. Krieg and J. Vollmer, "Toll-like receptors 7, 8, and 9: linking innate immunity to autoimmunity," *Immunological Reviews*, vol. 220, no. 1, pp. 251–269, 2007.

[90] E. D. Papadimitraki, G. K. Bertsias, and D. T. Boumpas, "Toll like receptors and autoimmunity: a critical appraisal," *Journal of Autoimmunity*, vol. 29, no. 4, pp. 310–318, 2007.

[91] D. Zipris, E. Lien, A. Nair et al., "TLR9-signaling pathways are involved in Kilham rat virus-induced autoimmune diabetes in the biobreeding diabetes-resistant rat," *The Journal of Immunology*, vol. 178, no. 2, pp. 693–701, 2007.

[92] T. Hayashi, C. S. Gray, M. Chan et al., "Prevention of autoimmune disease by induction of tolerance to toll-like receptor 7," *Proceedings of the National Academy of Sciences of the United States of America*, vol. 106, no. 8, pp. 2764–2769, 2009.

[93] M. Loiarro, F. Capolunghi, N. Fantò et al., "Inhibition of MyD88 dimerization and recruitment of IRAK1 and IRAK4 by a novel peptidomimetic compound," *Journal of Leukocyte Biology*, vol. 82, no. 4, pp. 801–810, 2007.

[94] T. Bartfai, M. M. Behrens, S. Gaidarova, J. Pemberton, A. Shivanyuk, and J. Rebek Jr., "A low molecular weight mimic of the Toll/IL-1 receptor/resistance domain inhibits IL-1 receptor-mediated responses," *Proceedings of the National Academy of Sciences of the United States of America*, vol. 100, no. 13, pp. 7971–7976, 2003.

[95] K. W. Song, F. X. Talamas, R. T. Suttmann et al., "The kinase activities of interleukin-1 receptor associated kinase (IRAK)-1 and 4 are redundant in the control of inflammatory cytokine expression in human cells," *Molecular Immunology*, vol. 46, no. 7, pp. 1458–1466, 2009.

[96] B. Skaug, J. Chen, F. Du, J. He, A. Ma, and Z. J. Chen, "Direct, noncatalytic mechanism of IKK inhibition by A20," *Molecular Cell*, vol. 44, no. 4, pp. 559–571, 2011.

[97] J.-M. Yuk, D.-M. Shin, H.-M. Lee et al., "The orphan nuclear receptor SHP acts as a negative regulator in inflammatory signaling triggered by Toll-like receptors," *Nature Immunology*, vol. 12, no. 8, pp. 742–751, 2011.

[98] T. Kondo, T. Kawai, and S. Akira, "Dissecting negative regulation of Toll-like receptor signaling," *Trends in Immunology*, vol. 33, no. 9, pp. 449–458, 2012.

[99] M. Shi, W. Deng, E. Bi et al., "TRIM30α negatively regulates TLR-mediated NFκB activation by targeting TAB2 and TAB3 for degradation," *Nature Immunology*, vol. 9, no. 4, pp. 369–377, 2008.

[100] T. Saitoh, A. Tun-Kyi, A. Ryo et al., "Negative regulation of interferon-regulatory factor 3-dependent innate antiviral response by the prolyl isomerase Pin1," *Nature Immunology*, vol. 7, no. 6, pp. 598–605, 2006.

[101] E. M. Palsson-McDermott, S. L. Doyle, A. F. McGettrick et al., "TAG, a splice variant of the adaptor TRAM, negatively regulates the adaptor MyD88-independent TLR4 pathway," *Nature Immunology*, vol. 10, no. 6, pp. 579–586, 2009.

[102] C. Han, J. Jin, S. Xu, H. Liu, N. Li, and X. Cao, "Integrin CD11b negatively regulates TLR-triggered inflammatory responses by activating Syk and promoting degradation of MyD88 and TRIF via Cbl-b," *Nature Immunology*, vol. 11, no. 8, pp. 734–742, 2010.

[103] M. Carty, R. Goodbody, M. Schröder, J. Stack, P. N. Moynagh, and A. G. Bowie, "The human adaptor SARM negatively regulates adaptor protein TRIF-dependent Toll-like receptor signaling," *Nature Immunology*, vol. 7, no. 10, pp. 1074–1081, 2006.

[104] N. Kayagaki, Q. Phung, S. Chan et al., "DUBA: a deubiquitinase that regulates type I interferon production," *Science*, vol. 318, no. 5856, pp. 1628–1632, 2007.

[105] A. Asari, T. Kanemitsu, and H. Kurihara, "Oral administration of high molecular weight hyaluronan (900 kDa) controls immune system via toll-like receptor 4 in the intestinal epithelium," *The Journal of Biological Chemistry*, vol. 285, no. 32, pp. 24751–24758, 2010.

[106] K. Matsushita, O. Takeuchi, D. M. Standley et al., "Zc3h12a is an RNase essential for controlling immune responses by regulating mRNA decay," *Nature*, vol. 458, no. 7242, pp. 1185–1190, 2009.

[107] O. Duramad, K. L. Fearon, B. Chang et al., "Inhibitors of TLR-9 act on multiple cell subsets in mouse and man in vitro and prevent death in vivo from systemic inflammation," *The Journal of Immunology*, vol. 174, no. 9, pp. 5193–5200, 2005.

[108] A. M. Krieg, T. Wu, R. Weeratna et al., "Sequence motifs in adenoviral DNA block immune activation by stimulatory CpG motifs," *Proceedings of the National Academy of Sciences of the United States of America*, vol. 95, no. 21, pp. 12631–12636, 1998.

[109] H. Yamada, I. Gursel, F. Takeshita et al., "Effect of suppressive DNA on CpG-induced immune activation," *The Journal of Immunology*, vol. 169, no. 10, pp. 5590–5594, 2002.

[110] F.-G. Zhu, C. F. Reich, and D. S. Pisetsky, "Inhibition of murine dendritic cell activation by synthetic phosphorothioate oligodeoxynucleotides," *Journal of Leukocyte Biology*, vol. 72, no. 6, pp. 1154–1163, 2002.

[111] L. L. Stunz, P. Lenert, D. Peckham et al., "Inhibitory oligonucleotides specifically block effects of stimulatory CpG oligonucleotides in B cells," *European Journal of Immunology*, vol. 32, pp. 1212–1222, 2002.

[112] P. P. Ho, P. Fontoura, P. J. Ruiz, L. Steinman, and H. Garren, "An immunomodulatory GpG oligonucleotide for the treatment of autoimmunity via the innate and adaptive immune systems," *Journal of Immunology*, vol. 171, no. 9, pp. 4920–4926, 2003.

[113] I. Gursel, M. Gursel, H. Yamada, K. J. Ishii, F. Takeshita, and D. M. Klinman, "Repetitive elements in mammalian telomeres suppress bacterial DNA-induced immune activation," *The Journal of Immunology*, vol. 171, no. 3, pp. 1393–1400, 2003.

[114] R. A. Zeuner, K. J. Ishii, M. J. Lizak et al., "Reduction of CpG-induced arthritis by suppressive oligodeoxynucleotides," *Arthritis Rheumatology*, vol. 46, pp. 2219–2224, 2002.

[115] L. Dong, S. Ito, K. J. Ishii, and D. M. Klinman, "Suppressive oligonucleotides protect against collagen-induced arthritis in mice," *Arthritis Rheumatology*, vol. 50, pp. 1686–1689, 2004.

[116] F. Grela, A. Aumeunier, E. Bardel et al., "The TLR7 agonist R848 alleviates allergic inflammation by targeting invariant NKT cells to produce IFN-γ," *The Journal of Immunology*, vol. 186, no. 1, pp. 284–290, 2011.

[117] A. M. Krieg, S. M. Efler, M. Wittpoth, M. J. Al Adhami, and H. L. Davis, "Induction of systemic TH1-like innate immunity in normal volunteers following subcutaneous but not intravenous administration of CPG 7909, a synthetic B-class CpG oligodeoxynucleotide TLR9 agonist," *Journal of Immunotherapy*, vol. 27, no. 6, pp. 460–471, 2004.

[118] J. W. Friedberg, H. Kim, M. McCauley et al., "Combination immunotherapy with a CpG oligonucleotide (1018 ISS) and rituximab in patients with non-Hodgkin lymphoma: increased interferon-α/ β-inducible gene expression, without significant toxicity," *Blood*, vol. 105, no. 2, pp. 489–495, 2005.

[119] G. M. Gauvreau, E. M. Hessel, L.-P. Boulet, R. L. Coffman, and P. M. O'Byrne, "Immunostimulatory sequences regulate interferon-inducible genes but not allergic airway responses," *American Journal of Respiratory and Critical Care Medicine*, vol. 174, no. 1, pp. 15–20, 2006.

[120] L. Bennett, A. K. Palucka, E. Arce et al., "Interferon and granulopoiesis signatures in systemic lupus erythematosus blood,"

The Journal of Experimental Medicine, vol. 197, no. 6, pp. 711–723, 2003.

[121] E. C. Baechler, F. M. Batliwalla, G. Karypis et al., "Interferon-inducible gene expression signature in peripheral blood cells of patients with severe lupus," *Proceedings of the National Academy of Sciences of the United States of America*, vol. 100, no. 5, pp. 2610–2615, 2003.

[122] E. Monnet, L. Shang, G. Lapeyre et al., "Translational data and phase 1 study results of a new monoclonal antibody targeting Toll like receptor 4 (TLR4) developed for rheumatoid arthritis (RA) treatment with a potential for personalized medicine," *Arthritis & Rheumatology*, vol. 67, abstract 1661, pp. 2051–2052, 2015.

[123] Y.-W. Wu, W. Tang, and J.-P. Zuo, "Toll-like receptors: Potential targets for lupus treatment," *Acta Pharmacologica Sinica*, vol. 36, no. 12, pp. 1395–1407, 2015.

19

Psoriatic Arthritis Is an Indicator of Significant Renal Damage in Patients with Psoriasis

Abidullah Khan, Iqbal Haider, Maimoona Ayub, and Mohammad Humayun

KTH, Peshawar, Pakistan

Correspondence should be addressed to Abidullah Khan; dr.abidk@yahoo.com

Academic Editor: Han J. Moshage

Background. Psoriasis affects joints in around 30% of the patients. Recent studies have demonstrated an increased risk of essential hypertension, ischemic heart disease, and stroke in psoriatic patients. However, the prevalence of renal disease in patients with psoriasis has not been evaluated properly. *Objectives.* Objectives were to evaluate renal functions in patients with psoriasis and to assess any possible relationship of renal failure with psoriasis and psoriatic arthritis. *Methods.* In this cross-sectional study, 30 participants were recruited into the following three groups: group-A, psoriatic arthritis; group-B, psoriasis without arthritis; and group-C, healthy subjects. Renal function tests were performed for every participant of each group. The data was analyzed by using SPSS version 16. Chi-squared and one-way ANOVA tests were applied, considering a P value of less than 0.05 as a standard criterion. *Results.* Serum creatinine, urea, and phosphate were the highest in group-A, higher in group-B, and normal in group-C, $P < 0.05$. Similarly, GFR was the lowest in group-A, lower in group-B, and normal in group-C. The difference in mean GFR values was statistically significant, $F(2) = 355$, $P < 0.001$. Moreover, proteinuria (gm/day) was seen in 96.7% of the patients with psoriatic arthritis, ($M = 1.18 \pm 0.55$, $P < 0.05$) against 10% of the psoriatic patients without arthritis ($M = 0.41 \pm 0.10$, $P < 0.05$). *Conclusion.* Derangement of renal function is more prevalent in psoriatic patients, especially in those with concomitant psoriatic arthritis. Therefore, each psoriatic patient must be routinely screened for an underlying renal failure.

1. Introduction

Psoriasis which affects around 5% of the general population is a chronic autoimmune inflammatory condition of the skin and/or joints. This disease peaks in adulthood and is one of the common causes of increased morbidity worldwide [1, 2]. Recent studies have demonstrated a link between psoriasis and other systemic disorders like diabetes mellitus, metabolic syndrome, cardiovascular, and cerebrovascular diseases [1, 3–6]. The pathogenesis of association of psoriasis with these disorders is attributed to a chronic inflammatory state, driven by activated T-cells and cytokines such as, tumor necrosis factor-α (TNF-α) [1]. Although, a link between renal impairment and psoriasis has been proposed on the basis of case reports of kidney disease in patients with psoriasis, the association between the two entities still remains largely unclear [7].

Studies examining the possible association between psoriasis and kidney disease have shown paradoxical results. In a study by Yang et al., derangement of renal function was more prevalent in patients with severe psoriasis than in the age and sex matched controls [8]. Similarly, other studies demonstrated a greater incidence of proteinuria and elevated creatinine in patients suffering from psoriasis [9–12]. However, contrarily to the aforementioned research work, other studies failed to show a link between psoriasis and the renal involvement [13–15].

Although, the risk of renal failure in patients with psoriasis has been studied occasionally, renal involvement in subjects with psoriatic arthritis has scarcely been evaluated. Therefore, we investigated the risk of renal involvement in patients with psoriasis, generally, and in those with arthritis psoriatica, specifically. We hypothesized that renal failure would be more frequent in patients with psoriatic arthritis

TABLE 1: Group specific demographic details.

Variable	Group-A	Group-B	Group-C
Males	63.3%	66.7%	70%
Females	36.7%	33.3%	30%
Occupations with maximum sun exposure (>8 hours/day)	80%	63.3%	26.7%
Occupations with minimum sun exposure (<8 hours/day)	20%	36.7%	73.3%
Age (years)	36.43 ± 6.26	34.6 ± 6.68	36.10 ± 7.76

Group-A: patients with psoriatic arthritis, group-B: psoriasis without arthritis, and group-C: healthy controls.

than in those without arthritis. Similarly, we hypothesized that deranged renal function would be more prevalent in patients with psoriasis without arthritis than the age and sex matched normal population.

2. Methods

This observational study was conducted in the departments of Dermatology of the three tertiary level hospitals of Peshawar, Pakistan, between February and December 2016, and included 90 subjects. Five of these participants, diagnosed with psoriatic arthritis, were recruited from Medical Unit "A" of Khyber Teaching Hospital (KTH), Peshawar, Pakistan, as well. The participants were divided into three equal groups as follows: group-A, patients with psoriasis and concomitant psoriatic arthritis; group-B, patients with psoriasis without arthritis; and group-C, healthy individuals without either psoriasis or psoriatic arthritis. This study was approved by the relevant hospital's ethics' review board. Furthermore, an informed written consent was obtained from every participant before the conduction of this study.

The inclusion criteria included (1) any gender, (2) age range of 18–70 years, (3) patients with psoriasis and/or psoriatic arthritis irrespective of severity of psoriasis itself for inclusion in either of group-A or group-B, and (4) thirty, age and sex matched healthy individuals for comparison in group-C, as a control group. The diagnosis of psoriasis was made on the basis of clinical grounds, expert opinion of the senior dermatologist, and/or skin biopsy in difficult cases. Similarly, patients were labeled as having psoriatic arthritis on the basis of clinical suspicion and detailed assessment by a senior rheumatologist and/or physician, supported by imaging and synovial fluid analysis in difficult cases.

Those who had preexisting kidney disease were excluded from the study. Similarly, those with risk factors for renal disease like hypertension, hyperlipidemia, diabetes, smoking, lupus, renovascular stenosis, recurrent urinary tract infections (UTIs), vasculitides like Wegner's granulomatosis or Churg-Strauss syndrome, and polyarteritis nodosa were also excluded from the study. Those with a history of intake of nonsteroidal anti-inflammatory drugs (NSAIDs), antibiotics like aminoglycosides, and other nephrotoxic medications in the preceding three months were also excluded. Moreover, patients with psoriasis who either previously received or were currently on potentially nephrotoxic medications for their disease like disease modifying antirheumatic drugs (DMARDs), biologic treatment, and so forth were also excluded from the study.

Initially, 200 individuals were assessed for their suitability in the final study. However, only 90 of them fulfilled the inclusion/exclusion criteria and were, thus, the subjects of final study. Each included participant was worked up with a detailed history, clinical examination, and a thorough review of the previous medical record. Serum creatinine, urea, and urinary protein estimation were done through enzymatic colorimetric assays on the automated biochemistry analyzer, ABX Pentra-400, Horiba Medical, France. Moreover, serum calcium and phosphate levels were measured through direct potentiometry through ion-selective electrodes (ISE) method by using the same biochemistry analyzer. Blood hemoglobin (Hb) was determined by using spectrophotometry on an automated 19-parameter hematology analyzer, Counter-19, provided by Weiner lab, Argentina. Similarly, glomerular filtration rate (GFR) and 24-hour urinary protein were measured for every participant. GFR was calculated by using Modification of Diet in Renal Disease (MDRD) criteria. Those who had significant proteinuria, defined as more than 0.5 gm protein per day, were subjected to a renal biopsy for histological evaluation.

All the data was obtained on a structured questionnaire specifically designed for this purpose. The questionnaire included questions regarding demography, disease duration, past medical and surgical history, drug history, and the study variables mentioned above. All the data was entered into and analyzed by the SPSS version 16. One-way ANOVA, with Turkey-HSD, and Chi-squared tests were used for the statistical analysis. A P value of less than 0.05 was considered as a standard criterion.

3. Results

Mean age of all the 90 participants was 35.71 ± 6.90 years. The male population made 66.70% of the sample while females were 33.30%. Majority of individuals with psoriasis or psoriatic arthritis worked in occupations with maximum sun exposure (more than 8 hours/day), such as outdoor hard labor, public driving, and farming. However, most of the healthy participants had minimum sun exposure. Occupation, age, and genderwise descriptive statistics for each group are given below (Table 1).

The results of Chi-squared test revealed that although psoriasis was more common in people belonging to occupations with maximum sun exposure (more than 8 hours/day), such as laborers, drivers, and farmers (N = 19 (37.3%), Z-score = 0.9), than those who were least exposed to sun, such as bankers and health professionals (N = 11 (28.2%), Z-score

TABLE 2: An overview of the different parameters of renal functions.

Variable	Group-A	Group-B	Group-C	P value
Creatinine (mg/dl)	3.36 ± 0.60	2.30 ± 0.53	1.03 ± 0.18	<0.001
Urea (mg/dl)	51.43 ± 12.29	41.03 ± 4.62	28.07 ± 4.77	<0.001
GFR (ml/minute/1.73 m^2)	57.57 ± 6.90	86.67 ± 7.49	106.33 ± 6.95	<0.001
Urinary protein (mg/day)	1182 ± 549	416 ± 102	170 ± 46	<0.001
Phosphate (mg/dl)	5.50 ± 0.63	3.97 ± 0.49	2.87 ± 0.57	<0.001
Calcium (mg/dl)	8.50 ± 0.63	9.93 ± 0.64	10.37 ± 0.61	<0.001
Hemoglobin (gm/dl)	11.20 ± 1.18	12.47 ± 0.57	14.33 ± 0.99	<0.001
Uric acid (mg/dl)	7.7 ± 0.91	6.9 ± 1.11	5.3 ± 1.23	<0.05

Group-A: patients with psoriatic arthritis, group-B: psoriasis without arthritis, group-C: healthy controls, and GFR: glomerular filtration rate.

TABLE 3: An overview of the pattern of histological involvement of the kidneys in 32 patients with proteinuria of more than 0.5 gm/day.

Histology	Group-A	Group-B	Total (n)
Membranous glomerulonephritis (MGN)	25 (92.6%)	2 (7.4%)	27
Focal segmental glomerulosclerosis (FSGS)	3 (75%)	1 (25%)	4
Membranoproliferative glomerulonephritis (MPGN)	1 (100%)	0 (0%)	1
	29	3	32

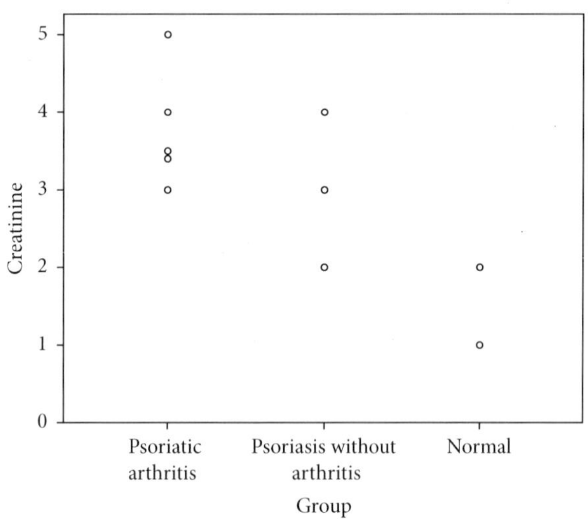

FIGURE 1: Scatter dot plot demonstrating groupwise distribution of serum creatinine (mg/dl).

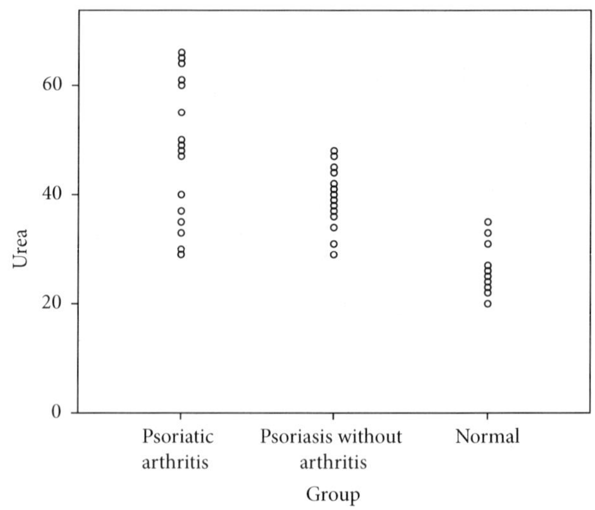

FIGURE 2: Scatter dot plot demonstrating groupwise distribution of serum urea (mg/dl).

= 0.9), the difference was not significant statistically, $P > 0.05$. Nevertheless, psoriatic arthritis was more prevalent in patients with maximum sun exposure than those less exposed to sun, and at a statistically significant level, Chi-squared (2) = 18.19, $P < 0.001$. The likelihood ratio (LR) for having psoriatic arthritis in patients with maximum sun exposure was statistically significant as well, LR (2) = 18.91, $P < 0.001$. Similarly, although, both psoriasis and psoriatic arthritis were seen to be more prevalent in males, but the impact of gender on having psoriasis or psoriatic arthritis was not found to be significant statistically, Chi-squared (2) = 0.30, $P = 0.86$, and LR (2) = 0.30, $P = 0.86$, respectively.

Assessment of renal function revealed that patients with psoriatic arthritis had significantly elevated creatinine [(mg/dl), ($M = 3.36 \pm 0.60$, $P < 0.001$)] and urea [(mg/dl), ($M = 51.43 \pm 12.29$, $P < 0.001$)]. Similarly, patient with psoriasis but without concomitant psoriatic arthritis still had significant derangement of creatinine ($M = 2.30 \pm 0.53$, $P < 0.001$) and urea ($M = 41.03 \pm 4.62$, $P < 0.001$), compared with the normal control group (Table 2). Groupwise distribution of serum creatinine and urea is given below (Figures 1 and 2).

Nevertheless, clinically significant proteinuria, defined as more than 500 mg of protein in 24-hour urine sample, was seen in 96.70% ($n = 29$) of the participants of group-A (patients with both psoriasis and psoriatic arthritis), 10% ($n = 3$) of the participants of group-B, (patients with psoriasis without arthritis), and none of the participants of group-C (the healthy subjects), as demonstrated below (Figure 3). All the 32 patients (35.6%), with clinically significant proteinuria, had renal biopsies; the results are as shown (Table 3). The

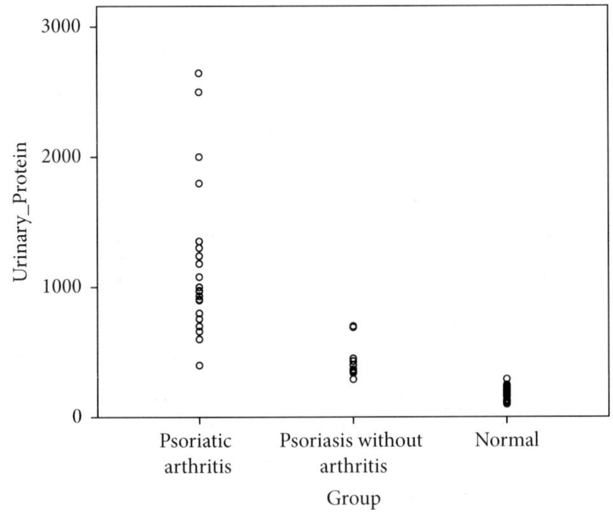

FIGURE 3: Scatter dot plot demonstrating groupwise distribution of daily proteinuria (mg/day).

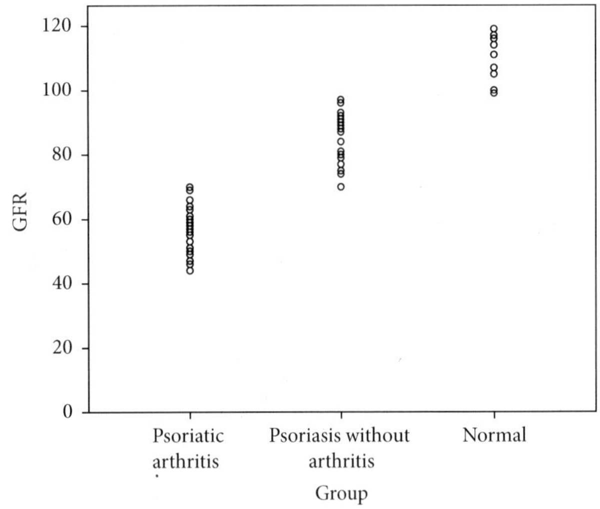

FIGURE 4: Scatter dot plot demonstrating groupwise distribution of e-GFR (ml/min).

predominant histological pattern of renal damage was that of membranous glomerulonephritis (MGN). No one had any evidence of renal tubular damage.

As can be seen in Table 2, the renal functions were impaired more in patients with psoriatic arthritis than those with psoriasis only. Similarly, the healthy controls had normal renal parameters. Furthermore, the GFR (ml/minute) was the lowest in group-A ($M = 57.57$, SD = 6.90), intermediate in group-B ($M = 86.67$, SD = 7.49), and the highest in group-C ($M = 106.33$, SD = 6.95). In order to compare mean values of GFR across these three groups, one-way ANOVA was run. The assumption of homogeneity of variance was tested and was found tenable; Levene's statistic (2, 87) = 0.10, $P = 0.90$. Similarly, the assumption of normality was satisfied (skewness = −0.19, kurtosis = −1.21). The results of one-way ANOVA demonstrated a statistically significant difference in mean GFR of the three study groups, $F(2) = 355$, $P < 0.001$. Post hoc analysis via Turkey-HSD showed that all the three groups were different from each other at a statistically significant level, $P < 0.001$ (Figures 4 and 5). Thus it can be concluded that there is enough evidence of significant renal impairment in patients with either psoriatic arthritis or psoriasis, compared with the age and sex matched unaffected individuals. This manifests in the form of raised creatinine, urea, and phosphate and a concomitant decline in GFR, Hb, and calcium, $P < 0.05$ (Table 2).

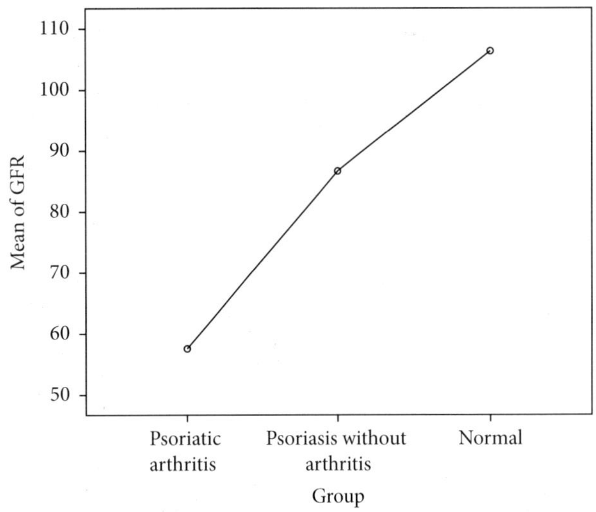

FIGURE 5: Mean plot demonstrating variation in e-GFR (ml/min) across the three study groups.

4. Discussion

We observed that both psoriasis and psoriatic arthritis are common in men in their 3rd to 4th decade of life. Moreover, they are more prevalent in persons exposed maximally to sunlight, such as farmers, laborers, sewerage worker, and drivers, and are relatively uncommon in people who remain or work indoors like bankers and health professionals. Our study demonstrated that patients with psoriatic arthritis are more likely to have deranged renal functions than those with psoriasis but without concomitant joint disease. However, such patients still have more incidence of renal disease than the normal people. Although, clinically significant proteinuria is more common in arthritis psoriatica, its prevalence in patients with psoriasis only is still significantly higher than the healthy controls. The most common renal abnormality in such people is that of membranous glomerulonephritis (MGN).

It is worth mentioning that a limited number of studies have demonstrated a link between psoriasis and kidney disease. The most commonly encountered renal problems in patients with psoriasis are IgA nephropathy, focal segmental glomerulosclerosis (FSGS), and membranous nephropathy [9, 16–19]. It is noteworthy that membranous glomerulonephritis (MGN) and focal segmental glomerulosclerosis

(FSGS) were the most common histological patterns on renal biopsies in our study group.

There is some emerging evidence that immunologic mechanisms such as chronic T-cell activation and increased levels of immune complexes and cytokines cause glomerular injury in psoriasis [7, 20]. However, other studies have demonstrated that direct tubular injury resulting from hyperuricemia in people with psoriasis could be another probable mechanism [21]. It should be noted that although we observed high uric acid levels in psoriatic patients with concomitant renal involvement, none had histologically proven renal tubular necrosis.

The extent of psoriasis is an independent risk factor for systemic involvement. In a study by Kurd and Gelfand, chronic kidney disease was more prevalent in patients with moderate-severe psoriasis than in those with mild disease [2]. However, it must be noted that one of the limitations of our study was the nonaccounting for the extent of psoriasis in terms of body surface area (BSA) involved.

Gelfand et al. observed that the risk of kidney disease was higher in the young than the elderly psoriatic patients [3]. This finding is in sharp contrast to our observation of a positive association between the risk of renal involvement and age of the patients. However, our finding of positive association between increasing age and the risk of renal disease in patients with psoriasis is supported by other relevant studies [22]. It has been argued that aging leads to a higher activity of inflammation-associated transcription factors, namely, NFκB, STAT1, and STAT3. This ultimately leads to an escalated action of TNF- α, causing renal injury [23]. Moreover, one recent study concluded that psoriasis accounted for one extra case of chronic kidney disease per 134 patients per year in patients aged 40–50, and in those aged 50–60, the incidence was even higher at one additional case per 62 patients per year [24].

Although we excluded all those patients who had received potentially nephrotoxic drugs for the treatment of psoriasis, Corden et al. reported a case of acute tubular necrosis (ATN), developing secondary to the topical use of vitamin-D in a psoriatic patient [25]. Hence, studies recommend rigorous monitoring of the renal function in patients treated for psoriasis with any potentially nephrotoxic medication [25, 26].

It is worth mentioning that the results of this study were according to our expectations. This study demonstrated an increased incidence of renal impairment in psoriasis and especially in psoriatic arthritis. However, this study still had a few limitations. The foremost was that of a smaller sample size. Second limitation was the cross-sectional study design. Thirdly, not all the patient had renal histological examination. Therefore, we recommend future cohort studies to throw more light on the possible link of psoriasis and psoriatic arthritis with kidney disease.

5. Conclusion

Renal function is impaired in people with psoriasis and psoriatic arthritis. Furthermore, psoriatic arthritis is an independent predictor of renal damage in patients with psoriasis. Therefore, every patient with psoriasis and/or psoriatic arthritis should be screened for an underlying renal damage.

Abbreviations

GFR:	Glomerular filtration rate
MGN:	Membranous glomerulonephritis
FSGS:	Focal segmental glomerulosclerosis
Hb:	Hemoglobin
ATN:	Acute tubal necrosis
DMARDs:	Disease modifying antirheumatic drugs
TNF-α:	Tumor necrosis factor-α
MDRD:	Modification of diet in renal disease.

Authors' Contributions

Abidullah Khan, Iqbal Haider, Maimoona Ayub, and Mohammad Humayun conceived the idea and promulgated the study design. Abidullah Khan and Maimoona Ayub drafted the manuscript. All the authors approved the final version before submission.

References

[1] C. E. Griffiths and J. N. Barker, "Pathogenesis and clinical features of psoriasis," *The Lancet*, vol. 370, no. 9583, pp. 263–271, 2007.

[2] S. K. Kurd and J. M. Gelfand, "The prevalence of previously diagnosed and undiagnosed psoriasis in US adults: results from NHANES 2003-2004," *Journal of the American Academy of Dermatology*, vol. 60, no. 2, pp. 218–224, 2009.

[3] J. M. Gelfand, A. L. Neimann, D. B. Shin, X. Wang, D. J. Margolis, and A. B. Troxel, "Risk of myocardial infarction in patients with psoriasis," *Journal of the American Medical Association*, vol. 296, no. 14, pp. 1735–1741, 2006.

[4] K. Abuabara, R. S. Azfar, D. B. Shin, A. L. Neimann, A. B. Troxel, and J. M. Gelfand, "Cause-specific mortality in patients with severe psoriasis: a population-based cohort study in the U.K.," *British Journal of Dermatology*, vol. 163, no. 3, pp. 586–592, 2010.

[5] R. S. Azfar, N. M. Seminara, D. B. Shin, A. B. Troxel, D. J. Margolis, and J. M. Gelfand, "Increased risk of diabetes mellitus and likelihood of receiving diabetes mellitus treatment in patients with psoriasis," *Archives of Dermatology*, vol. 148, no. 9, pp. 995–1000, 2012.

[6] S. M. Langan, N. M. Seminara, D. B. Shin et al., "Prevalence of metabolic syndrome in patients with psoriasis: a population-based study in the United Kingdom," *Journal of Investigative Dermatology*, vol. 132, no. 3, pp. 556–562, 2012.

[7] N. P. Singh, A. Prakash, S. Kubba et al., "Psoriatic nephropathy—does an entity exist?" *Renal Failure*, vol. 27, no. 1, pp. 123–127, 2005.

[8] Y.-W. Yang, J. J. Keller, and H.-C. Lin, "Medical comorbidity associated with psoriasis in adults: a population-based study," *British Journal of Dermatology*, vol. 165, no. 5, pp. 1037–1043, 2011.

[9] E. Dervisoglu, A. S. Akturk, K. Yildiz, R. Kiran, and A. Yilmaz, "The spectrum of renal abnormalities in patients with psoriasis," *International Urology and Nephrology*, vol. 44, no. 2, pp. 509–514, 2012.

[10] J. C. Szepietowski, E. Bielicka, F. Wasik, W. Kopec, and T. Szepietowski, "Microalbuminuria as a subclinical marker of renal impairment in subjects with psoriasis vulgaris," *Journal of the European Academy of Dermatology and Venereology*, vol. 14, no. 6, pp. 513–514, 2000.

[11] R. Cecchi, G. Seghieri, A. Gironi, F. Tuci, and A. Giomi, "Relation between urinary albumin excretion and skin involvement in patients with psoriasis," *Dermatology*, vol. 185, no. 2, pp. 93–95, 1992.

[12] P. Madeddu, P. Ena, N. Glorioso, D. Cerimele, and A. Rappelli, "High prevalence of microproteinuria, an early index of renal impairment, in patients with diffuse psoriasis," *Nephron*, vol. 48, no. 3, pp. 222–225, 1988.

[13] D. J. Pearce, A. E. Morrison, K. B. Higgins et al., "The comorbid state of psoriasis patients in a university dermatology practice," *Journal of Dermatological Treatment*, vol. 16, no. 5-6, pp. 319–323, 2005.

[14] O. Kaftan, B. Kaftan, M. F. Toppare, and M. Eksioglu, "Renal involvement in psoriasis," *Dermatology*, vol. 192, no. 2, pp. 189–190, 1996.

[15] N. Cassano, M. Vestita, M. Panaro, M. Carbonara, and G. A. Vena, "Renal function in psoriasis patients," *European Journal of Dermatology*, vol. 21, no. 2, pp. 264–265, 2011.

[16] H. Imai, T. Kodama, T. Ishino et al., "IgA nephropathy associated with hyper IgAnemia, psoriasis or pustulosis and ossification," *Clinical Nephrology*, vol. 44, no. 1, pp. 64–68, 1995.

[17] J. Zadrazil, B. Tichy, P. Horak et al., "IgA nephropathy associated with psoriasis vulgaris: a contribution to the entity of 'psoriatic nephropathy'," *Journal of Nephrology*, vol. 19, no. 3, pp. 382–386, 2006.

[18] T. S. Ahuja, M. Funtanilla, J. J. de Groot, A. Velasco, J. Badalamenti, and S. Wilson, "IgA nephropathy in psoriasis," *American Journal of Nephrology*, vol. 18, no. 5, pp. 425–429, 1998.

[19] T. Kaji, Y. Tsukada, A. Shimada et al., "Membranous nephropathy associated with psoriasis vulgaris," *Clinical Nephrology*, vol. 42, no. 1, pp. 63–64, 1994.

[20] M. Kim, Y. Ko, U. C. Yeo, Y. Kim, and H. Oh, "Psoriasis and glomerulonephritis," *Clinical and Experimental Dermatology*, vol. 23, no. 6, pp. 295–296, 1998.

[21] I. N. Bruce, C. T. Schentag, and D. D. Gladma, "Hyperuricemia in psoriatic arthritis: prevalence and associated features," *Journal of Clinical Rheumatology*, vol. 6, no. 1, pp. 6–9, 2000.

[22] Z. K. O'Brown, E. L. Van Nostrand, J. P. Higgins, and S. K. Kim, "The inflammatory transcription factors NFκB, STAT1 and STAT3 drive age-associated transcriptional changes in the human kidney," *PLoS Genetics*, vol. 11, no. 12, Article ID e1005734, 2015.

[23] D. Bolignano, F. Mattace-Raso, E. J. G. Sijbrands, and C. Zoccali, "The aging kidney revisited: a systematic review," *Ageing Research Reviews*, vol. 14, no. 1, pp. 65–80, 2014.

[24] J. Wan, S. Wang, K. Haynes, M. R. Denburg, D. B. Shin, and J. M. Gelfand, "Risk of moderate to advanced kidney disease in patients with psoriasis: population based cohort study," *The British Medical Journal*, vol. 347, Article ID f5961, 2013.

[25] E. Corden, E. Higgins, and C. Smith, "Hypercalcaemia-induced kidney injury caused by the vitamin D analogue calcitriol for psoriasis: a note of caution when prescribing topical treatment," *Clinical and Experimental Dermatology*, vol. 41, no. 8, pp. 899–901, 2016.

[26] P. Gisondi and G. Girolomoni, "Glomerular filtration rate in patients with psoriasis treated with etanercept," *Journal of International Medical Research*, vol. 44, no. 2, supplement, pp. 106–108, 2016.

20

Hyperexcitability in Spinal WDR Neurons following Experimental Disc Herniation Is Associated with Upregulation of Fractalkine and Its Receptor in Nucleus Pulposus and the Dorsal Root Ganglion

Daniel Pitz Jacobsen,[1] Aurora Moen,[1,2] Fred Haugen,[1] and Johannes Gjerstad[1,2]

[1]*National Institute of Occupational Health, Oslo, Norway*
[2]*Department of Biosciences, University of Oslo, Norway*

Correspondence should be addressed to Daniel Pitz Jacobsen; dpja@stami.no

Academic Editor: David A. Hart

Introduction. Lumbar radicular pain following intervertebral disc herniation may be associated with a local inflammatory response induced by nucleus pulposus (NP) cells. *Methods.* In anaesthetized Lewis rats, extracellular single unit recordings of wide dynamic range (WDR) neurons in the dorsal horn and qPCR were used to explore the effect of NP application onto the dorsal nerve roots (L3–L5). *Results.* A clear increase in C-fiber response was observed following NP conditioning. In the NP tissue, the expression of interleukin-1β (IL-1β), colony stimulating factor 1 (Csf1), fractalkine (CX3CL1), and the fractalkine receptor CX3CR1 was increased. Minocycline, an inhibitor of microglial activation, inhibited the increase in neuronal activity and attenuated the increase in IL-1β, Csf1, CX3L1, and CX3CR1 expression in NP tissue. In addition, the results demonstrated an increase in the expression of TNF, CX3CL1, and CX3CR1 in the dorsal root ganglions (DRGs). *Conclusion.* Hyperexcitability in the pain pathways and the local inflammation after disc herniation may involve upregulation of CX3CL1 signaling in both the NP and the DRG.

1. Introduction

Earlier studies show that leakage of nucleus pulposus (NP) out of the disc after intervertebral disc herniation is associated with a local release of many substances including interleukin-1β (IL-1β), tumor necrosis factor (TNF), and colony stimulating factor 1 (Csf1) [1–4]. Such cytokines released after intervertebral disc herniation may induce increased neuronal excitability in the primary afferent nerve fibers and reduced axonal speed of conduction and may also promote nerve injury [1, 5, 6]. Thus, intervertebral disc herniation has adverse effects on the sensory pathways.

Peripheral inflammation in animals may be associated with activation of satellite glial cells in the dorsal root ganglion (DRG) [7]. Nerve injury and release of inflammatory substances may also activate microglia in the spinal cord [8–10]. For instance, previous data show that soluble fractalkine (CX3CL1) activates glia and leukocytes through its receptor CX3CR1 [11, 12]. Furthermore, spinal upregulation of CX3CL1 may be associated with mechanical allodynia and thermal hyperalgesia [13]. Thus, one important inflammatory molecule possibly influencing the sensory pathways may be CX3CL1.

Evidence exists that the local inflammation associated with disc herniation as well as microglial activation is dependent on phosphorylation of MAPK p38 [14, 15]. Thus, drugs targeting this kinase may attenuate inflammatory pain [10, 16, 17]. Here, in an animal model mimicking clinical intervertebral disc herniation, we investigate the effect of NP on neuronal activity in the spinal cord and examine the local gene expression. We hypothesize that the interaction between NP cells and neuronal tissue may induce a local upregulation of CX3CL1 signaling and increased nociceptive activity in the pain pathways.

2. Materials and Methods

2.1. Animals and Surgery. A total of 87 adult inbred female Lewis rats (170–215 g) were used in the present study. Female rats were preferred because allergens are more potent in males. Before use, all rats were initially sedated with isoflurane gas (Baxter International Inc., USA) followed by intraperitoneal administration of 250 mg/mL~2.1 g/kg body weight urethane (Sigma-Aldrich Co., Germany). Absence of hind paw withdrawal and ear wriggling to pinch indicated adequate surgical anesthesia. The rat's core temperature was maintained at 36-37°C by a feedback heating pad.

To expose the sciatic nerve, a 1-2 cm incision was made above the pelvic girdle and a bipolar silver hook electrode was placed proximal to the main branches of the sciatic nerve for electrical stimulation. As previously described [1], a laminectomy, with a 1 mm lateral expansion on the left side for the application of NP, was performed at vertebrae Th13-L1, corresponding to the spinal cord segments L3-S1. The vertebral column was rigidly fixed by clamps rostral and caudal to the exposed spinal cord segments. The meninges, that is, dura mater and arachnoidea, were punctured by a cannula and carefully removed by two tweezers. The animals were euthanized by an overdose of pentobarbital.

2.2. In Vivo Electrophysiology. A parylene-coated tungsten microelectrode with impedance 2–4 MΩ (Frederick Haer & Co., USA) was lowered vertically into the left dorsal horn of the spinal cord by an electrically controlled micromanipulator (Märzhäuser Wetzlar GmbH & Co. KG, Germany). The spinal cord segments L3-S1 were identified by the neuronal response to left hind paw finger tapping and pinching. Extracellular single cell recordings of wide dynamic range (WDR) neurons were performed at depths of 50–700 μm from the surface of the spinal cord. Only one cell was studied in each animal. The recorded signals from the headstage were amplified (×5000) with an AC preamplifier, band-pass filtered with half amplitude cut of 500–1250 Hz (NeuroLog by Digitimer Ltd, UK), digitalized with interface CED Micro1401, and displayed on a computer screen by the software CED Spike 2.2 (Cambridge Electronic Design, UK). The sampling frequency was 20 kHz.

The software Spike 2.2 was also used to control the electrical stimuli frequency given to the sciatic nerve by the hook electrode, while a pulse buffer connected to a stimulus isolator unit (NeuroLog System, Digitimer Ltd, UK) controlled the stimuli intensities. Single cell recordings were ensured by examining spike shape and amplitude. Spikes 50–300 ms after stimulus were defined as C-fiber responses. The C-fiber threshold was defined at the beginning of each experiment as the lowest stimulus intensity capable of eliciting a single visible spike in the defined C-fiber timeframe. Every fourth minute a single test stimuli (2 ms rectangular pulse, 1.5x C-fiber threshold) was applied to the sciatic nerve. Six stable recordings varying less than 20% served as a baseline for the subsequent experiments. Only cells with baseline responses of 5–20 spikes were included in the study.

To study the effect of NP conditioning on neuronal activity, NP was harvested from 3 to 4 caudal intervertebral discs of a genetically identical donor rat and applied 0.5–2 mm caudally to the recording electrode, covering the incoming left dorsal nerve roots. Minocycline (MC, M9511, Sigma-Aldrich Co., Germany) was chosen to target MAPKp38 in the glial cells. MC was dissolved in 0.9% NaCl, diluted to a concentration of 5 μg/μL, and topically administered onto the nerve roots (25 μL before and 25 μL after NP application). Four series of electrophysiological experiments were performed: (I) NP conditioning ($n = 7$), (II) NP conditioning together with MC ($n = 7$), (III) MC ($n = 5$), and (IV) NaCl control ($n = 5$). The C-fiber response was followed for 180 minutes after conditioning. In addition, 14 animals were used as donor rats.

2.3. Parallel NP Gene Expression Experiments. In order to investigate changes in the expression of our candidate genes in NP tissue, four series of experiments were performed and defined as (I) NP, (II) NP+MC, (III) NP^{fat}, and (IV) NP^{native}. The tissue in the NP group ($n = 7$) had been in contact with the dorsal nerve roots for 180 minutes, as had the tissue in the NP+MC group ($n = 7$) together with minocycline. Tissue samples for these two groups were harvested directly following the electrophysiological experiments described above. The NP^{fat} group ($n = 9$), which was applied onto neck fat tissue for 180 minutes, served as a control group to investigate whether any possible gene expression changes in the NP group were caused by the tissue-specific properties of the nerve roots or surrounding tissues. NP^{native} tissue ($n = 10$) was frozen directly after isolation from the caudal intervertebral discs of the donor rats and served as control. In addition, 9 extra animals were used for the fat controls.

2.4. Ipsi- and Contralateral Dorsal Root Ganglion Gene Expression. We also wanted to investigate the gene expression changes in the DRG following experimental disc herniation. Thus, lumbar DRG L3–L5, giving input to TH13 and L1 through their dorsal nerve roots, were dissected out and frozen on liquid nitrogen. The DRG isolation protocol has been described elsewhere [18]. Two series of DRG experiments were performed: NP ($n = 7$) and native ($n = 7$). In both groups, a laminectomy exposing the dorsal nerve roots was performed three hours before isolation of DRG. In the NP group, NP tissue from the caudal intervertebral discs of a donor rat was applied onto the left dorsal nerve roots immediately after the laminectomy. In total, 7 donor rats were used for DRG gene expression experiments. Both the left and the right dorsal root ganglia were isolated. Left L3, L4, and L5 and right L3, L4, and L5 were pooled separately before gene expression analyses.

2.5. qPCR. As previously described [19], total RNA was extracted from frozen (−80°C) NP and DRG tissue by the TRIzol reagent (Life technologies, Inc., Rockville, Maryland, USA), chloroform (Sigma-Aldrich, St. Louis, MO, USA), and isopropanol (Merck, Darmstadt, Germany). RNA

Table 1: Primer sequences.

Primer	Sequence 5′ → 3′	Bp	% GC	Tm °C
IL1β forward	CGT GGA GCT TCC AGG ATG AG	20	60.0	59.4
IL1β reverse	CGT CAT CAT CCC ACG AGT CA	20	50.0	59.1
TNF forward	GCC ACC ACG CTC TTC TGT CTA	21	57.1	59.1
TNF reverse	TGA GAG GGA GCC CAT TTG G	19	57.9	59.6
Csf1 forward	GGG AAT GGA CAC CTA CAG ATT TTG	24	45.8	59.6
Csf1 reverse	AAA TTT ATA TTC GAT CAG GCA TGCA	25	32.0	59.7
CX3CL1 forward	TTG CAC AGC CCA GAT CAT TC	21	47.6	54.3
CX3CL1 reverse	CTG CGC TCT CAG ATG TAG GAA A	22	50.0	55.7
CX3CR1 forward	GTG GCC TTT GGG ACC ATC T	19	57.9	56.7
CX3CR1 reverse	CCA CCA GAC CGA ACG TGA A	19	57.9	56.6
β-actin forward	CTA AGG CCA ACC GTG AAA AGA	21	47.6	58.0
β-actin reverse	ACA ACA CAG CCT GGA TGG CTA	21	52.4	59.2

was reversibly transcribed by aid of the first-strand cDNA Synthesis Kit for reverse-transcriptase polymerase chain reaction (RT-PCR) (AMV) (Roche Diagnostic, Mannheim, Germany). The qPCR analysis was then performed in two parallels on a StepOnePlus qPCR machine (Applied Biosciences, USA). Primers were designed using Primer Express 2.0 (Applied Biosystems, California, USA) and checked for specificity by performing a BLAST search. Effort was made to design primers without nonspecific binding (the melting curves indicated no biproducts). For more details about the primers (Risskov, Denmark), see Table 1. Target genes were normalized to β-actin (internal reference).

2.6. Statistics. The spinal nociceptive activity, that is, the C-fiber response, was presented as percent of baseline. The 6 baseline recordings were converted to 2 baseline values (each an average of 3 consecutive responses), and the 45 postbaseline recordings were converted to 9 values (each an average of 5 consecutive responses). To examine the effect of the four types of intervention, NP, NP+MC, MC, and control, on spinal nociceptive response, an analysis of variance, repeated-measure design (rmANOVA), was performed. Because the assumption of sphericity was not met, the degrees of freedom were corrected using a Greenhouse–Geisser correction. The average C-fiber responses from 60 to 180 minutes after conditioning were compared using one-way ANOVA and Tukey's honestly significant difference (HSD) post hoc comparisons. Regarding the gene expression, fold change values for each sample were defined by the expression of the target gene normalized to the expression of the reference gene β-actin and the level of the corresponding native tissue. Group means of NP expression values were compared using one-way ANOVA and Tukey's HSD post hoc comparisons, while DRG expressions were compared with an unpaired Student's t-test. Statistical analyses were performed by use of SPSS 21 (IBM SPSS inc., USA). A P value <0.05 was set as the level of statistical significance. Data are given as representative examples and means ± SEM.

3. Results

We here report that IL-1β (red), TNF (green), Csf1 (blue), but also CX3CL1 (brown), and CX3CR1 (yellow) were expressed in the native NP tissue (Figure 1(a)). Moreover, NP applied onto the dorsal nerve roots induced a rapid increase in the C-fiber response (Figure 1(b)), but this was in most cases blocked by minocycline (Figure 1(c)). The observed increase in C-fiber response was evident already 10–20 minutes after NP administration (Figure 2(a)), whereas no clear increase in the C-fiber response was seen following application of NP together with minocycline (Figure 2(b)). Application of minocycline alone caused a short lasting decrease in C-fiber response (Figure 2(c)). No clear changes in the C-fiber response were observed in the vehicle control experiments (Figure 2(d)).

The average C-fiber response 60–180 minutes after NP conditioning was 136.1% ± 13.9 of baseline, but after NP conditioning together with minocycline only 99.9% ± 6.5 of baseline. Moreover, the average C-fiber response after minocycline alone was 92.0% ± 8.6 of baseline, and in the corresponding vehicle control 91.7% ± 7.4 of baseline (Figure 2(e)). The C-fiber response after conditioning with NP alone was significantly higher than the C-fiber response after conditioning with NP plus minocycline, minocycline alone or in the corresponding vehicle control.

Moreover we observed a clear increase in the expression of IL1β in NP samples, but no change in the expression of TNF, and a minor increase in the expression of macrophage colony stimulating factor Csf1 180 minutes after application onto the nerve roots (fold expression: IL-1β; 13.47±3.03, TNF 2.89 ± 2.08, Csf1; 3.13 ± 1.21). Notably, a significant increase in the gene expression of CX3CL1 and its cognate receptor CX3CR1 was also observed in the NP tissue (fold expression: CX3CL1; 7.32 ± 1.89, CX3CR1; 7.32 ± 1.89).

Interestingly, the NP-induced changes in expression were almost completely blocked when NP was applied together with minocycline, the inhibitor of glial cells and macrophage activation (fold expression: IL1β; 5.19±2.08, TNF; 1.55±0.43, Csf1; 0.92 ± 0.15, CX3CL1; 2.01 ± 0.51, CX3CR1; 1.95 ± 0.45).

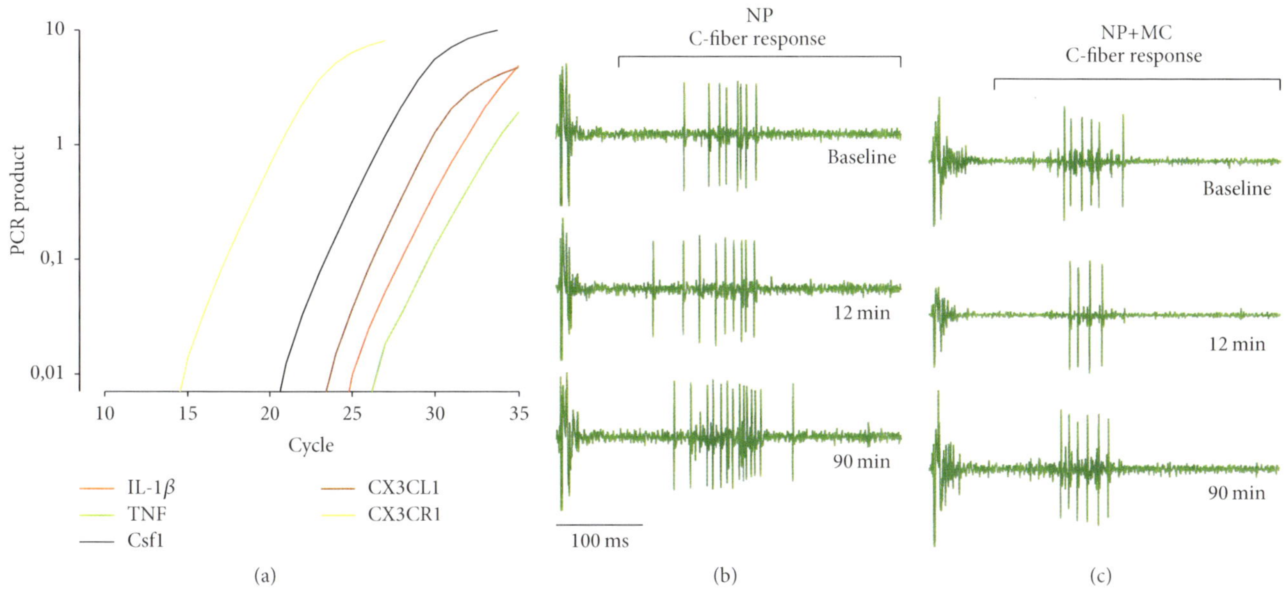

Figure 1: (a) Examples of qPCR amplification plots demonstrating the presence IL-1β (red), TNF (green), Csf1 (blue), CX3CL1 (brown), and CX3CR1 (yellow) in native NP tissue. (b) Examples of single cell recordings at baseline, 12 minutes and 90 minutes after nucleus pulposus conditioning alone. (c) Examples of single cell recordings at baseline, 12 minutes and 90 minutes after nucleus pulposus conditioning together with minocycline.

No clear changes in expression were observed in the corresponding fat control experiments where the NP was applied onto the intrascapular adipose tissue (fold expression: IL1β; 3.68 ± 0.54, TNF; 1.99 ± 0.32, Csf1; 1.53 ± 0.25, CX3CL1; 2.51 ± 0.33, CX3CR1; 2.66 ± 0.47). Thus, the increase in expression, which was dependent on the contact between the NP tissue and the dorsal nerve roots, was attenuated by minocycline (Figures 3(a)–3(e)).

After 3 hours, NP applied onto the left dorsal nerve roots induced an ipsilateral increase in the expressions of TNF, CX3CL1, and CX3CR1 in the DRGs (fold expression in ipsilateral DRGs: TNF; 1.91 ± 0.56, CX3CL1; 1.88 ± 0.13, CX3CR1; 1.86 ± 0.26; fold expression in contralateral DRGs: TNF; 1.47 ± 0.56, CX3CL1; 1.23 ± 0.27, CX3CR1; 1.33 ± 0.47) (Figures 4(a)–4(e)). Although NP was applied 5–15 mm proximal to the DRG, this seemed to have a clear effect on the DRG cells. The fold expressions of IL1-β and Csf1, however, were not increased (ipsilateral DRGs: IL-1β; 1.08 ± 0.16, Csf1; 1.03 ± 0.07; contralateral DRGs: IL-1β; 1.10 ± 0.28, Csf1; 1.08 ± 0.09).

4. Discussion

Our results showed that application of NP onto the dorsal nerve roots within minutes increased the C-fiber response in the dorsal horn. The changes in gene expression in the DRG suggest that the primary afferent nerve fibers may be affected by NP. In addition, proinflammatory cytokines released near the dorsal nerve roots could diffuse to the dorsal horn and affect postsynaptic cells and spinal microglia. Thus, the increase in excitability at the spinal level may be due to direct effects of NP on the primary nerve fibers, but also secondary changes induced by molecules from NP in postsynaptic WDR neurons. Previous findings indicate that the rapid effects of NP are induced by IL-1β and TNF action on dorsal horn lamina II ion channels and suppressed spinal GABA and glycine-induced currents [20, 21]. The effect of NP on nociceptive signaling has also been demonstrated in behavioral studies [22].

Previous observations show that application of NP onto the dorsal nerve roots may affect the expression of cytokines like IL-1β and TNF in the NP tissue [1]. In accordance with these earlier findings, the present data show a significant upregulation of IL-1β after application of NP onto the dorsal nerve roots in the NP tissue. However, in contrast to the observation of our earlier report, no clear upregulation of TNF was observed in the NP tissue this time. On the other hand, the present data showed a significant upregulation of TNF in the DRG.

Anyway, several lines of evidence suggest that IL-1β and TNF, but also Csf1, may be upregulated in NP or surrounding tissue following disc herniation [1, 3, 4, 23]. Therefore, it seems likely that persistent hyperexcitability in the pain pathways after disc herniation is associated with a local inflammatory process including activation of macrophages close to the nerve roots. Moreover, previous data show that IL-1β [24, 25], Csf1 [26–28], and CX3CL1 [22, 29, 30] can induce M1 microglia activation. For the first time, however, we showed that application of NP onto the dorsal nerve roots also increased the gene expression of CX3CL1 and CX3CR1 in the NP cells and in the ipsilateral DRGs. These observations suggest that local upregulation of IL-1β, Csf1, and CX3CL1 following disc herniation may activate microglia and induce pain [21]. Interestingly, no change in gene expression was

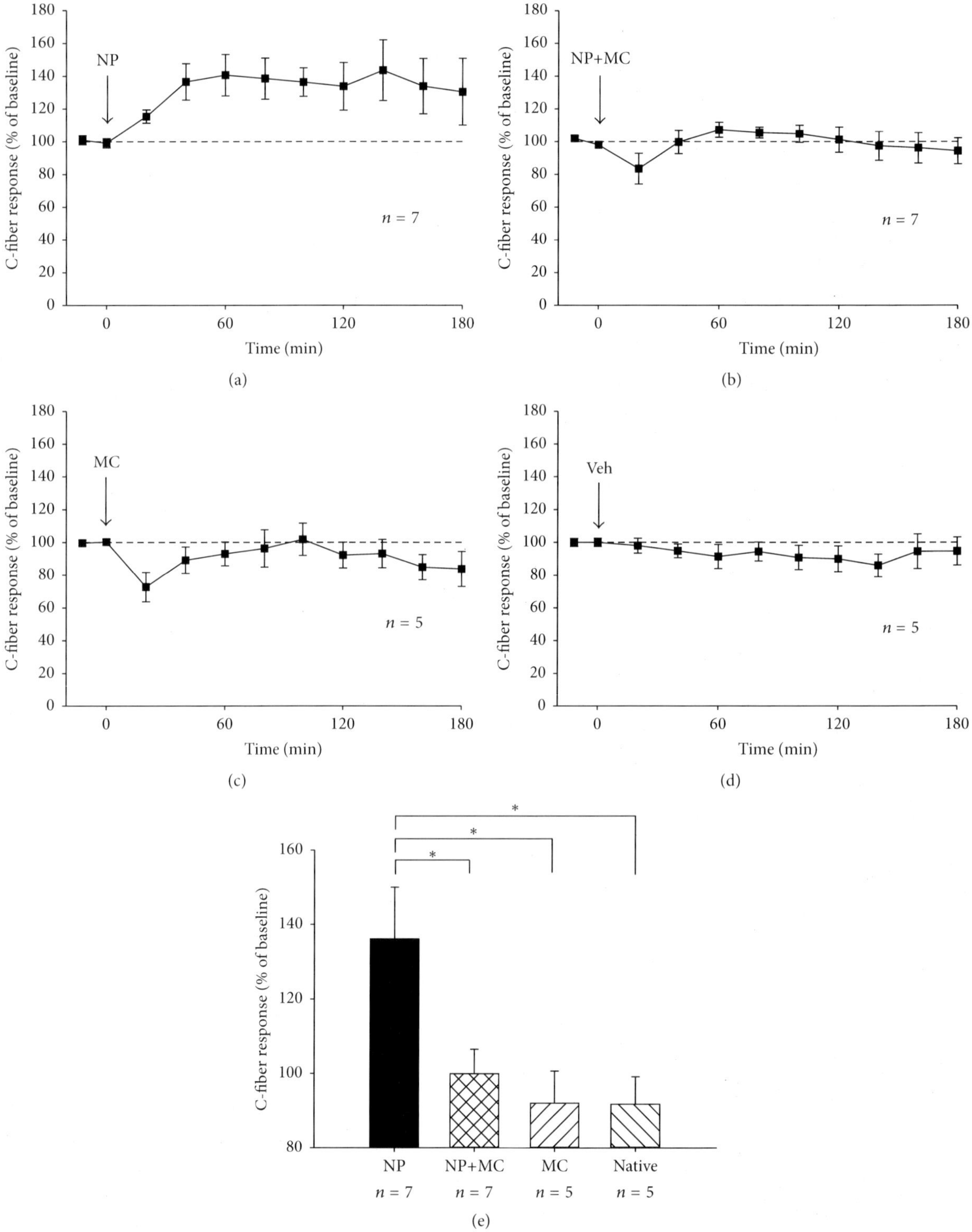

FIGURE 2: C-fiber response in percent of baseline after application of (a) NP (NP), (b) NP and minocycline (NP+MC), (c) minocycline (MC), and (d) Vehicle (Veh). (e) The mean value 60 to 180 minutes after baseline in the four groups. $P = 0.018$, rmANOVA, four groups; NP, NP+MC, MC, Veh. $^{*}P < 0.05$, one-way ANOVA, Tukey's post hoc test.

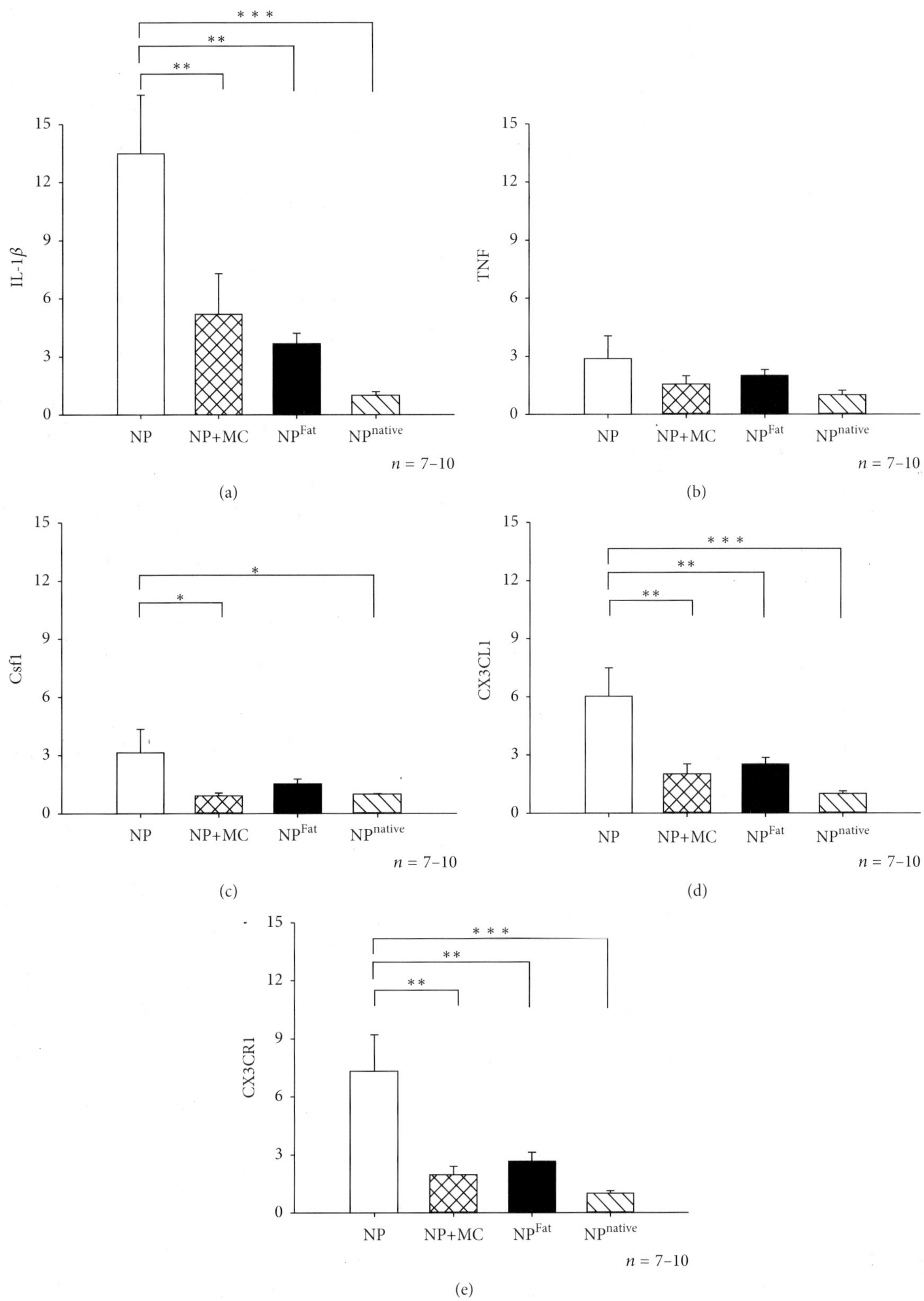

FIGURE 3: Fold expression of (a) IL-1β, (b) TNF, (c) Csf1, (d) CX3CL1, and (e) CX3CR1 in NP in the three groups: NP in contact with dorsal nerve roots for 180 minutes (NP), NP in contact with dorsal nerve roots for 180 minutes together with minocycline (NP+MC), NP in contact with neck fat tissue for 180 minutes (NP^{Fat}), and native nucleus pulposus (NP^{native}). $^{*}P < 0.05$, $^{**}P < 0.01$, $^{***}P < 0.001$, one-way ANOVA, Tukey's post hoc test.

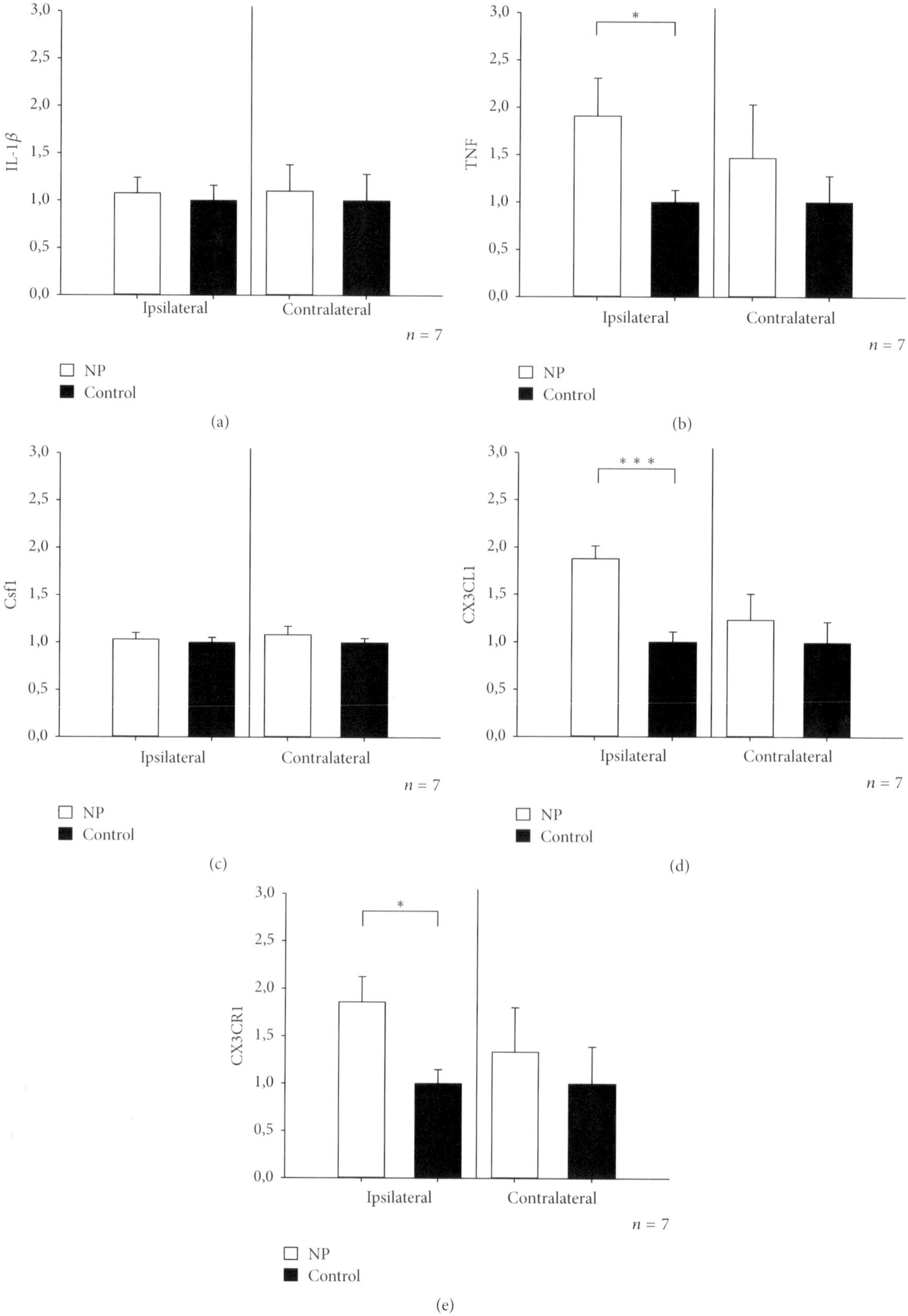

FIGURE 4: Fold expression of (a) IL-1β, (b) TNF, (c) Csf1, (d) CX3CL1, and (e) CX3CR1 in the ipsi- and contralateral DRG after NP application onto the dorsal nerve roots. $^{*}P < 0.05$, $^{***}P < 0.001$, Student's t-test.

observed in NP tissue following contact with intrascapular adipose tissue, suggesting a specific interaction between NP cells and neuronal tissue.

In accordance with the earlier observation that microglial inhibition may prevent hyperalgesia [16, 17, 31], minocycline attenuated the increase in nociceptive signaling induced by NP in the present study. Data from earlier in vitro studies also suggest that inhibition of MAPK p38 in human NP cells inhibits inflammation [14]. Hence, it is tempting to speculate that the antinociceptive effects of minocycline may be a result of reduced MAPK p38 phosphorylation in microglia.

However, the anti-inflammatory effect of minocycline may be due to other mechanisms as well, not only by inhibition of p38 phosphorylation. For instance, minocycline is reportedly an inhibitor of nitric oxide synthase [32] and 5-lipoxygenase [33] attenuates TNF expression [34] and suppresses NF-kappa B activity [35]. In addition, minocycline may directly affect Na^+-channels in primary afferent neurons [36], which could explain the short lasting drop in C-fiber response following minocycline administration. Minocycline also attenuated the increase in the gene expression of IL-1β, Csf1, CX3CL1, and CX3CR1 in NP tissue. The alleviating effect of minocycline on nociceptive signaling following application of NP onto the dorsal nerve roots may therefore be related to this anti-inflammatory processes in NP.

The changes in gene expression were less pronounced in the DRG than in the NP tissue itself. Still, a significant increase in the expression of TNF, CX3CL1, and CX3CR1 was demonstrated, supporting the previous observation that local application of NP onto the primary afferents may change the gene expression in the DRGs [37]. The changes in gene expression were only observed on the ipsilateral side. This supports the hypothesis that the observed nociceptive effect is dependent on contact between NP tissue and the dorsal nerve roots.

Increased expression of CX3CL1 and its receptor CX3CR1 has previously been shown in the DRG after nerve injury [38]. Our observation that hyperexcitability in the pain pathways after application of NP may involve an upregulation of CX3CL1 signaling in the DRG supports these previous findings. Moreover, evidence exists that CX3CL1 mediates inflammatory pain through activation of DRG satellite glial cells [7]. However, recent discoveries challenge the previous notion that CX3CL1 is expressed in DRG neurons [39]. Thus, it seems likely that the observed CX3CL1 upregulation takes place in endothelial cells, possibly facilitating infiltration of monocytes or other leukocytes into the DRG [40].

The distance from the NP graft to the DRG in our animal model may be larger than the distance from the NP to the DRG in lumbar disc herniation in patients. Still, our data show that application of NP onto the dorsal nerve roots induces a significant upregulation of several genes in the ipsilateral DRG tissue, emphasizing the clinical relevance of our animal model. Moreover, previous data show that peripheral inflammation through circulating IL-1β may increase the expression, of, for example, Cox 2, in the spinal cord [41]. Notably, circulating mediators released in the peripheral tissue may therefore also influence central secondary WDR neurons.

5. Conclusion

In summary, the present data suggest that hyperexcitability in the pain pathways and the local inflammation after disc herniation may involve upregulation of CX3CL1 signaling in both the NP and the DRG. The molecular consequence of the upregulation of CX3CL1 remains to be investigated.

Ethical Approval

All animal experiments were approved by the Norwegian Animal Research Authority and were performed in conformity with the laws and regulations controlling experiments and procedures on live animals in Norway.

Competing Interests

The authors declare that there are no competing interests regarding the publication of this paper.

Authors' Contributions

Daniel Pitz Jacobsen, Aurora Moen, Fred Haugen, and Johannes Gjerstad designed research; Daniel Pitz Jacobsen, Aurora Moen, Fred Haugen, and Johannes Gjerstad performed research; Daniel Pitz Jacobsen, Aurora Moen, and Johannes Gjerstad analyzed data; Aurora Moen and Fred Haugen contributed to the drafting of the manuscript; Daniel Pitz Jacobsen and Johannes Gjerstad wrote the paper.

Acknowledgments

The work was funded by the Norwegian Research Council (NFR).

References

[1] N. G. Egeland, A. Moen, L. M. Pedersen, H. Brisby, and J. Gjerstad, "Spinal nociceptive hyperexcitability induced by experimental disc herniation is associated with enhanced local expression of Csf1 and FasL," *Pain*, vol. 154, no. 9, pp. 1743–1748, 2013.

[2] J. M. Cuéllar, P. M. Borges, V. G. Cuéllar, A. Yoo, G. J. Scuderi, and D. C. Yeomans, "Cytokine expression in the epidural space: a model of noncompressive disc herniation-induced inflammation," *Spine*, vol. 38, no. 1, pp. 17–23, 2013.

[3] J. M. Cuellar, P. X. Montesano, and E. Carstens, "Role of TNF-alpha in sensitization of nociceptive dorsal horn neurons induced by application of nucleus pulposus to L5 dorsal root ganglion in rats," *Pain*, vol. 110, no. 3, pp. 578–587, 2004.

[4] N. J. Rothwell and P. J. L. M. Strijbos, "Cytokines in neurodegeneration and repair," *International Journal of Developmental Neuroscience*, vol. 13, no. 3-4, pp. 179–185, 1995.

[5] K. Olmarker, C. Nordborg, K. Larsson, and B. Rydevik, "Ultrastructural changes in spinal nerve roots induced by autologous nucleus pulposus," *Spine*, vol. 21, no. 4, pp. 411–414, 1996.

[6] K. Olmarker, B. Rydevik, and C. Nordborg, "Autologous nucleus pulposus induces neurophysiologic and histologic changes in porcine cauda equina nerve roots," *Spine*, vol. 18, no. 11, pp. 1425–1432, 1993.

[7] G. R. Souza, J. Talbot, C. M. Lotufo, F. Q. Cunha, T. M. Cunha, and S. H. Ferreira, "Fractalkine mediates inflammatory pain through activation of satellite glial cells," *Proceedings of the National Academy of Sciences of the United States of America*, vol. 110, no. 27, pp. 11193–11198, 2013.

[8] D. E. Coyle, "Partial peripheral nerve injury leads to activation of astroglia and microglia which parallels the development of allodynic behavior," *GLIA*, vol. 23, no. 1, pp. 75–83, 1998.

[9] Z.-Y. Zhuang, P. Gerner, C. J. Woolf, and R.-R. Ji, "ERK is sequentially activated in neurons, microglia, and astrocytes by spinal nerve ligation and contributes to mechanical allodynia in this neuropathic pain model," *Pain*, vol. 114, no. 1-2, pp. 149–159, 2005.

[10] H. Ikeda, T. Kiritoshi, and K. Murase, "Contribution of microglia and astrocytes to the central sensitization, inflammatory and neuropathic pain in the juvenile rat," *Molecular Pain*, vol. 8, article 43, 2012.

[11] T. Imai, K. Hieshima, C. Haskell et al., "Identification and molecular characterization of fractalkine receptor CX3CR1, which mediates both leukocyte migration and adhesion," *Cell*, vol. 91, no. 4, pp. 521–530, 1997.

[12] A. Nishiyori, M. Minami, Y. Ohtani et al., "Localization of fractalkine and CX_3CR1 mRNAs in rat brain: does fractalkine play a role in signaling from neuron to microglia?" *FEBS Letters*, vol. 429, no. 2, pp. 167–172, 1998.

[13] H. W. Park, S. H. Ahn, S. J. Kim et al., "Changes in spinal cord expression of fractalkine and its receptor in a rat model of disc herniation by autologous nucleus pulposus," *Spine*, vol. 36, no. 12, pp. E753–E760, 2011.

[14] R. K. Studer, A. M. Aboka, L. G. Gilbertson et al., "p38 MAPK inhibition in nucleus pulposus cells: a potential target for treating intervertebral disc degeneration," *Spine*, vol. 32, no. 25, pp. 2827–2833, 2007.

[15] J. Huoyan, W. Huimin, Z. Fupeng, L. Xiaohong, X. Lu, and A. Shen, "PPARγ agonist pioglitazone inhibits microglia inflammation by blocking p38 mitogen-activated protein kinase signaling pathways," *Inflammation Research*, vol. 59, no. 11, pp. 921–929, 2010.

[16] A. Ledeboer, E. M. Sloane, E. D. Milligan et al., "Minocycline attenuates mechanical allodynia and proinflammatory cytokine expression in rat models of pain facilitation," *Pain*, vol. 115, no. 1-2, pp. 71–83, 2005.

[17] X. Zhang, Y. Xu, J. Wang et al., "The effect of intrathecal administration of glial activation inhibitors on dorsal horn BDNF overexpression and hind paw mechanical allodynia in spinal nerve ligated rats," *Journal of Neural Transmission*, vol. 119, no. 3, pp. 329–336, 2012.

[18] S. A. Malin, B. M. Davis, and D. C. Molliver, "Production of dissociated sensory neuron cultures and considerations for their use in studying neuronal function and plasticity," *Nature Protocols*, vol. 2, no. 1, pp. 152–160, 2007.

[19] L. M. Pedersen, L. M. Jacobsen, S. Mollerup, and J. Gjerstad, "Spinal cord long-term potentiation (LTP) is associated with increased dorsal horn gene expression of IL-1β, GDNF and iNOS," *European Journal of Pain*, vol. 14, no. 3, pp. 255–260, 2010.

[20] H. Brisby and I. Hammar, "Thalamic activation in a disc herniation model," *Spine*, vol. 32, no. 25, pp. 2846–2852, 2007.

[21] Y. Kawasaki, L. Zhang, J.-K. Cheng, and R.-R. Ji, "Cytokine mechanisms of central sensitization: distinct and overlapping role of interleukin-1β, interleukin-6, and tumor necrosis factor-α in regulating synaptic and neuronal activity in the superficial spinal cord," *Journal of Neuroscience*, vol. 28, no. 20, pp. 5189–5194, 2008.

[22] Z.-Y. Zhuang, Y. Kawasaki, P.-H. Tan, Y.-R. Wen, J. Huang, and R.-R. Ji, "Role of the CX3CR1/p38 MAPK pathway in spinal microglia for the development of neuropathic pain following nerve injury-induced cleavage of fractalkine," *Brain, Behavior, and Immunity*, vol. 21, no. 5, pp. 642–651, 2007.

[23] K. Olmarker and K. Larsson, "Tumor necrosis factor α and nucleus-pulposus-induced nerve root injury," *Spine*, vol. 23, no. 23, pp. 2538–2544, 1998.

[24] K. Y. Yang, W. S. Bae, M. J. Kim et al., "Participation of the central p38 and ERK1/2 pathways in IL-1beta-induced sensitization of nociception in rats," *Progress in Neuro-Psychopharmacology & Biological Psychiatry*, vol. 46, pp. 98–104, 2013.

[25] X.-H. Wei, T. Yang, Q. Wu et al., "Peri-sciatic administration of recombinant rat IL-1β induces mechanical allodynia by activation of src-family kinases in spinal microglia in rats," *Experimental Neurology*, vol. 234, no. 2, pp. 389–397, 2012.

[26] B. Shafit-Zagardo, N. Sharma, J. W. Herman, M. B. Bornstein, and C. F. Brosnan, "CSF-1 expression is upregulated in astrocyte cultures by IL-1 and TNF and affects microglial proliferation and morphology in organotypic cultures," *International Journal of Developmental Neuroscience*, vol. 11, no. 2, pp. 189–198, 1993.

[27] G. Gowing, M. Lalancette-Hébert, J.-N. Audet, F. Dequen, and J.-P. Julien, "Macrophage colony stimulating factor (M-CSF) exacerbates ALS disease in a mouse model through altered responses of microglia expressing mutant superoxide dismutase," *Experimental Neurology*, vol. 220, no. 2, pp. 267–275, 2009.

[28] M. Sawada, A. Suzumura, H. Yamamoto, and T. Marunouchi, "Activation and proliferation of the isolated microglia by colony stimulating factor-1 and possible involvement of protein kinase C," *Brain Research*, vol. 509, no. 1, pp. 119–124, 1990.

[29] M. Kiyomoto, M. Shinoda, A. Okada-Ogawa et al., "Fractalkine signaling in microglia contributes to ectopic orofacial pain following trapezius muscle inflammation," *The Journal of Neuroscience*, vol. 33, no. 18, pp. 7667–7680, 2013.

[30] A. K. Clark, A. A. Staniland, and M. Malcangio, "Fractalkine/CX3CR1 signalling in chronic pain and inflammation," *Current Pharmaceutical Biotechnology*, vol. 12, no. 10, pp. 1707–1714, 2011.

[31] C.-S. Sung, C.-H. Cherng, Z.-H. Wen et al., "Minocycline and fluorocitrate suppress spinal nociceptive signaling in intrathecal IL-1β-induced thermal hyperalgesic rats," *Glia*, vol. 60, no. 12, pp. 2004–2017, 2012.

[32] A. R. Amin, M. G. Attur, G. D. Thakker et al., "A novel mechanism of action of tetracyclines: effects on nitric oxide synthases," *Proceedings of the National Academy of Sciences of the United States of America*, vol. 93, no. 24, pp. 14014–14019, 1996.

[33] Y. Song, E.-Q. Wei, W.-P. Zhang, L. Zhang, J.-R. Liu, and Z. Chen, "Minocycline protects PC12 cells from ischemic-like injury and inhibits 5-lipoxygenase activation," *NeuroReport*, vol. 15, no. 14, pp. 2181–2184, 2004.

[34] S. M. Lee, T. Y. Yune, S. J. Kim et al., "Minocycline inhibits apoptotic cell death via attenuation of TNF-α expression following iNOS/NO induction by lipopolysaccharide in neuron/glia co-cultures," *Journal of Neurochemistry*, vol. 91, no. 3, pp. 568–578, 2004.

[35] P. Ataie-Kachoie, S. Badar, D. L. Morris, and M. H. Pourgholami, "Minocycline targets the NF-κB nexus through suppression of TGF-β1-TAK1-IκB signaling in ovarian cancer," *Molecular Cancer Research*, vol. 11, no. 10, pp. 1279–1291, 2013.

[36] T. H. Kim, H. I. Kim, J. Kim, M. Park, and J.-H. Song, "Effects of minocycline on Na^+ currents in rat dorsal root ganglion neurons," *Brain Research*, vol. 1370, pp. 34–42, 2011.

[37] K. Takahashi Sato, K. Satoh, M. Sekiguchi et al., "Local application of nucleus pulposus induces expression OF P2X3 in rat dorsal root ganglion cells," *Fukushima Journal of Medical Science*, vol. 58, no. 1, pp. 17–21, 2012.

[38] W. Zhu, C. Acosta, B. Macneil et al., "Elevated expression of fractalkine (CX3CL1) and fractalkine receptor (CX3CR1) in the dorsal root ganglia and spinal cord in experimental autoimmune encephalomyelitis: implications in multiple sclerosis-induced neuropathic pain," *BioMed Research International*, vol. 2013, Article ID 480702, 14 pages, 2013.

[39] K.-W. Kim, A. Vallon-Eberhard, E. Zigmond et al., "In vivo structure/function and expression analysis of the CX3C chemokine fractalkine," *Blood*, vol. 118, no. 22, pp. e156–e167, 2011.

[40] E. A. Old, S. Nadkarni, J. Grist et al., "Monocytes expressing CX3CR1 orchestrate the development of vincristine-induced pain," *The Journal of Clinical Investigation*, vol. 124, no. 5, pp. 2023–2036, 2014.

[41] T. A. Samad, K. A. Moore, A. Sapirstein et al., "Interleukin-1β-mediated induction of Cox-2 in the CNS contributes to inflammatory pain hypersensitivity," *Nature*, vol. 410, no. 6827, pp. 471–475, 2001.

21

Transcriptional and Molecular Pathways Activated in Mesenteric Adipose Tissue and Intestinal Mucosa of Crohn's Disease Patients

Andressa Coope,[1] Lívia Bitencourt Pascoal,[1] Francesca Aparecida Ramos da Silva,[1] José Diego Botezelli,[1] Maria de Lourdes Setsuko Ayrizono,[1] Marciane Milanski,[2] Michel Gardere Camargo,[1] Núria Planell,[3] Mariana Portovedo,[2] Cilene Bicca Dias,[1] João José Fagundes,[1] and Raquel Franco Leal[1]

[1]*IBD Research Laboratory, Surgery Department, University of Campinas (UNICAMP), Medical School, Campinas, SP, Brazil*
[2]*Laboratory of Metabolic Disorders, Faculty of Applied Sciences, University of Campinas (UNICAMP), Campinas, SP, Brazil*
[3]*Department of Gastroenterology and Bioinformatics Platform, CIBER-EHD, Barcelona, Spain*

Correspondence should be addressed to Raquel Franco Leal; rafranco.unicamp@gmail.com

Academic Editor: Jean-Marc Cavaillon

Crohn's disease (CD) is a chronic inflammatory disorder, characterized by cytokine imbalance and transcription signaling pathways activation. In addition, the increase of mesenteric adipose tissue (MAT) near the affected intestinal area is a hallmark of CD. Therefore, we evaluated the transcription signaling pathways and cytokines expression in intestinal mucosa and MAT of active CD patients. Ten patients with ileocecal CD and eight with noninflammatory diseases were studied. The biopsies of intestinal mucosa and MAT were snap-frozen and protein expression was determined by immunoblotting. RNA levels were measured by qPCR. The pIkB/IkB ratio and TNFα level were significantly higher in intestinal mucosa of CD when compared to controls. However, STAT1 expression was similar between intestinal mucosa of CD and controls. Considering the MAT, the pIkB/IkB ratio was significantly lower and the anti-inflammatory cytokine IL10 was significantly higher in CD when compared to controls. Finally, the protein content of pSTAT1 was higher in MAT of CD compared to controls. These findings reinforce the predominance of the proinflammatory NF-kB pathway in CD intestinal mucosa. For the first time, we showed the activation of STAT1 pathway in MAT of CD patients, which may help to understand the physiopathology of this immune mediated disease.

1. Introduction

Crohn's disease (CD) is characterized by mucosal immune cell activation and cytokine imbalance. The tumor necrosis factor alfa (TNFα) is one of the most important proinflammatory cytokines involved in this process, and its transcription depends on the activation of the transcription factor known as nuclear factor kB (NF-kB) [1]. Besides, some members of the signal transducer and activator of transcription (STAT) family have been involved in this process. STAT1 is upregulated in response to interferons and when activated (pSTAT1) binds to the promoter region of interferon-stimulated genes. All the transcription factors translocate into the nucleus and interact with conserved regulatory DNA sequences resulting in the transcription of genes like chemokines, cytokines, receptors, signaling regulatory genes, among others. Those molecules have been studied in several gastrointestinal disorders. However, the most common data about them comes from analysis of intestinal tissue, rarer than from the mesenteric adipose tissue (MAT) nearby the affected intestinal area [2]. The increase of the MAT is a common feature of the disease and may involve the small and large bowels; thus this tissue may represent a relevant role in the pathogenesis of CD [3, 4]. Histological analyses reveal abnormalities in the adipose tissue, including infiltration of macrophages and fibrosis [5]. Adipose tissue is able to release hormones which can lead to pro- or anti-inflammatory pathways, such as leptin that has been shown to increase the secretion of TNFα and IL6, as well as activate NF-kB [6, 7] and such as adiponectin and anti-inflammatory factors which attenuate the proinflammatory response.

TNFα has several functions, which are generally counterbalanced by anti-inflammatory pathways, such as IL10. There is an exacerbation of TNFα expression along with other inflammatory mediators in the intestinal *lamina propria* of the inflammatory bowel diseases (IBD). The intraluminal stimuli lead to the increased expression of interleukins such as IL1β, IL6, and IL8, which stimulate the proliferation and activation of lymphocytes, by a mechanism not completely understood [8].

Studies of immunological differences between CD and ulcerative colitis (UC), the two major IBD, have shown that the activation of NF-kB is more common in CD than in UC; conversely, expression and activation of STAT1 are predominantly high in UC. Indeed, STAT1 is activated by an intracytoplasmic pathway activated by the transmembrane receptor of IFNγ [9, 10] and can be blocked by SOCS3, which play an important role in the regulation of this pathway [11, 12].

This study aimed to investigate if the intestinal mucosa and MAT of CD patients activate different molecular and transcriptional pathways, which could lead to different tissue-specific drugs response in patients and, also, to establishing potential pharmacologic targets to treat CD. Thus, we evaluated molecules involved in the activation of NF-kB and STAT1 pathways and consequent cytokine expression in intestinal mucosa and MAT of active CD patients. Finally, the correlation between intestinal mucosa and MAT of CD patients may help towards a better understanding of the pathophysiology of this chronic inflammatory disorder.

2. Materials and Methods

2.1. Chemicals and Reagents. All the reagents for SDS-polyacrylamide gel electrophoresis and immunoblotting were from Bio-Rad Laboratories (Richmond, CA, USA). HEPES, phenylmethylsulfonyl fluoride, aprotinin, dithiothreitol, Triton X-100, Tween 20, glycerol, and BSA (fraction V) were purchased from Sigma Chemical Co. (St. Louis, MO, USA). Nitrocellulose paper (BA85, 0.2 μm) and the reagents for chemoluminescence protein labeling in immunoblots were purchased from Amersham (Aylesbury, UK). The antibodies against IL10 (sc1783), IκBα (sc1643), pIkK (sc7977), pSTAT1 (sc7988), TNFα (sc8301), and SOCS3 (sc7009) were from Santa Cruz Biotechnology (Santa Cruz, CA, USA). IL6 (ab 6672), IL17 (ab 79056), and IL23 (ab45420) antibodies were from Abcam (Cambridge, MA). The antibody against IL1β (503502) was obtained from Biolegend (San Diego, CA). The protein molecular weight was assessed by the PageRulerTM from Fermentas (Glenburnie, MD). Reagents for real-time PCR analysis were from Invitrogen (Carlsbad, CA, USA) and Applied Biosystems (Foster City, CA, USA). Taqman Primers for *TNFα* (Mm00443258_m1), *IL1β* (Mm00434228_m1), *IL6* (Mm00446190_m1), *IL10* (Mm01288386_m1), and glyceraldehyde-3-phosphate dehydrogenase (*GAPDH*) (#4352339E) were obtained from Applied Biosystems and Integrated DNA Technologies (IDT).

2.2. Experimental Protocols. Biopsies from intestinal mucosa (ICD Group) and from mesenteric adipose tissue (ACD Group) were taken from 10 patients with ileocecal CD who underwent surgical resection. The presence of disease activity was assessed by colonoscopy one day before surgery and all patients had Crohn's disease activity index (CDAI) [13] more than 250 points. Patients with CD in other locations were excluded. The control group of ileal tissue was composed of eight patients who underwent ileocolonoscopy and the examination was normal (intestinal mucosa tissue control group–IC Group). The control group of MAT was composed of eight patients who underwent rectosigmoidectomy for noninflammatory disease with normal distal ileum (ileum mesenteric adipose tissue control group–AC Group). The study was performed in accordance with the Declaration of Helsinki and was approved by the Ethical Committee of the University of Campinas. All samples were taken after informed consent from the patients. The study was carried out at the University of Campinas, IBD Research Laboratory of the Colorectal Surgery Unit, Surgery Department, and at the Laboratory of Cell Signaling of the Department of Internal Medicine.

2.3. Western Blot. Biopsies were snap-frozen in liquid nitrogen and stored at −80°C until use. For total protein extract preparation, the fragments were homogenized in solubilizing buffer at 4°C [1% Triton X-100, 100 mM Tris-HCl (pH 7.4), 100 mM sodium pyrophosphate, 100 mM sodium fluoride, 10 mM EDTA, 10 mM sodium orthovanadate, 2.0 mM phenylmethylsulfonyl fluoride (PMSF), and 0.1 mg aprotinin/ml] with a Polytron PTA 20S generator (model PT 10/35; Brinkmann Instruments, Westbury, NY) operated at maximum speed for 30 sec. Insoluble material was removed by centrifugation (12000 rpm at 4°C for 40 min). The protein concentration of the supernatants was determined by BCA method (Pierce™ BCA Protein Assay Kit. Catalog number 23225). Aliquots of the supernatants containing 50 μg total proteins were separated by SDS-PAGE, transferred to nitrocellulose membranes and blotted with indicated antibodies as described in the results. Specific bands were labeled by a chemiluminescence reaction (SuperSignal West Pico Chemiluminescent Substrate from Pierce Biotechnology, Inc. Rockford, IL) and quantified by optical densitometry (Un-Scan-It Program). We have applied Ponceau staining to check equal loading of gels and membrane transfer (see Supplementary Figure S1 in Supplementary Material available online at https://doi.org/10.1155/2017/7646859) [14, 15].

2.4. RNA Extraction and Quantitative Real-Time PCR (qPCR). Total RNA was extracted using a commercially available acid-phenol reagent Trizol (Invitrogen Corp.) according to the manufacturer's instructions. The RNA concentration, purity, and integrity were confirmed spectrophotometrically using a

Nanodrop (ND-1000; Nanodrop Technologies, Wilmington, DE). RNA was treated with RNase-free Dnase (RQ1 RNase-free Dnase, Promega) and then reverse transcribed using oligo (dT) primers and reverse transcriptase (RevertAid™ Kit, Fermentas). The reaction mixture (20 μl) was incubated at 42°C for 60 min and then 10 min at 70°C and cooled on ice. qPCR was performed on resulting cDNA, using the manufacturer's protocol. Amplification was performed in a 10 μL final volume containing 40–50 ng of reverse-transcribed RNA according to the manufacturer's recommendations using the TaqMan PCR master mix.

Real-time PCR amplification consisted of an initial denaturation step (50°C for 2 min and 95°C for 10 min), 40 cycles of denaturation (95°C for 15 s), annealing (53°C for 20 s), and extension (72°C for 20 s), followed by a final incubation at 60°C for 1 minute. All measurements were normalized by the expression of *GAPDH* gene, considered as a stable housekeeping gene. Gene expression was determined using the delta-delta Ct method [16].

Real-time PCR analysis of gene expression was carried out in an ABI Prism 7500 sequence detection system (Applied Biosystems). The optimal concentration of complementary DNA (cDNA) and primers, as well as the maximum efficiency of amplification, were obtained through five-point, twofold dilution curve analysis for each gene. Amplification was performed in a 20 μL final volume containing 40–50 ng of cDNA according to the manufacturer's recommendations using the TaqMan PCR master mix. Real-time data were analyzed using the Sequence Detector System 1.7 (Applied Biosystems). Results were expressed as relative transcript amount as previously optimized [16].

2.5. Histological Analysis: Hematoxylin and Eosin (H&E) Staining. Biopsies from the intestinal mucosa and from MAT near the affected intestinal area were embedded in paraffin blocks for histological analysis. Sections of 5 μm were cut and stained with H&E dye. Photomicrographs were taken using a Zeiss Axiophot microscope and Cannon Power Shot G5 digital camera system (Cannon Inc., Tokyo). Fields of higher magnification (20x) were scanned and random fields were analyzed.

2.6. Statistical Analysis. All results are reported as means ± SEM. Data were analyzed by the Mann-Whitney Test, comparing the MAT of the CD group and its respective adipose control group and comparing, separately, the intestinal tissue of the CD group and its respective intestinal control group. The level of significance was set at $p < 0.05$.

3. Results

3.1. Morphometric Analysis of the Intestinal and MAT of CD Patients. H&E staining of CD intestinal mucosa showed thickening of the bowel wall associated with inflammation and deep linear ulcerations (Figure 1(b)) when compared to control (Figure 1(a)). In addition, we demonstrated that the area and the perimeter of the MAT were lower (Figure 1(d)) in CD patients when compared to the control group (Figure 1(c)).

3.2. Evaluation of the Inflammatory Markers in Intestinal Mucosa of CD Patients. Patients with CD showed increased mRNA levels of inflammatory markers such as *IL6, IL8, IL23,* and *IL10* ($p < 0.05$; Figures 2(a), 2(b), 2(c), and 2(d), resp.) in the intestinal mucosa when compared to control. However, no difference in *TNFα* gene expression was detected between ICD and IC groups (Figure 2(e)). On the other hand, the protein level of TNFα, IL1β, and IL23 ($p < 0.05$; Figures 2(f), 2(g), and 2(h), resp.) was significantly higher in the ICD Group when compared to control.

3.3. Evaluation of the Inflammatory Markers in MAT of CD Patients. TNFα, IL6, IL8, IL23, and *IL10* gene expressions (Figures 3(a), 3(b), 3(c), 3(d), and 3(e), resp.) were similar among the MAT groups, as well as protein expressions of TNFα, IL17, and IL23 (Figures 3(f), 3(g), and 3(h), resp.). The anti-inflammatory cytokine IL10 was increased in MAT of CD patients when compared to respective control ($p > 0.05$; Figure 3(i)).

3.4. Modulation of Nuclear Transcription Factors in the Intestinal Mucosa and MAT of CD Patients. We evaluated the pIkB/IkB ratio by immunoblotting and it was significantly higher in the ICD Group when compared to control ($p < 0.05$; Figure 4(a)). Conversely, the pIkB/IkB ratio was lower in MAT of CD patients when compared to control group ($p > 0.05$; Figure 5(a)), showing a different pattern in the inflammatory signaling response compared to the intestinal mucosa.

Despite the increased gene expression of *STAT1* in the intestinal mucosa of CD patients compared to control group ($p < 0.05$ Figure 4(c)), no differences in the phosphorylated and activated form of STAT1 (pSTAT1) were observed among the groups in intestinal mucosa (Figure 4(b)). Indeed, the SOCS3 protein, which is a downregulator of STAT pathways, was also significantly higher in ICD Group when compared to IC Group ($p < 0.05$; Figure 4(d)).

Interestingly, although there were no differences in *STAT1* gene expression, the protein content of the activated form of STAT1 (pSTAT1) was higher in ACD Group compared to AC Group ($p < 0.05$), showing that the STAT1 transcriptional pathway is activated in MAT of CD patients. Figures 5(c) and 5(b), respectively, illustrate these findings.

4. Discussion

The predominance of NF-kB activation in CD and STAT1 activation in UC has been reported in the literature [9, 10, 17]. Schreiber et al. [9] studied patients with active IBD and compared the expression and activation of STAT1 in endoscopic colonic biopsies. They concluded that STAT1 expression and activation are higher in UC compared to CD and controls. However, there are no studies of STAT1 activation in MAT. Schreiber et al. [10] revealed that NF-kB activation was detected in intestinal mucosa of both diseases, CD and UC, but the highest levels were seen in the *lamina propria* biopsy samples from CD patients. NF-kB is found in cytoplasm and is bound to IkBα, which prevents it from going into the nucleus [18]. Once this signaling pathway is activated,

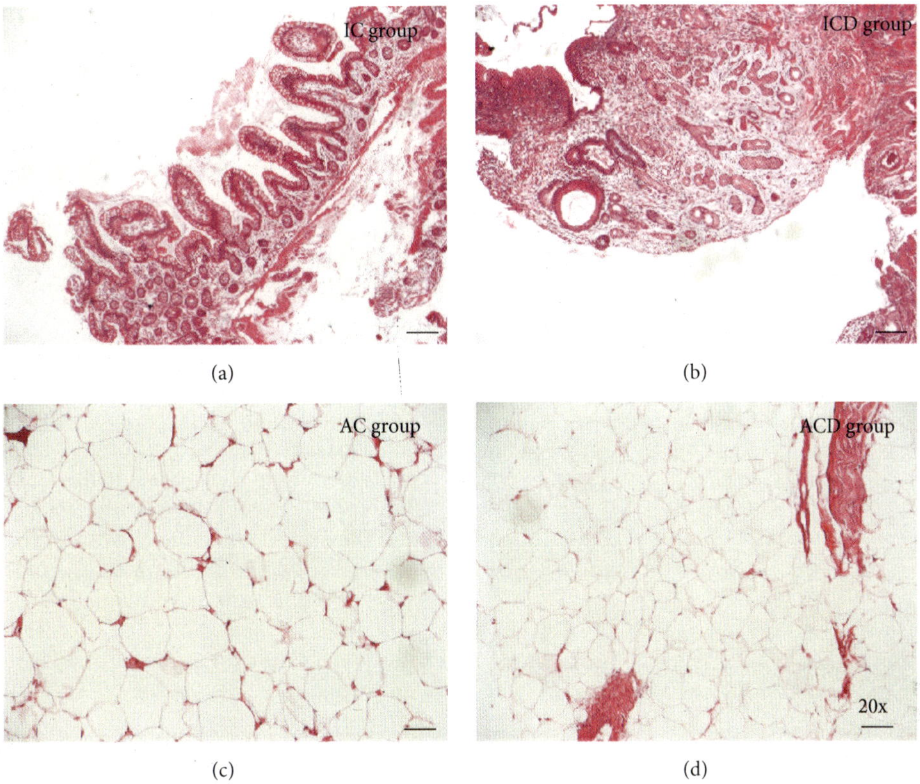

FIGURE 1: Haematoxylin and Eosin (H&E) staining of intestinal mucosa and mesenteric adipose tissues segments of a representative Crohn's disease patient. (a) Intestinal mucosa of a normal control subject (IC Group). (b) Intestinal mucosa of CD patient (ICD Group), showing crypt distortion, ulcers, and inflammatory infiltrate. (c) Mesenteric adipose tissue of a normal control subject (AC Group). (d) Mesenteric adipose tissue of CD patient (ACD Group) revealing characteristic morphometric features, with reduced adipocyte size. Nuclear counterstaining: Mayer's haematoxylin. Original magnification ×20.

the protein IkBα is phosphorylated and degraded by the ubiquitin-proteasome pathway, releasing the NF-kB, which binds to specific DNA sequences in the nucleus, activating target genes involved in the proinflammatory response [18].

In the present study, we show that TNFα expression and the NF-kB signaling pathway are activated in the intestinal mucosa of CD patients when compared to controls, whereas no differences were observed in STAT1 pathway, as demonstrated by the lack of pSTAT1 modulation in ICD and IC groups. This finding can be explained by the increased levels of SOCS3 in ICD Group, which may inhibit the STAT1 activation [19] and reinforce the predominance of NF-kB pathway in CD. At least in experimental models [20], NF-kB inhibitors ameliorate colonic inflammation.

Additionally, several other proinflammatory cytokines were found to be increased in intestinal mucosa of CD. Furthermore, although higher TNFα protein levels were noticed in the intestinal mucosa of CD, no differences were observed in its transcriptional expression, probably due to increased stability of the gene promoter [21]. Another possibility is that high TNFα protein expression could induce a negative feedback of TNFα gene transcription. Conversely, higher STAT1 gene expression in intestinal mucosa of CD and no differences in pSTAT1 expression were observed and could be explained by a higher protein stability and protection from ubiquitination and degradation outcomes.

The increase of MAT is usually shown as a marker of an active and more aggressive CD [22–26]. MAT can have an important role in the maintenance of CD, since the altered balance between proinflammatory and anti-inflammatory factors in adipocytes could lead to the activation of the innate and adaptive immune response [27, 28]. Previous studies have demonstrated the controversy expression of important inflammatory markers in MAT of CD patients. Desreumaux and coworkers published in 1999 a study showing an increased expression of TNFα in the MAT of the small bowel mesentery in CD patients, suggesting the adipocytes as one of the source of TNFα production [29]. Our results seem controversial to the literature, once we show no differences in TNFα expression, along with decreased NF-kB pathway activation demonstrated by decreased pIKB/IKB ratio and increased IL10 expression in MAT of CD patients. Besides, there were no differences in IL17 and IL23 protein expressions in this tissue.

Furthermore, a study conducted by Yamamoto and collaborators [3] in 2005 showed an increase of adiponectin secretion and tissue concentration in hypertrophied MAT of CD patients. Although, in this study, the comparison was made with normal MAT from IBD patients, differently of our controls, they concluded that the MAT could serve as a barrier that prevents the spread of inflammation into the intra-abdominal space. Conversely, Rodrigues and

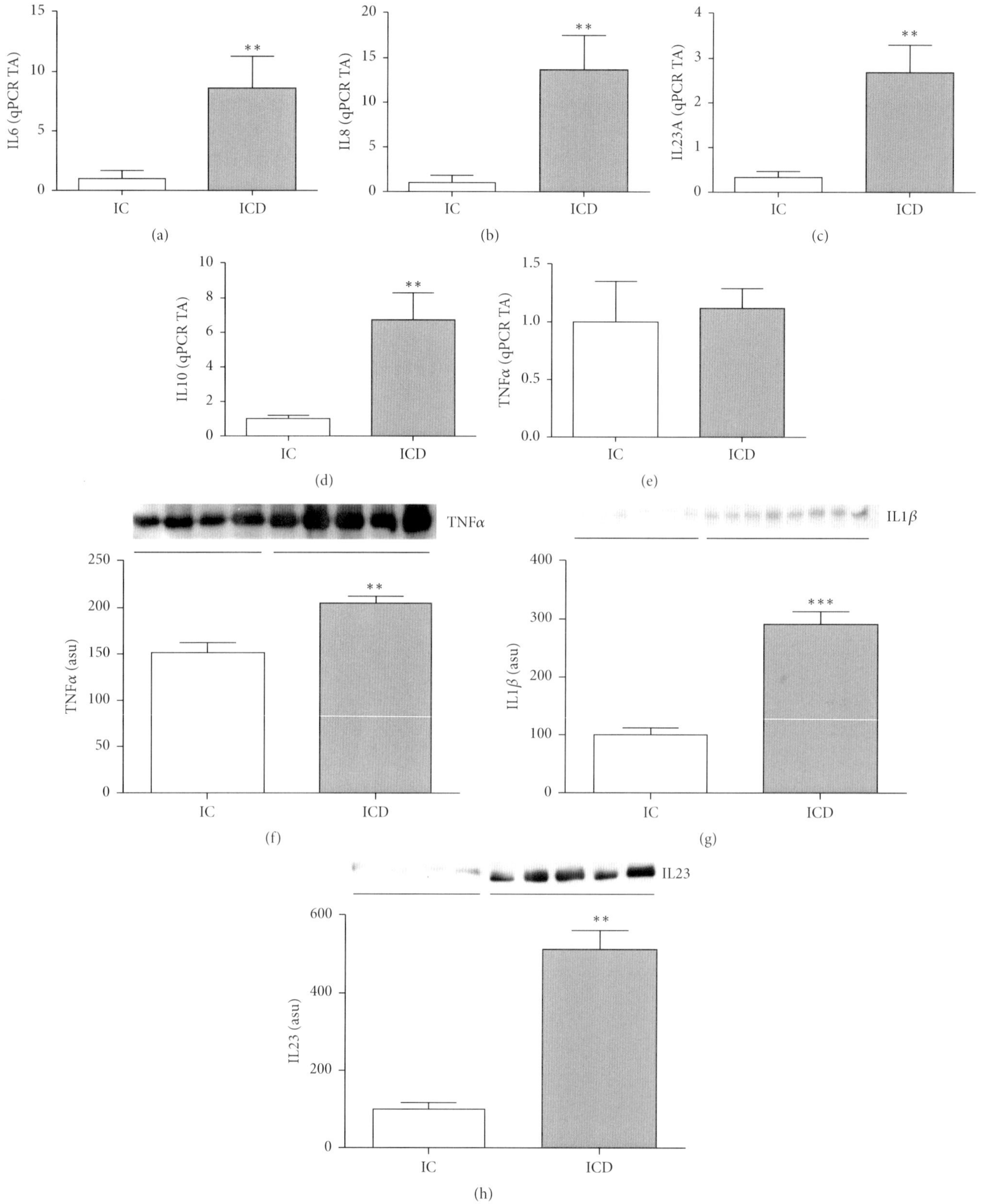

FIGURE 2: Evaluation of cytokines gene expressions in the intestinal mucosa of Crohn's disease patients. Inflammatory signaling proteins reveal a proinflammatory pattern in the intestinal mucosa of Crohn's disease patients. mRNA levels (qRT-PCR) of *IL6* (a), *IL8* (b), *IL23A* (c), *IL10* (d), and *TNFα* (e), in intestinal mucosa of CD patients (ICD Group) compared to controls (IC Group). Western blot analysis of TNFα (f), IL1β (g), and IL23 (h) in intestinal mucosa of CD patients (ICD Group) compared to controls (IC Group). Each band represents one patient. For ICD, $n = 10$; for IC, $n = 8$, $^{*}p < 0.05$, $^{**}p < 0.01$, and $^{***}p < 0.001$ versus control. TA: transcription amount. ASU: arbitrary scanning unit.

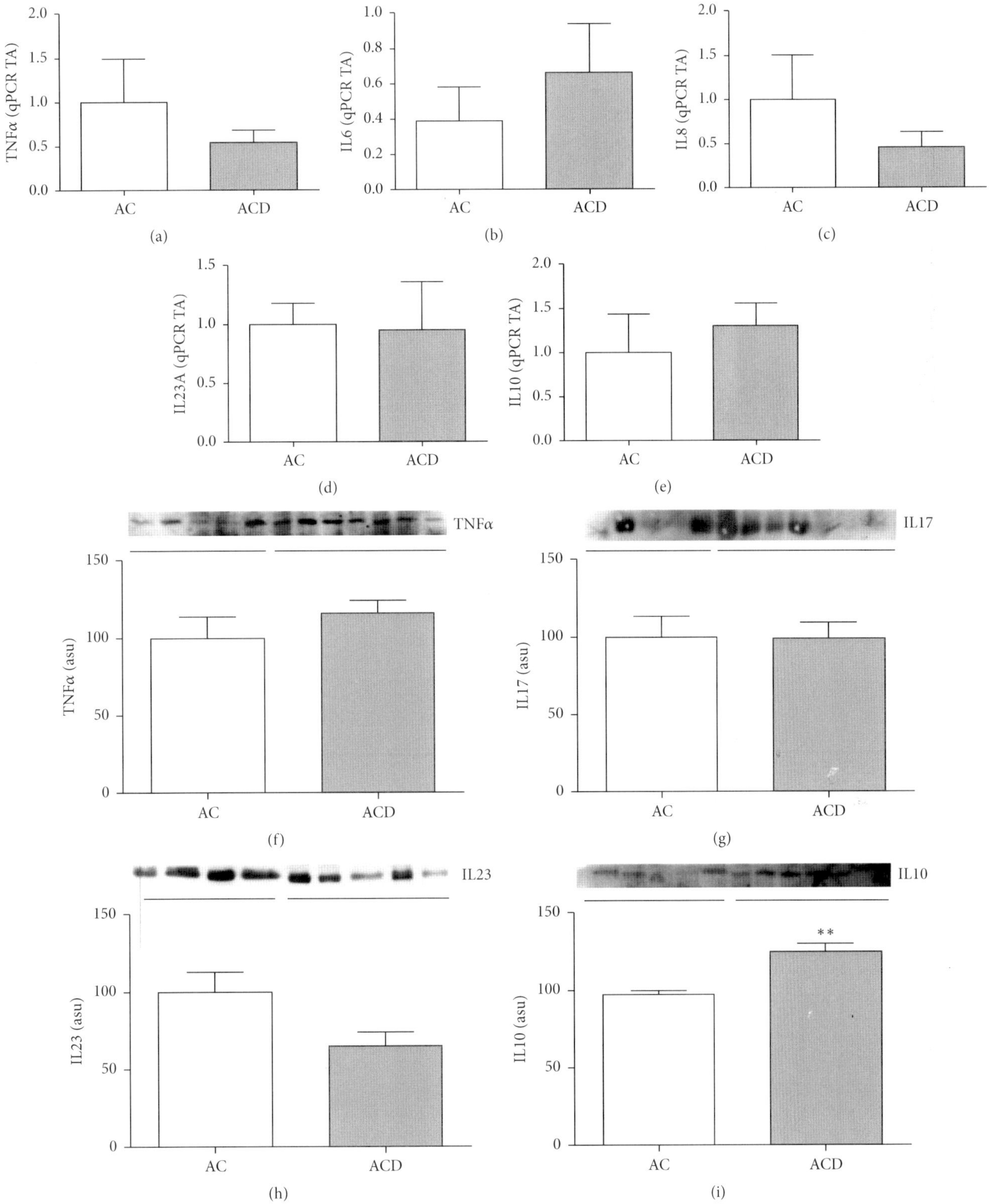

FIGURE 3: Evaluation of cytokines gene expressions in the mesenteric adipose tissue of Crohn's disease patients. Inflammatory signaling pattern in the mesenteric adipose tissue of Crohn's disease patients. mRNA levels (qRT-PCR) of *TNFα* (a), *IL6* (b), *IL8* (c), *IL23A* (d), and *IL10* (e) in the mesenteric adipose tissue (MAT) of CD patients (ACD Group) compared to controls (AC Group). Western blot analysis of TNFα (f), IL17 (g), IL23 (h), and IL10 (i) in the mesenteric adipose tissue (MAT) of CD patients (ACD Group) compared to controls (AC Group). Each band represents one patient. For ACD, $n = 10$; for AC, $n = 8$, $^{*}p < 0.05$, $^{**}p < 0.01$, and $^{***}p < 0.001$ versus control. TA: transcription amount. ASU: arbitrary scanning unit.

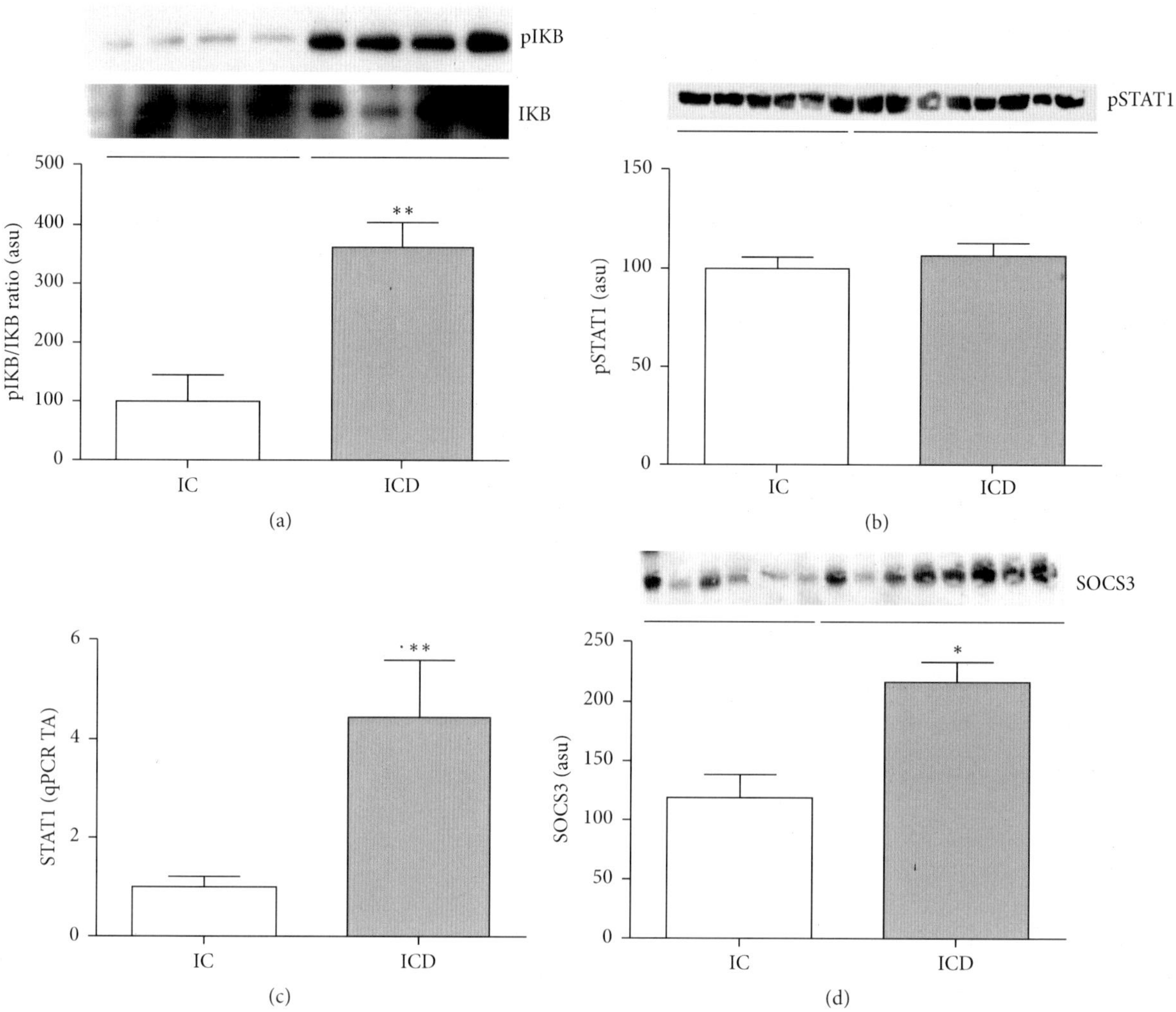

FIGURE 4: Intestinal mucosa of Crohn's disease patients shows inflammation driven by NF-KB. Higher SOCS3 protein expression counterbalances the STAT1 activation. Western blot analysis of pIκB/IκB ratio (a), pSTAT1 (b), and SOCS3 (d) in intestinal mucosa of CD patients (ICD Group) compared to controls (IC Group). mRNA levels (qRT-PCR) of *STAT1* (c) in intestinal mucosa of CD patients (ICD Group) compared to controls (IC Group). Each band represents one patient. For ICD, $n = 10$; for IC, $n = 8$; $^{*}p < 0.05$, $^{**}p < 0.01$, and $^{***}p < 0.001$ versus control. ASU: arbitrary scanning unit; TA: transcription amount.

collaborators [30] in 2012 revealed low expression of adiponectin in MAT of CD patients, which may show a deficiency in the anti-inflammatory mechanism in intestinal mesentery near the affected intestinal area during the late stages of this chronic disease, and this could help to perpetuate a state of chronic inflammation. Our results showing the increased protein levels of IL10 in MAT of CD patients corroborate with Yamamoto study; however, the controversy persists.

Additionally, our results showed no differences among protein and gene expression of TNFα or other proinflammatory cytokines in AC and ACD groups. Also, the pIkB/IkB ratio was lower in ACD Group compared to AC Group. No difference in STAT1 gene expression was observed in MAT; however the pSTAT1 was higher in MAT of CD patients, similar to the increase found in UC patients, as reported in the literature [31]. Although we found higher IL10 and pSTAT1 protein expression in MAT of CD, there were no differences in the transcriptional levels. This discrepancy of transcription and protein levels may be also explained by an increased stability of the gene promoter or a negative feedback of IL10 and STAT1 gene transcription induced by their respective higher protein expressions [21].

The role of MAT is still controversial in the literature as discussed above. The small diameter of MAT adipocytes of CD, as seen in severe obese patients, suggests a latent inflammatory condition in MAT [22]. Morphometric features of the adipocytes from CD MAT were already verified in the literature [4, 32]. Dias and collaborators [32] also correlated the lower diameter and area of the adipocytes with lower apoptosis, which could explain the higher number of adipocytes per field of higher magnification. Indeed, they did not find proliferation in this tissue as expected in nonobese individuals. Mature adipocytes are not able to do cell division; we can only see adipocyte proliferation in severe obesity. However, another mechanism that can lead

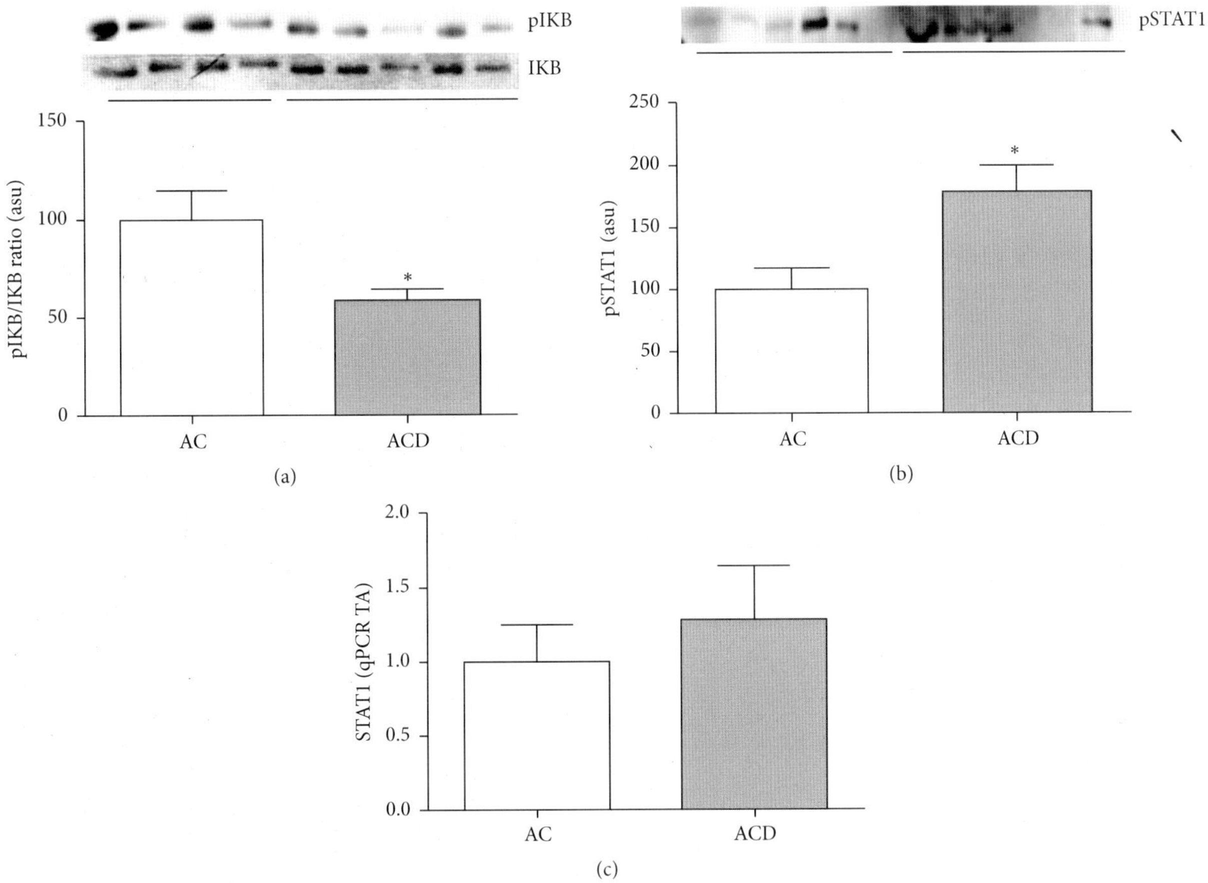

FIGURE 5: Mesenteric adipose tissue of Crohn's disease patients shows activation of STAT1 transcriptional pathway. Western blot analysis of pIκB/IκB ratio (a) and pSTAT1 (b) in the mesenteric adipose tissue (MAT) of CD patients (ACD Group) compared to controls (AC Group). mRNA levels (qRT-PCR) of *STAT1* (c) in MAT of CD patients (ACD Group) when compared to controls (AC Group). Each band represents one patient. For ACD, $n = 10$; and, for AC, $n = 8$, $^{*}p < 0.05$, $^{**}p < 0.01$, and $^{***}p < 0.001$ versus control. ASU: arbitrary scanning unit; TA: transcription amount.

to adipocyte number increase is by cell differentiation. This occurs through the adipogenesis pathway initiated by adipose stem cells [33, 34], which could explain the morphological and metabolic alterations in CD MAT. Recently, paracrine functions of the adipose-derived stromal vascular fraction (AD-SVF) have been studied and heterogeneous populations of undifferentiated mononuclear elements were also verified [34, 35]. Thus, in light of our results, it is still hard to confirm if MAT have an anti-inflammatory role that could attenuate the inflammation in CD patients or if a mild proinflammatory response is activated as seen in UC patients. The interaction between cytokines, adipokines, transcription factors, adipose stem cells, vascular endothelia, and adipocyte plasticity may be implicated in MAT remodeling, which certainly influences CD physiopathology.

Therefore the results of the present study reinforce the predominance of proinflammatory NF-KB pathway in the intestinal mucosa of CD patients. Additionally, for the first time, we showed that the inflammatory status of MAT in CD is mediated by STAT1 activation. On the other hand, this activation may lead to increase of anti-inflammatory cytokines, such as IL10. According to this study, MAT may play an important role in the pathophysiology and/or activity of CD. Indeed, the knowledge of the molecular signaling activated, along with the transcription factors and cytokine expression in different tissues, such as MAT and intestinal mucosa, is important to understand the physiopathology of CD and also to search for new drugs that address tissue-specific differences.

Authors' Contributions

Andressa Coope and Lívia Bitencourt Pascoal contributed equally to this study.

Acknowledgments

The authors thank FAPESP (Fundação de Amparo à Pesquisa do Estado de São Paulo) and FAEPEX (Fundo de Apoio ao Ensino, à Pesquisa e Extensão) for financial support. The authors are grateful to Dr. Nicola Conran and Professor Tristan Torriani for English grammar revision.

References

[1] J. H. Cho, "The genetics and immunopathogenesis of inflammatory bowel disease," *Nature Reviews Immunology*, vol. 8, no. 6, pp. 458–466, 2008.

[2] A. Mencarelli, E. Distrutti, B. Renga et al., "Probiotics modulate intestinal expression of nuclear receptor and provide counter-regulatory signals to inflammation-driven adipose tissue activation," *PLoS ONE*, vol. 6, no. 7, Article ID e22978, 2011.

[3] K. Yamamoto, T. Kiyohara, Y. Murayama et al., "Production of adiponectin, an anti-inflammatory protein, in mesenteric adipose tissue in Crohn's disease," *Gut*, vol. 54, no. 6, pp. 789–796, 2005.

[4] L. Peyrin-Biroulet, M. Chamaillard, F. Gonzalez et al., "Mesenteric fat in Crohn's disease: a pathogenetic hallmark or an innocent bystander?" *Gut*, vol. 56, no. 4, pp. 577–583, 2007.

[5] A. L. Sheehan, B. F. Warren, M. W. L. Gear, and N. A. Shepherd, "Fat-wrapping in Crohn's disease: pathological basis and relevance to surgical practice," *British Journal of Surgery*, vol. 79, no. 9, pp. 955–958, 1992.

[6] M. Barbier, H. Vidal, P. Desreumax et al., "Overexpression of leptin mRNA in mesenteric adipose tissue in inflammatory bowel diseases," *Gastroentérologie Clinique et Biologique*, vol. 27, pp. 1–5, 2005.

[7] S. Sitaraman, X. Liu, L. Charrier et al., "Colonic leptin: source of a novel proinflammatory cytokine involved in IBD," *The FASEB Journal*, vol. 18, no. 6, pp. 696–698, 2004.

[8] H.-C. Reinecker, M. Steffen, T. Witthoeft et al., "Enhanced secretion of tumour necrosis factor-alpha, IL-6, and IL-1 beta by isolated lamina propria mononuclear cells from patients with ulcerative colitis and Crohn's disease," *Clinical and Experimental Immunology*, vol. 94, no. 1, pp. 174–181, 1993.

[9] S. Schreiber, P. Rosenstiel, J. Hampe et al., "Activation of signal transducer and activator of transcription (STAT) 1 in human chronic inflammatory bowel disease," *Gut*, vol. 51, no. 3, pp. 379–385, 2002.

[10] S. Schreiber, S. Nikolaus, and J. Hampe, "Activation of nuclear factor κB in inflammatory bowel disease," *Gut*, vol. 42, no. 4, pp. 477–484, 1998.

[11] A. Sasaki, H. Yasukawa, A. Suzuki et al., "Cytokine-inducible SH2 protein-3 (CIS3/SOCS3) inhibits Janus tyrosine kinase by binding through the N-terminal kinase inhibitory region as well as SH2 domain," *Genes to Cells*, vol. 4, no. 6, pp. 339–351, 1999.

[12] T. Naka, M. Narazaki, M. Hirata et al., "Structure and function of a new STAT-induced STAT inhibitor," *Nature*, vol. 387, no. 6636, pp. 924–929, 1997.

[13] W. R. Best, J. M. Becktel, J. W. Singleton, and F. Kern Jr., "Development of a Crohn's disease activity index. National cooperative Crohn's disease study," *Gastroenterology*, vol. 70, no. 3, pp. 439–444, 1976.

[14] I. Romero-Calvo, B. Ocón, P. Martínez-Moya et al., "Reversible Ponceau staining as a loading control alternative to actin in Western blots," *Analytical Biochemistry*, vol. 401, no. 2, pp. 318–320, 2010.

[15] M. A. S. Fortes, G. N. Marzuca-Nassr, K. F. Vitzel, C. H. Da Justa Pinheiro, P. Newsholme, and R. Curi, "Housekeeping proteins: how useful are they in skeletal muscle diabetes studies and muscle hypertrophy models?" *Analytical Biochemistry*, vol. 504, pp. 38–40, 2016.

[16] K. J. Livak and T. D. Schmittgen, "Analysis of relative gene expression data using real-time quantitative PCR and the 2–$\Delta\Delta$CT method," *Methods*, vol. 25, no. 4, pp. 402–408, 2001.

[17] I. Russo, A. Luciani, P. de Cicco, E. Troncone, and C. Ciacci, "Butyrate attenuates lipopolysaccharide-induced inflammation in intestinal cells and Crohn's mucosa through modulation of antioxidant defense machinery," *PLoS ONE*, vol. 7, no. 3, Article ID e32841, 2012.

[18] Y. Takada, A. Mukhopadhyay, G. C. Kundu, G. H. Mahabeleshwar, S. Singh, and B. B. Aggarwal, "Hydrogen peroxide activates NF-κB through tyrosine phosphorylation of IκBα and serine phosphorylation of p65. Evidence for the involvement of IκBα kinase and Syk protein-tyrosine kinase," *The Journal of Biological Chemistry*, vol. 278, no. 26, pp. 24233–24241, 2003.

[19] Y. Li, C. de Haar, M. P. Peppelenbosch, and C. J. van der Woude, "SOCS3 in immune regulation of inflammatory bowel disease and inflammatory bowel disease-related cancer," *Cytokine and Growth Factor Reviews*, vol. 23, no. 3, pp. 127–138, 2012.

[20] T. Funakoshi, K. Yamashita, N. Ichikawa et al., "A novel NF-κB inhibitor, dehydroxymethylepoxyquinomicin, ameliorates inflammatory colonic injury in mice," *Journal of Crohn's and Colitis*, vol. 6, no. 2, pp. 215–225, 2012.

[21] J. Lin, J.-Q. Hou, H.-D. Xiang et al., "Stabilization of G-quadruplex DNA by C-5-methyl-cytosine in bcl-2 promoter: implications for epigenetic regulation," *Biochemical and Biophysical Research Communications*, vol. 433, no. 4, pp. 368–373, 2013.

[22] A. Zulian, R. Cancello, G. Micheletto et al., "Visceral adipocytes: old actors in obesity and new protagonists in Crohn's disease?" *Gut*, vol. 61, no. 1, pp. 86–94, 2012.

[23] I. Olivier, V. Théodorou, P. Valet et al., "Is Crohn's creeping fat an adipose tissue?" *Inflammatory Bowel Diseases*, vol. 17, no. 3, pp. 747–757, 2011.

[24] A. Schäffler and H. Herfarth, "Creeping fat in Crohn's disease: travelling in a creeper lane of research," *Gut*, vol. 54, no. 6, pp. 742–744, 2005.

[25] E. D. A. Westcott, C. A. Mattacks, A. C. J. Windsor, S. C. Knight, and C. M. Pond, "Perinodal adipose tissue and fatty acid composition of lymphoid tissues in patients with and without Crohn's disease and their implications for the etiology and treatment of CD," *Annals of the New York Academy of Sciences*, vol. 1072, pp. 395–400, 2006.

[26] B. Erhayiem, R. Dhingsa, C. J. Hawkey, and V. Subramanian, "Ratio of visceral to subcutaneous fat area is a biomarker of complicated Crohn's Disease," *Clinical Gastroenterology and Hepatology*, vol. 9, no. 8, pp. 684–687.e1, 2011.

[27] S. P. Weisberg, D. McCann, M. Desai, M. Rosenbaum, R. L. Leibel, and A. W. Ferrante Jr., "Obesity is associated with macrophage accumulation in adipose tissue," *The Journal of Clinical Investigation*, vol. 112, no. 12, pp. 1796–1808, 2003.

[28] C. A. Curat, A. Miranville, C. Sengenès et al., "From blood monocytes to adipose tissue-resident macrophages: induction of diapedesis by human mature adipocytes," *Diabetes*, vol. 53, no. 5, pp. 1285–1292, 2004.

[29] P. Desreumaux, O. Ernst, K. Geboes et al., "Inflammatory alterations in mesenteric adipose tissue in Crohn's disease," *Gastroenterology*, vol. 117, no. 1, pp. 73–81, 1999.

[30] V. S. Rodrigues, M. Milanski, J. J. Fagundes et al., "Serum levels and mesenteric fat tissue expression of adiponectin and leptin in patients with Crohn's disease," *Clinical and Experimental Immunology*, vol. 170, no. 3, pp. 358–364, 2012.

[31] G. P. Christophi, R. Rong, P. G. Holtzapple, P. T. Massa, and S. K. Landas, "Immune markers and differential signaling networks in ulcerative colitis and Crohn's disease," *Inflammatory Bowel Diseases*, vol. 18, no. 12, pp. 2342–2356, 2012.

[32] C. B. Dias, M. Milanski, M. Portovedo et al., "Defective apoptosis in intestinal and mesenteric adipose tissue of Crohn's disease patients," *PLoS ONE*, vol. 9, no. 6, Article ID e98547, 2014.

[33] M. S. Rodeheffer, K. Birsoy, and J. M. Friedman, "Identification of white adipocyte progenitor cells in vivo," *Cell*, vol. 135, no. 2, pp. 240–249, 2008.

[34] R. W. Alexander, "Understanding adipose-derived stromal vascular fraction (AD-SVF) cell biology and use on the basis of cellular, chemical, structural and paracrine components: a concise review," *Journal of Prolotherapy*, vol. 4, no. 1, pp. e855–e869, 2012.

[35] D. Alderman and R. W. Alexander, "Advances in regenerative medicine: highdensity platelet-rich plasma and stem cell prolotherapy," *Practical Pain Management*, vol. 10, pp. 58–75, 2011.

22

The Difference in Interleukin-19 Serum on Degrees of Acne Vulgaris Severity

Moerbono Mochtar,[1] Alamanda Murasmita,[1] M. Eko Irawanto,[1] Indah Julianto,[1] Harijono Kariosentono,[1] and Fajar Waskito[2]

[1] *Dermatovenerology Department, Sebelas Maret University, Dr. Moewardi General Hospital, Surakarta, Indonesia*
[2] *Dermatovenerology Department, Gadjah Mada University, Dr. Sardjito' General Hospital, Yogyakarta, Indonesia*

Correspondence should be addressed to Alamanda Murasmita; dottalamanda@gmail.com

Academic Editor: B. L. Slomiany

Introduction. Acne vulgaris is a multifactorial disease. Recent study showed that inflammation does have a central role in the formation of both inflammatory and noninflammatory lesions in acne vulgaris. There are various findings of proinflammatory cytokines related to acne vulgaris, but no previous study correlate interleukin- (IL-) 19 to acne vulgaris. This pilot study aims to look at difference in IL-19 serum concentration on degrees of severity of acne vulgaris. *Methods.* This is an analytical observational cross-sectional study. Sample subjects were patients with acne vulgaris who met the inclusion criteria. Enzyme-linked immunosorbent assay (ELISA) study was applied to measure IL-19 serum. *Result.* Analysis test found statistically significant difference between IL-19 serum concentration of group of patients with mild acne vulgaris and that of group of patients with severe acne vulgaris. Moreover, analysis revealed significant difference between IL-19 serum concentration of group of patients with moderate acne vulgaris and that of group of patients with severe acne vulgaris. *Conclusions.* There are differences in serum levels of IL-19 on the severity of acne vulgaris. The significant difference might show that inflammation has a core role in severity of acne vulgaris, and IL-19 might potentially be related to acne vulgaris.

1. Introduction

Acne vulgaris is a multifactorial disease which is associated with pilosebaceous follicle and results in inflammatory and noninflammatory lesions [1]. The pathogenesis of acne is attributed to increased sebum production, inflammatory processes, follicular hyperproliferation, and the proliferation of *Propionibacterium acnes (P. acnes)* [2]. Nowadays, it is stated that inflammation continuous to happen in early stage and late stage of acne vulgaris [3]; therefore, the inflammation does have a central role in the formation of both inflammatory and noninflammatory lesions in acne vulgaris [4].

The inflammation in acne vulgaris itself linked with *P. acnes. Propionibacterium acnes* stimulates keratinocytes through the Toll-like receptors (TLRs) to produce proinflammatory cytokines. An example of proinflammatory cytokines that are already known is interleukin- (IL-) 1β [5]. The other cytokines related to pathogenesis of acne vulgaris are IL-6, IL-8, IL-10, and IL-12 [6]. There is no study about IL-19 cytokines related to acne vulgaris or acne vulgaris severity.

Interleukin- (IL-) 19 is a cytokine expressed by epithelial cells with proinflammatory stimulation [7]. A distinctive feature of IL-19 is their ability of giving positive feedback loop to amplify themselves [8]; once they are activated in inflammatory process, they will continuously produce the cytokine. The present research sought to find out the difference in IL-19 serum concentration on degrees of severity of acne vulgaris; this is the pilot study of IL-19 serum in acne vulgaris patients.

The research belongs to an observational analytical study with cross-sectional study design. The target population includes acne vulgaris patients in Surakarta, while the accessible population involves acne vulgaris patients in Dr. Moewardi General Hospital of Surakarta and private specialist

TABLE 1: Grading classification Lehmann.

Grading	Comedones	Inflammatory lesions*	Cyst	Total
Mild	<20	<15	-	<30
Moderate	20–100	15–50	<5	30-125
Severe	>100	>50	>5	>125

*Inflammatory lesions: example, papule/pustule/nodules.

TABLE 2: Detecting the difference in means of IL-19 serum concentration among samples.

Detecting the difference in means	Mann–Whitney test	
	Value of Z-MW	p
Degrees of severity of acne vulgaris: mild-moderate	−1.011	0.312
Degrees of severity of acne vulgaris: mild-severe	−2.586	0.010*
Degrees of severity of acne vulgaris: moderate-severe	−1.974	0.048*

Source. Primary data 2017, processed; *Annotation.* *Significant at significance level of 5%.

clinics which meet the inclusion criteria. Samples were taken using purposive sampling.

2. Method

The number of samples was determined using unpaired numerical analytical test. The inclusion criteria include subjects between the ages of 16 and 30 years clinically diagnosed with acne vulgaris who were willing to participate in the research and to fill in a questionnaire and a statement of willingness. Meanwhile, the exclusion criteria involve acne vulgaris patients undergoing systemic and topical treatment in the last two weeks and patients with other conditions related to an increase in IL-19 expression in serum or skin lesions such as psoriasis [9, 10], atopic dermatitis [10, 11], and asthma [12, 13].

To determine the degree of severity of acne vulgaris, anamnesis, clinical checkup, and picture taking were carried out. We used acne severity grading systems from Lehmann recommended in Indonesian acne expert meeting 2012 (Table 1) [14].

A 6 mL blood sample was drawn from every subject for an examination of IL-19 serum concentration. Such procedures which applied human IL-19 immunoassay with quantitative sandwich enzyme-linked immunosorbent assay (ELISA) (Quantikine ELISA Kits: R&D systems; ELISA reader 680 Bio-Rad) conform to the laboratory protocols. A number of 66 subjects comprising 3 groups (a group of patients with mild acne vulgaris, of patients with moderate acne vulgaris, and of patients with severe acne vulgaris) were obtained. The average ages of a group of patients with mild acne vulgaris, of patients with moderate acne vulgaris, and of patients with severe acne vulgaris are 21.55 ± 3.74 years, 22.18 ± 2.70 years, and 21.18 ± 3.90 years, respectively.

3. Results

The mean of IL-19 serum concentration of group of patients with mild acne vulgaris is 18.38 ± 9.59 pg/ml, that of group of patients with moderate acne vulgaris is 21.23 ± 11.99 pg/ml, and that of group of patients with severe acne vulgaris is 31.19 ± 20.36 pg/ml. The mean of IL-19 serum concentration of all groups is 23.60 ± 15.51 pg/ml. Figure 1 presents the difference in means of IL-19 serum concentration among the groups.

Analysis of independent samples t-test using Mann–Whitney test found statistically significant difference between IL-19 serum concentration of group of patients with mild acne vulgaris and that of group of patients with severe acne vulgaris ($p = 0.010$) and no significant difference between IL-19 serum concentration of group of patients with mild acne vulgaris and that of group of patients with moderate acne vulgaris ($p = 0.312$). Moreover, analysis of dependent samples t-test revealed significant difference between IL-19 serum concentration of group of patients with moderate acne vulgaris and that of group of patients with severe acne vulgaris ($p = 0.048$) (Table 2).

4. Discussion

Acne vulgaris belongs to a complex and multifactorial disease of pilosebaceous unit. Acne pathogenesis cannot be viewed as impartial since its etiologies influence each other. Pathogenesis of acne vulgaris recently emphasizes inflammatory process. The latest finding indicates role of *P. acnes* as a triggering factor of inflammatory responses which exerts an influence on severity of acne vulgaris. Pathways underlying the formation of papules, pustules, and nodulocystic acne which involve cytokines were detected [15]. *Propionibacterium acnes* proliferates in lipid-rich environment contribute to formation of inflammation, by inducing TLR-2 to release such proinflammatory cytokines as IL-1β [16]. The present research was intended to find out the difference in IL-19 serum concentration on various degrees of severity of acne vulgaris. The study from Kunz et al. stated that IL-1β could induce expression of IL-19 in keratinocytes both in vitro and in vivo [10]. Epithelial cells such as keratinocytes will

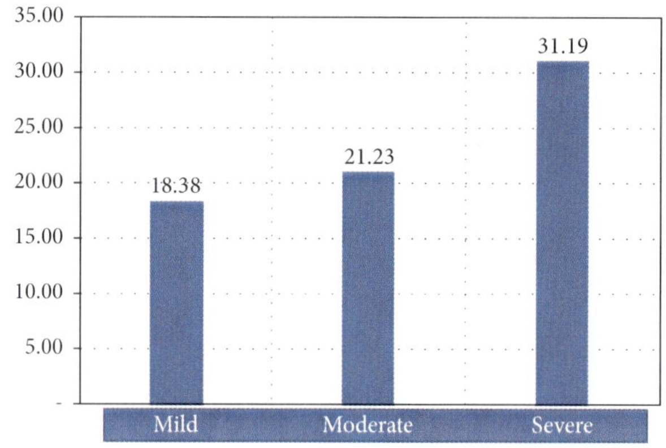

FIGURE 1: The difference in means of IL-19 serum (pg/ml).

produce IL-19 after being stimulated by IL-1β [17, 18]. It is found out that the release of proinflammatory cytokines of IL-1β may lead to the release of IL-19 despite the unknown special activation signal between IL-1β and IL-19 [11]. Such mechanism ends up with inflammatory processes and tissue damage in acne vulgaris patients and an increase in incidence and severity of acne vulgaris. Such cytokines are related and influence degrees of severity of acne vulgaris.

The research finding which signified the difference in IL-19 serum concentration on various degrees of severity of acne vulgaris is in line with a study conducted by Li et al., measuring IL-19 in patients with psoriasis, which emphasizes that, with reference to etiopathogenesis, the severity of both diseases is indicated by an increase in concentration of proinflammatory cytokines [19].

The measurement of IL-19 using serum was carried out by Li et al. to find out the correlation between IL-19 serum concentration and diabetic nephropathy. The measurement conducted on healthy control subjects revealed smaller IL-19 concentration (mean = 13.2 pg/ml) than on subjects with type 2 diabetes (mean = 40.5 pg/ml) [20], since IL-19 is only expressed in inflammatory location and condition. The present research detected proportional increase in IL-19 serum and degrees of severity of acne vulgaris. It may indicate inflammatory condition of acne vulgaris which can lead to an increase in IL-19, as detected in serum.

The measurement of expression of proinflammatory cytokines in acne vulgaris through serum was also carried out in several studies. Maulinda et al. examined IL-17 serum concentration on patients with papulopustular acne and comedonal acne with total subjects of 24 persons [21]. Another study was carried out by Liu et al. measuring IL-6 serum to predict effectivity of acupuncture for severe acne vulgaris [22].

Enzyme-Linked Immunosorbent Assay was applied in the research to measure IL-19 serum on research subjects. Enzyme-Linked Immunosorbent Assay refers to the most commonly used proteomic method with the best validity. The method enables us to detect antigens or cytokines through an antibody, while another antibody linked to an enzyme provides detection and an amplification factor. Due to accurate and sensitive detection of the antigen, ELISA has been considered the standard cytokine measurement method and is widely utilized in clinical laboratories and biomedical research [23].

The research results indicated the significant difference between moderate and severe acne vulgaris. The more the severe inflammation is, the bigger the detected IL-19 serum concentration will be. Such finding is in accordance with a research conducted by Yahil which shows that IL-19 production depends very much on the involved cells and expressing cell microenvironment, and therefore the more severe inflammation is, the higher expression of IL-19 will be [24].

5. Conclusion

There are differences in means of IL-19 serum concentration in acne vulgaris patients. The significant difference between IL-19 serum concentration of group of patients with moderate acne vulgaris and patients with severe acne vulgaris might show that inflammation has a core role in severity of acne vulgaris. This may lead to another research to find out that IL-19 might relate more to acne vulgaris inflammation and severity due to its unique features.

References

[1] S. Younis and Q. Javed, "The Interleukin-6 and Interleukin-1A gene promoter polymorphism is associated with the pathogenesis of acne vulgaris," *Arch Dermatol Res*, vol. 307, pp. 365–370, 2015.

[2] A. S. Karadag, D. T. Ertugrul, S. G. Bilgili, Z. Takci, K. O. Akin, and O. Calka, "Immunoregulatory effects of isotretinoin in patients with acne," *British Journal of Dermatology*, vol. 167, no. 2, pp. 433–435, 2012.

[3] E. A. Tanghetti, "The Role of Inflammation in the Pathology of Acne Clin Aesth Derm," *The Journal of Clinical Aesthet Dermatol*, vol. 6, p. 27, 2013.

[4] M. J. Rico, "The Role of Inflammation in Acne Vulgaris," *Practical Dermatology*, vol. 8, pp. 22–33, 2013.

[5] P. A. Grange, B. Weill, N. Dupin, and F. Batteux, "Does inflammatory acne result from imbalance in the keratinocyte innate immune response?" *Microbes and Infection*, vol. 12, no. 14-15, pp. 1085–1090, 2010.

[6] S. Das and R. V. Reynolds, "Recent advances in acne pathogenesis: implications for therapy," *American Journal of Clinical Dermatology*, vol. 15, pp. 479–488, 2014.

[7] C. A. Fielding, "Interleukin-19: A new target to aim for?" *Rheumatology*, vol. 51, no. 3, Article ID ker174, pp. 399-400, 2012.

[8] W. J. Jordan, J. Eskdale, M. Boniotto et al., "Human IL-19 regulates immunity through auto-induction of IL-19 and production of IL-10," *European Journal Immunology*, vol. 35, pp. 1576–1582, 2005.

[9] K. Otkjaer, K. Kragballe, A. T. Funding et al., "The dynamics of gene expression of interleukin-19 and interleukin-20 and their receptors in psoriasis," *British Journal of Dermatology*, vol. 153, no. 5, pp. 911–918, 2005.

[10] S. Kunz, K. Wolk, E. Witte et al., "Interleukin (IL)-19, IL-20 and IL-24 are produced by and act on keratinocytes and are distinct from classical ILs," *Experimental Dermatology*, vol. 15, no. 12, pp. 991–1004, 2006.

[11] L. Bao, J. B. Alexander, V. Y. Shi, G. C. Mohan, and L. S. Chan, "Interleukin-4 up-regulation of epidermal interleukin-19 expression in keratinocytes involves the binding of signal transducer and activator of transcription 6 (Stat6) to the imperfect Stat6 sites," *The Journal of Immunology*, vol. 143, no. 4, pp. 601–608, 2014.

[12] S. Liao, Y. Cheng, Y. Wang et al., "IL-19 Induced Th2 Cytokines and Was Up-Regulated in Asthma Patients," *The Journal of Immunology*, vol. 173, no. 11, pp. 6712–6718, 2004.

[13] G. Gallagher, "Interleukin-19: Multiple roles in immune regulation and disease," *Cytokine & Growth Factor Reviews*, vol. 21, no. 5, pp. 345–352, 2010.

[14] Indonesia Cosmetic Dermatology Study Group (KSDKI), *Indonesian acne expert meeting 2012: kelompok studi dermatologi kosmetik Indonesia*, Centra Communications, Jakarta, Indonesia, 2013.

[15] B. D. M. Ribeiro, L. M. C. Almeida, A. Costa, F. Francesconi, I. Follador, and J. R. Neves, "Etiopathogeny of acne vulgaris: A practical review for day-to-day dermatologic practice," *Surgical and Cosmetic Dermatology*, vol. 7, no. 3, pp. 20–26, 2015.

[16] E. Contassot and L. E. French, "New insights into acne pathogenesis: propionibacterium acnes activates the inflammasome," *Journal of Investigative Dermatology*, vol. 134, no. 2, pp. 310–313, 2014.

[17] G. F. Camarillo, J. F. Carballeda, J. Granados, and J. K. Y. Furusho, "Expression of interleukin (IL)-19 and IL-24 in inflammatory bowel disease patients: a cross-sectional study," *Clinical and Experimental Immunology*, pp. 64–75, 2014.

[18] S. Rutz, X. Wang, and W. Ouyang, "The IL-20 subfamily of cytokines–from host defence to tissue homeostasis," *Nature Review Immunology*, vol. 14, pp. 783–795, 2014.

[19] H. H. Li, Y. C. Lin, P. J. Chen et al., "Interleukin-19 upregulates keratinocyte growth factor and is associated with psoriasis," *British Journal of Dermatology*, vol. 153, pp. 591–595, 2005.

[20] L. Li, X. G. Jiang, J. Y. Hu et al., "The association between interleukin-19 concentration and diabetic nephropathy," *BMC Nephrol*, vol. 18, p. 65, 2017.

[21] S. Maulinda, R. Hindritiani, K. Ruchiatan, and O. Suwarsa, "Perbandingan Kadar IL-17 Serum Pasien Akne Vulgaris Tipe Papulopustular dengan Komedonal," *Majalah Kedokteran Bandung*, vol. 48, pp. 160–163, 2016.

[22] C.-Z. Liu, B. Lei, and J.-F. Zheng, "Randomized control study on the treatment of 26 cases of acne conglobata with encircling acupuncture combined with venesection and cupping," *Zhen Ci Yan Jiu*, vol. 33, no. 6, pp. 406–408, 2008.

[23] S. X. Leng, J. E. Mcelhaney, J. D. Walston, D. Xie, N. S. Fedarko, and G. A. Kuchel, "ELISA and multiplex technologies for cytokine measurement in inflammation and aging research," *The Journals of Gerontology: Series A*, vol. 63, pp. 879–884, 2008.

[24] R. J. Yahil, "The role of Interleukin-19 in Interleukin-10 production by regulatory macrophages," in *Cell Biology and Molecular Genetics Thesses and Dissertations*, University of Maryland, Maryland , Md, USA, 2010.

23

S-Equol, a Major Isoflavone from Soybean, Inhibits Nitric Oxide Production in Lipopolysaccharide-Stimulated Rat Astrocytes Partially via the GPR30-Mediated Pathway

Mitsuaki Moriyama, Ayano Hashimoto, Hideyo Satoh, Kenji Kawabe, Mizue Ogawa, Katsura Takano, and Yoichi Nakamura

Laboratory of Integrative Physiology in Veterinary Sciences, Osaka Prefecture University, Izumisano, Osaka, Japan

Correspondence should be addressed to Mitsuaki Moriyama; moriyama@vet.osakafu-u.ac.jp

Academic Editor: Ke-Wu Zeng

Cumulative evidence indicates that estrogen receptor (ER) agonists attenuate neuroinflammation. Equol, a major isoflavone from soybean, exhibits estrogen-like biological activity, but their effect on inflammatory response has not been well established. Here, we investigated the effect of S-equol on nitric oxide (NO) production, well-known inflammatory change in astrocytes stimulated by LPS. S-Equol attenuated LPS-induced NO production with a concomitant decrease in expression of inducible NO synthase (iNOS). S-Equol did not affect LPS-induced increase in intracellular ROS production. Intracellular ER blocker ICI 182.780 had no effect on S-equol-induced decrease in NO production. Addition of G-15, antagonist of G protein-coupled receptor 30 which is nongenomic ER and located on cell surface, partially recovered S-equol-induced attenuation of NO production. These findings suggest that attenuation of NO production by S-equol may mitigate LPS-induced neuroinflammation in astrocytes. S-Equol may exert a glioprotective effect, at least in part, via a nongenomic effect.

1. Introduction

Recently the crucial role has been recognized for neuroinflammation which is complicated in the pathogenesis of several neurodegenerative diseases such as Alzheimer's disease (AD), Parkinson's disease (PD), and stroke [1, 2]. In these pathological states, microglia and astrocytes are activated; they produce proinflammatory cytokines, such as tumor necrosis factor-α (TNFα), interleukin-1β (IL-1β), and interferon-γ (IFNγ), as well as nitric oxide (NO) and reactive oxygen species (ROS), resulting in neuronal damage; all these changes contribute to CNS disorder [1–3]. Several lines of evidence indicate that estrogen receptor (ER) agonists attenuate neuroinflammation [4–6]. Systemic injection of estrogen inhibits microglial activation induced by intraventricular injection of lipopolysaccharide (LPS) [7]. An ER agonist also reduces TNFα and IL-1β secretion in cultured astrocytes following LPS treatment [8]. Reduced estrogen level potentiates β amyloid peptide deposition in AD model mice [9]. These results suggest that estrogen can alleviate neuroinflammation due to suppressing microglial and astrocyte activation. ER agonists modulate transcriptional activities *via* nuclear ER signaling [10]. In addition to this "genomic" effects, estrogen also acts "nongenomically" on the receptor which is located on plasma membrane, activating multiple signaling pathways that regulate cellular functions [11]. G protein-coupled receptor 30 (GPR30) acts as plasma membrane receptor and shows biological activities of estrogen [12, 13]. GPR30 expressed in microglia contributes to neuroprotective roles in a model of PD and ischemic stroke [14, 15]. However, the roles of genomic and nongenomic effect of ER on neuroinflammation remain to be fully elucidated.

Isoflavones are natural polyphenolic compounds, which act as phytoestrogens [16] and have several activities such as antioxidant, anti-inflammatory, and antitumor properties [17]. Equol is a major isoflavone compound from soybean. Intestinal bacteria such as *Lactococcus garvieae* metabolize daidzein to S-equol [18]. Similar to other isoflavones such as

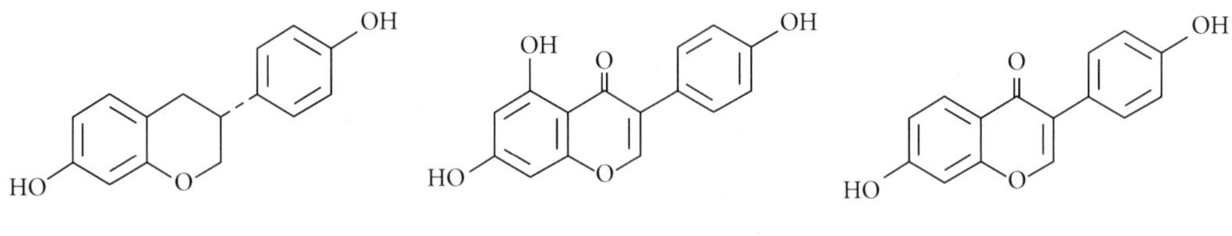

S-Equol Genistein Daidzein

FIGURE 1: Chemical structures of *S*-equol, genistein, and daidzein.

genistein and daidzein, equol exhibits antioxidant property [19]. Because of its similar conformational structure (see Figure 1), *S*-equol shows an affinity of ER and exhibits estrogen-like biological activity [19]. In peripheral, equol inhibits prostate carcinogenesis [20] and also protects and reduces UV-induced skin aging [21]. Such effects are thought to be due to antioxidative effects and induction of apoptosis. In CNS cells, soy isoflavones such as genistein, daidzein, and equol have been reported to be neuroprotective against hypoxia in primary cortical neurons [22]. In glial cells, most of previous work has paid attention to the effect of isoflavones on microglia; genistein [23] and daidzein [24] suppress LPS-induced microglial activation and this is also true for equol [25]. Compared to microglia, there are few reports concerning the effects of isoflavones on astrocytes; genistein suppresses neuroinflammatory changes induced by hemolysate [26] or amyloid β [27]. Since the effect of equol on inflammatory responses in astrocytes has not been investigated until now, the role of equol on neuroinflammation is not clear.

LPS, gram-negative bacteria's outer membrane component, directly binds and activates toll-like receptors (TLRs) and its signaling cascades, generating several inflammatory mediators including proinflammatory cytokines such as TNFα, IL-1β, and IFNγ. The LPS-induced changes are thought to mimic those under neurodegenerative diseases [28, 29]. Here, we investigated the effect of *S*-equol on NO production, well-known inflammatory change in astrocytes activated by LPS.

2. Materials and Methods

2.1. Chemicals and Antibodies. Unless otherwise stated, all chemicals and reagents used in the present study were of analytical grade. Chemicals and antibodies used were as follows: horse serum and Dulbecco's modified Eagle medium (DMEM) from Gibco BRL, Grand Island, NY, USA; LPS from *Escherichia coli* 0127:B8, protease inhibitor cocktail, fetal bovine serum (FBS), trypsin, 2′,7′-dichlorodihydrofluorescein diacetate (H_2DCFDA), ICI 182.780 (7α,17β-[9-(4,4,5,5,5-pentafluoropentylsulfinyl)nonyl]estra-1,3,5(10)-triene-3,17-diol), antibodies of anti-β-actin and anti-GFAP, and horseradish peroxidase-conjugated goat anti-rabbit IgG (whole molecule) antibody from Sigma Aldrich Corp, St. Louis, MO, USA; *S*-(-)equol from Toronto Research Chemicals, Toronto, ON, Canada; genistein and daidzein from Wako Pure Chemical Co., Osaka, Japan; 2,3-Diaminonaphthalene (DAN), 4′,6-diamidino-2-phenylindole (DAPI), and 3-(4,5-dimethyl-2-thiazolyl)-2,5-diphenyl-tetrazolium bromide (MTT) from Dojindo, Kumamoto, Japan; G-1 (1-[(3a*R**,4*S**,9b*S**)-4-(6-Bromo-1,3-benzodioxol-5-yl)-3a,4,5,9b-tetrahydro-3*H*-cyclopenta[*c*]quinolin-8-yl]-ethanone) from Tocris Bioscience, Bristol, UK; G-15 (3aS,4R,9bR)-4-(6-bromo-1,3-benzodioxol-5-yl)-3a,4,5,9b-tetrahydro-3H-cyclopenta[c]quinolone from Cayman Chemical, Ann Arbor, MI, USA; antibodies of anti-extracellular signal-regulated kinase (ERK)1/2, anti-dual phospho-ERK1/2, anti-p38-mitogen activated protein kinase (MAPK), and anti-phospho-p38-MAPK from Cell Signaling Technology, Inc., Danvers, MA, USA; anti-CD11b antibody from AbD Serotec, Oxford, UK; Immobilon™ Western Chemiluminescent horseradish peroxidase substrate from Millipore Corp., Billerica, MA, USA. iNOS antibody was provided as mentioned previously [30].

2.2. Astrocyte Preparation and Cell Culture. This study was approved by the Ethical Committees for Animal Experimentation at Osaka Prefecture University. Rat primary cortical astrocytes were prepared and maintained in DMEM containing 10% FBS, 100 μg/ml streptomycin, and 50 units/ml penicillin in a humidified atmosphere of 95% air and 5% CO_2 as described previously [31]. For the experiments, astrocytes were replated on day 14 or later into culture dishes or plates (cell density: 4×10^5 cells/ml). In our experiments, there were more than 95% astrocytes as determined by GFAP immunohistochemistry (Figure 2).

2.3. NO Measurement. The production of nitrite which is a stable metabolite of NO was measured as previously mentioned [31]. Astrocytes, seeded in 96-well plates, were stimulated with 1 μg/ml LPS for 24 h with or without isoflavones. The concentration of nitrite in cell-free supernatant was determined fluorometrically using DAN reagents with ARVO 1420 Multilabel counter (Wallac, Turuk, Finland; excitation/emission: 355/460 nm).

2.4. Cell Viability Assay. The viability of astrocytes was measured using colorimetric MTT assay as mentioned previously [31]. Absorbance at 585 nm was measured using ARVO 1420 Multilabel counter.

2.5. Measurement of Intracellular ROS. Intracellular ROS generation was estimated by H_2DCFDA, the cell-permeable fluorescent dye, as previously described [31]. Briefly, 96-well

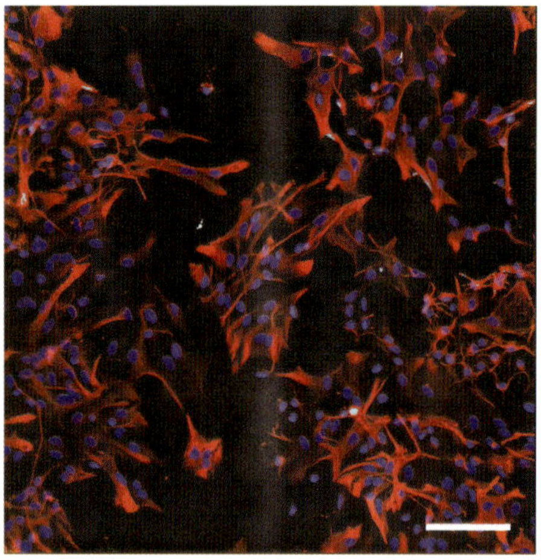

FIGURE 2: Representative immunohistochemical staining for GFAP (astrocyte, red), CD11b (microglia, green), and DAPI staining (nuclei, blue) in rat primary cortical astrocytes. Scale bar = 20 μm.

plated astrocytes were stimulated with 1 μg/ml LPS with or without 50 μM each isoflavones for 3, 6, and 24 h. After that, 5 μM H_2DCFDA was added to the cells in serum-free medium and incubated for 30 min at 37°C. Dichlorofluorescein (DCF) fluorescent intensity in the cells was measured to estimate ROS generation with ARVO 1420 Multilabel counter, excitation/emission 485/535 nm.

2.6. Western Blotting. Cultured astrocytes in 60-mm dishes were stimulated with LPS with or without 50 μM *S*-equol, and subjected to gel electrophoresis followed by immunoblotting as previously described [31].

Immunoblotting was performed using antibodies to iNOS (1 : 10,000), ERK1/2 (1 : 1,000), phosphorylated ERK1/2 (*p*-ERK 1/2; 1 : 1,000), p38-MAPK (1 : 1,000), phosphorylated p38-MAPK (*p*-p38-MAPK; 1 : 1,000), or β-actin (1 : 100,000). Protein detection was performed with the aid of enhanced chemiluminescence detection reagents and quantified with LAS-4000 lumino-imaging analyzer (Fujifilm, Tokyo, Japan).

2.7. Data Analysis. For estimation of NO and ROS, each group consisting of six culture plates per experiment was studied. Experiments were carried out using five separate seedings of the cells. Data are presented as means ± SEM. The differences between treatments were analyzed by one-way ANOVA followed by the Tukey-Kramer multiple comparison procedure or Student's *t*-test and considered statistically significant when value of $p < 0.05$.

3. Results and Discussion

3.1. S-Equol Attenuated Both Protein Expression of iNOS and NO Production in LPS-Stimulated Astrocytes. It is widely accepted that immune response in the CNS plays critical roles in several neurodegenerative diseases such as AD, PD, and stroke [1, 2]. Under these pathological conditions, inflammatory responses have been employed to stimulate astrocytes and microglia, resulting in activation of pattern recognition receptors including TLRs. Such activation generates inflammatory mediators including proinflammatory cytokines such as TNFα and IL-1β, free radicals, and NO. LPS directly binds and activates TLR4 and its signaling cascades are thought to mimic those under neurodegenerative diseases [28, 29]. Therefore, stimulating astrocytes with LPS is a useful model to investigate neuroinflammation.

We first examined whether *S*-equol has an inhibitory effect on LPS-stimulated NO production. Cultured astrocytes were treated with 1 μg/ml LPS in the presence of various concentrations of *S*-equol for 24 h, and NO production in the medium was determined. In the presence of *S*-equol LPS-induced NO production was attenuated in a dose-dependent manner (Figure 3(a)). Significant inhibitory effects were observed with *S*-equol concentration of 25 μM or higher. *S*-Equol, in concentrations up to 100 μM used in this study, did not affect the cell viability (Figure 3(b)).

To explore the mechanism by which *S*-equol inhibits LPS-induced NO production, we next investigated iNOS expression with western blotting. Astrocytes were treated with LPS with or without 50 μM *S*-equol for 24 h; the expressions of iNOS levels were compared. Similar to NO production, *S*-equol significantly inhibited LPS-induced iNOS expression (Figure 3(c)).

We also examined the effect of other isoflavones on NO production. Genistein and daidzein are popular isoflavones found in soybean that also act as phytoestrogens [16, 17]. Similar to *S*-equol, both genistein and daidzein significantly inhibited LPS-induced NO production (Figure 3(d)). This result of genistein confirmed the previous reports that genistein prevents neuroinflammatory changes in astrocytes [26, 27]. These results suggest that these isoflavones reduce neuroinflammatory changes such as NO production in LPS-stimulated cultured astrocytes.

3.2. S-Equol Had No Effect on LPS-Induced Intracellular ROS Production. The antioxidant property of *S*-equol is well documented in several lines of cells such as macrophages [32] and aortic endothelial cells [33] during inflammation. In addition, treatment of astrocytes with LPS leads to ROS production followed by induction of iNOS expression [34, 35]. Thus, reduced NO production by *S*-equol (Figure 3(a)) might be due to decreased ROS production. To test this, we investigated intracellular ROS generation in *S*-equol-treated astrocytes. Treatment with LPS to astrocytes increased ROS production at 3, 6, and 24 h (Figure 4(a)), as reported previously [31]. Addition of 50 μM *S*-equol failed to decrease LPS-induced ROS production at least within 24 h. Moreover, applying *S*-equol of 100 μM, most effective dose in attenuating NO production in this study (Figure 3(a)), did not mitigate LPS-induced ROS production at 6 h when ROS production was highest in the present study (*S*-equol, 113.2 ± 3.1; LPS, 156.1 ± 5.5; *S*-equol + LPS, 173.7 ± 10.1 in % of control, resp.). Similar results were obtained by using other isoflavones, genistein and daidzein, although each of these isoflavones alone had no significant effect on ROS production (Figure 4(b)). It is unlikely that isoflavones, at least examined in the present study, scavenge ROS and mitigate oxidative stress in astrocytes.

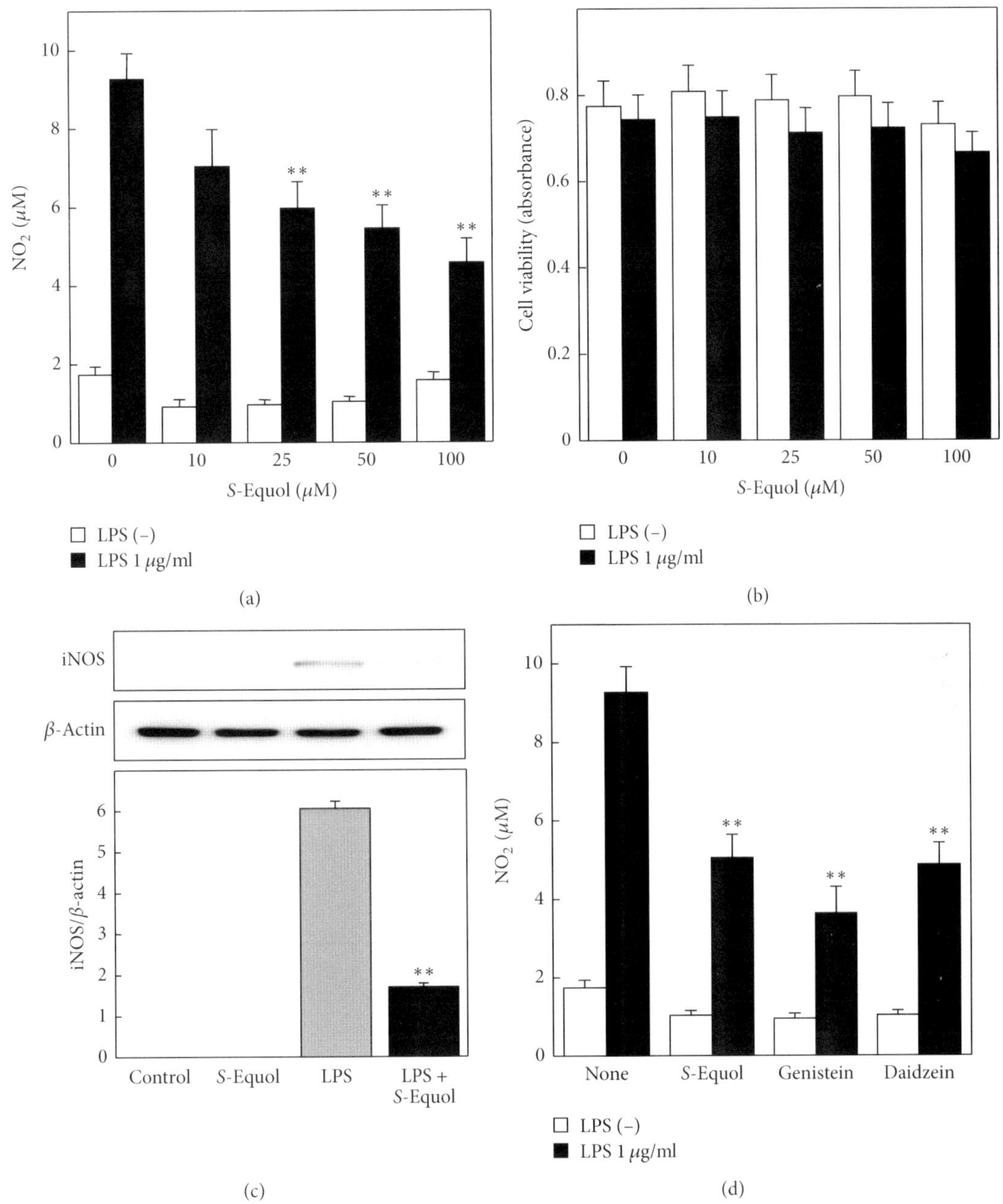

FIGURE 3: Effect of *S*-equol on LPS-induced NO production, cell viability, and expression of iNOS protein. Cultured astrocytes were stimulated with 1 μg/ml LPS for 24 h in the presence of various concentrations of *S*-equol. The nitrite concentration in the medium was measured fluorometrically (a), and cell viability was evaluated with the MTT assay (b). The cells were treated with 1 μg/ml LPS in the absence or presence of 50 μM *S*-equol for 24 h. The expression of iNOS protein was detected with western blotting (c). Effect of isoflavones (*S*-equol, genistein, and daidzein, each concentration of 50 μM) on LPS-induced NO production (d). Data are the mean ± SEM of 5-6 samples. $^{**}p < 0.01$ significantly different from 1 μg/ml LPS.

It is well known that LPS activates MAPKs which mediate intracellular signaling cascades associated with a variety of cellular activities such as cell proliferation, differentiation, survival, and death [36, 37]. To clarify the possible mechanism of *S*-equol-induced suppression of NO production, we checked the effect of *S*-equol on MAPK activation. Astrocytes were stimulated by LPS in the presence or absence of *S*-equol for different time periods (1, 3, and 6 h), and we determined the changes in total and phosphorylated (activated) p38-MAPK and ERK1/2 by western blotting. LPS significantly increased the p38-MAPK phosphorylation at 1, 3, and 6 h. Cotreatment with *S*-equol and LPS had no effect on p38-MAPK activation (Figures 5(a)–5(c)). Also, trend toward increased phosphorylation of ERK1/2 induced by LPS was not affected by the addition of *S*-equol at 1, 3, and 6 h (Figures 5(d)–5(f)). These results suggest that factors other than ROS

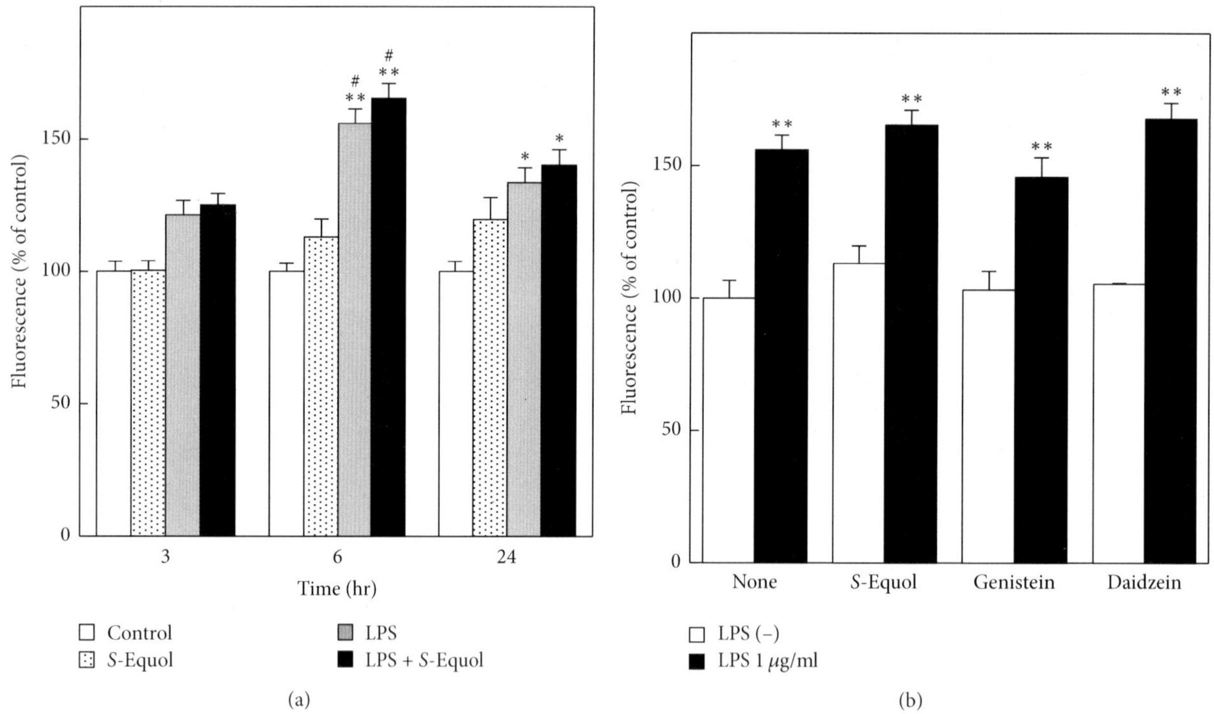

FIGURE 4: Effect of S-equol on LPS-induced ROS production. Cultured astrocytes were treated with LPS (1 μg/ml) in the absence or presence of 50 μM S-equol for 3, 6, and 24 h, and the intracellular ROS levels were evaluated using the DCFDA method (a). Effect of isoflavones (S-equol, genistein, and daidzein, each concentration of 50 μM) on LPS-induced ROS production at 6 h after LPS treatment (b). Data are the mean ± SEM of 5 samples. $^{*}p < 0.05$; $^{**}p < 0.01$ significantly different from the nontreated control. $^{\#}p < 0.05$ significantly different from S-equol.

or MAPKs such as p38-MAPK and ERK may be responsible for the reduction of NO production by S-equol. Additional work is necessary to clarify this issue.

3.3. S-Equol Exerted Its Effect via a Nongenomic Pathway. It is well known that estrogen exerts genomic effects through intracellular nuclear receptor family, ERα and ERβ, that are located in the cytoplasm or on the nuclear membrane [10]. To investigate the molecular mechanism of NO inhibition by S-equol in LPS-activated astrocytes, we next examined the effect of ICI 182.780, an intracellular ER antagonist, on NO production. Addition of 1 μM ICI 182.780 had no effect on S-equol-induced decrease in NO production (Figure 6).

Recently several lines of evidence reveal that estrogen also acts on the receptor which is located on plasma membrane, activating multiple signaling pathways that regulate cellular function [11–13]. To ascertain whether these nongenomic pathways are responsible for S-equol-induced inhibition of NO production, we investigated the effect of agonist/antagonist of GPR30. Addition of 1 μM G-15, antagonist of GPR30, partially recovered S-equol-induced attenuation of NO production. Moreover, cotreatment of LPS with GPR30 agonist G-1 (100 nM), instead of S-equol, significantly inhibited NO production, although its effect was lesser than that of S-equol. These results suggest that S-equol attenuates LPS-induced NO production, at least in part, via GPR30-mediated pathway.

The effect of equol on astrocyte function has not been fully investigated previously. In the present study, we revealed, for the first time, that S-equol attenuated LPS-induced NO production in astrocytes. Since excessive production of NO aggravates neuronal damage in neurodegenerative diseases [1–3], our results indicate the role of S-equol in the attenuation of inflammatory response in CNS. In general, isoflavones are known to be an antioxidant, and, indeed, daidzein has been reported to suppress ROS production in microglia during LPS-induced neuroinflammation [24]. In addition, LPS-induced NO production was inhibited by estrogen which was antagonized in the presence of ICI 182.780 in macrophage [38], indicating that these effects are mediated by classical genomic pathway. In contrast, S-equol failed to show antioxidative effect in astrocytes (Figure 4). Therefore, the differences in the effects of S-equol on astrocytes and microglia may be attributed to the expression of ER. Moreover, GPR30 antagonist did not completely recover the S-equol-induced suppressive effect of NO production, suggesting that other nongenomic pathways such as PI3 kinase-Akt signaling may also be responsible for the effect of S-equol [39, 40]. Additional studies are needed to reveal the precise mechanism induced by S-equol. Because equol is thought to be easier to pass through BBB than other isoflavones due to its chemical structure [22, 41], our results show new insight into the idea that intake of S-equol may be used for managing CNS diseases.

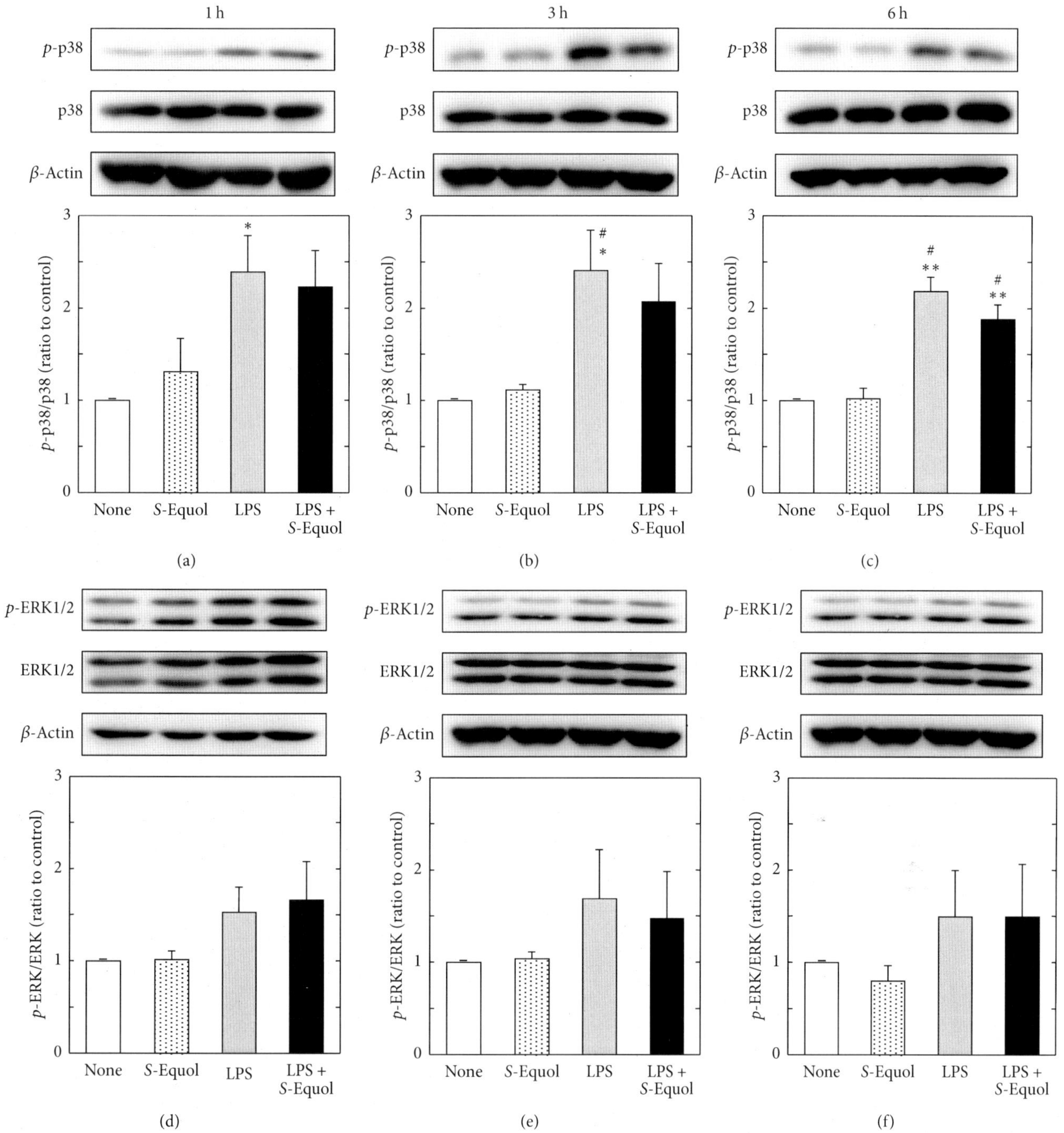

FIGURE 5: Effect of S-equol on LPS-induced MAPK expression. Cultured astrocytes were treated with LPS (1 μg/ml) with or without S-equol (50 μM) for 1, 3, and 6 h, and then the expressions of phosphorylated and total p38-MAPK (a–c) and ERK1/2 (d–f) proteins were detected with western blotting. In case of ERK1/2, total density of two bands was analyzed. Data are the mean ± SEM of 4 samples. $^{*}p < 0.05$; $^{**}p < 0.01$ significantly different from the nontreated control. $^{\#}p < 0.05$ significantly different from S-equol.

4. Conclusions

In summary, our study demonstrates that a soybean isoflavone S-equol is a key factor in modulating neuroinflammation induced by the glial activation. S-Equol exerts its effect, at least in part, via a nongenomic pathway.

Abbreviations

AD: Alzheimer's disease
DAPI: 4′,6-Diamidino-2-phenylindole
DCF: Dichlorofluorescein
DMEM: Dulbecco's modified Eagle medium

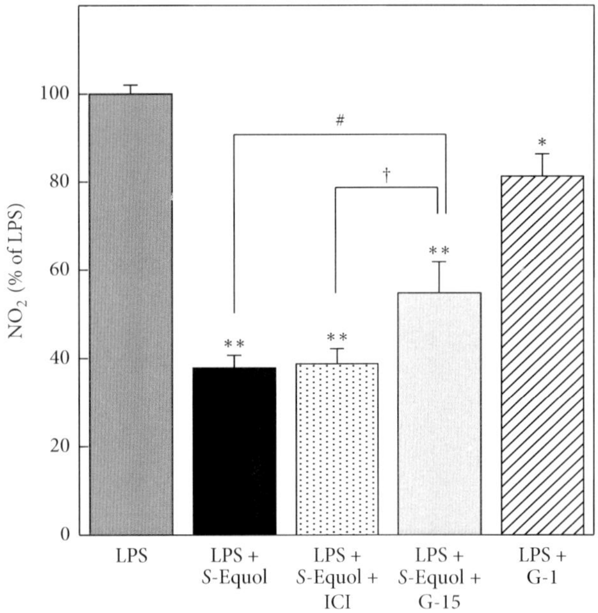

FIGURE 6: Effect of ER antagonist/agonist on LPS-induced NO production. Cultured astrocytes were treated with LPS (1 μg/ml) and *S*-equol (50 μM) in the presence of ICI 182.780 (an intracellular ER antagonist; 1 μM) or G-15 (a GPR30 antagonist; 1 μM) for 24 h, and NO production was evaluated as described in Figure 3. Some cultures were treated with LPS (1 μg/ml) and G-1 (a GPR30 agonist; 100 nM) for 24 h, and NO production was determined. Data are the mean ± SEM of 5 samples. $^{*}p < 0.05$; $^{**}p < 0.01$ significantly different from LPS. $^{\#}p < 0.05$ statistical difference between LPS + *S*-equol and LPS + *S*-equol + G-15. $^{\dagger}p < 0.05$ statistical difference between LPS + *S*-equol + ICI and LPS + *S*-equol + G-15.

ER:	Estrogen receptor
ERK:	Extracellular signal-regulated kinase
FBS:	Fetal bovine serum
GPR30:	G protein-coupled receptor 30
H_2DCFDA:	2′,7′-Dichlorodihydrofluorescein diacetate
IFNγ:	Interferon-γ
IL-1β:	Interleukin-1β
iNOS:	Inducible nitric oxide synthase
LPS:	Lipopolysaccharide
MAPK:	Mitogen activated protein kinase
MTT:	3-(4,5-Dimethyl-2-thiazolyl)-2,5-diphenyl-tetrazolium bromide
NO:	Nitric oxide
PD:	Parkinson's disease
ROS:	Reactive oxygen species
TLRs:	Toll-like receptors
TNFα:	Tumor necrosis factor-α.

Disclosure

The present address of Kenji Kawabe is Department of Regenerative Science, Okayama University Graduate School of Medicine, Dentistry and Pharmaceutical Sciences, Okayama, Japan.

Authors' Contributions

Mitsuaki Moriyama conceived and designed the experiments; Mitsuaki Moriyama, Ayano Hashimoto, Kenji Kawabe, Mizue Ogawa, and Hideyo Satoh performed the experiments; Mitsuaki Moriyama, Katsura Takano, and Yoichi Nakamura analyzed the data; Mitsuaki Moriyama and Yoichi Nakamura wrote the paper.

Acknowledgments

This work was supported in part by JSPS KAKENHI Grants nos. 7K08127 (to Mitsuaki Moriyama), 15K07768 (to Yoichi Nakamura), and 17K15390 (to Katsura Takano).

References

[1] S.-M. Lucas, N. J. Rothwell, and R. M. Gibson, "The role of inflammation in CNS injury and disease," *British Journal of Pharmacology*, vol. 147, supplement 1, pp. S232–S240, 2006.

[2] E. Czirr and T. Wyss-Coray, "The immunology of neurodegeneration," *The Journal of Clinical Investigation*, vol. 122, no. 4, pp. 1156–1163, 2012.

[3] V. Calabrese, C. Mancuso, M. Calvani, E. Rizzarelli, D. A. Butterfield, and A. M. G. Stella, "Nitric oxide in the central nervous system: neuroprotection versus neurotoxicity," *Nature Reviews Neuroscience*, vol. 8, no. 10, pp. 766–775, 2007.

[4] M. Chakrabarti, A. Haque, N. L. Banik, P. Nagarkatti, M. Nagarkatti, and S. K. Ray, "Estrogen receptor agonists for attenuation of neuroinflammation and neurodegeneration," *Brain Research Bulletin*, vol. 109, pp. 22–31, 2014.

[5] A. Villa, E. Vegeto, A. Poletti, and A. Maggi, "Estrogens, Neuroinflammation, and Neurodegeneration," *Endocrine Reviews*, vol. 37, no. 4, pp. 372–402, 2016.

[6] E. Acaz-Fonseca, R. Sanchez-Gonzalez, I. Azcoitia, M. A. Arevalo, and L. M. Garcia-Segura, "Role of astrocytes in the neuroprotective actions of 17β-estradiol and selective estrogen receptor modulators," *Molecular and Cellular Endocrinology*, vol. 389, no. 1-2, pp. 48–57, 2014.

[7] E. Vegeto, S. Belcredito, S. Etteri et al., "Estrogen receptor-alpha mediates the brain antiinflammatory activity of estradiol," *Proceedings of the National Acadamy of Sciences of the United States of America*, vol. 100, no. 16, pp. 9614–9619, 2003.

[8] D. K. Lewis, A. B. Johnson, S. Stohlgren, A. Harms, and F. Sohrabji, "Effects of estrogen receptor agonists on regulation of the inflammatory response in astrocytes from young adult and middle-aged female rats," *Journal of Neuroimmunology*, vol. 195, no. 1-2, pp. 47–59, 2008.

[9] X. Yue, M. Lu, T. Lancaster et al., "Brain estrogen deficiency accelerates Aβ plaque formation in an Alzheimer's disease animal model," *Proceedings of the National Academy of Sciences of the United States of America*, vol. 102, no. 52, pp. 19198–19203, 2005.

[10] N. Heldring, A. Pike, S. Andersson et al., "Estrogen receptors: How do they signal and what are their targets," *Physiological Reviews*, vol. 87, no. 3, pp. 905–931, 2007.

[11] E. R. Levin, "Plasma membrane estrogen receptors," *Trends in Endocrinology & Metabolism*, vol. 20, no. 10, pp. 477–482, 2009.

[12] Y.-C. Hsieh, H.-P. Yu, M. Frink et al., "G protein-coupled receptor 30-dependent protein kinase A pathway is critical in nongenomic effects of estrogen in attenuating liver injury after trauma-hemorrhage," *The American Journal of Pathology*, vol. 170, no. 4, pp. 1210–1218, 2007.

[13] E. R. Prossnitz, L. A. Sklar, T. I. Oprea, and J. B. Arterburn, "GPR30: a novel therapeutic target in estrogen-related disease," *Trends in Pharmacological Sciences*, vol. 29, no. 3, pp. 116–123, 2008.

[14] J. Guan, B. Yang, Y. Fan, and J. Zhang, "GPER agonist G1 attenuates neuroinflammation and dopaminergic neurodegeneration in Parkinson disease," *Neuroimmunomodulation*, vol. 24, no. 1, pp. 60–66, 2017.

[15] T.-Z. Zhao, Q. Ding, J. Hu, S.-M. He, F. Shi, and L.-T. Ma, "GPER expressed on microglia mediates the anti-inflammatory effect of estradiol in ischemic stroke," *Brain and Behavior*, vol. 6, no. 4, p. e00449, 2016.

[16] J. Rodríguez-Morató, M. Farré, C. Pérez-Maná et al., "Pharmacokinetic comparison of soy isoflavone extracts in human plasma," *Journal of Agricultural and Food Chemistry*, vol. 63, no. 31, pp. 6946–6953, 2015.

[17] J. Yu, X. Bi, B. Yu, and D. Chen, "Isoflavones: anti-inflammatory benefit and possible caveats," *Nutrients*, vol. 8, no. 12, p. 361, 2016.

[18] K. D. R. Setchell and C. Clerici, "Equol: history, chemistry, and formation," *Journal of Nutrition*, vol. 140, no. 7, pp. 1355s–1362s, 2010.

[19] K. D. R. Setchell and C. Clerici, "Equol: Pharmacokinetics and biological actions," *Journal of Nutrition*, vol. 140, no. 7, pp. 1363s–1368s, 2010.

[20] A. M. Mahmoud, W. Yang, and M. C. Bosland, "Soy isoflavones and prostate cancer: a review of molecular mechanisms," *The Journal of Steroid Biochemistry and Molecular Biology*, vol. 140, pp. 116–132, 2014.

[21] E. D. Lephart, "Skin aging and oxidative stress: Equol's anti-aging effects via biochemical and molecular mechanisms," *Ageing Research Reviews*, vol. 31, pp. 36–54, 2016.

[22] D. A. Schreihofer and L. Redmond, "Soy phytoestrogens are neuroprotective against stroke-like injury in vitro," *Neuroscience*, vol. 158, no. 2, pp. 602–609, 2009.

[23] J.-W. Jeong, H. H. Lee, M. H. Han, G.-Y. Kim, W.-J. Kim, and Y. H. Choi, "Anti-inflammatory effects of genistein via suppression of the toll-like receptor 4-mediated signaling pathway in lipopolysaccharide-stimulated BV2 microglia," *Chemico-Biological Interactions*, vol. 212, no. 1, pp. 30–39, 2014.

[24] S. J. Chinta, A. Ganesan, P. Reis-Rodrigues, G. J. Lithgow, and J. K. Andersen, "Anti-inflammatory role of the isoflavone diadzein in lipopolysaccharide-stimulated microglia: implications for Parkinson's disease," *Neurotoxicity Research*, vol. 23, no. 2, pp. 145–153, 2013.

[25] L. Subedi, E. Ji, D. Shin, J. Jin, J. H. Yeo, and S. Y. Kim, "Equol, a dietary daidzein gut metabolite attenuates microglial activation and potentiates neuroprotection in vitro," *Nutrients*, vol. 9, no. 3, p. 207, 2017.

[26] H. Lu, J.-X. Shi, D.-M. Zhang et al., "Inhibition of hemolysate-induced iNOS and COX-2 expression by genistein through suppression of NF-κB activation in primary astrocytes," *Journal of the Neurological Sciences*, vol. 278, no. 1-2, pp. 91–95, 2009.

[27] S. L. Valles, P. Dolz-Gaiton, J. Gambini et al., "Estradiol or genistein prevent Alzheimer's disease-associated inflammation correlating with an increase PPARγ expression in cultured astrocytes," *Brain Research*, vol. 1312, pp. 138–144, 2010.

[28] S. Amor, L. A. N. Peferoen, D. Y. S. Vogel et al., "Inflammation in neurodegenerative diseases—an update," *The Journal of Immunology*, vol. 142, no. 2, pp. 151–166, 2014.

[29] J. Drouin-Ouellet and F. Cicchetti, "Inflammation and neurodegeneration: the story 'retolled'," *Trends in Pharmacological Sciences*, vol. 33, no. 10, pp. 542–551, 2012.

[30] Y. Nakamura, T. Kitagawa, H. Ihara, S. Kozaki, M. Moriyama, and Y. Kannan, "Potentiation by high potassium of lipopolysaccharide-induced nitric oxide production from cultured astrocytes," *Neurochemistry International*, vol. 48, no. 1, pp. 43–49, 2006.

[31] M. Moriyama, R. Kurebayashi, K. Kawabe, K. Takano, and Y. Nakamura, "Acetate attenuates lipopolysaccharide-induced nitric oxide production through an anti-oxidative mechanism in cultured primary rat astrocytes," *Neurochemical Research*, vol. 41, no. 11, pp. 3138–3146, 2016.

[32] G.-C. Yen and H.-H. Lai, "Inhibition of reactive nitrogen species effects in vitro and in vivo by isoflavones and soy-based food extracts," *Journal of Agricultural and Food Chemistry*, vol. 51, no. 27, pp. 7892–7900, 2003.

[33] J.-E. Chung, S. Y. Kim, H. H. Jo et al., "Antioxidant effects of equol on bovine aortic endothelial cells," *Biochemical and Biophysical Research Communications*, vol. 375, no. 3, pp. 420–424, 2008.

[34] S. Y. Lee, D. J. Son, Y. K. Lee et al., "Inhibitory effect of sesaminol glucosides on lipopolysaccharide-induced NF-κB activation and target gene expression in cultured rat astrocytes," *Neuroscience Research*, vol. 56, no. 2, pp. 204–212, 2006.

[35] S. Pawate, Q. Shen, F. Fan, and N. R. Bhat, "Redox regulation of glial inflammatory response to lipopolysaccharide and interferonγ," *Journal of Neuroscience Research*, vol. 77, no. 4, pp. 540–551, 2004.

[36] M. Raman, W. Chen, and M. H. Cobb, "Differential regulation and properties of MAPKs," *Oncogene*, vol. 26, no. 22, pp. 3100–3112, 2007.

[37] Y. Zhang and C. Dong, "Regulatory mechanisms of mitogen-activated kinase signaling," *Cellular and Molecular Life Sciences*, vol. 64, no. 21, pp. 2771–2789, 2007.

[38] L. Liu and Z. Wang, "Estrogen attenuates lipopolysaccharide-induced nitric oxide production in macrophages partially via the nongenomic pathway," *Cellular Immunology*, vol. 286, no. 1-2, pp. 53–58, 2013.

[39] G. Han, H. Ma, R. Chintala et al., "Nongenomic, endothelium-independent effects of estrogen on human coronary smooth muscle are mediated by type I (neuronal) NOS and PI3-kinase-Akt signaling," *American Journal of Physiology-Heart and Circulatory Physiology*, vol. 293, no. 1, pp. H314–H321, 2007.

[40] A.-M. Jaubert, N. Mehebik-Mojaat, D. Lacasa, D. Sabourault, Y. Giudicelli, and C. Ribière, "Nongenomic estrogen effects on nitric oxide synthase activity in rat adipocytes," *Endocrinology*, vol. 148, no. 5, pp. 2444–2452, 2007.

[41] G. R. Sareddy, B. C. Nair, V. K. Gonugunta et al., "Therapeutic significance of estrogen receptor β agonists in gliomas," *Molecular Cancer Therapeutics*, vol. 11, no. 5, pp. 1174–1182, 2012.

Potential Pitfalls of the Humanized Mice in Modeling Sepsis

Krzysztof Laudanski,[1] Michael Stentz,[2] Matthew DiMeglio,[3] William Furey,[3] Toby Steinberg,[1] and Arpit Patel[1]

[1]*Department of Anesthesiology and Critical Care, University of Pennsylvania, Philadelphia, PA 19104, USA*
[2]*Department of Anesthesiology and Intensive Care, Emory University, Atlanta, GA 30322, USA*
[3]*Philadelphia College of Osteopathic Medicine, Philadelphia, PA 19131, USA*

Correspondence should be addressed to Krzysztof Laudanski; klaudanski@gmail.com

Academic Editor: Jean-Marc Cavaillon

Humanized mice are a state-of-the-art tool used to study several diseases, helping to close the gap between mice and human immunology. This review focuses on the potential obstacles in the analysis of immune system performance between humans and humanized mice in the context of severe acute inflammation as seen in sepsis or other critical care illnesses. The extent to which the reconstituted human immune system in mice adequately compares to the performance of the human immune system in human hosts is still an evolving question. Although certain viral and protozoan infections can be replicated in humanized mice, whether a highly complex and dynamic systemic inflammation like sepsis can be accurately represented by current humanized mouse models in a clinically translatable manner is unclear. Humanized mice are xenotransplant animals in the most general terms. Several organs (e.g., bone marrow mesenchymal cells, endothelium) cannot interact with the grafted human leukocytes effectively due to species specificity. Also the interaction between mice gut flora and the human immune system may be paradoxical. Often, grafting is performed utilizing an identical batch of stem cells in highly inbred animals which fails to account for human heterogeneity. Limiting factors include the substantial cost and restricting supply of animals. Finally, humanized mice offer an opportunity to gain knowledge of human-like conditions, requiring careful data interpretation just as in nonhumanized animals.

1. Introduction

Animal models are frequently employed as a precursor to clinical trials and even more broadly in research investigations. Despite their enormous contribution to the development of scientific knowledge, there is a well-funded and accepted appreciation of their limitations [1–3]. Animal and human physiology may be similar, but this is not a universal rule [4]. For example, the toll-like receptor pathway is relatively conserved in both humans and *Drosophila*, but the clinical response to ligands varies between animals and humans [5]. These differences are sufficiently profound to prevent the successful, direct translation of discoveries in mice into human clinical trials. However, the high prevalence and mortality resulting from sepsis necessitate further research in the field of critical care inflammation using animal models [2, 6].

Some of the issues hampering clinical implementation of discoveries in animal models are related to the shortcomings of the general methodology of animal experimentation [3]. Animals are often inbred and kept in sterile conditions, leading to high homogeneity. While reducing interindividual variability is helpful in pure laboratory research, the applicability of the research may be compromised by the lack of diversity typical of human patients. It is also questionable how well the environment of the animal facility resembles natural conditions. Stable temperature, rigorously controlled diet, multiple barriers to prevent infection, and limitations on animal mobility due to housing constraints are far from typical clinical environments [2, 7]. Furthermore, disease models are only an approximation of illness and may not correspond well to clinical scenarios [8]. For example, cecal ligation and puncture are a widely employed model of sepsis in rodents, but they have been criticized for not adequately reflecting typical clinical conditions and treatment [3, 9]. In particular, antibiotic and fluid management are dramatically different between lab animals and clinical settings [2, 10]. Lastly, rodent models offer only limited efficacy in testing several higher-order neurological functions such as cognition, memory, and emotional regulation which makes modeling of inflammation-induced dysfunction of central nervous system somewhat difficult.

Numerous papers have been published debating the utility of animal models [3, 4, 8, 9]. There is little doubt that animal models are essential research tools, but increased concerns have triggered a search for alternative methods to investigate important clinical questions [3, 4, 8, 11]. With the National Institutes of Health (NIH) emphasizing "translational research," there is added impetus to look for these alternatives.

One promising approach to bridging this translational gap is the application of "humanized mice." Here, we will review the basic understanding of their immunology and their applicability to human disease in the context of acute critical care illness. Our review discusses certain characteristics of the humanized mice model that are potentially limiting their capacity for direct translation of research findings into clinical therapy [9, 12].

2. Development of "the Ideal" Humanized Mice

Humanized mice can be defined simply as mice carrying human genes or tissues such as leukocytes, stem cells, organs, and tumors [12]. In this review, we will focus only on animals with a reconstituted immune system and not mice with transplanted human neoplastic tissues, human pancreatic islets, cardiomyocytes, or other biological materials. A viable humanized mouse model is contingent on the successful development of an immunodeficient host enabling the native immune system to combat the transplanted one. Consequently, the primary goal of humanized mice development is to engineer mice with increasingly deficient native immune systems to curb the rejection of the transplanted immune system [13–15]. The secondary goal is aimed at providing the grafted cells with a specific microenvironment in which they can successfully settle and thrive [16].

2.1. Development of Immunocompromised Host. The earliest model consisted of CB17 mice strain carrying the $Prkdc^{scid}$ mutation leading to severe combined immunodeficiency (SCID) [13, 16]. The first attempt was a simple transplant of human peripheral leukocytes into mice [14]. HIV-1 was the primary impetus for the development of this model, notwithstanding issues with efficient grafting and graft stability with overrepresentation of NK cell activity. The development of nonobese diabetic- (NOD-) *scid* mice further improved the engraftment in comparison to previous immunodeficient host types [17]. The success of this subsequent model was attributed to its decreased NK cell activity and the emergence of additional defects of innate immunity, which allowed for higher levels of engraftment [10, 18]. Null mutations in the IL-2 receptor γ chain ($IL2rg^{null}$) were particularly successful in attaining this goal. Consequently, mouse strains including IL-2 receptor γ chain mutations such as NOD/Shi-$scid/IL2r\gamma^{-/-}$ (NOG), NOD-$Ragl^{-/-}IL2r\gamma^{-/-}$ (NRG), NOD-$scid/IL2r\gamma^{-/-}$ (NSG), or BALB/c/$Rag2^{-/-}IL2r\gamma^{-/-}$ (BRG) were widely adapted for their best hosting capability [15, 18–20]. The deletion of β2-microglobulin (NOD-*said* $B2m^{-/-}$), a critical component of MHC I, further improved engraftment compared to NOD-*SCID* mice [16]. The most unique feature of the NOD-$Ragl^{-/-}$ mice was generation of the first radiation-resistant strain, though engraftment was less efficient as compared to previous strains [19, 21]. Progress continued in developing mice strains with increasingly deficient native immune systems improving graft success and stability. Subsequently, the newest types of humanized mice have satisfactory recovery of T cells, B cells, and NK cells despite some variability [22–24]. At the same time, they suffer from diminished monocyte and dendritic cell counts coupled with frequently underperforming function of their humanized leukocytes [25–27]. High variability in emergence of the human mononuclear component results from the variable expression of signal regulatory protein-α (SIRP-α) [28].

The immunocompromised host retains a significant part of the native immune system despite all aforementioned interventions. Consequently, all models are at risk of developing graft versus host disease (GVHD) since transplanted $CD8^+$ cells will interact with MHC class I of the host [15, 28, 29]. Incomplete eradication of the native immune system results in the development of lymphomas whereby more advanced humanized models have had much longer lag time and a lower propensity allowing for prolonged longitudinal studies [30].

2.2. Evolution of Grafting. First, researchers observed that human peripheral blood mononuclear cells (PBMCs) could engraft successfully [14, 31]. While injecting mice with PBMCs resulted in the reconstitution of T cells, the high risk of graft versus host disease limited such models to short-term experiments [14]. In next step human fetal thymus and liver were implanted into the kidney capsule and $CD34^+$ cells from bone marrow (BLT model) [32]. This system preserved the complex interaction between antigen presenting cells (APCs) and T cells, which is critical in the resolution of acute inflammation [8, 10, 32]. MHC restricted selection of T cells took place in this model. Furthermore, a secondary lymphatic system developed along the human mucosal immune system. In the next step, $CD34^+$ stem cells were used for grafting allowing for even more complete restoration of the immune system (HIS model) [33, 34]. This model featured high graft stability and diversity, proportional to the number of cells used for grafting [33–36].

Due to a lack of species-specific cytokines and inefficient ability of host mesenchymal cells to support function of the leukocytes, an emergence of a more complete human immune system was impaired [23, 37, 38]. Lack of interlocking cytokine networks contributed to the poor regulation of leukocyte populations [39]. Nanoparticles, plasmids, and lentiviruses were tried to boost the supportive environment of mice bone marrow since optimal cytokine environment is pivotal for the emergence of a complete immune system [21, 38, 39]. Despite these efforts and several other modifications, the development of most specialized cells was hampered [40, 41]. Even more alarming was the emergence of unintended consequences of genetic manipulation aimed at boosting the production of human cytokines. For example, Billerbeck et al. found that increased expression of stem cells factor, IL-3, and GM-CSF led not only to the increased expression of monocytes but also to the significant skewness of the circulating T cells toward Fox3(+) T cells [37]. Aberration of composition of leukocyte population is one of the critical phenomena of sepsis. Consequently, an introduction of any bias may affect the validity of results and their translation into clinical practice. Currently, engineering of MIRTG mice, which can produce four human cytokines endogenously, is the most sophisticated model even among similar models [23, 40, 41]. Assessment of MIRTG mice performance in sepsis follows.

2.3. Additional Techniques. Ancillary techniques surrounding grafting procedures have evolved as well. Initially, all animals were subjected to irradiation to remove the native immune system [15–17, 19, 33, 34, 36, 40]. However, collateral damage to supportive structures of bone marrow and organs was often present. Humanized mice with *Rag2* mutations appeared to be less sensitive to the effects of radiation [19, 41]. Some mice strains such as those carrying the *c-kit* mutation did not need irradiation, but they have not been evaluated in sepsis studies [42]. Finally, chemical ablation can be used, but it appears to have a detrimental effect on animal survival [34].

Since murine monocytes and other indigenous phagocytic cells are responsible for poor engraftment, several targeted techniques aimed at their eradication were developed such as the use of anti-murine SIRPα, CD47, or Ncf1 knockout, and clodronate liposomes [42–44].

Additionally, reconstitution of the immune system was found to be more efficient and better tolerated in newborn versus adult mice especially if augmented by the injection of human grafting factors [12].

3. The Performance of Immune System Components in Humanized Mice

Reconstitution of the human immune system is a relatively slow process that may take up to 3 months [53]. B cells are the earliest leukocytes to reconstitute, followed by T cells [18]. B cells in humanized mice produce all classes of immunoglobulins [22, 53, 58–60]. These data should be viewed with caution since the maturation of B cells and antibody class switching from IgM to IgG are particularly inefficient as compared to the human system [61, 62]. Effective immunoglobulin class switching is critical for recovery from an acute infectious process. The lack of human IL-6 is considered one of the most important reasons for this inefficiency. Only recently, a novel model of humanized mice with active human IL-6 gene was described. Interestingly, while the immunoglobulin switch was more efficient in this model, the maturation of B cells remained impaired [63]. Evaluation of these IL-6 boosted mice should be noteworthy as IL-6 is one of the critical cytokines in the development of sepsis. Additionally, the introduction of human stem cell factor, granulocyte macrophage stimulating factor, and IL-3 into the BLT model resulted in more efficient maturation and optimized immunoglobulin production at baseline and after viral infection [38].

T cells obtained from humanized mice after reconstitution are proficient as measured by the delayed hypersensitivity reaction, but their ability to respond to antigen was suboptimal [45]. Introduction of the BLT model partially resolved this problem as human T cells rely on grafted fetal thymus for clonal selection [53]. The performance of T cells depended on several factors but was mostly mediated by stimulation via MHC class II or IL-2R [22]. Since humanized mice are xenotransplanted animals, it is unclear how a state of tolerance to different MHC antigens affects their performance. Lack of MHC-matched APCs would impair that process [25, 33, 64]. Conversely, an additional transplant of sensitized dendritic cells alleviated the problem and presented an interesting opportunity for future research [54]. Altering the cytokine environment was another way to improve the presence of APCs like dendritic cells (DCs) [33, 54, 65–67]. In critical care illnesses, like sepsis, dendritic cells emerge from circulating monocytes that stimulate optimal T cell responses [10, 32]. Recently, only one study has investigated monocyte function in sepsis using humanized mice [55]. Other T cell populations may encounter similar difficulties as well. Reconstitution of the T cells in mucosal membranes depends on the presence of $\gamma\delta$ chain, but its expression was variable in humanized mice [68]. Since this subtype of T cells plays a critical role in the emergence of the tolerance and the modulation of complex T cell responses, it is unclear how the deficit will affect the evolution of the immune response in the setting of critical care illness. T cells with regulatory properties (T_{reg}) are present in humanized mice, but their role seems to be conflicting in terms of function and number, and it is greatly influenced by the cytokine environment [37, 69]. It is also worth mentioning that balance between different T cell populations may be abnormal in humanized mice and was linked to a deficiency of the human cytokine network [22, 29, 37, 45, 48].

Myeloid cells are the last to reconstitute after grafting. Stem cell factor, M-CSF, GM-CSF, and IL-4 are supportive in speed and efficiency of the recovery as well as in functional maturation [23, 70]. Slow and incomplete reconstitution of the myeloid line results in the inability of T cells to mount a proficient response to antigen challenges. Enhanced recovery of the myeloid compartment was seen in MISTRG and MITRG mice [23]. MO obtained from humanized mice resemble neonatal cells in their ability to upregulate CD80/CD86, two critical factors in modulating T cell function [25]. MO from humanized animals were shown to generate a robust T cell response and cytokine production after sepsis [35, 55]. Supplementation of the humanized mice with *in vitro* generated allogeneic DCs can restore T cell responsiveness [46, 64, 65]. DCs emerge in some humanized models on their own or after Flt3 supplementation [46, 49].

TABLE 1: Pitfalls of humanized models and the means to compensate them.

Problem definition	*Impact on progress in research*	*Ways to overcome limitations*	*Ref.*
The artificial condition of housing	Increased susceptibility of the animals to infection, decreased immunity,	Creating a more realistic environment for housing	[2, 4, 7, 12]
Clinical relevance of septic model in general	Separation of the research outcome from clinical reality.	Developing more clinically relevant model by introducing fluid resuscitation and antibiotics, comparisons between humanized and non-humanized animals.	[2, 8, 10]
Homogeneity of animals	Decrease robustness of the findings.	Increasing diversity, developing models with different strains, engaging in cross-species research, grafting with different stem cells.	
Preservation of mice native immune system	Incomplete or inefficient grafting, GVHD, the emergence of lymphomas	Development of more profoundly immunosuppressed hosts, eradication of the residual immune system, knock-out of SIRP-α.	[13, 16, 17, 19, 24, 28, 30, 34, 45–47]
Lack of supportive human cytokine environment	Inefficient grafting, inefficient cytokine network and immune system regulation	Supplementation of human cytokines via various means	[31, 37, 48–52]
Poor recovery of certain leukocyte population	Incomplete restoration of the immune system, ineffective and clinically irrelevant responses	Introduction of HIS, BLT, MITGR models, supplementation of human cytokines via genetic engineering,	[10, 16, 19, 22, 24, 25, 33, 34, 36, 44, 53]
Immunoglobulin switching	Inability to mimic humoral responses	Development of human IL-6 producing mice, introduction of additional cytokine modification	[38, 54]
Functional immaturity of human leukocytes	The inappropriate response, difficulties in translating	Supplementation of adequate cytokine environment, ex vivo cell maturation, and supplementation	[35, 51, 55]
Poor inter-organ communication	Difficulty mimicking complex interaction between organs in sepsis	Additional transplantation to better mimic inter-organ interaction in the autologous/allogeneic system, the introduction of human intestinal flora	[35, 54–57]

Such *in vivo*-generated and antigen-sensitive DCs can trigger T cell response to a specific antigen [49].

In summary, these studies show that the function of several leukocyte populations can be restored during reconstitution of the immune system. However, the complex nature of the process, dependence on numerous interventions, and unclear functional competency of leukocytes undermine the robustness of the humanized model.

4. Current Studies of Humanized Mice and Sepsis

Humanized mice were used successfully to study HIV [19, 30]. Most recently, several other viral infections were successfully modeled in humanized mice including Zika and West Nile virus [59, 71]. Introduction of Epstein-Barr virus reproduced several traits of the infection with high fidelity in humanized mice [40]. The ability to replicate the trajectory of viral hepatitis, longevity, and mimicry of response to subsequent infections made humanized mice especially suitable for finding the optimal drug to cure hepatitis C [71]. The endothelial inflammation of the highly lethal dengue virus and other pathological agents causing hemorrhagic fever were investigated in humanized mice, but concerns were raised regarding the accuracy of the model [60, 72, 73]. Of primary concern was the ability of the xenotransplant to mimic vasculitis and interactions between mice endothelium and human immune system [55, 74–76]. This illustrates a typical shortcoming of humanized mice when the interaction between two organs encounters an interspecies difference that can be overcome only through further modification of the models (Table 1). Whether these modifications make the model closer to reality or more artificial remains to be ascertained.

The success of humanized mice in mimicking viral infections established high expectations for using them to study sepsis [2, 32].

Sepsis is a highly prevalent and serious condition that has a profound and prolonged impact on morbidity and mortality [6, 40, 55, 74–77]. Unsinger et al. demonstrated that humanized mice replicate several key features of the septic process, including apoptosis and exaggerated cytokine production [10]. Bone marrow suppression closely resembling the natural history of sepsis was seen as well [77]. The critical role of HMGB1, TLR4, and Notch in sepsis and apoptosis was also demonstrated using humanized mice [67, 76–78]. However, the degree to which these processes replicate the complexity of the septic response is difficult to assess fully. For example, IL-15, a critical cytokine for the development of sepsis-related apoptosis, can be studied in humanized mice only after modification of the model still resulting in production of age-dependent IL-15 [32, 39, 78]. Introduction of several human cytokines improved cell recovery but introduced artificially skewed populations [37]. It was demonstrated that extended depression in bone marrow function is mediated by methylation changes in the PU.1 gene, and retransplantation of the postsepsis surviving mice with allogeneic stem cells partially restored immune reactivity [55]. However, M-CSF production and biological activities were limited to transplanted stem cells since the mice environment did not provide indigenously produced cross-reactive cytokines [66, 70]. It becomes evident that these observations may not reflect clinical reality with so many features absent from the model.

Other humans disease models successfully mimicked in humanized mice include Toxic Shock Syndrome Toxin-1-(TSST-1-) mediated shock and staphylococcal infections [40, 76]. To date, only a few research investigations have focused on sepsis in humanized mice [10, 27, 55, 67, 76, 77]. The CLP model of sepsis is by far the most popular for studying sepsis despite several shortcomings of the CLP itself and some unique features of humanized mice undergoing sepsis.

Further studies with humanized mice tested clinical compounds for the treatment of sepsis. Wang et al. tested the potential of curcumin analogs to reverse lung injury secondary to sepsis in humanized mice [27]. Autologous stem cell transplants showed a potential to reverse some of the postseptic immune system aberrations, but clinical relevance remains to be seen [55]. In another example, antibodies to human-specific toxins were tested [79]. Finally, a researcher utilized humanized mice to test indomethacin as the modulator of the immune response in neonatal sepsis under the assumption that the functional immaturity of the grafted immune system was a good model of neonatal immunity [79, 80]. These results are guarded due to insufficient evidence as to whether immature humanized mice and neonatal immunology are in fact equivalent.

5. Limitations of Humanized Mice Models to Study Sepsis

Humanized mice seem to be an appealing choice to investigate the pathology and treatment of sepsis [2, 10, 32, 75]. However, interest remains relatively low. PubMed cites approximately 90 publications for which "*sepsis*" and "*humanized mice*" are keywords. Many of the authors assume that several limitations of humanized mice prevent broader implementation into mainstream septic research (Table 1). Humanized mice earned justifiable praise from several researchers. However, the inherited problems of this model have been acknowledged by a few [8, 10, 12, 29, 42, 62, 77, 81].

First, there exist fundamental differences between human and mice physiology [11]. More specifically, humanized mice exhibit several differences in the natural history of sepsis. Weight loss and mortality are greater in humanized mice than wild-type mice when short-term and long-term data are analyzed [35, 55, 67, 81]. Only the introduction of extensive measures (antibiotics, fluid resuscitation, and diet modification) resulted in animal survival exceeding a couple days [35, 55]. Prolonged studies were complicated by the emergence of GVHD and lymphomas as well as the suppressive effect of preserved components of the indigenous mice immune system [15, 29, 82]. Additionally, the recovery of the granulocyte compartment required supplementation of human G-CSF [50]. Considering that granulocytes are a pivotal defense against microbial infections, this need for supplementation is a shortcoming of humanized mice in mimicking their function and heterogeneity significantly limiting that model [2, 32]. The deficit in the granulocyte compartment may also underlie early mortality in sepsis and require a more aggressive therapeutic approach [55]. Furthermore, all leukocyte types demonstrate a sign of functional immaturity unless remedial measures are implemented [25, 31, 36, 46, 66]. The corrective modification may create an artificial condition on its own or only be partially effective [37, 38]. In the example of T_{reg} expansion in humanized cells, the imbalance may not reflect the natural history of sepsis or postseptic leukocyte population changes [37]. Other shifts in T cell population composition were reported, but virtually no study investigated population heterogeneity of monocytes, NK, and B cells in the context of the response to infection [35, 45, 55]. Finally, another limitation exists in that some of the pivotal cells of the immune system are not replaced in grafting. Particularly, microglia are not part of the humanized grafted system with potentially profound negative effects on the modeling of the central nervous system's effects from sepsis.

Second, the time after grafting is critical for modulating immune responses. A minimum of 8 weeks is required for NSG grafting but longer periods are related to the emergence of lymphoma and GVHD [28, 50, 60, 82]. The question of how to measure the age of humanized mice remains. Possible measurements include host's age, grafting time, or the age of the grafted human immune system. This important question has some biological underpinnings since the production of cytokines in response to pathogens has been reported as a variable dependent on the amount of time after grafting [78]. Since sepsis disproportionally affects the lower and upper extremes of age, younger mice are still reconstituting their immune system while older ones are at higher risk of immune system disorders; humanized mice may not be the most suitable model in age-related studies of sepsis [2, 6, 32, 83].

To improve grafting, animals are frequently irradiated. Despite wide acceptance of this process, the effect of irradiation on humanized mouse physiology and sepsis remains complex and extends beyond just the immune system [56, 84]. Certain humanized models do not require irradiation, but none of them have been evaluated in septic conditions [19, 24, 85].

Third, gut flora has a significant effect on the performance of the immune system and is increasingly perceived as one of the modifiers for sepsis trajectory [2, 32]. Humanized mice have mouse gut flora interacting with the human immune system, but significant alterations are also introduced by irradiation [41, 84]. Some attempts to establish human-specific flora in humanized animals have been tried to increase the fidelity of the models since gut immune interaction is gaining increased recognition in the pathology of sepsis [72].

Fourth, sepsis is a multiorgan disease with poorly defined etiologies. The multiple interactions between pathogen and host organs as well as between the host organs themselves are crucial for understanding the clinical trajectory [2, 32, 85]. Mesenchymal cells, the central nervous system, and endothelium are frequently quoted culprits of unfavorable outcomes in sepsis [57, 85, 86]. Several deficits in the crosstalk between the grafted human immune system and mice organs may create a translation barrier for implementation of humanized mice into sepsis research [73]. Their xenotransplant nature inherently limits their usefulness as it was already suggested in studies of hemorrhagic fever or meningitis [57, 86]. Additionally, the endothelium is critical for immune system performance, and humanized mice are deemed a less favorable model for them unless significant modification is introduced [57]. Moreover, on the level of immune system interaction between APC and effector cells is notably ineffective. Vagal nerve or subcortical structures have also been suggested as playing a role in sepsis outcomes [2, 32, 86]. Meanwhile, it is unclear how the murine nervous system interacts with the human immune system during critical care illness. Lastly, mesenchymal cells are not able to have crosstalk efficiently with the grafted human immune system unless modified [51].

These are significant limitations of humanized mice as a model of sepsis due to the xenotransplant nature of these animals. In contrast, humanized mice are robust models to study pathogen cycles or relatively simple, most likely conservative, immunological processes since these illnesses trigger very specific immune system response or have a life cycle that is independent of the immune system [40, 59, 71, 72, 82].

Fifth, one often-overlooked limitation of the humanized mouse model is the statistical approach to the grafted animals. For example, several mice can be injected with the same stem cell. It is then debatable whether these mice represent one organism/ecosystem repeated several times or if they are independent experiments. Using the same cells in highly modified NSG mice would intuitively support the former conclusion. On the other hand, the interaction of the immune system with the mouse body results in unavoidable (and perhaps desirable) stochastic variation in the characteristics of the immune system.

Finally, one cannot ignore the costly nature of the humanized mice model. The high initial cost derives from the cost of stem cells used for grafting since the efficiency of grafting is proportional to the cells used for grafting. Furthermore, the animals must be housed in exceptionally protective conditions and may require a special maintenance regimen. Often, mice production is lengthy and, in some cases, restricted by patents.

6. Conclusions

In conclusion, humanized mice promise a better approximation of human physiology and are often recommended as a tool to bridge the gap between rodent models and clinical scenarios. However, such a view is potentially oversimplified. Our review shows that humanized mice have several unclear biases, which may profoundly affect their ability to mimic clinically relevant scenarios of sepsis. Furthermore, the significant cost and limitations associated with this model may not justify their use. There is little doubt that humanized mice are a useful tool to study the partial mechanism of sepsis, but the complexity of this disease demands more sophisticated models whereby several complex systems may interact with each other.

Acknowledgments

The authors would like to express appreciation to Lucia DiNapoli for proofreading this manuscript. This work is supported by the National Institute of Health NIGMS 1K23GM120630-01A1.

References

[1] Á. González-Fernández, J. Faro, and C. Fernández, "Immune responses to polysaccharides: Lessons from humans and mice," *Vaccine*, vol. 26, no. 3, pp. 292–300, 2008.

[2] R. P. Dellinger, M. M. Levy, A. Rhodes et al., "Surviving sepsis campaign: international guidelines for management of severe sepsis and septic shock: 2012. Surviving Sepsis Campaign Guidelines Committee including the Pediatric Subgroup," *Intensive Care Medicine*, vol. 41, no. 2, pp. 580–637, 2013.

[3] M. F. Osuchowski, D. G. Remick, J. A. Lederer et al., "Abandon the mouse research ship? Not just yet!," *Shock*, vol. 41, no. 6, pp. 463–475, 2014.

[4] J. Mestas and C. C. W. Hughes, "Of mice and not men: differences between mouse and human immunology," *The Journal of Immunology*, vol. 172, no. 5, pp. 2731–2738, 2004.

[5] E. P. McCarron, D. P. Williams, D. J. Antoine et al., "Exploring the translational disconnect between the murine and human inflammatory response: Analysis of LPS dose–response relationship in murine versus human cell lines and implications for translation into murine models of sepsis," *Journal of Inflammation Research*, vol. 8, pp. 201–209, 2015.

[6] H. E. Wang, R. S. Devereaux, D. M. Yealy, M. M. Safford, and G. Howard, "National variation in United States sepsis mortality: A descriptive study," *International Journal of Health Geographics*, vol. 9, article no. 9, 2010.

[7] D. Masopust, C. P. Sivula, and S. C. Jameson, "Of mice, dirty mice, and men: Using mice to understand human immunology," *The Journal of Immunology*, vol. 199, no. 2, pp. 383–388, 2017.

[8] P. McGonigle and B. Ruggeri, "Animal models of human disease: Challenges in enabling translation," *Biochemical Pharmacology*, vol. 87, no. 1, pp. 162–171, 2014.

[9] J. Seok, HS. Warren, AG. Cuenca, MN. Mindrinos, HV. Baker, W. Xu et al., "Genomic responses in mouse models poorly mimic human inflammatory diseases," *Proceedings of the National Acadamy of Sciences of the United States of America*, vol. 110, no. 9, pp. 3507–3512, 2013.

[10] J. Unsinger, J. S. McDonough, L. D. Shultz, T. A. Ferguson, and R. S. Hotchkiss, "Sepsis-induced human lymphocyte apoptosis

and cytokine production in "humanized" mice," *Journal of Leukocyte Biology*, vol. 86, no. 2, pp. 219–227, 2009.

[11] J. P. Sundberg, A. Berndt, B. A. Sundberg et al., "The mouse as a model for understanding chronic diseases of aging: the histopathologic basis of aging in inbred mice," *Pathobiology of Aging & Age-related Diseases*, vol. 1, article 7179, 2011.

[12] M. A. Brehm, A. Cuthbert, C. Yang et al., "Parameters for establishing humanized mouse models to study human immunity: Analysis of human hematopoietic stem cell engraftment in three immunodeficient strains of mice bearing the IL2rγnull mutation," *Clinical Immunology*, vol. 135, no. 1, pp. 84–98, 2010.

[13] G. C. Bosma, R. P. Custer, and M. J. Bosma, "A severe combined immunodeficiency mutation in the mouse," *Nature*, vol. 301, no. 5900, pp. 527–530, 1983.

[14] D. E. Mosier, R. J. Gulizia, S. M. Baird, and D. B. Wilson, "Transfer of a functional human immune system to mice with severe combined immunodeficiency," *Nature*, vol. 335, no. 6187, pp. 256–259, 1988.

[15] M. A. King, L. Covassin, M. A. Brehm et al., "Human peripheral blood leucocyte non-obese diabetic-severe combined immunodeficiency interleukin-2 receptor gamma chain gene mouse model of xenogeneic graft-versus-host-like disease and the role of host major histocompatibility complex," *Clinical & Experimental Immunology*, vol. 157, no. 1, pp. 104–118, 2009.

[16] S. W. Christianson, D. L. Greiner, R. A. Hesselton et al., "Enhanced human CD4+ T cell engraftment in beta2-microglobulin-deficient NOD-scid mice," *Journal of immunology (Baltimore, Md)*, vol. 158, no. 8, pp. 3578–3586, 1950.

[17] M. Ito, H. Hiramatsu, K. Kobayashi et al., "NOD/SCID/γcnull mouse: An excellent recipient mouse model for engraftment of human cells," *Blood*, vol. 100, no. 9, pp. 3175–3182, 2002.

[18] P. Lan, N. Tonomura, A. Shimizu, S. Wang, and Y.-G. Yang, "Reconstitution of a functional human immune system in immunodeficient mice through combined human fetal thymus/liver and CD34+ cell transplantation," *Blood*, vol. 108, no. 2, pp. 487–492, 2006.

[19] L. D. Shultz, P. A. Lang, S. W. Christianson et al., "NOD/LtSz-Rag1(null) mice: An immunodeficient and radioresistant model for engraftment of human hematolymphoid cells, HIV infection, and adoptive transfer of NOD mouse diabetogenic T cells," *The Journal of Immunology*, vol. 164, no. 5, pp. 2496–2507, 2000.

[20] S. P. McDermott, K. Eppert, E. R. Lechman, M. Doedens, and J. E. Dick, "Comparison of human cord blood engraftment between immunocompromised mouse strains," *Blood*, vol. 116, no. 2, pp. 193–200, 2010.

[21] L. D. Shultz, P. A. Schweitzer, S. W. Christianson et al., "Multiple defects in innate and adaptive immunologic function in NOD/LtSz-scid mice," *Journal of immunology (Baltimore, Md)*, vol. 154, no. 1, pp. 180–191, 1950.

[22] Y. Watanabe, T. Takahashi, A. Okajima et al., "The analysis of the functions of human B and T cells in humanized NOD/shi-scid/γcnull (NOG) mice (hu-HSC NOG mice)," *International Immunology*, vol. 21, no. 7, pp. 843–858, 2009.

[23] A. Rongvaux, T. Willinger, J. Martinek et al., "Development and function of human innate immune cells in a humanized mouse model," *Nature Biotechnology*, vol. 32, no. 4, pp. 364–372, 2014.

[24] B. E. McIntosh, M. E. Brown, B. M. Duffin et al., "Nonirradiated NOD,B6.SCID Il2rγ-/- kitW41/W41 (NBSGW) mice support multilineage engraftment of human hematopoietic cells," *Stem Cell Reports*, vol. 4, no. 2, pp. 171–180, 2015.

[25] C. Gille, T. W. Orlikowsky, B. Spring et al., "Monocytes derived from humanized neonatal NOD/SCID/IL2Rγ null mice are phenotypically immature and exhibit functional impairments," *Human Immunology*, vol. 73, no. 4, pp. 346–354, 2012.

[26] C. S. Netherby, M. N. Messmer, L. Burkard-Mandel et al., "The granulocyte progenitor stage is a key target of irf8-mediated regulation of myeloid-derived suppressor cell production," *The Journal of Immunology*, vol. 198, no. 10, pp. 4129–4139, 2017.

[27] Y. Wang, X. Shan, Y. Dai et al., "Curcumin Analog L48H37 Prevents Lipopolysaccharide-Induced TLR4 Signaling Pathway Activation and Sepsis via Targeting MD2," *The Journal of Pharmacology and Experimental Therapeutics*, vol. 353, no. 3, pp. 539–550, 2015.

[28] N. Hilger, J. Glaser, C. Müller et al., " Attenuation of graft-versus-host-disease in NOD scid IL-2Rγ ," *Cytometry Part A*, vol. 89, no. 9, pp. 803–815, 2016.

[29] N. Ali, B. Flutter, R. Sanchez Rodriguez et al., "Xenogeneic Graft-versus-Host-Disease in NOD-scid IL-2Rγnull Mice Display a T-Effector Memory Phenotype," *PLoS ONE*, vol. 7, no. 8, p. e44219, 2012.

[30] B. K. Berges and M. R. Rowan, "The utility of the new generation of humanized mice to study HIV-1 infection: Transmission, prevention, pathogenesis, and treatment," *Retrovirology*, vol. 8, article no. 65, 2011.

[31] T. Lapidot, F. Pflumio, M. Doedens, B. Murdoch, D. E. Williams, and J. E. Dick, "Cytokine stimulation of multilineage hematopoiesis from immature human cells engrafted in SCID Mice," *Science*, vol. 255, no. 5048, pp. 1137–1141, 1992.

[32] J. Cohen, J. L. Vincent, and N. K. Adhikari, "Sepsis: a roadmap for future research," *The Lancet Infectious Diseases*, vol. 15, no. 5, pp. 581–614, 2015.

[33] A. K. Palucka, J. Gatlin, J. P. Blanck et al., "Human dendritic cell subsets in NOD/SCID mice engrafted with CD34 + hematopoietic progenitors," *Blood*, vol. 102, no. 9, pp. 3302–3310, 2003.

[34] S. Watanabe, S. Ohta, M. Yajima et al., "Humanized NOD/SCID/IL2Rγnull mice transplanted with hematopoietic stem cells under nonmyeloablative conditions show prolonged life spans and allow detailed analysis of human immunodeficiency virus type 1 pathogenesis," *Journal of Virology*, vol. 81, no. 23, pp. 13259–13264, 2007.

[35] K. Laudanski, N. Lapko, M. Zawadka, B. X. Zhou, G. Danet-Desnoyers, and G. S. Worthen, "The clinical and immunological performance of 28 days survival model of cecal ligation and puncture in humanized mice," *PLoS ONE*, vol. 12, no. 7, 2017.

[36] M. C. André, A. Erbacher, C. Gille et al., "Long-term human CD34+ stem cell-engrafted nonobese diabetic/SCID/IL-2Rγnull mice show impaired CD8+ T cell maintenance and a functional arrest of immature NK cells," *The Journal of Immunology*, vol. 185, no. 5, pp. 2710–2720, 2010.

[37] E. Billerbeck, W. T. Barry, K. Mu, M. Dorner, C. M. Rice, and A. Ploss, "Development of human CD4+FoxP3+ regulatory T cells in human stem cell factor-, granulocyte-macrophage colony-stimulating factor-, and interleukin-3-expressing NOD-SCID IL2Rγnull humanized mice," *Blood*, vol. 117, no. 11, pp. 3076–3086, 2011.

[38] S. Jangalwe, L. D. Shultz, A. Mathew, and M. A. Brehm, "Improved B cell development in humanized NOD-scid IL2Rγnull mice transgenically expressing human stem cell factor, granulocyte-macrophage colony-stimulating factor and interleukin-3," *Immunity, Inflammation and Disease*, vol. 4, no. 4, pp. 427–440, 2016.

[39] Q. Chen, M. Khoury, and J. Chen, "Expression of human cytokines dramatically improves reconstitution of specific

human-blood lineage cells in humanized mice," *Proceedings of the National Acadamy of Sciences of the United States of America*, vol. 106, no. 51, pp. 21783–21788, 2009.

[40] M. W. Melkus, J. D. Estes, A. Padgett-Thomas et al., "Humanized mice mount specific adaptive and innate immune responses to EBV and TSST-1," *Nature Medicine*, vol. 12, no. 11, pp. 1316–1322, 2006.

[41] J. S. Knibbe-Hollinger, N. R. Fields, T. R. Chaudoin et al., "Influence of age, irradiation and humanization on NSG mouse phenotypes," *Biology Open*, vol. 4, no. 10, pp. 1243–1252, 2015.

[42] Z. Hu, N. Van Rooijen, and Y.-G. Yang, "Macrophages prevent human red blood cell reconstitution in immunodeficient mice," *Blood*, vol. 118, no. 22, pp. 5938–5946, 2011.

[43] T. Yamauchi, K. Takenaka, S. Urata et al., "Polymorphic Sirpa is the genetic determinant for NOD-based mouse lines to achieve efficient human cell engraftment," *Blood*, vol. 121, no. 8, pp. 1316–1325, 2013.

[44] K. J. Lavender, R. J. Messer, B. Race, and K. J. Hasenkrug, "Production of bone marrow, liver, thymus (BLT) humanized mice on the C57BL/6 Rag2-/-γc-/-CD47-/- background," *Journal of Immunological Methods*, vol. 407, pp. 127–134, 2014.

[45] D. Rajesh, Y. Zhou, E. Jankowska-Gan et al., "Th1 and Th17 immunocompetence in humanized NOD/SCID/IL2rγnull mice," *Human Immunology*, vol. 71, no. 6, pp. 551–559, 2010.

[46] E. R. Jarman, K. Perschke, E. Montermann et al., "Deficient cytokine response of human allergen-specific T lymphocytes from humanized SCID mice and reconstitution by professional antigen- presenting cells," *The Journal of Allergy and Clinical Immunology*, vol. 105, no. 5, pp. 967–974, 2000.

[47] K. Takenaka, T. K. Prasolava, J. C. Y. Wang et al., "Polymorphism in Sirpa modulates engraftment of human hematopoietic stem cells," *Nature Immunology*, vol. 8, no. 12, pp. 1313–1323, 2007.

[48] A. Kimura and T. Kishimoto, "IL-6: Regulator of Treg/Th17 balance," *European Journal of Immunology*, vol. 40, no. 7, pp. 1830–1835, 2010.

[49] Y. Ding, A. Wilkinson, A. Idris et al., "FLT3-ligand treatment of humanized mice results in the generation of large numbers of CD141+ and CD1c+ dendritic cells in vivo," *The Journal of Immunology*, vol. 192, no. 4, pp. 1982–1989, 2014.

[50] A. M. Coughlan, C. Harmon, S. Whelan et al., "Myeloid engraftment in humanized mice: Impact of granulocyte-colony stimulating factor treatment and transgenic mouse strain," *Stem Cells and Development*, vol. 25, no. 7, pp. 530–541, 2016.

[51] M. Carretta, B. de Boer, J. Jaques et al., "Genetically engineered mesenchymal stromal cells produce IL-3 and TPO to further improve human scaffold-based xenograft models," *Experimental Hematology*, vol. 51, pp. 36–46, 2017.

[52] J. Bergounioux, M. Coureuil, E. Belli et al., "Experimental evidence of bacterial colonization of human coronary microvasculature and myocardial tissue during meningococcemia," *Infection and Immunity*, vol. 84, no. 10, pp. 3017–3023, 2016.

[53] A. K. Wege, M. W. Melkus, P. W. Denton, J. D. Estes, and J. V. Garcia, "Functional and phenotypic characterization of the humanized BLT mouse model," *Current Topics in Microbiology and Immunology*, vol. 324, pp. 149–165, 2008.

[54] G. Salguero, A. Daenthanasanmak, C. Münz et al., "Dendritic cell-mediated immune humanization of mice: Implications for allogeneic and xenogeneic stem cell transplantation," *The Journal of Immunology*, vol. 192, no. 10, pp. 4636–4647, 2014.

[55] N. Lapko, M. Zawadka, J. Polosak et al., "Long-term Monocyte Dysfunction after sepsis in humanized mice is related to persisted activation of macrophage-colony stimulation factor (M-CSF) and demethylation of PU.1, and it can be reversed by blocking m-csf in vitro or by transplanting naïve autologous stem cells in vivo," *Frontiers in Immunology*, vol. 8, no. 401, 2017.

[56] I. Brook, R. I. Walker, and T. J. Macvittie, "Effect of antimicrobial therapy on bowel flora and bacterial infection in irradiated mice," *International Journal of Radiation Biology*, vol. 53, no. 5, pp. 709–716, 1988.

[57] K. Melican, F. Aubey, and G. Duménil, "Humanized mouse model to study bacterial infections targeting the microvasculature," *Journal of Visualized Experiments*, no. 86, 2014.

[58] H. D. Brightbill, S. Jeet, Z. Lin et al., "Antibodies specific for a segment of human membrane IgE deplete IgE-producing B cells in humanized mice," *The Journal of Clinical Investigation*, vol. 120, no. 6, pp. 2218–2229, 2010.

[59] S. Biswas, H. Chang, P. T. N. Sarkis, E. Fikrig, Q. Zhu, and W. A. Marasco, "Humoral immune responses in humanized BLT mice immunized with West Nile virus and HIV-1 envelope proteins are largely mediated via human CD5 + B cells," *The Journal of Immunology*, vol. 134, no. 4, pp. 419–433, 2011.

[60] S. Jaiswal, K. Smith, A. Ramirez et al., "Dengue virus infection induces broadly cross-reactive human IgM antibodies that recognize intact virions in humanized BLT-NSG mice," *Experimental Biology and Medicine*, vol. 240, no. 1, pp. 67–78, 2015.

[61] D. M. Brainard, E. Seung, N. Frahm et al., "Induction of robust cellular and humoral virus-specific adaptive immune responses in human immunodeficiency virus-infected humanized BLT mice," *Journal of Virology*, vol. 83, no. 14, pp. 7305–7321, 2009.

[62] J. Villaudy, R. Schotte, N. Legrand, and H. Spits, "Critical assessment of human antibody generation in humanized mouse models," *Journal of Immunological Methods*, vol. 410, pp. 18–27, 2014.

[63] H. Yu, C. Borsotti, J.-N. Schickel et al., "A novel humanized mouse model with significant improvement of class-switched, antigen-specific antibody production," *Blood*, vol. 129, no. 8, pp. 959–969, 2017.

[64] A. Harui, S. M. Kiertscher, and M. D. Roth, "Reconstitution of huPBL-NSG mice with donor-matched dendritic cells enables antigen-specific T-cell activation," *Journal of Neuroimmune Pharmacology*, vol. 6, no. 1, pp. 148–157, 2011.

[65] M. A. M. Willart, K. Deswarte, P. Pouliot et al., "Interleukin-1α controls allergic sensitization to inhaled house dust mite via the epithelial release of GM-CSF and IL-33," *The Journal of Experimental Medicine*, vol. 209, no. 8, pp. 1505–1517, 2012.

[66] Y. Peretz, Z. F. Zhou, F. Halwani, and G. J. Prud'homme, "In vivo generation of dendritic cells by intramuscular codelivery of FLT3 ligand and GM-CSF plasmids," *Molecular Therapy*, vol. 6, no. 3, pp. 407–414, 2002.

[67] C. Ye, J.-G. Choi, S. Abraham et al., "Human macrophage and dendritic cell-specific silencing of high-mobility group protein B1 ameliorates sepsis in a humanized mouse model," *Proceedings of the National Acadamy of Sciences of the United States of America*, vol. 109, no. 51, pp. 21052–21057, 2012.

[68] P. W. Denton, T. Nochi, A. Lim et al., "IL-2 receptor γ-chain molecule is critical for intestinal T-cell reconstitution in humanized mice," *Mucosal Immunology*, vol. 5, no. 5, pp. 555–566, 2012.

[69] T. Onoe, H. Kalscheuer, N. Danzl et al., "Human Natural Regulatory T Cell Development, Suppressive Function, and Postthymic Maturation in a Humanized Mouse Model," *The Journal of Immunology*, vol. 187, no. 7, pp. 3895–3903, 2011.

[70] Y. Li, Q. Chen, D. Zheng et al., "Induction of functional human macrophages from bone marrow promonocytes by M-CSF in humanized mice," *The Journal of Immunology*, vol. 191, no. 6, pp. 3192–3199, 2013.

[71] M. Dorner, J. A. Horwitz, B. M. Donovan et al., "Completion of the entire hepatitis C virus life cycle in genetically humanized mice," *Nature*, vol. 501, no. 7466, pp. 237–241, 2013.

[72] J. G. Kuruvilla, R. M. Troyer, S. Devi, and R. Akkina, "Dengue virus infection and immune response in humanized RAG2-/-γc-/- (RAG-hu) mice," *Virology*, vol. 369, no. 1, pp. 143–152, 2007.

[73] J. Mota and R. Rico-Hesse, "Humanized mice show clinical signs of dengue fever according to infecting virus genotype," *Journal of Virology*, vol. 83, no. 17, pp. 8638–8645, 2009.

[74] S. J. Libby, M. A. Brehm, D. L. Greiner et al., "Humanized nonobese diabetic-scid IL2r null mice are susceptible to lethal Salmonella Typhi infection," *Proceedings of the National Acadamy of Sciences of the United States of America*, vol. 107, no. 35, pp. 15589–15594, 2010.

[75] W. Ernst, N. Zimara, F. Hanses, D. N. Männel, B. Seelbach-Göbel, and A. K. Wege, "Humanized mice, a new model to study the influence of drug treatment on neonatal sepsis," *Infection and Immunity*, vol. 81, no. 5, pp. 1520–1531, 2013.

[76] J. Knop, F. Hanses, T. Leist et al., "Staphylococcus aureus Infection in Humanized Mice: A New Model to Study Pathogenicity Associated with Human Immune Response," *The Journal of Infectious Diseases*, vol. 212, no. 3, pp. 435–444, 2015.

[77] T. Skirecki, J. Kawiak, E. Machaj et al., "Early severe impairment of hematopoietic stem and progenitor cells from the bone marrow caused by CLP sepsis and endotoxemia in a humanized mice model," *Stem Cell Research & Therapy*, vol. 6, no. 1, article no. 142, 2015.

[78] A. Rodewohl, J. Scholbach, A. Leichsenring, M. Köberle, and F. Lange, "Age-dependent cellular reactions of the human immune system of humanized NOD scid gamma mice on LPS stimulus," *Journal of Innate Immunity*, vol. 23, no. 3, pp. 258–275, 2017.

[79] W. Ernst, E. Kusi, S. Fill Malfertheiner, E. Reuschel, L. Deml, and B. Seelbach-Göbel, "The effect of Indomethacin and Betamethasone on the cytokine response of human neonatal mononuclear cells to gram-positive bacteria," *Cytokine*, vol. 73, no. 1, pp. 91–100, 2015.

[80] F. Schlieckau, D. Schulz, S. Fill Malfertheiner, K. Entleutner, B. Seelbach-Goebel, and W. Ernst, " A novel model to study neonatal ," *American Journal of Reproductive Immunology*, vol. 80, no. 1, p. e12859, 2018.

[81] A. Prince, H. Wang, K. Kitur, and D. Parker, "Humanized mice exhibit increased susceptibility to staphylococcus aureus pneumonia," *The Journal of Infectious Diseases*, vol. 215, no. 9, pp. 1386–1395, 2017.

[82] K. Schmitt and R. Akkina, "Ultra-Sensitive HIV-1 Latency Viral Outgrowth Assays Using Humanized Mice," *Frontiers in Immunology*, vol. 9, 2018.

[83] I. R. Turnbull, J. J. Wlzorek, D. Osborne, R. S. Hotchkiss, C. M. Coopersmith, and T. G. Buchman, "Effects of age on mortality and antibiotic efficacy in cecal ligation and puncture.," *Shock (Augusta, Ga.)*, vol. 19, no. 4, pp. 310–313, 2003.

[84] K.-H. Song, S.-Y. Jung, S.-H. Kho et al., "Effects of low-dose irradiation on mice with Escherichia coli-induced sepsis," *Toxicology and Applied Pharmacology*, vol. 333, pp. 17–25, 2017.

[85] M. Schouten, W. J. Wiersinga, M. Levi, and T. van der Poll, "Inflammation, endothelium, and coagulation in sepsis," *Journal of Leukocyte Biology*, vol. 83, no. 3, pp. 536–545, 2008.

[86] G. Peña, B. Cai, L. Ramos, G. Vida, E. A. Deitch, and L. Ulloa, "Cholinergic regulatory lymphocytes re-establish neuromodulation of innate immune responses in sepsis," *The Journal of Immunology*, vol. 187, no. 2, pp. 718–725, 2011.

Administration of Protein Kinase D1 Induces a Protective Effect on Lipopolysaccharide-Induced Intestinal Inflammation in a Co-Culture Model of Intestinal Epithelial Caco-2 Cells and RAW264.7 Macrophage Cells

Ditte Søvsø Gundelund Nielsen,[1] Marlene Fredborg,[1] Vibeke Andersen,[2,3] and Stig Purup[1]

[1]*Department of Animal Science, Aarhus University, Blichers Allé 20, 8830 Tjele, Denmark*
[2]*Hospital of Southern Jutland, 6200 Aabenraa, Denmark*
[3]*Institute of Regional Health Research and Institute of Molecular Medicine, University of Southern Denmark, 5000 Odense, Denmark*

Correspondence should be addressed to Ditte Søvsø Gundelund Nielsen; ditteg.nielsen@anis.au.dk

Academic Editor: Jian-Dong Li

Inflammatory bowel diseases (IBD) are chronic inflammatory diseases involving all or part of the gastrointestinal tract. The stress-activated serine-threonine protein kinase D1 (PKD1) protein has previously been implicated in intestinal immune regulation. The objective of this study was to evaluate the effects of human PKD1 in relation to intestinal inflammation, using a co-culture model of intestinal epithelial Caco-2 cells and RAW264.7 macrophages. An inflammatory response was induced in the macrophages by lipopolysaccharide (LPS), upregulating the expression of tumour necrosis factor alpha (TNF-α), interleukin- (IL-) 1β, and IL-6 besides increasing the secretion of TNF-α protein. The effect of administering PKD1 to Caco-2 was evaluated in relation to both amelioration of inflammation and the ability to suppress inflammation initiation. Administration of PKD1 (10–100 ng/ml) following induction of inflammation induced downregulation of TNF-α expression in RAW264.7 cells. In addition, PKD1 administered for 3 h prior to LPS stimulation reduced the subsequent inflammatory response through downregulation of TNF-α, IL-1β, and IL-6 in RAW264.7 cells. These results demonstrate a potential role of PKD1 in the intercellular communication between intestinal epithelial and immune cells, proposing a protective effect of PKD1 on the induction of an inflammatory response in macrophages, an important aspect during the pathogenesis of IBD.

1. Introduction

IBD including Crohn's disease (CD) and ulcerative colitis (UC) are characterized by an impaired intestinal barrier function and enhanced intestinal inflammation. IBD has emerged as global diseases with increasing incidence rates specifically in newly industrialized countries [1]. The pathogenesis of IBD is related to a decreased intestinal barrier function, impeding the segregation between the intestinal epithelial cells (IECs) and the intestinal milieu. Specifically, an impaired intestinal barrier function is associated with disease severity in IBD patients [2] as microbes infiltrate the underlying tissue, inducing inappropriate and excessive activation of the mucosal immune system [3]. Indeed, inappropriate responses to these external stimuli by immune cells including dendritic cells and macrophages contribute to the pathogenesis of IBD as immune and tissue homeostasis is disturbed [4]. Reducing inflammation is of utmost importance in IBD patients and specifically proinflammatory mediators such as IL-6 and TNF-α are enhanced in both CD and UC [5]. Indeed, the immune-regulatory nuclear transcription factor-kappaB (NF-κB) is strongly activated in IECs and macrophages during the course of IBD, augmenting the secretion of proinflammatory cytokines as TNF-α, IL-1, IL-6, IL-12, and IL-23 [6]. However, beneficial effects of the proinflammatory cytokines such as IL-1β, IL-6, and TNF-α are also observed in relation to both inflammation and reepithelialization of wounded intestinal tissue, emphasizing

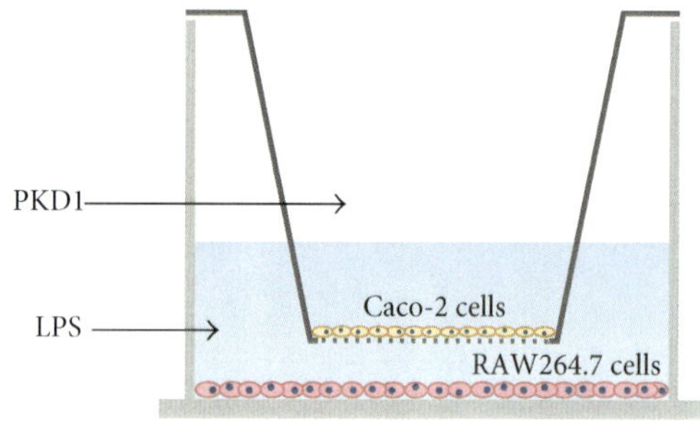

FIGURE 1: Schematic illustration of the co-culture system. Protein kinase D1 (PKD1) was administered to Caco-2 cells grown for 21 days in transwell inserts, while lipopolysaccharide (LPS) was administered to RAW264.7 macrophage cells to induce an inflammatory response.

the importance of temporal control of their expression to balance appropriate responses to intestinal damage and inflammation [7–9].

Human PKD1 is a stress-activated protein kinase implicated in signal transduction, cell proliferation, differentiation, migration, and immune regulation [10]. PKD1 is expressed in B- and T-cells [11] and activated in RAW264.7 macrophage cells upon recognition of bacterial pathogen DNA, inducing activation of NF-κB and subsequent expression of the proinflammatory cytokines, TNF-α, IL-6, IL-8, and IL-12 [12]. Also, PKD1 induces activation of NF-κB in response to oxidative stress [13], protecting IECs against oxidative-stress-induced apoptosis [14]. This suggests an important role for PKD1 in relation to intestinal inflammation. In the present study we investigated two important questions: (1) Can administration of human recombinant PKD1 to IECs ameliorate an already established inflammatory response in macrophages? (2) Can administration of human recombinant PKD1 to IECs suppress initiation of a subsequent LPS-induced inflammatory response in macrophages? To study these effects, we employed an *in vitro* intestinal inflammation model using a co-culture system with intestinal epithelial Caco-2 cells and RAW264.7 macrophage cells (Figure 1) [15].

2. Materials and Methods

2.1. Cell Lines and Culturing. The human epithelial colorectal adenocarcinoma cell line, Caco-2, was kindly donated by Jan Trige Rasmussen (Aarhus University, Denmark). Cells were cultivated in Dulbecco's Modified Eagle Medium (DMEM, Life Technologies, Denmark) supplemented with 10% fetal calf serum (FCS, Bio-Whittaker, Denmark), HEPES (10 mM, Life Technologies), GlutaMax (2 mM, Life Technologies), and penicillin-streptomycin (1% v/v, Sigma-Aldrich, Denmark). RAW264.7 macrophage cells (ATCC, Germany) were cultivated in DMEM supplemented with 10% FCS, 2 mM GlutaMax, and 1% v/v penicillin-streptomycin. Cells were maintained at 37°C and 5% CO_2. Caco-2 cells were passaged using 0.05% Trypsin-EDTA (Life Technologies) and RAW264.7 cells were passaged by scraping off cells when reaching 80–90% confluence.

2.2. Co-Culture Model. Caco-2 cells (passages 10 to 12) were seeded at a density of 4.76×10^5 cells/cm^2 in polyethylene terephthalate cell culture inserts with a pore size of 0.4 μm (BD Falcon, VWR, Denmark) and placed in 6-well cell culture plates (BD Falcon, VWR, Denmark). Cells were cultured for 21 days. On day 20, RAW264.7 cells (passages 5 to 8) were seeded in 6-well cell culture plates at a density of 1.04×10^5 cells/cm^2 in 10% FCS cell culture media. To establish the co-culture model, Caco-2 inserts were transferred to RAW264.7 wells on day 21. RAW264.7 cells were stimulated with 1 μg/ml LPS (*Escherichia coli* O127:B8, Sigma-Aldrich) whereas 0.001, 0.1, 10, and 100 ng/ml PKD1 (129.3 kDa, Thermo Fisher Scientific, Denmark) were added apically to Caco-2 cells (Figure 1). Two studies were performed, either LPS was administered for 3 h followed by PKD1 for 3 h or PKD1 was administered for 3 h followed by LPS for 6 h. Supernatants were collected and stored at −80°C for ELISA analysis, while cells were harvested and stored in RNAlater at −80°C for qPCR analysis. Three biological replicas were performed.

2.3. Transepithelial Electrical Resistance. Triplicate measurements were performed using a Millicell-ERS volt-ohm meter combined with a MERSSTX03 electrode (Millipore, Denmark) according to the manufacturer's guidelines. Caco-2 cells were considered fully differentiated once reaching a stable reading of around 700 Ωcm^2.

2.4. Enzyme-Linked Immunosorbent Assay. Quantikine ELISA analysis of murine TNF-α was performed on supernatant from RAW264.7 cells. Samples were analysed in duplicate according to the manufacturer's guidelines (R&D systems, AH diagnostics, Denmark). Absorbance was measured at 450 nm and wavelength corrected at 540 nm using an EnVision 2103 Multilabel Reader (PerkinElmer, USA).

2.5. Real-Time Reverse-Transcription PCR. Total RNA was isolated and purified using the NucleoSpin RNA II kit according to the manufacturer's guidelines (Macherey-Nagel, Germany). Total RNA concentration and purity was assessed by measuring the absorbance at 260 and 280 nm using a NanoDrop spectrophotometer. Purified RNA was reverse transcribed using oligo(dT) 12–18 primers, random primers, and SuperScript III Reverse Transcriptase (Invitrogen, Denmark). cDNA synthesis was performed at 42°C for 60 minutes followed by reaction inactivation at 70°C for 15 minutes on an Esco Swift MaxPro Thermal Cycler (Holm & Halby, Denmark). cDNA samples were diluted 1:10 and standard samples were diluted 1:5. For real-time PCR quantitation a standard dilution series of 1:4 was prepared and analysed in triplicate, while cDNA samples were analysed in duplicate. The housekeeping gene, hypoxanthine phosphoribosyl transferase (HPRT1), was quantitated by SYBR GREEN PCR master mix (Applied Biosystems, Sweden) using the forward primer: 5′-CAGTCAACGGGCGATATAAAAGTA-3′ and 5′-CCAGTGTCAATTATATCTTCAACAATCAA-3′

Table 1: Primers used during PCR quantitation of selected genes in Caco-2 and RAW264.7 cells.

Analysed in the following	Gene symbol	Gene name	Life-Tech. Id. number	Organism
Caco-2	*TNF-α*	Tumor necrosis factor alpha	Hs01113624_g1	*Homo sapiens*
	PPARG	Peroxisome proliferator-activated receptor gamma	Hs01115513_m1	*Homo sapiens*
	IL-10	Interleukin 10	Hs00961622_m1	*Homo sapiens*
	IL-8	C-X-C motif chemokine ligand 8	Hs00174103_m1	*Homo sapiens*
	CTNNB1	Catenin beta 1	Hs00355049_m1	*Homo sapiens*
RAW264.7	*Gapdh*	Glyceraldehyde-3-phosphate dehydrogenase	Mm99999915_g1	*Mus musculus*
	Tnf-α	Tumor necrosis factor alpha	Mm00443258_m1	*Mus musculus*
	Il-6	Interleukin 6	Mm00446190_m1	*Mus musculus*
	Il-1β	Interleukin 1 beta	Mm00434228_m1	*Mus musculus*

as the reverse primer. The other selected genes were analysed by TaqMan™ Gene Expression Assays consisting of predesigned unlabelled PCR primers (Table 1), TaqMan MGB probes labelled with fluorescein amidite (FAM), and TaqMan Universal Master Mix (Applied Biosystems, Sweden). Fluorescence was detected using the Viaa7 Real-Time PCR System (Applied Biosystems, Sweden) with 40 cycles as follows: 1.6°C/s to 95°C held for 15 sec followed by 1.6°C/s to 60°C for 1 min. GAPDH and HPRT1 were chosen as the housekeeping genes for RAW264.7 and Caco-2 cells, respectively.

2.6. Statistical Analyses. Data were analysed using the MIXED procedure of Statistical Analysis Software (SAS Institute Inc., USA, version 9.3). Mean Ct values of GAPDH or HPRT1 were used to normalize transcription of the target genes for RAW264.7 and Caco-2 cells, respectively. Real-time RT-PCR data are presented as LSMEANS with 95% confidence intervals, relative to the unstimulated negative control (=1) of replicate experiments. Results from ELISA are presented as LSMEANS ± standard error of the mean (SEM) of replicate experiments. Significant differences were judged at $P < 0.05$.

3. Results

3.1. PKD1 Stimulates Secretion of TNF-α from RAW264.7 Cells. To evaluate the immunological response of PKD1 we employed the already established co-culture model with intestinal epithelial Caco-2 cells and RAW264.7 macrophage cells [15–18]. Caco-2 cells were grown for 21 days until forming a confluent monolayer of enterocyte-like cells [19], at which point a co-culture with RAW264.7 macrophages were established, enabling crosstalk between the two individual cell monolayers (Figure 1). RAW264.7 macrophages were stimulated with LPS at a concentration of 1 μg/ml for 6 h, reaching maximum TNF-α secretion within a 24 h period (data not shown). Various concentrations of PKD1 protein were administered apically to Caco-2 cells either before or after stimulation of RAW264.7 cells with LPS. This enabled us to study the ability of PKD1 to ameliorate an already established inflammatory response as well as the ability to suppress initiation of an inflammatory response subsequently induced by LPS.

Stimulation with LPS induced an inflammatory response in RAW264.7 cells within 6 h as observed by secretion of TNF-α at a concentration of approximately 11.5 ng/ml into the basolateral compartment (Figure 2). During this 6 h period of LPS stimulation, the integrity of the Caco-2 monolayer remained stable (data not shown). Administration of PKD1 to Caco-2 cells prior to stimulation with LPS induced TNF-α secretion at all concentrations ($P < 0.05$). In contrast, PKD1 administered following stimulation with LPS induced TNF-α secretion at only 0.1 ng/ml of PKD1.

3.2. Effect of PKD1 on the Expression of Inflammatory Markers. To evaluate the effect of the various treatments, mRNA from Caco-2 and RAW264.7 cells were isolated and the expression of selected genes was evaluated by real-time RT-PCR. The inflammatory response induced by LPS in RAW264.7 cells was confirmed by upregulated expression of IL-1β, IL-6, and TNF-α when compared with the unstimulated control (Figures 3(a)–3(c)). Specifically, a considerable upregulation of both IL-6 and IL-1β expression levels was observed (>5,000 times).

Treatment with PKD1 in the LPS-stimulated Caco-2/RAW264.7 co-culture caused alterations in the expression of TNF-α, whereas IL-1β and IL-6, in RAW264.7 cells, remained unchanged during treatment with PKD1 (Figures 3(a)–3(c)). A concentration-dependent effect on TNF-α was observed with low concentrations of PKD1 (0.001–0.1 ng/ml) upregulating TNF-α expression and high concentrations of PKD1 (10–100 ng/ml) downregulating the expression of TNF-α when compared with the LPS control ($P < 0.05$, Figure 3(c)). Interestingly, the observed effect on TNF-α expression levels was independent on the order of PKD1, as a similar concentration-dependent effect was seen, when administering PKD1 prior to LPS stimulation in RAW264.7 cells. Similarly, administration of PKD1 prior to LPS downregulated the expression of IL-1β (100 ng/ml) and IL-6 (0.001–100 ng/ml), when compared with the LPS control ($P < 0.05$) in RAW264.7 cells (Figures 3(a) and 3(b)).

Whereas the inflammatory response initiated in RAW264.7 cells stimulated an immune response in the Caco-2 cells as observed by an upregulated expression of IL-8 and TNF-α, only minor differential effects were observed with PKD1 (Figures 4(a)–4(d)). The effect of PKD1 on the expression of IL-8, β-catenin, and PPAR-γ in Caco-2 cells was nonsignificantly affected, whereas treatment with 0.1 ng/ml of PKD1 after stimulation with LPS upregulated the expression

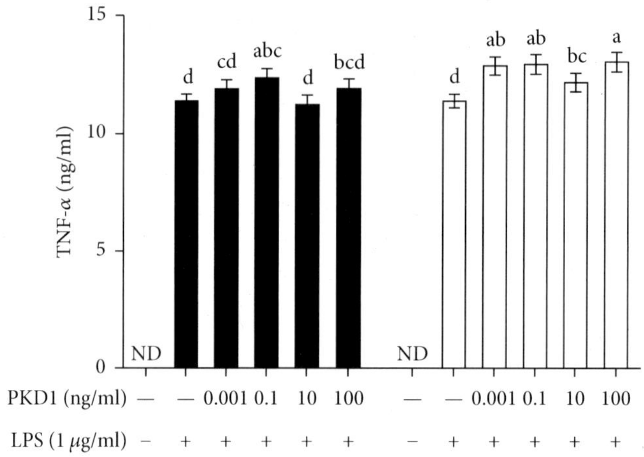

FIGURE 2: PKD1 stimulate secretion of TNF-α from LPS-stimulated RAW264.7 cells. Protein kinase D1 (PKD1; 0.001, 0.1, 10, 100 ng/ml) was administered apically to Caco-2 cells in co-culture with RAW264.7 cells. An inflammatory response was induced in RAW264.7 cells with 1 μg/ml lipopolysaccharide (LPS, *E. coli*: O127). Effects of PKD1 on secretion of TNF-α from RAW264.7 cells were evaluated in two different situations: (■) LPS was administered to RAW264.7 cells for 3 h, followed by PKD1 to Caco-2 cells for 3 h to investigate whether PKD1 can ameliorate an already induced inflammation. (□) PKD1 was administered to Caco-2 cells for 3 h at which point RAW264.7 cells were stimulated with LPS for 6 h to evaluate whether PKD1 can suppress inflammation initiation. TNF-α level in controls (no LPS stimulation) was undetectable (ND). Data are presented as means ± SEM ($n = 3$). Significant differences ($P < 0.05$) within concentrations of PKD1 are indicated by the lowercase letters.

of TNF-α when compared with the LPS control in Caco-2 cells ($P < 0.05$).

4. Discussion

4.1. LPS Stimulated an Inflammatory Response in Caco-2 and RAW264.7 Cells. To evaluate the effect of PKD1 in relation to intestinal inflammation we employed a co-culture model with intestinal epithelial Caco-2 cells and LPS-stimulated RAW264.7 macrophages to resemble gut inflammation, as previously observed [16–18]. Tanoue et al. demonstrated crosstalk between these cells, as LPS-stimulated RAW264.7 cells secrete TNF-α, thereby inducing IL-8 mRNA expression in Caco-2 cells [15]. In agreement, we observed LPS-induced secretion of TNF-α (11.5 ng/ml) in RAW264.7 cells when RAW264.7 cells were stimulated with 1 μg/ml of LPS (*E. coli* O127, Figure 2). Also, an upregulated expression of TNF-α, IL-6, and IL-1β was observed in RAW264.7 cells (Figures 3(a)–3(c)). Varying concentrations of LPS have been used for inducing an inflammatory response. Tanoue et al. reported the secretion of 50 ng/ml of TNF-α when stimulating with 100 ng/ml of LPS (*E. coli* O127) for 3 h [15], whereas 5 ng/ml of LPS (*E. coli* O127) for 3 h induced secretion of TNF-α levels at 350 pg/ml [16]. These differential responses might be explained by varying cell densities as well as different passages of RAW264.7 cells employed in the studies, potentially influencing the responses to LPS stimulation. Concomitantly, LPS stimulation of RAW264.7 cells induced an upregulated expression of IL-8 and TNF-α in Caco-2 cells (Figures 4(a)-4(b)). Specifically expression of IL-8 in Caco-2 cells was induced by almost 4-fold when stimulated with 1 μg/ml of LPS, a substantial increase compared to the 2-fold induction observed by Tanoue et al., when stimulating with 100 ng/ml of LPS [15]. Since previous studies have identified Caco-2 cells as unresponsive to LPS [20], these results strongly indicate that RAW264.7 macrophage cells stimulated with LPS induce an inflammatory response in the Caco-2 cells through crosstalk between the two individual cell layers.

4.2. PKD1 Displays a Concentration-Dependent Effect in the Amelioration of Intestinal Inflammation. To test the ability of PKD1 protein to ameliorate intestinal inflammation, RAW264.7 cells were stimulated with LPS for 3 h. This was followed by administration of PKD1 to Caco-2 monolayers for 3 h. Whereas no effects were observed on IL-1β and IL-6 in RAW264.7 cells, a concentration-dependent effect on TNF-α expression levels were observed. Here administration of 10–100 ng/ml of PKD1 downregulated TNF-α, whereas lower concentrations (0.001–0.1 ng/ml) caused upregulation of TNF-α in RAW264.7 cells. However, a comparable effect was not observed on the secretion of TNF-α (Figure 2), indicating that the observed transcriptional effects did not directly translate into corresponding effects at the protein level during this 6 h time period. Since anti-TNF-α treatment has emerged as the central target to ameliorate IBD [21], this emphasizes the potential importance of the observed PKD1-induced downregulation of TNF-α in RAW264.7 cells. However, PKD1 (0.1 ng/ml) upregulated the expression of TNF-α in Caco-2 cells (Figure 4(b)), demonstrating a detrimental effect to the IECs when treated with PKD1. However, due to the limited effects observed in Caco-2 cells, other potential mediators induced upon PKD1 treatment might exert the effects observed in the RAW264.7 cells.

4.3. PKD1 Affects the Initiation of Intestinal Inflammation. The ability of PKD1 to hamper inflammation initiation was investigated by administering PKD1 to Caco-2 cells for

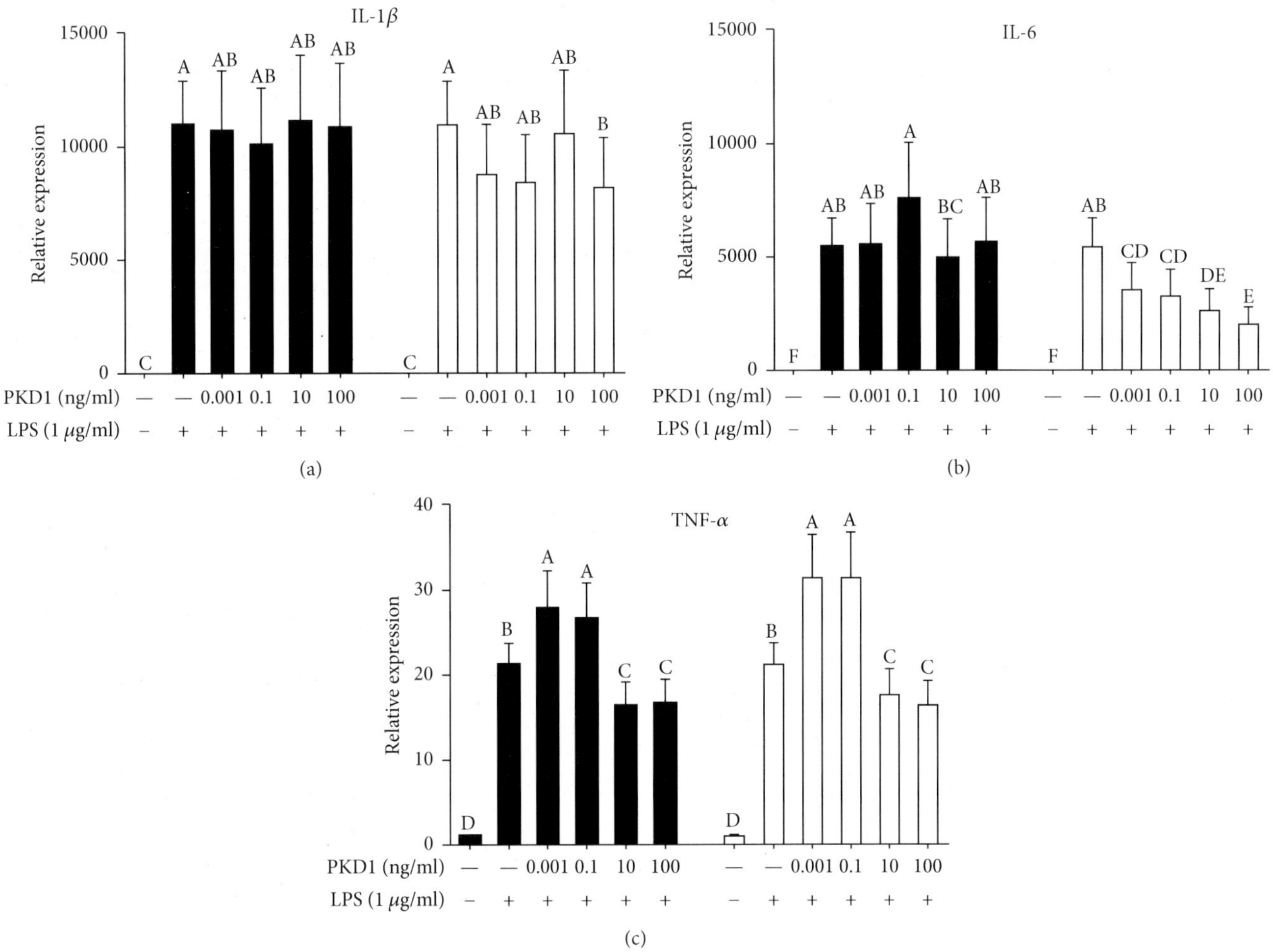

FIGURE 3: Effect of PKD1 on IL-1β, IL-6, and TNF-α mRNA expression in RAW264.7 cells. Protein kinase D1 (PKD1; 0.001, 0.1, 10, 100 ng/ml) was administered apically to Caco-2 cells in co-culture with RAW264.7 cells. An inflammatory response was induced in RAW264.7 cells with 1 μg/ml lipopolysaccharide (LPS, *E. coli*: O127). Effects of PKD1 on IL-1β, IL-6, and TNF-α expression levels were evaluated in two different situations: (■) LPS was administered to RAW264.7 cells for 3 h, followed by PKD1 to Caco-2 cells for 3 h to investigate whether PKD1 can ameliorate an already established inflammation. (□) PKD1 was administered to Caco-2 cells for 3 h at which point RAW264.7 cells were stimulated with LPS for 6 h to evaluate whether PKD1 can suppress inflammation initiation. Data are presented as mean transcriptional levels relative to the negative control (0% FCS, unstimulated) with 95% confidence intervals ($n = 3$). Significant differences ($P < 0.05$) within concentrations of PKD1 and LPS are indicated by the uppercase letters.

3 h prior to a 6 h LPS stimulation in RAW264.7 cells. In RAW264.7 cells, administration of PKD1 to Caco-2 cells suppressed the LPS-induced inflammatory response as IL-1β (100 ng/ml PKD1), IL-6 (0.001–100 ng/ml PKD1), and TNF-α (10–100 ng/ml PKD1) expression levels were downregulated. Specifically, a concentration-dependent downregulation of IL-6 was observed. The proinflammatory cytokine IL-6 is augmented in acute and chronic wounds [7] and implicated in the course of IBD [22]. This PKD1-dependent downregulation therefore demonstrates a potential important effect of PKD1 in hampering intestinal inflammation. The TNF-α response observed in RAW264.7 cells with low PKD1 levels upregulating and high levels downregulating TNF-α mRNA levels signifies this concentration-dependent effect of PKD1 observed. Interestingly, secretion of TNF-α was induced significantly from the LPS control with no dependency on the concentration of PKD1 (Figure 2). Administration of PKD1 to Caco-2 cells induced TNF-α secretion from RAW264.7 cells, while downregulating the mRNA expression at 10–100 ng/ml of PKD1. Hence, the observed effects on the mRNA and protein levels did not directly associate with each other. Since TNF-α mRNA and protein levels were evaluated at identical times, these variations might be seen as transcriptional alterations translate into effects at the protein level with a certain delay, limiting the comparability between the two analyses. Interestingly, PKD1 has previously been found to induce the expression of TNF-α and IL-6 in RAW264.7 cells upon stimulation with bacterial DNA [12]. The downregulation observed in this study therefore represents a differential effect of PKD1 once administered to the Caco-2 cells prior to initiation of inflammation.

Prostaglandin from LPS-stimulated macrophages induces stimulation of PPAR-γ and late activation of IL-10 at 72 h in IECs [23].Here, changes in the TEER (data not shown)

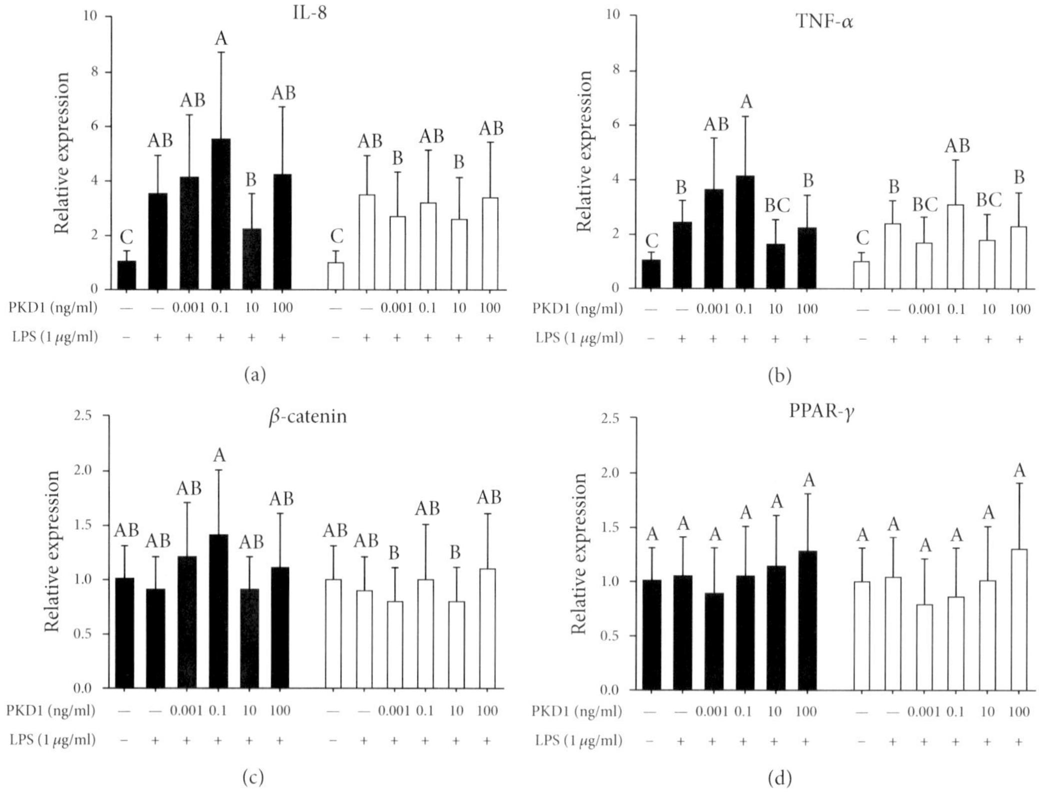

Figure 4: Effect of PKD1 on IL-8, TNF-α, β-catenin, and PPAR-γ mRNA expression in Caco-2 cells. Protein kinase D1 (PKD1; 0.001, 0.1, 10, 100 ng/ml) was administered apically to Caco-2 cells in co-culture with RAW264.7 cells. An inflammatory response was induced in RAW264.7 cells with 1 μg/ml lipopolysaccharide (LPS, *E. coli*: O127). Effects of PKD1 on IL-8, TNF-α, β-catenin, and PPAR-γ expression levels were evaluated in two different situations: (■) LPS was administered to RAW264.7 cells for 3 h, followed by PKD1 to Caco-2 cells for 3 h to investigate whether PKD1 can ameliorate an already established inflammation. (□) PKD1 was administered to Caco-2 cells for 3 h at which point RAW264.7 cells were stimulated with LPS for 6 h to evaluate whether PKD1 can suppress inflammation initiation. Data are presented as mean transcriptional levels relative to the negative control (0% FCS, unstimulated) with 95% confidence intervals ($n = 3$). Significant differences ($P < 0.05$) within concentrations of PKD1 and LPS are indicated by the uppercase letters.

and the expression of PPAR-γ in Caco-2 cells remained unchanged. Similarly, β-catenin, a major component in the formation of adherens junctions (AJs) [24], remained unaffected during the various treatments, despite previous observations of crosstalk between PKD1 and β-catenin [25, 26]. Consequently, the studies presented here indicate that a 6 h treatment period with LPS is insufficient for evaluating inflammation-induced effects on β-catenin and PPAR-γ in Caco-2 cells. Importantly, we did not evaluate the level of PKD1 in the RAW264.7 cell supernatant. The effects observed in the macrophages might therefore be caused by either an indirect or a direct effect, depending on whether PKD1 penetrated the Caco-2 cells and the transwell inserts, entering the lower compartment.

Expression of IL-8 and TNF-α in Caco-2 cells was unaffected by the various treatments, implying that either the expression was affected during other time periods or other cellular mediators might be affected by PKD1. Importantly, from these studies it seems that PKD1 has limited effects once an inflammatory response has been initiated. This indicates that the potential anti-inflammatory effect of PKD1 is unable to affect the severe proinflammatory response initiated in RAW264.7 cells upon stimulation with LPS. Oppositely, it seems that a preventive treatment with PKD1 has the ability to hamper a subsequent proinflammatory response induced in the macrophages. However, we have to consider the difference between the periods of PKD1 treatment in the two studies. Whereas the preventive PKD1 treatment was administered for 3 h prior to the 6 h LPS stimulation, giving a total of 9 h treatment with PKD1, Caco-2 cells were only treated with PKD1 for a total of 3 h when studying the ability to ameliorate an already established inflammatory response. Since the inflammation was initiated 3 h prior to the treatment with PKD1, the inflammatory response initiated might be too strong for PKD1 to cause significant effects during a 3 h period.

In conclusion, PKD1 ameliorated an on-going intestinal inflammation in the Caco-2/RAW264.7 co-culture at high concentrations of PKD1, through downregulation of the principal proinflammatory cytokine, TNF-α. In contrast, PKD1 administered prior to initiation of an inflammatory response revealed a concentration-dependent anti-inflammatory effect through downregulation of the proinflammatory mediators, IL-6 and TNF-α. The studies provide evidence for a potential beneficial and protective effect of PKD1 in relation to intestinal inflammation.

Acknowledgments

The authors wish to thank Janne B. Funch Adamsen and Kasper Vrangstrup Poulsen for laboratory assistance and Mihai V. Curtasu for providing the illustration of the co-culture system. This work was supported by the Danish Council for Independent Research [Grant no. 1335-00116].

References

[1] G. G. Kaplan, "The global burden of IBD: from 2015 to 2025, Nature reviews," *Gastroenterology & Hepatology*, vol. 12, pp. 720–727, 2015.

[2] V. A. Gerova, S. G. Stoynov, D. S. Katsarov, and D. A. Svinarov, "Increased intestinal permeability in inflammatory bowel diseases assessed by iohexol test," *World Journal of Gastroenterology*, vol. 17, no. 17, pp. 2211–2215, 2011.

[3] Y. Huang and Z. Chen, "Inflammatory bowel disease related innate immunity and adaptive immunity," *American Journal of Translational Research*, vol. 8, pp. 2490–2497, 2016.

[4] E. C. Steinbach and S. E. Plevy, "The role of macrophages and dendritic cells in the initiation of inflammation in IBD," *Inflammatory Bowel Diseases*, vol. 20, no. 1, pp. 166–175, 2014.

[5] R. Atreya and M. F. Neurath, "Chemokines in infammatory bowel diseases," *Digestive Diseases*, vol. 28, no. 3, pp. 386–394, 2010.

[6] I. Atreya, R. Atreya, and M. F. Neurath, "NF-κB in inflammatory bowel disease," *Journal of Internal Medicine*, vol. 263, no. 6, pp. 591–596, 2008.

[7] S. Barrientos, O. Stojadinovic, M. S. Golinko, H. Brem, and M. Tomic-Canic, "Growth factors and cytokines in wound healing," *Wound Repair and Regeneration*, vol. 16, no. 5, pp. 585–601, 2008.

[8] I. I. Singer, D. W. Kawka, S. Schloemann, T. Tessner, T. Riehl, and W. F. Stenson, "Cyclooxygenase 2 is induced in colonic epithelial cells in inflammatory bowel disease," *Gastroenterology*, vol. 115, no. 2, pp. 297–306, 1998.

[9] J. O'Brien, "Nonsteroidal anti-inflammatory drugs in patients with inflammatory bowel disease," *The American Journal of Gastroenterology*, vol. 95, pp. 1859–1861, 2000.

[10] E. Rozengurt, "Protein kinase D signaling: Multiple biological functions in health and disease," *Physiology Journal*, vol. 26, no. 1, pp. 23–33, 2011.

[11] S. A. Matthews, T. Iglesias, E. Rozengurt, and D. Cantrell, "Spatial and temporal regulation of protein kinase D (PKD)," *The EMBO journal*, vol. 19, pp. 2935–2945, 2000.

[12] J. E. Park, Y. I. Kim, and A. K. Yi, "Protein kinase D1: a new component in TLR9 signaling," *Journal of Immunology*, vol. 181, no. 3, pp. 2044–2055, 2008.

[13] P. Storz and A. Toker, "Protein kinase D mediates a stress-induced NF-κB activation and survival pathway," *EMBO Journal*, vol. 22, no. 1, pp. 109–120, 2003.

[14] J. Song, J. Li, A. Lulla, B. M. Evers, and D. H. Chung, "Protein kinase D protects against oxidative stress-induced intestinal epithelial cell injury via Rho/ROK/PKC-δ pathway activation," *American Journal of Physiology-Cell Physiology*, vol. 290, no. 6, pp. C1469–C1476, 2006.

[15] T. Tanoue, Y. Nishitani, K. Kanazawa, T. Hashimoto, and M. Mizuno, "In vitro model to estimate gut inflammation using co-cultured Caco-2 and RAW264.7 cells," *Biochemical and Biophysical Research Communications*, vol. 374, no. 3, pp. 565–569, 2008.

[16] A. Olejnik, K. Kowalska, M. Kidon et al., "Purple carrot anthocyanins suppress lipopolysaccharide-induced inflammation in the co-culture of intestinal Caco-2 and macrophage RAW264.7 cells," *Food & Function*, vol. 7, pp. 557–564, 2016.

[17] K.-M. Kim, Y.-S. Kim, J. Y. Lim et al., "Intestinal anti-inflammatory activity of sasa quelpaertensis leaf extract by suppressing Lipopolysaccharide-Stimulated inflammatory mediators in intestinal epithelial Caco-2 cells co-cultured with RAW 264.7 macrophage cells," *Nutrition Research and Practice*, vol. 9, no. 1, pp. 3–10, 2015.

[18] X. Xu, J. Yang, Z. Luo, and X. Zhang, "Lentinula edodes-derived polysaccharide enhances systemic and mucosal immunity by spatial modulation of intestinal gene expression in mice," *Food & Function*, vol. 6, pp. 2068–2080, 2015.

[19] M. R.-L. Pinto, S. Appay, M. Kedinger et al., "Enterocyte-like differentiation and polarization of the human colon carcinoma cell line caco-2 in culture," *Biol. Cell*, vol. 47, pp. 323–330, 1983.

[20] L. Eckmann, H. C. Jung, C. Schürer-Maly, A. Panja, E. Morzycka-Wroblewska, and M. F. Kagnoff, "Differential cytokine expression by human intestinal epithelial cell lines: Regulated expression of interleukin 8," *Gastroenterology*, vol. 105, no. 6, pp. 1689–1697, 1993.

[21] M. F. Neurath, "Cytokines in inflammatory bowel disease," *Nature Reviews Immunology*, vol. 14, no. 5, pp. 329–342, 2014.

[22] K. Mitsuyama, M. Sata, and K. Tanikawa, "Significance of interleukin-6 in patients with inflammatory bowel disease," *Gastroenterologia Japonica*, vol. 26, pp. 20–28, 1991.

[23] J. Hyun, L. Romero, R. Riveron et al., "Human intestinal epithelial cells express interleukin-10 through Toll-like receptor 4-mediated epithelial-macrophage crosstalk," *Journal of Innate Immunity*, vol. 7, no. 1, pp. 87–101, 2015.

[24] K. Ebnet, "Organization of multiprotein complexes at cell-cell junctions," *Histochemistry and Cell Biology*, vol. 130, no. 1, pp. 1–20, 2008.

[25] J. Wang, L. Han, J. Sinnett-Smith et al., "Positive cross talk between protein kinase D and β-catenin in intestinal epithelial cells: Impact on β-catenin nuclear localization and phosphorylation at ser552," *American Journal of Physiology-Cell Physiology*, vol. 310, no. 7, pp. C542–C557, 2016.

[26] C. Du, M. Jaggi, C. Zhang, and K. C. Balaji, "Protein kinase D1-mediated phosphorylation and subcellular localization of β-catenin," *Cancer Research*, vol. 69, no. 3, pp. 1117–1124, 2009.

26

Impaired mRNA Expression of the Migration Related Chemokine Receptor CXCR4 in Mesenchymal Stem Cells of COPD Patients

K. Karagiannis,[1,2] A. Proklou,[1,2] E. Tsitoura,[1] I. Lasithiotaki,[1] C. Kalpadaki,[3] D. Moraitaki,[2] I. Sperelakis,[4] G. Kontakis,[4] K. M. Antoniou,[1,2] and N. Tzanakis[2]

[1]*School of Medicine, Laboratory of Molecular and Cellular Pneumonology, University of Crete, Heraklion, Crete, Greece*
[2]*Department of Respiratory Medicine, University Hospital of Heraklion, Heraklion, Crete, Greece*
[3]*Department of Haematology, University Hospital of Heraklion, Heraklion, Crete, Greece*
[4]*Department of Orthopedics, University Hospital of Heraklion, Heraklion, Crete, Greece*

Correspondence should be addressed to K. Karagiannis; k.karagiannis@med.uoc.gr

Academic Editor: Sarah Howie

Defective tissue repair and remodeling are main aspects of Chronic Obstructive Pulmonary Disease (COPD) pathophysiology. Bone marrow mesenchymal stem cells (BM-MSCs) have been implicated in this direction, as their functional impairment and recruitment could possibly contribute to disease development and progression. The present study characterizes for the first time the expression of migration related chemokine receptors and their ligands in BM-MSCs from COPD patients. CXCR4/SDF1a and CCR7/CCL19-CCL21 mRNA levels were evaluated in BM-MSCs obtained from twelve COPD patients and seven healthy donors. SDF1a protein levels in sera and BM-MSCs' conditioned media were also evaluated. CXCR4, SDF1a, CCL19, and CCL21 mRNA levels were significantly reduced in COPD BM-MSCs while CCR7 levels were undetectable. Notably, SDF1a protein levels were marginally elevated in both patient sera and BM-MSCs' conditioned media while the increase in SDF1a serum levels significantly correlated with disease severity in COPD. Our findings show posttranscriptional regulation of SDF1a levels in BM-MSCs of COPD patients and significant downregulation of SDF1a and CXCR4 mRNA indicating an involvement of the SDF1a signaling pathway in the disease pathophysiology.

1. Background

Chronic Obstructive Pulmonary Disease (COPD) is defined as a "common preventable and treatable disease characterized by persistent airflow limitation that is usually progressive and associated with an enhanced chronic inflammatory response in the airways and the lung to noxious particles or gases." Exacerbations and comorbidities contribute to the overall severity in individual patients [1]. COPD is one of the leading causes of death globally, with huge social and economic burden [2]. Thus, it is estimated to be the fifth most common cause of morbidity and the third leading cause of death worldwide by 2030 [3]. Tobacco smoking, being well established as the main etiological factor for the development of COPD, induces a vicious circle of epithelial damage, impaired tissue repair, and remodeling. However, despite the plethora of research studies in COPD, the exact pathophysiological mechanisms are not yet fully understood.

Mesenchymal stem (stromal) cells (MSCs) are multipotent stromal cells that can be isolated from bone marrow, skeletal muscle, amniotic fluid, and adipose tissue, among others tissues. They are plastic adherent cells with a differentiation potential towards adipocytes, chondrocytes, and osteoblasts [4]. Waterman et al. have recently proposed that MSCs may be polarized into a proinflammatory MSC1 population or immunosuppressive MSC2 phenotype, dependent on their exposure to specific stimuli [5]. Therefore, it is likely that MSCs play a crucial role in both the maintenance of epithelial integrity and the pathogenesis of lung diseases. During the last few years a number of experimental data on animal models have showed MSCs' contribution to tissue regeneration in certain lung diseases such as elastase-induced emphysema, homing to sites of asbestos-induced lung injury, tissue remodeling in pulmonary hypertension, decrease in chronic airway inflammation in asthma, and restoration of alveolar and lung fluid balance after endotoxin-induced acute lung injury [6–11]. Consequently, great interest in the therapeutic potential of ex vivo expanded MSC has been noticed for the treatment of many disease states [12–14]. Bone marrow–derived MSCs are activated and migrate to sites of injury via mechanisms that have not yet been fully elucidated. The proposed mechanism of attraction at the sites of lung injury is via the production of soluble factors such as granulocyte colony-stimulating factor and granulocyte-macrophage colony-stimulating factor, which lead to MSC proliferation and migration via the stromal cell derived factor- (SDF-) 1–CXCR4 axis [15, 16]. Similarly, previous data from Antoniou et al. showed overexpression of CXCR4 in patients with Idiopathic Pulmonary Fibrosis (IPF) [17]. Additionally, CCR7 and its ligands CCL19 and CCL21 have recently been suggested as another chemotactic axis for MSCs [18, 19]. Hence, changes in chemokines and their receptors expression by stem cells can represent defects on the migratory ability of those cells.

The aim of the current study is to investigate the possible involvement of BM-MSCs in the pathophysiology of COPD by evaluating the expression of genes involved in proliferation/migration process, namely, the CXCL12a/CXCR4 and CCR7/CCL19, CCL21 ligand/receptor dyad.

2. Methods

2.1. Ethics and Patient Data. This study was conducted in accordance with the amended Declaration of Helsinki. The Research Ethics Committee of the University of Crete approved the study protocol and written informed consent was obtained from the 19 subjects before entering the study (Decision 412, 18/06/2014 protocol number 14724). Of these, the 12 participants diagnosed as having COPD, according to the GOLD guidelines, were current or ex-smokers who had at least a 20-pack-year smoking history and had an FEV1/FVC ratio of <70% and reversibility to an inhaled beta-2 agonist of <10% or <200 mls absolute improvement [20]. Six healthy smoking individuals, defined as smokers without airflow limitation, and one healthy ex-smoker, with an FEV1 predicted above 80%, were recruited and matched for age and for smoking history, as closely as possible.

2.2. Lung Function Tests. Lung function testing, including spirometry with a bronchodilation test and DLCO measurement, was performed by all participants with a computerized system (MasterLab; 2.12, Jaeger, Wuerzburg, Germany) according to standardized guidelines.

2.3. Blood Samples Collection. Peripheral blood samples and serum were obtained from all participants and were stored at −80°C, after appropriate preparation, according to standard procedures.

2.4. BM-MSCs Collection and Culture. BM-MSCs were obtained from posterior iliac crest aspirates and cultured in vitro as previously described [17, 21]. In brief, BM mononuclear cells (BMMCs) isolated with Histopaque-1077 (Sigma, Saint Louis MO) were cultured in Dulbecco's Modified Eagle Medium-Low Glucose (DMEM-LG; Gibco Invitrogen, Paisley Scotland)/10% fetal calf serum (FCS; Hyclone, Logan, Utah, USA)/100 IU/ml penicillin-streptomycin (PS, Gibco) (MSC medium) at a concentration of 2×10^5 cells/cm^2 in 25 cm^2 culture flasks in 37°C temperature/5% CO2 humidified atmosphere. One to three days after seeding, floating cells were removed and the medium was replaced by fresh MSC medium. Cells were passaged when 70–90% confluence was reached, using 0.25% trypsin-1 mM EDTA (Gibco). MSCs were identified by their morphologic and immunophenotypic characteristics and their potential to differentiate towards three different pathways, namely, adipocytes, osteocytes, and chondrocytes.

2.5. Immunophenotypic Characteristics of MSCs. BM-MSCs from second passage (P2) were immunophenotypically characterized by flow cytometry using anti-human monoclonal antibodies against anti-CD73 (AD2; Becton Dickinson-Pharmingen, San Diego, CA), anti-CDw90 (F15.42; Immunotech/Coulter), anti-CD105 (SN6; Caltag, Burlingame, CA), anti-CD45 (IMMU19.2; Immunotech/Coulter), anti-CD14 (IM2580U; Beckman-Coulter), and antiCD34 (QBend10; Beckman-Coulter). Data were processed in an Epics Elite flow cytometer (Coulter, Miami, FL).

2.6. Real-Time Reverse Transcriptase-Polymerase Chain Reaction Assay. BM-MSCs at P2 were homogenized in TRIzol reagent (Invitrogen, Carlsbad, CA), total RNA was extracted, and cDNA was synthesized by reverse transcription (RT) with the Thermoscript RT kit (Invitrogen). mRNA expression was measured using a real-time RT-PCR assay with SYBR-Green I. Glyceraldehyde-3-phosphate dehydrogenase (GAPDH) was used as the internal control, in order to normalize SDF-1a, CXCR4, CCR7, CCL19, and CCL21 expression levels. Relative expression levels per sample were calculated as $2^{-(\text{Ct of gene of interest}-\text{Ct of GAPDH})}$. The mRNA-specific primers used are listed in Table 1.

2.7. Chemokine Protein Levels in Serum and BM-MSCs Conditioned Media. SDF-1a levels in MSC conditioned media at P2 and sera were evaluated by means of ELISA (Quantikine; R&D Systems, Minn., MN).

2.8. Statistical Analysis. Results were analyzed using IBM SPSS statistics v21.0. Nonparametric Mann–Whitney statistical test was used and values were expressed as medians (interquartile range). Spearman's rank coefficient (rho) was used to evaluate correlations between severity of the disease (FEV1% pred) and chemokines expression. A value of $p < 0.05$ was considered as statistically significant.

Table 1: Primer sequences used for real-time RT-PCR.

Gene		Primer sequence (5′-3′)	Annealing temperature
CXCR4	FOR	GGTGGTCTATGTTGGCGTCT	55°C
	REV	TGGAGTGTGACAGCTTGGAG	
SDF1a	FOR	TGAGAGCTCGCTTTGAGTGA	55°C
	REV	CACCAGGACCTTCTGTGGAT	
CCR7	FOR	GGTGGTGGCTCTCCTTGTCATTTT	55°C
	REV	AGTTCCGCACGTCCTTCTT	
CCL19	FOR	GGACTTCCCCAGCCCCAACTCT	62°C
	REV	TAACTGCTGCGGCGCTTCATCTT	
CCL21	FOR	CCTCAGCTCTGGCCTCTTAC	57°C
	REV	GGGGCAAGAACAGGATAGCTG	
GAPDH	FOR	AGCCACATCGCTCAGACA	53°C
	REV	CCAATACGACCAAATCCGTT	

Table 2: Patient's demographic data.

	COPD patients (N = 12)	Controls (N = 7)	p value
Age (years)	65.5 (55.3–72)	58 (33–63)	NS
Gender (m/f)	11/1	6/1	NS
BMI	30.1 (259–31.8)	27.8 (25.5–31.1)	NS
Smoking status (c/ex)	7/5	6/1	NS
PY	53 (40–78.8)	30 (12–80)	NS
COPD Gold stage			
Stage 1	2		
Stage 2	4		
Stage 3	5		
Stage 4	1		

Values are expressed as median (interquartile range) or frequencies; p value < 0.05 as statistically significant; m/f = male/female; BMI = Body Mass Index; c/ex = current/ex-smokers; PY = pack years.

3. Results

3.1. Demographics and Lung Function. Table 2 displays patients' data. There were no significant differences between COPD and control group in age, gender, smoking status, and history and Body Mass Index (BMI). Lung function testing results are shown in Table 3. As expected, there were statistically significant differences between COPD patients and controls in forced expiratory volume in one second (FEV1%, 49% versus 107%, resp., $p < 0.001$), forced vital capacity (FVC%, 64% versus 103%, resp., $p = 0.001$), and FEV1/FVC ratio (60% versus 79%, $p < 0.001$).

Table 3: Lung function test results.

	COPD patients (N = 12)	Controls (N = 7)	p value
FEV1%	49 (35–72)	107 (80–120)	<0.001
FVC%	64 (56–81)	103 (87–120)	0.001
FEV1/FVC ratio	60 (45–70)	79 (75–83)	<0.001
RV%	165 (141–204)	105 (79–139)	0.045
TLC%	112 (99–123)	98 (94–112)	NS
RV/TLC ratio	56 (50–69)	37 (28–45)	0.001
DLCO%	65 (27–94)	82 (72–96)	NS
KCO%	84 (43–110)	90 (77–106)	NS

Values are expressed as median (interquartile range); p value < 0.05 as statistically significant; FEV1 = forced expiratory volume in 1 second; FVC = forced vital capacity; TLCOc = transfer factor of the lung for carbon monoxide; KCO = transfer coefficient; RV = residual volume; TLC = total lung capacity.

3.2. BM-MSCs Identification and Immunophenotypic Characteristics. BM-MSCs from both COPD and healthy subjects were cultured to P2 and subsequently were characterized by their immunophenotypic characteristics and differentiation capacity. Immunophenotypic analysis demonstrated the presence of a homogenous cell population positive for CD73, CD90, and CD105 and negative for CD45, CD14, and CD34 antigens (Table 4). Additionally, MSCs were found capable of differentiating towards the adipogenic, osteogenic, and chondrogenic lineages.

3.3. SDF1a/CXCR4 Axis. CXCR4 mRNA levels were reduced in BM-MSCs of COPD patients, as Figure 1(a) displays. Particularly, a significant downregulation of CXCR4 expression was detected in COPD in comparison with control group

TABLE 4: Flow cytometry results.

	CD 73	CD 90	CD 105	CD 45	CD 14	CD 34
MSCs	98.2 (1.6)	97.8 (1.65)	97.8 (1.9)	0.4 (1.77)	0.3 (1.45)	0 (0)

Values are expressed as median (interquartile range).

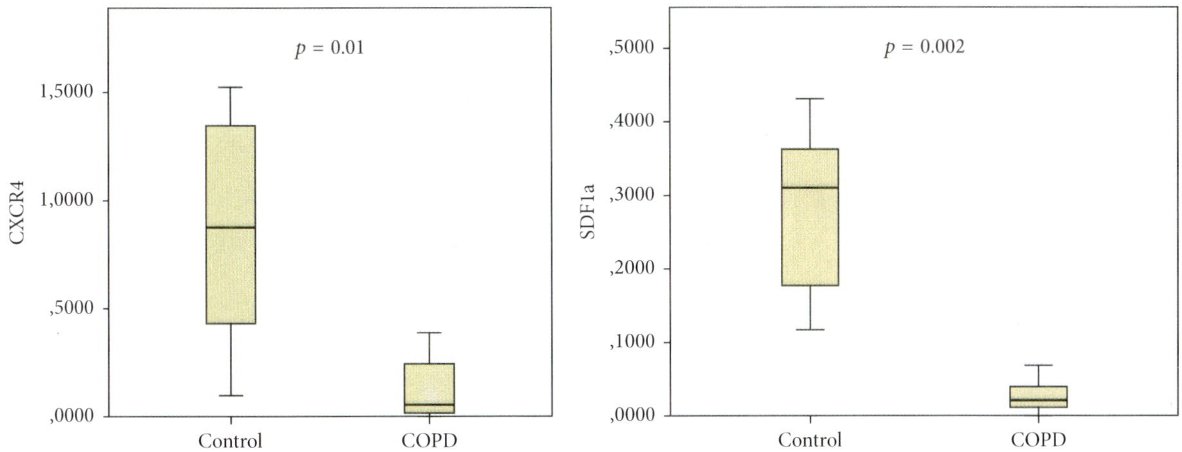

(a) CXCR4 mRNA expression by BM-MSCs

(b) SDF1a mRNA expression by BM-MSCs

FIGURE 1

TABLE 5: Real-time RT-PCR results.

	COPD patients ($N = 12$)	Controls ($N = 7$)	p value
CXCR4	0.05 (0.01–0.31)	0.87 (0.34–1.35)	0.01
SDF1a	0.03 (0.01–0.06)	0.32 (0.18–0.43)	0.002
CCL19	0.001 (0.00–0.03)	0.02 (0.004–0.04)	0.01
CCL21	0.00 (0.00–0.04)	0.04 (0.04–0.19)	0.02
CCR7	No expression	No expression	NS

Values are expressed as median (interquartile range); p value < 0.05 as statistically significant; measurements are 2^{-DCT}; DCT= Ctgene – Ctgapdh.

(0.05 versus 0.87 relative expression levels, resp., $p = 0.01$, Table 5).

BM-MSCs SDF1a mRNA levels were also significantly reduced in COPD relative to healthy subjects (0.03 versus 0.32 relative expression levels, resp., $p = 0.005$, Figure 1(b), Table 5). Interestingly, SDF1a protein levels in the BM-MSCs conditioned media were found increased in the COPD group, albeit nonstatistically significant (5570 versus 2995 pg/ml, $p = 0.053$).

Additionally, serum SDF1a levels were higher in COPD patients as compared to healthy subjects; however, our results did not reach statistical significance (6358 versus 3941 pg/ml, $p = 0.079$, Figure 2).

Notably, both SDF1a mRNA expression by BM-MSCs and serum protein levels were positively correlated to the severity of disease (GOLD stages) (rho = 0.59, $p = 0.04$ and rho = 0.63, $p = 0.03$, resp.). Expectedly, SDF1a mRNA levels were inversely correlated to FEV1% predicted of COPD patients (rho = −0.57, $p = 0.05$, Figure 3).

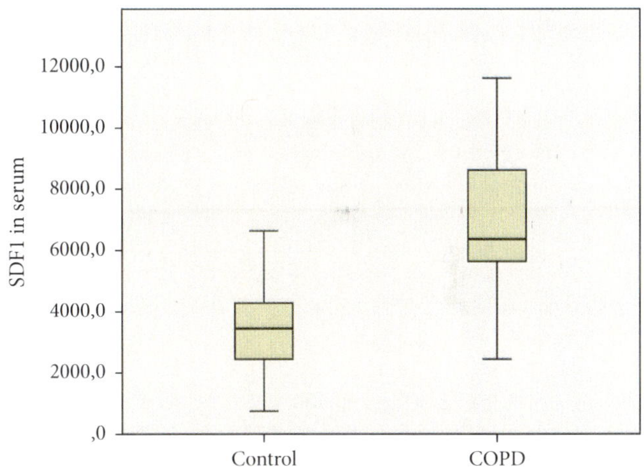

FIGURE 2: SDF1a protein levels in serum.

3.4. CCR7/CCL19-CCL21 Axis. Real-time RT-PCR showed no detectable CCR7 mRNA expression in both groups. Nevertheless, its ligands' expression was downregulated in BM-MSCs of COPD patients. Specifically, CCL19 (0.001 versus 0.02, $p = 0.01$, Figure 4(a)) and CCL21 (0.00 versus 0.04, $p = 0.02$, Figure 4(b)) mRNA levels were significantly reduced in COPD BM-MSCs compared to controls (Table 5).

4. Discussion

Our study aims to characterize the expression of chemokines and chemokine receptors involved in the migration of mesenchymal stem cells such as the SDF1/CXCR4 and CCR7/CCL19 CCL21 axes, in BM-MSCs of COPD patients in

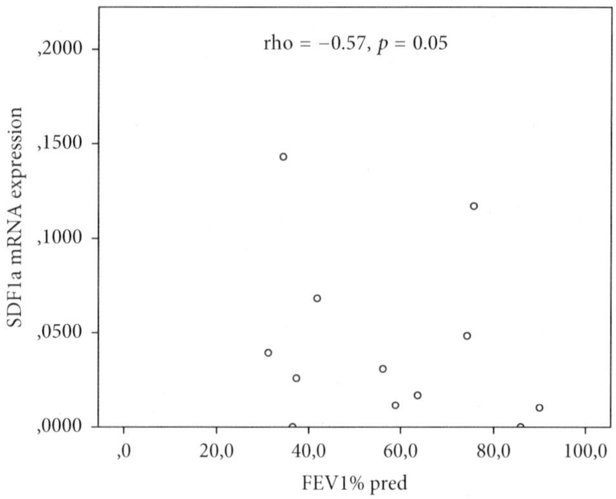

FIGURE 3: Correlations between SDF1a levels and severity of disease.

comparison to healthy subjects with similar age and smoking histories. Interestingly, our results showed decreased CXCR4 mRNA expression by BM-MSCs obtained from COPD patients suggesting a possible impairment of their migratory capacity. Similarly, mesenchymal cells from the COPD group expressed lower mRNA levels of SDF1a, CCL19, and CCL21 compared to controls; however, within the patient group SDF1a mRNA positively correlated with disease severity. Additionally, SDF1a serum protein levels were found elevated in the patient group and positively correlated to the severity of disease (GOLD stages) suggesting activation of SDF1a pathway in COPD. Our study suggests therefore a role of CXCR4/SDF1a axis in COPD pathophysiology that may lead to deregulation of the migration ability of stem cells from bone marrow.

Chronic inflammation and defects in repair mechanisms are considered key mechanisms in COPD development and progression of [22, 23]. Recently, mesenchymal stem cells have been used in several animal and human studies as a potential therapeutic option for the disease, due to their anti-inflammatory and repair effect [24–27]. Our team has previously investigated the role of SDF1/CXCR4 axis in migration of BM-MSCs in Idiopathic Pulmonary Fibrosis and Rheumatoid Arthritis with Usual Interstitial Pneumonia [17, 28]. Adachi et al. showed that bone marrow transplantation had curative effect in mice with emphysema while transplantation from emphysematous mice induced the disease in normal ones, indicating a major role of bone marrow in the pathophysiology of this disease [29].

Stem cell exhaustion and senescence are considered potential pathogenetic mechanisms in COPD [30]. It could be hypothesized that an impairment of the migratory capacity of BM-MSCs could have a proinflammatory effect in COPD patients. Our results show a reduced expression of CXCR4 mRNA in BM-MSCs of COPD patients compared to healthy subjects. However, we did not find an inverse correlation between CXCR4 mRNA expression and COPD stage. Several researchers have demonstrated the importance of CXCR4 expression by mesenchymal stem cells for the mediation of their trafficking [31–33]. Recently, Yang et al. have demonstrated that CXCR4 overexpression by MSCs improves homing and colonization of damaged lung tissue and additionally suppresses the acute lung injury in animal models [31]. In another study, Bustos et al. showed that aged BM-MSCs have reduced migratory and anti-inflammatory capacity and CXCR4 is one of the genes that are downregulated in these cells [32]. The reduced mRNA expression of CXCR4 in BM-MSCs of COPD patients in our study may therefore provide evidence of a defect in migratory properties of these cells and therefore a reduced ability to mobilize and play their protective role. Liu and Xie have demonstrated that endothelial progenitor cells from COPD patients decrease in numbers and show impaired migration ability, specifically lower levels of CXCR4 expression [34]. To the best of our knowledge, the present study is the first study providing evidence that COPD affects CXCR4 mRNA expression of BM-MSCs.

Our results also showed an increase in SDF1a serum levels of COPD patients, although statistical significance was not reached. Activation of the SDF1a pathway could be expected due to inflammation and tissue damage in the lung of COPD patients and our finding of elevated SDF1a levels could point to this direction; however this hypothesis requires further investigation. This assumption, further supported by the positive correlation of SDF1a serum levels with COPD stages, indicates an association of protein levels to the severity of the disease. SDF1 secretion from sites of tissue injury results in the increased migratory rates of progenitor cells and BM-MSCs [18, 35, 36]. Zhang et al. have demonstrated that SDF1 and Hypoxia Inducible Factor-1a (HIF-1a) are involved in regulation of MSCs function and homing to the lungs of COPD rat models [37]. Our study demonstrates that SDF1a is also induced in COPD in humans.

Findings for SDF1a expression by cultured BM-MSCs are intriguing. SDF1a mRNA expression by COPD mesenchymal cells was significantly reduced compared to controls but protein levels in conditioned media were higher in COPD group. Our data imply the presence of a posttranscriptional regulation of SDF1a production by BM-MSCs in COPD. It is known that MSCs are expressing SDF1 but its role has not yet been fully elucidated [38]. Lisignoli et al. have demonstrated an inverse correlation between CXCR4 and SDF1 expression by MSCs, suggesting a suppressive autocrine loop for CXCR4 expression [39]. A similar finding was reported by Pelekanos et al. in their study of fetal MSCs, but autocrine loop for CXCR4 expression was not adequate to fully explain their results [40]. It seems that there are multiple molecular pathways implicated in SDF1a expression and secretion by MSCs. Interestingly, SDF1a mRNA expression within the COPD group showed a positive correlation with severity of the disease similarly to the serum levels of SDF1a. This result is confirmed, as expected, by a significant inverse correlation of SDF1a mRNA levels with FEV1% predicted. Both mRNA expression and secretion of SDF1a by MSCs are affected in COPD patients, according to the aforementioned data; it appears though that further characterization of the regulation of SDF1a expression is required.

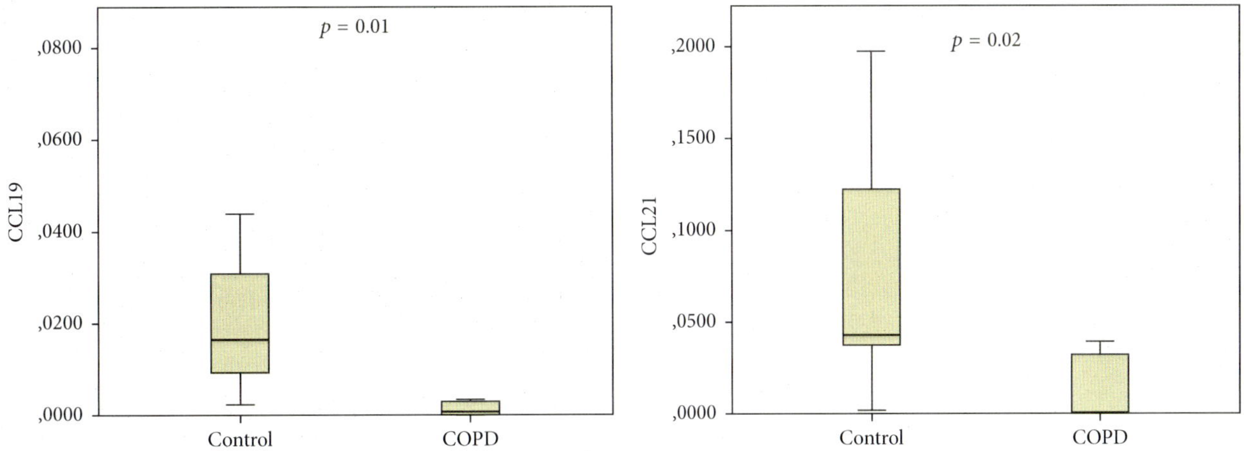

(a) CCL19 mRNA expression by BM-MSCs

(b) CCL21 mRNA expression by BM-MSCs

FIGURE 4

Another chemotactic axis that has been studied as a possible regulator of mesenchymal stem cell migration is CCR7 and its ligands CCL19 and CCL21 [41]. Our results showed downregulation of both CCL19 and CCL21 mRNA transcripts in COPD patients similarly to SDF1a, whereas there was no detectable expression of CCR7 in both COPD and control BM-MSCs. Although not extensively investigated, CCR7/CCL19/CCL21 axis has been also implicated in MSCs chemotaxis and tissue repair [18]. Demoor et al. have demonstrated that CCR7 plays a major role in modulating inflammatory responses in airways in COPD, and cigarette smoking upregulated CCR7, CCL19, and CCL21 mRNA expression in lymph nodes of wild-type mice [42]. CCL19 and CCL21 mRNA levels were found significantly lower in COPD BM-MSCs, similarly to the CXCR4 and SDF1a mRNAs. This reduction in mRNA levels may also be associated with the senescence of BM-MSCs previously suggested as a pathogenic mechanism in COPD [30].

There are limitations in our study, which need mentioning. First, the limited sample size due to the practical difficulties of patient recruitment is noteworthy. However, this was a pilot/guide study, investigating ex vivo BM-MSCs from COPD patients which, based on our results, should be expanded to a larger patient group. Additionally, since COPD is a heterogeneous disease, different disease stages may be reflected on BM-MSCs properties and should be taken into consideration in future studies. Considering that cigarette smoking may affect the migration of BM-MSCs even in subjects without COPD, another limitation of our study is the lack of a group of healthy nonsmokers. A future study comparing the migratory capacity of BM-MSCs between smokers and nonsmokers could provide new knowledge about the effect of cigarette smoking on stem cells.

In conclusion, our study demonstrates a downregulation of the CXCR4 mRNA expression by BM-MSCs in COPD patients, providing for the first time evidence from a human study that CXCR4/SDF1 axis is dysregulated in COPD. Additionally, it shows that COPD also affects SDF1a levels in serum and BM-MSCs. Although further studies are needed, we suggest that potential defects in migratory capacity of BM-MSCs may compromise their protective role, leading to development and progression of COPD.

Acknowledgments

The present study protocol has been awarded a grant from Hellenic Thoracic Society in 2008.

References

[1] "Global Initiative for Chronic Obstructive Lung Disease," GOLD Update, 2015.

[2] A. D. Lopez, C. D. Mathers, M. Ezzati, D. T. Jamison, and C. J. Murray, "Global and regional burden of disease and risk factors, 2001: systematic analysis of population health data," *The Lancet*, vol. 367, no. 9524, pp. 1747–1757, 2006.

[3] C. D. Mathers and D. Loncar, "Projections of global mortality and burden of disease from 2002 to 2030," *PLoS Medicine*, vol. 3, no. 11, article e442, 2006.

[4] M. E. Bernardo, F. Locatelli, and W. E. Fibbe, "Mesenchymal stromal cells," *Annals of the New York Academy of Sciences*, vol. 1176, pp. 101–117, 2009.

[5] R. S. Waterman, S. L. Tomchuck, S. L. Henkle, and A. M. Betancourt, "A new mesenchymal stem cell (MSC) paradigm: polarization into a pro-inflammatory MSC1 or an immunosuppressive MSC2 phenotype," *PLoS ONE*, vol. 5, no. 4, Article ID e10088, 2010.

[6] K. Ishizawa, H. Kubo, M. Yamada et al., "Bone marrow-derived cells contribute to lung regeneration after elastase-induced pulmonary emphysema," *FEBS Letters*, vol. 556, no. 1-3, pp. 249–252, 2004.

[7] J. L. Spees, D. A. Pociask, D. E. Sullivan et al., "Engraftment of bone marrow progenitor cells in a rat model of asbestos-induced pulmonary fibrosis," *American Journal of Respiratory and Critical Care Medicine*, vol. 176, no. 4, pp. 385–394, 2007.

[8] V. Sueblinvong, R. Loi, P. L. Eisenhauer et al., "Derivation of lung epithelium from human cord blood-derived mesenchymal stem cells," *American Journal of Respiratory and Critical Care Medicine*, vol. 177, no. 7, pp. 701–711, 2008.

[9] T. L. Bonfield, M. Koloze, D. P. Lennon, B. Zuchowski, S. E. Yang, and A. I. Caplan, "Human mesenchymal stem cells suppress chronic airway inflammation in the murine ovalbumin asthma model," *The American Journal of Physiology—Lung Cellular and Molecular Physiology*, vol. 299, no. 6, pp. L760–L770, 2010.

[10] J. W. Lee, X. Fang, N. Gupta, V. Serikov, and M. A. Matthay, "Allogeneic human mesenchymal stem cells for treatment of E. coli endotoxin-induced acute lung injury in the ex vivo perfused human lung," *Proceedings of the National Academy of Sciences of the United States of America*, vol. 106, no. 38, pp. 16357–16362, 2009.

[11] N. Gupta, X. Su, B. Popov, W. L. Jae, V. Serikov, and M. A. Matthay, "Intrapulmonary delivery of bone marrow-derived mesenchymal stem cells improves survival and attenuates endotoxin-induced acute lung injury in mice," *Journal of Immunology*, vol. 179, no. 3, pp. 1855–1863, 2007.

[12] K. Sinclair, S. T. Yerkovich, and D. C. Chambers, "Mesenchymal stem cells and the lung," *Respirology*, vol. 18, no. 3, pp. 397–411, 2013.

[13] X. Liu, Q. Fang, and H. Kim, "Preclinical studies of mesenchymal stem cell (MSC) administration in chronic obstructive pulmonary disease (COPD): a systematic review and meta-analysis," *PLoS ONE*, vol. 11, no. 6, Article ID e0157099, 2016.

[14] Z. Jin, X. Pan, K. Zhou et al., "Biological effects and mechanisms of action of mesenchymal stem cell therapy in chronic obstructive pulmonary disease," *Journal of International Medical Research*, vol. 43, no. 3, pp. 303–310, 2015.

[15] M. Rojas, J. Xu, C. R. Woods et al., "Bone marrow-derived mesenchymal stem cells in repair of the injured lung," *American Journal of Respiratory Cell and Molecular Biology*, vol. 33, no. 2, pp. 145–152, 2005.

[16] J. Xu, A. Mora, H. Shim, A. Stecenko, K. L. Brigham, and M. Rojas, "Role of the SDF-1/CXCR4 axis in the pathogenesis of lung injury and fibrosis," *The American Journal of Respiratory Cell and Molecular Biology*, vol. 37, no. 3, pp. 291–299, 2007.

[17] K. M. Antoniou, H. A. Papadaki, G. Soufla et al., "Investigation of bone marrow mesenchymal stem cells (BM MSCs) involvement in idiopathic pulmonary fibrosis (IPF)," *Respiratory Medicine*, vol. 104, no. 10, pp. 1535–1542, 2010.

[18] A. M. Hocking, "The role of chemokines in mesenchymal stem cell homing to wounds," *Advances in Wound Care*, vol. 4, no. 11, pp. 623–630, 2015.

[19] S. J. Baek, S. K. Kang, and J. C. Ra, "*In vitro* migration capacity of human adipose tissue-derived mesenchymal stem cells reflects their expression of receptors for chemokines and growth factors," *Experimental & Molecular Medicine*, vol. 43, no. 10, pp. 596–603, 2011.

[20] "Global Initiative for Chronic Obstructive Lung Disease," GOLD Report, 2012.

[21] M.-C. Kastrinaki, P. Sidiropoulos, S. Roche et al., "Functional, molecular and proteomic characterisation of bone marrow mesenchymal stem cells in rheumatoid arthritis," *Annals of the Rheumatic Diseases*, vol. 67, no. 6, pp. 741–749, 2008.

[22] C. Noujeim and P. Bou-Khalil, "Copd updates: what's new in pathophysiology and management?" *Expert Review of Respiratory Medicine*, vol. 7, no. 4, pp. 429–437, 2013.

[23] M. Tsoumakidou and N. M. Siafakas, "Novel insights into the aetiology and pathophysiology of increased airway inflammation during COPD exacerbations," *Respiratory Research*, vol. 22, no. 7, article 80, 2006.

[24] S. Murakami, N. Nagaya, T. Itoh et al., "Adrenomedullin regenerates alveoli and vasculature in elastase-induced pulmonary emphysema in mice," *American Journal of Respiratory and Critical Care Medicine*, vol. 172, no. 5, pp. 581–589, 2005.

[25] N. Shigemura, M. Okumura, S. Mizuno et al., "Lung tissue engineering technique with adipose stromal cells improves surgical outcome for pulmonary emphysema," *American Journal of Respiratory and Critical Care Medicine*, vol. 174, no. 11, pp. 1199–1205, 2006.

[26] K. S. Schweitzer, B. H. Johnstone, J. Garrison et al., "Adipose stem cell treatment in mice attenuates lung and systemic injury induced by cigarette smoking," *American Journal of Respiratory and Critical Care Medicine*, vol. 183, no. 2, pp. 215–225, 2011.

[27] D. J. Weiss, R. Casaburi, R. Flannery, M. LeRoux-Williams, and D. P. Tashkin, "A placebo-controlled, randomized trial of mesenchymal stem cells in COPD," *Chest*, vol. 143, no. 6, pp. 1590–1598, 2013.

[28] G. A. Margaritopoulos, K. M. Antoniou, I. Lasithiotaki, A. Proklou, G. Soufla, and N. M. Siafakas, "Expression of SDF-1/CXCR4 axis in bone marrow mesenchymal stem cells derived from rheumatoid arthritis-usual interstitial pneumonia," *Clinical and Experimental Rheumatology*, vol. 31, no. 4, pp. 610-611, 2013.

[29] Y. Adachi, H. Oyaizu, S. Taketani et al., "Treatment and transfer of emphysema by a new bone marrow transplantation method from normal mice to Tsk mice and vice versa," *Stem Cells*, vol. 24, no. 9, pp. 2071–2077, 2006.

[30] N. Mercado, K. Ito, and P. J. Barnes, "Accelerated ageing of the lung in COPD: new concepts," *Thorax*, vol. 70, no. 5, pp. 482–489, 2015.

[31] J.-X. Yang, N. Zhang, H.-W. Wang, P. Gao, Q.-P. Yang, and Q.-P. Wen, "CXCR4 overexpression in mesenchymal stem cells facilitates treatment of acute lung injury in rats," *The Journal of Biological Chemistry*, 2014.

[32] M. L. Bustos, L. Huleihel, M. G. Kapetanaki et al., "Aging mesenchymal stem cells fail to protect because of impaired migration and antiinflammatory response," *The American Journal of Respiratory and Critical Care Medicine*, vol. 189, no. 7, pp. 787–798, 2014.

[33] R. J. Miller, G. Banisadr, and B. J. Bhattacharyya, "CXCR4 signaling in the regulation of stem cell migration and development," *Journal of Neuroimmunology*, vol. 198, no. 1-2, pp. 31–38, 2008.

[34] X. Liu and C. Xie, "Human endothelial progenitor cells isolated from COPD patients are dysfunctional," *Molecular and Cellular Biochemistry*, vol. 363, no. 1-2, pp. 53–63, 2012.

[35] M. Kucia, J. Ratajczak, R. Reca, A. Janowska-Wieczorek, and M. Z. Ratajczak, "Tissue-specific muscle, neural and liver stem/progenitor cells reside in the bone marrow, respond to an SDF-1 gradient and are mobilized into peripheral blood during stress and tissue injury," *Blood Cells, Molecules, and Diseases*, vol. 32, no. 1, pp. 52–57, 2004.

[36] A. Kortesidis, A. Zannettino, S. Isenmann, S. Shi, T. Lapidot, and S. Gronthos, "Stromal-derived factor-1 promotes the growth, survival, and development of human bone marrow stromal stem cells," *Blood*, vol. 105, no. 10, pp. 3793–3801, 2005.

[37] W.-G. Zhang, L. He, X.-M. Shi et al., "Regulation of transplanted mesenchymal stem cells by the lung progenitor niche in rats with chronic obstructive pulmonary disease," *Respiratory Research*, vol. 15, no. 1, article 33, 2014.

[38] N. Van Overstraeten-Schlögel, Y. Beguin, and A. Gothot, "Role of stromal-derived factor-1 in the hematopoietic-supporting activity of human mesenchymal stem cells," *European Journal of Haematology*, vol. 76, no. 6, pp. 488–493, 2006.

[39] G. Lisignoli, S. Cristino, A. Piacentini, C. Cavallo, A. I. Caplan, and A. Facchini, "Hyaluronan-based polymer scaffold modulates the expression of inflammatory and degradative factors in mesenchymal stem cells: involvement of Cd44 and Cd54," *Journal of Cellular Physiology*, vol. 207, no. 2, pp. 364–373, 2006.

[40] R. A. Pelekanos, M. J. Ting, V. S. Sardesai et al., "Intracellular trafficking and endocytosis of CXCR4 in fetal mesenchymal stem/stromal cells," *BMC Cell Biology*, vol. 15, article 15, 2014.

[41] M. Sasaki, R. Abe, Y. Fujita, S. Ando, D. Inokuma, and H. Shimizu, "Mesenchymal stem cells are recruited into wounded skin and contribute to wound repair by transdifferentiation into multiple skin cell type," *The Journal of Immunology*, vol. 180, no. 4, pp. 2581–2587, 2008.

[42] T. Demoor, K. R. Bracke, K. Y. Vermaelen, L. Dupont, G. F. Joos, and G. G. Brusselle, "CCR7 modulates pulmonary and lymph node inflammatory responses in cigarette smoke-exposed mice," *Journal of Immunology*, vol. 183, no. 12, pp. 8186–8194, 2009.

27

Is Neutrophil-to-Lymphocyte Ratio a Predictor of Coronary Artery Disease

Kamal Sharma,[1] Alap K. Patel,[1] Komal H. Shah,[2] and Ashwati Konat[2]

[1]*Department of Cardiology, U. N. Mehta Institute of Cardiology and Research Centre, Ahmedabad, Gujarat, India*
[2]*Department of Research, U. N. Mehta Institute of Cardiology and Research Centre, Ahmedabad, Gujarat, India*

Correspondence should be addressed to Kamal Sharma; kamalsharma1975@gmail.com

Academic Editor: Marla R. Wolfson

Introduction. The current study was designed to evaluate the association of neutrophil-to-lymphocyte ratio (NLR) with coronary artery disease (CAD) presence. We also aimed to propose a suitable cut-off of NLR for diagnosis of CAD in Western Indians. *Methods.* Total 324 patients undergoing coronary angiography were enrolled and were subdivided into two groups: group 1 ($n = 99$; population without CAD) and group 2 ($n = 225$; population with CAD). *Results.* The results indicated significant ($p < 0.05$) positive association between elevated levels of WBC, neutrophil, monocyte, NLR, hs-CRP, CPK-MB, and troponin I and disease presence. According to subgroup analysis, the association was more profound in male and older population. Among all the markers NLR showed the strongest predictive potential for CAD with highest odds ratio (1.495; 95% CI: 0.942–2.371; $p < 0.048$). Optimum cut-off of NLR for diagnosis of CAD was 2.13 (AUC-0.823; $p < 0.001$; sensitivity: 83.64%; specificity: 63.46%). Association of NLR with other biochemical markers such as hs-CRP, CPK-MB, and troponin I was also observed in quartile analysis. *Conclusion.* NLR is a simple indicator that could be effectively used for the diagnosis of CAD with a cut-off of 2.13 in Western Indian population.

1. Introduction

The relationship between various inflammatory markers and coronary artery disease (CAD) has been established long ago [1]. Among them, white blood cell (WBC) subtypes have immerged as a community of inflammatory markers playing a crucial role in the pathogenesis of atherogenesis and atherothrombosis [2]. Neutrophil-to-lymphocyte ratio (NLR)—a new addition to the long list of markers—is an inexpensive, easy to obtain, widely available marker of inflammation, which can aid in the risk stratification of patients with various cardiovascular diseases in addition to the traditionally used markers. Ample research databases from Indian subcontinents have supported a potential of NLR as a prognostic and diagnostic index of coronary artery disease (CAD) and disease associated mortality [3–5]. An elevated NLR, irrespective of other biomarker levels, independently indicates an increased long term risk of mortality not only in patients with stable CAD but also in acute coronary syndrome (ACS) patients [6, 7].

These studies substantiate the negative impact of elevated NLR, and hence effort had been made to propose a suitable cut-off of it with effective clinical usage in various patient population. However the reference values for NLR vary with age and ethnicity. Misumida et al. in 2015 had also demonstrated an independent association between race and NLR in patients with NSTEMI, suggesting that a tailored cut-off value according to race would provide more precise prognostic information. These variations need to be considered while using NLR for predictive and prognostic purposes and before proposing a diagnostic cut-off in particular race. While some studies categorized their patients according to NLR intervals (e.g., tertiles, quartiles, and quintiles) [8–10], other studies used definite NLR cut-off points (e.g., NLR ≥ 2.5, NLR ≥ 2.7, NLR ≥ 3, NLR ≥ 4), and others used NLR ≥ 5 [11–16]. In fact, studies report different timing for the collection of blood used to calculate NLR; some collect the blood sample on admission [7], and others use preoperative NLR [17], maximum NLR during hospitalization [18], or average NLR of three readings during hospitalization [19].

Herewith we aim to investigate the association of NLR with CAD and establish it as a useful diagnostic and prognostic tool for CAD in Western Indians. We also seek to propose a suitable cut-off of NLR with effective clinical usage in this population.

2. Materials and Method

2.1. Study Population. This prospective study was conducted at U. N. Mehta Institute of Cardiology and Research Centre and was approved by institutional ethics committee. Total 324 individuals of both genders were enrolled from March 2014 to January 2016. The patients admitted for coronary angiography (CAG), hospitalized with first-time chest pain, having myocardial infarction, and with ECG showing changes and patients admitted in emergency were included in this study. Exclusion criteria of the study were as follows: patients taking any lipid lowering drug (statin), recent major surgery, and rheumatic heart disease. All patients were evaluated by taking detailed history and physical examination. The variables included in the study were age, sex, hypertension (HTN), diabetes mellitus (DM), smoking, cardiac biomarkers (troponin I, CK-MB), hs-CRP and white blood cell (WBC) count, differential count, mean platelet volume (MPV), red cell distribution width (RDW), and erythrocyte sedimentation rate (ESR). Hypertension was defined as the active use of antihypertensive drugs or documentation of blood pressure more than 140/90 mmHg, and diabetes mellitus was defined as fasting plasma glucose (FPG) levels over 126 mg/dl or random plasma glucose level over 200 mg/dl or active use of antidiabetic treatment. Smoking was defined as current smoking status of an individual. Complete blood count and biochemical values were evaluated from blood samples obtained by antecubital vein puncture. The study population was divided into two groups based on angiographic findings: group 1 (n = 99; population without CAD – no/nonsignificant CAD) and group 2 (n = 225; population with CAD - stenosis >70%).

2.2. Biochemical Estimations. Blood samples for laboratory assessment were collected upon first point of patient contact to refrain from bias. Total leucocyte count and its subtypes including neutrophil and lymphocyte platelet count and MPV and RDW were analysed using an automated blood cell counter, CELLDYN Ruby (Abott). Troponin I, CPK-MB, and hs-CRP were analysed using counter ARCHITECT PLUS (ci 4100) (Abott). Erythrocytes sedimentation rate was assessed using E-VACC disposable ESR pipettes (matrix) at 1 hr. Troponin I, CPK-MB, hs-CRP, CBC, and ESR were assessed from the same sample.

2.3. Statistical Analysis. All statistical studies were carried out using SPSS program version 20. Neutrophil-to-lymphocyte ratio (NLR), WBC-to-platelet ratio (WBCPR), and platelet-to-lymphocyte ratio (PLR) were automatically calculated by loading all the data to the statistical program used. Quantitative variables were expressed as the mean ± standard deviation and qualitative variables were expressed as percentage (%). Univariate statistics between two groups were calculated using the t-test or Mann–Whitney U test whichever is applicable. Categorical variables were compared using the chi-square test. A correlation between the variables was determined by using Pearson's correlation test. Strength of an association of the markers with disease presence was assessed using logistic regression for the parameters showing association with disease presence on univariate analysis ($p < 0.05$). Receiver operating characteristics (ROC) curves were constructed and the most discriminating cut-off values were determined to assess the predictive value of the NLR. Distribution of NLR values in the quartile ranges of established cardiac biomarkers were also calculated. A level of significance was accepted as a two-tailed p value < 0.05.

3. Results

The comparative baseline details of all the biochemical parameters between the two groups are presented in Table 1. Elevated levels of WBC count and neutrophil and monocyte count were observed in group 2 patients as compared to group 1 population. Significantly ($p < 0.05$) low level of NLR was found in group 1 (4.3 ± 3.8) in contrast to group 2 (5.6 ± 4.5). Patients with significant CAD had higher RDW (12.9 ± 1.6) as compared to patients without CAD (12.4 ± 2). Raised hs-CRP (3.3±4.3 versus 1.8±4.2), CPK-MB (116.4±152.5 versus 51.4±76.7), and troponin I (14±18.8 versus 6.3±14.4) levels were also found in group 2 patients as compared to group 1 subjects. The relationship between CAD and biochemical markers according to age and gender are presented in Tables 2 and 3. NLR showed a significant association with CAD in male and comparatively older (>40 years) population. Nonsignificantly ($p = 0.333$) high mean NLR value was found in patients with ejection fraction (EF) of <50% (5.55 ± 5.04) as compared to patients with EF of ≥50% (4.75 ± 3.19) in CAD positive group.

Figure 1 shows correlation analysis of various markers with disease presence. Strong positive correlation was observed between increasing values of WBC, neutrophil, monocyte, NLR, and troponin I and CAD occurrence. The strength of association of the markers with CAD was assessed using regression analysis and is presented in Table 4. Among all the studied variables NLR was found to be the strongest predictor of CAD showing an odds ratio of 1.495 (95% CI: 0.942–2.371; p = 0.048). Following this the diagnostic potency of the significantly associated markers were investigated using ROC analysis (Table 5). As indicated NLR exhibited highest area under curve (AUC-0.823; p = 0.0001; 95% CI; 0.712–0.931), closely followed by neutrophil count (AUC-0.821; p = 0.0001; 95% CI; 0.714–0.932) and troponin I (AUC-0.820; p = 0.0001; 95% CI; 0.716–0.935). Based on ROC a suitable cut-off of NLR was found to be 2.13 showing sensitivity and specificity of 83.64% and 63.46%, respectively (Table 6). According to quartile analysis, as indicated in Table 7 with increasing quartile of ACS markers there is an increase in NLR mean value. The association between NLR and left ventricle ejection fraction (LVEF) was assessed using Pearson's correlation analysis in CAD patients and results showed that there is no significant correlation between both parameters (coefficient of correlation: −0.086; p = 0.234).

Table 1: Comparison of parameters between group 1 (population without CAD) and group 2 (population with CAD).

Variables	Groups	Mean	Standard deviation	Significance
WBC	Group 1	10175.6	3772.0	0.034
	Group 2	12045.8	4596.6	
Neutrophil	Group 1	7284.2	3924.9	0.041
	Group 2	9184.2	4532.9	
Lymphocyte	Group 1	2265.6	951.9	0.507
	Group 2	2191.0	922.6	
Eosinophil	Group 1	257.4	169.3	0.391
	Group 2	254.8	190.2	
Monocyte	Group 1	370.1	304.5	0.0001
	Group 2	476.9	209.1	
Basophil	Group 1	0.7	6.5	0.404
	Group 2	1.3	13.9	
Platelet	Group 1	308440.0	120954.6	0.818
	Group 2	318787.4	159314.1	
MPV	Group 1	6.6	1.3	0.150
	Group 2	6.9	1.5	
NLR	Group 1	4.3	3.8	0.001
	Group 2	5.6	4.5	
PLR	Group 1	163.4	107.9	0.751
	Group 2	190.8	266.4	
RDW	Group 1	12.4	2.0	0.002
	Group 2	12.9	1.6	
hs-CRP	Group 1	1.8	4.2	<0.0001
	Group 2	3.3	4.3	
CPK-MB	Group 1	51.4	76.7	<0.0001
	Group 2	116.4	152.5	
Troponin I	Group 1	6.3	14.4	<0.0001
	Group 2	14.0	18.8	
ESR	Group 1	22.4	8.3	0.227
	Group 2	23.6	8.5	

CAD: coronary artery disease, Group 1: population without CAD, group 2; population with CAD, WBC: white blood cell, MPV: mean platelet volume, NLR: neutrophil-to-lymphocyte ratio, PLR: platelet-to-lymphocyte ratio, PWBC: platelet white blood cell ratio, RDW: red cell distribution width, hs-CRP: high sensitivity C-reactive protein, CPK-MB: creatinine phosphokinase-MB, and ESR: erythrocyte sedimentation rate.

4. Discussion

To our knowledge, this study is the first to propose clinically most relevant cut-off of NLR with considerably high sensitivity and specificity of CAD in Western Indians. We herewith demonstrate that patients with abnormal CAG had significantly higher NLR compared to patients with normal CAG.

The NLR test, which can be derived from the WBC count, is a common, cheap, and reproducible test worldwide. Previous studies have shown that NLR is associated with poor clinical outcomes in various cardiovascular diseases [8, 20–22]. Through entire spectrum of CAD and its associated diseases, the role of NLR has been extensively studied in order to provide a cheap and easily accessible for screening of population at risk. Following global trend, from India too various studies have proposed NLR cut-off for diagnosis of CAD. Fernando et al. (2015) had studied the relation of NLR with CAD in diabetic population and found ≥ 2.26 as the best suitable cut-off to identify the presence of CAD in diabetic patients [4]. Among immune-inflammatory markers in non-ST-elevation acute coronary syndrome and stable angina patients also, neutrophil counts and NLR were significantly correlated with noncalcified plaques, suggesting the potency of these easily measured biomarkers in reflecting the burden of vulnerable plaques in CAD. Numerous imaging modalities such as invasive coronary angiography and calcium scoring by multidetector CT have also confirmed the role of NLR in the presence, severity, and progression of coronary atherosclerosis [23, 24]. Parallel to us Sari et al. (2015) have also reported that from all other systemic inflammatory markers only NLR is the predictor of CAD showing a strong odds ratio (1.576, confidence interval: 1.198–2.072, $p = 0.001$) [25]. Even in geriatric population too, the patients with CAD had higher NLR, where the cut-off of 1.96 was reported with 66.5% of sensitivity and 48.8% of specificity (AUC = 0.575) [26]. In addition, higher NLR has also been associated with increased cardiac mortality in clinically stable patients with CAD compared with total WBCs count [27]. In patients with chronic coronary total occlusion (CTO), the NLR was significantly higher showing a positive correlation with SYNTAX score. The cut-off identify for CTO disease by NLR was 2.09 with a sensitivity and specificity of 61% and 69.3%, respectively. Similarly in this study NLR was found to be the strongest predictor of CAD with highest odds ratio; however we are able to achieve greater degree of sensitivity and specificity as compared to previous reported studies. The improvement in sensitivity could be obtained by lowering the cut-off; however in that case we were compromising on specificity and hence the current cut-off of 2.13 was found to be most suitable for Western Indians.

The main role of neutrophilia in CAD may be explained by secretion of various inflammatory mediators such as elastase, myeloperoxidase, and oxygen free radicals which causes tissue damage. The probable cause of lymphopenia include decreased production as a result of increased steroid level due to CAD induced stress and increased apoptosis triggered by increased inflammation thereby resulting in elevated NLR in CAD (+) group [2, 28]. Increased number of neutrophils and decreased lymphocytes are risk indicators for future cardiovascular events. Therefore, elevated NLR integrates the predictive risk of the two leukocyte subtypes into a single risk factor. As the biomarkers used in this study predicted cardiac myocyte damage, the possibility of their association with LVEF was also evaluated in order to differentiate between heart failure patients with preserved EF and heart failure

TABLE 2: Comparison of parameters between group 1 (population without CAD) and group 2 (population with CAD) according to gender.

Variables	Groups	Male			Females		
		Mean	Standard deviation	Significance	Mean	Standard deviation	Significance
WBC	Group 1	10214.9	3783.8	0.002	10065.1	3810.9	0.032
	Group 2	12014.7	4598.9		12338.9	4479.7	
Neutrophil	Group 1	7337.3	3915.8	0.002	7135.2	4024.3	0.039
	Group 2	9168.0	4550.5		9293.0	4446.1	
Lymphocyte	Group 1	2241.2	972.0	0.667	2334.0	908.0	0.978
	Group 2	2184.7	928.7		2328.6	737.5	
Eosinophil	Group 1	285.2	164.1	0.272	266.6	141.0	0.838
	Group 2	277.8	184.1		276.0	180.3	
Monocyte	Group 1	380.6	171.9	0.477	435.8	525.5	0.008
	Group 2	409.1	214.1		443.9	175.7	
Basophil	Group 1	1.9	7.6	0.658	0.7	6.5	0.65
	Group 2	2.6	14.2		3.6	16.3	
Platelet	Group 1	293062.5	136846.6	0.979	335777.8	86389.8	0.953
	Group 2	276300.0	81127.3		320840.0	62082.4	
MPV	Group 1	6.7	1.4	0.382	6.4	1.0	0.145
	Group 2	6.9	1.5		7.0	1.5	
NLR	Group 1	4.5	4.0	0.011	3.9	3.4	0.055
	Group 2	5.2	3.7		4.5	2.8	
PLR	Group 1	153.1	104.8	0.431	181.8	117.2	0.626
	Group 2	157.2	79.3		146.7	52.3	
RDW	Group 1	12.7	2.1	0.89	11.7	1.4	0.006
	Group 2	12.5	1.5		12.4	1.6	
hs-CRP	Group 1	1.6	3.9	0.382	2.5	5.1	0.284
	Group 2	1.8	3.3		3.6	6.6	
CPK-MB	Group 1	48.9	57.4	<0.0001	58.5	116.2	<0.0001
	Group 2	111.6	141.8		106.9	136.4	
Troponin I	Group 1	6.0	13.8	<0.0001	7.0	16.3	0.001
	Group 2	13.4	18.7		15.8	19.0	
ESR	Group 1	22.5	9.1	0.243	22.1	6.0	0.803
	Group 2	23.6	8.4		23.5	9.2	

CAD: coronary artery disease, group 1: population without CAD, group 2; population with CAD, WBC: white blood cell, MPV: mean platelet volume, NLR: neutrophil lymphocyte ratio, PLR: platelet lymphocyte ratio, PWBC: platelet white blood cell ratio, RDW: red cell distribution width, hs-CRP: high sensitivity C-reactive protein, CPK-MB: creatinine phosphokinase-MB, and ESR: erythrocyte sedimentation rate.

patients with depressed EF. In concordance with other studies where higher NLR values were associated with lower EF [29], in our population also patients with low EF had elevated mean NLR value as compared to their counterparts, though in our case the difference could not reach a statistically significant level. Moreover the lack of association was also observed between overall EF and that of NLR values. This finding could be justified by the fact that greater number of the patients (≈60%) had compromised LVEF and hence more systematic randomized study is needed to evaluate association of LVEF with NLR in Indian CAD patients.

Diagnosis of CAD is principally based on CAG and other cardiovascular imaging modalities; however these tools are expensive and time consuming with potential unwanted effects such as exposure to radiation. Therefore, NLR, which is cheap and easily obtainable, could be used as an initial filter criterion, especially in small centres to determine the need for further imaging modalities in the assessment of CAD.

5. Conclusion

Keeping in mind the early acting immunological nature of neutrophils and lymphocytes and their presence in the blood circulation, we recommend the use of NLR as a biomarker of CAD because of their simple, easily measurable, and inexpensive method. Along with previous international recommendations, our study supports the use of NLR as a cost-effective biomarker to predict the future cardiovascular risk.

TABLE 3: Comparison of parameters between group 1 (population without CAD) and group 2 (population with CAD) according to age.

Variables	Groups	≤40 years Mean	≤40 years Standard deviation	≤40 years Significance	>40 years Mean	>40 years Standard deviation	>40 years Significance
WBC	Group 1	8795.7	2103.3	0.17	10280.6	3856.5	<0.0001
	Group 2	10804.9	3617.9		12267.8	4665.6	
Neutrophil	Group 1	5921.5	2256.7	0.168	7387.9	4012.5	<0.0001
	Group 2	7896.2	3511.4		9381.9	4623.7	
Lymphocyte	Group 1	2378.6	1018.8	0.889	2257.0	952.0	0.619
	Group 2	2316.5	1055.6		2200.6	868.1	
Eosinophil	Group 1	202.8	84.8	0.282	286.5	160.7	0.195
	Group 2	304.6	239.0		273.8	174.6	
Monocyte	Group 1	292.8	62.8	0.454	402.9	314.3	0.058
	Group 2	343.1	171.3		427.2	209.5	
Basophil	Group 1	0	0		1.2	12.7	0.653
	Group 2	9.8	37.6		3.9	56.9	
Platelet	Group 1	358000.0	141421.4	0.532	304130.4	121689.0	0.972
	Group 2	314909.1	79353.0		286001.4	77884.5	
MPV	Group 1	5.9	0.8	0.045	6.7	1.3	0.256
	Group 2	6.9	1.7		6.9	1.5	
NLR	Group 1	3.3	2.5	0.375	4.4	3.9	0.002
	Group 2	4.3	3.5		5.1	3.5	
PLR	Group 1	141.4	54.5	0.468	165.3	111.9	0.601
	Group 2	133.9	41.5		157.1	75.3	
RDW	Group 1	12.6	1.6	0.804	12.4	2.0	0.129
	Group 2	12.7	1.4		12.5	1.5	
hs-CRP	Group 1	0.3	0.5	0.011	2.0	4.4	0.382
	Group 2	2.2	4.2		2.2	4.3	
CPK-MB	Group 1	33.4	17.3	0.194	52.8	79.3	<0.0001
	Group 2	102.1	154.1		111.8	138.6	
Troponin I	Group 1	3.4	8.3	0.032	6.5	14.8	<0.0001
	Group 2	14.7	20.6		13.8	18.6	
ESR	Group 1	18.1	6.2	0.404	22.7	8.4	0.206
	Group 2	19.6	7.2		24.1	8.6	

CAD: coronary artery disease, group 1: population without CAD, group 2; population with CAD, WBC: white blood cell, MPV: mean platelet volume, NLR: neutrophil-to-lymphocyte ratio, PLR: platelet-to-lymphocyte ratio, PWBC: platelet white blood cell ratio, RDW: red cell distribution width, hs-CRP: high sensitivity C-reactive protein, CPK-MB: creatinine phosphokinase-MB, and ESR: erythrocyte sedimentation rate.

TABLE 4: Multivariate logistic regression analysis for coronary artery disease presence by various biochemical markers.

Variables	exp(*B*)	Significance	95% CI for exp(*B*) Lower	95% CI for exp(*B*) Upper
WBC	1.000	0.030	1.000	1.000
Neutrophil	1.044	0.436	0.936	1.165
Monocyte	1.101	0.133	0.971	1.249
NLR	1.495	0.048	0.942	2.371
RDW	1.116	0.186	0.948	1.314
hs-CRP	1.031	0.399	0.960	1.109
CPK-MB	0.993	0.034	0.986	0.999
Troponin I	0.994	0.669	0.966	1.022
Constant	0.001	0.219		

exp(*B*): exponentiation of the coefficients/odds ratios of the predictors, CI: confidence interval, WBC: white blood cell, NLR: neutrophil-to-lymphocyte ratio, RDW: red cell distribution width, hs-CRP: high sensitivity C-reactive protein, CPK-MB: creatinine phosphokinase-MB, and ESR: erythrocyte sedimentation rate.

Table 5: Receiver operative curve analysis of biochemical markers for CAD diagnosis.

Test result variable(s)	Area	Std. Error[a]	Asymptotic Sig.[b]	Asymptotic Sig.[b]	
				Lower bound	Upper bound
WBC	0.809	0.062	0.000	0.687	0.931
Neutrophil	0.821	0.056	0.000	0.714	0.932
Monocyte	0.697	0.064	0.022	0.572	0.823
NLR	0.823	0.056	0.000	0.712	0.931
RDW	0.713	0.064	0.014	0.587	0.839
hs-CRP	0.648	0.072	0.086	0.506	0.790
Troponin I	0.820	0.035	0.000	0.816	0.951

CAD: coronary artery disease, WBC: white blood cell, NLR: neutrophil-to-lymphocyte ratio, RDW: red cell distribution width, hs-CRP: high sensitivity C-reactive protein, CPK-MB: creatinine phosphokinase-MB, and ESR: erythrocyte sedimentation rate. [a]Under the nonparametric assumption. [b]Null hypothesis: true area = 0.5.

Table 6: Receiver operative curve analysis of NLR cut-off (2.13) for CAD diagnosis.

Statistic	Value	95% CI
Sensitivity	83.64%	78.67% to 87.86%
Specificity	63.46%	55.39% to 71.02%
Positive predictive value	79.79%	76.13% to 83.01%
Negative predictive value	69.23%	62.61% to 75.14%

CI: confidence interval.

Table 7: Association of acute coronary syndrome biomarkers with NLR.

Quartiles	hs-CRP	Mean NLR in hs-CRP quartile	CPK-MB	Mean NLR in CPK-MB quartile	Troponin I	Mean NLR in troponin I quartile
1st quartile	0.175	3.58	24	2.9	0.007	2.62
2nd quartile	0.45	4.88	40	4.07	0.974	4.31
3rd quartile	2.1	6.06	115	5.8	19.75	6.87

NLR, neutrophil-to-lymphocyte ratio; hs-CRP, high sensitivity C-reactive protein; CPK-MB, creatine phosphokinase-MB.

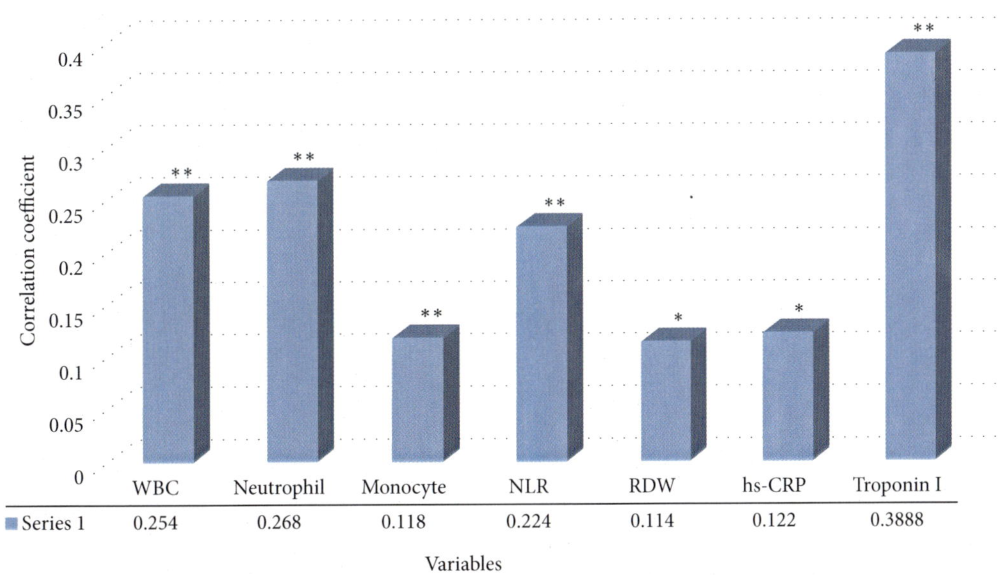

Figure 1: Correlation of biochemical markers with disease presence. **Correlation is significant at the 0.01 level (2-tailed). *Correlation is significant at the 0.05 level (2-tailed). WBC: white blood cell, NLR: neutrophil-to-lymphocyte ratio, RDW: red cell distribution width, and hs-CRP: high sensitivity C-reactive protein.

References

[1] A. H. Ateş, U. Canpolat, H. Yorgun et al., "Total white blood cell count is associated with the presence, severity and extent of coronary atherosclerosis detected by dual-source multislice computed tomographic coronary angiography," *Cardiology Journal*, vol. 18, no. 4, pp. 371–377, 2011.

[2] B. D. Horne, J. L. Anderson, J. M. John et al., "Which white blood cell subtypes predict increased cardiovascular risk?" *Journal of the American College of Cardiology*, vol. 45, no. 10, pp. 1638–1643, 2005.

[3] R. S. Allichandi and S. M. Khilari, "Association between neutrophil to lymphocyte ratio with presence and severity of coronary artery disease," *IOSR Journal of Dental and Medical Sciences*, vol. 15, no. 6, pp. 11–13, 2016.

[4] M. L. Fernando, S. Silambanan, and J. Malar, "Neutrophil to lymphocyte ratio as an indicator of presence of coronary artery disease in diabetic patients," *International Journal of Clinical Biochemistry and Research*, vol. 2, no. 3, pp. 143–147, 2015.

[5] J. H. Prajapati, S. Sahoo, T. Nikam, K. H. Shah, B. Maheriya, and M. Parmar, "Association of high density lipoprotein with platelet to lymphocyte and neutrophil to lymphocyte ratios in coronary artery disease patients," *Journal of Lipids*, vol. 2014, Article ID 686791, 8 pages, 2014.

[6] A. Papa, M. Emdin, C. Passino, C. Michelassi, D. Battaglia, and F. Cocci, "Predictive value of elevated neutrophil-lymphocyte ratio on cardiac mortality in patients with stable coronary artery disease," *Clinica Chimica Acta*, vol. 395, no. 1-2, pp. 27–31, 2008.

[7] J. Núñez, E. Núñez, V. Bodí et al., "Usefulness of the neutrophil to lymphocyte ratio in predicting long-term mortality in st segment elevation myocardial infarction," *American Journal of Cardiology*, vol. 101, no. 6, pp. 747–752, 2008.

[8] S. Uthamalingam, E. A. Patvardhan, S. Subramanian et al., "Utility of the neutrophil to lymphocyte ratio in predicting long-term outcomes in acute decompensated heart failure," *The American Journal of Cardiology*, vol. 107, no. 3, pp. 433–438, 2011.

[9] B. Azab, V. R. Bhatt, J. Phookan et al., "Usefulness of the neutrophil-to-lymphocyte ratio in predicting short- and long-term mortality in breast cancer patients," *Annals of Surgical Oncology*, vol. 19, no. 1, pp. 217–224, 2012.

[10] T. Yamanaka, S. Matsumoto, S. Teramukai, R. Ishiwata, Y. Nagai, and M. Fukushima, "The baseline ratio of neutrophils to lymphocytes is associated with patient prognosis in advanced gastric cancer," *Oncology*, vol. 73, no. 3-4, pp. 215–220, 2008.

[11] Y. Ohno, J. Nakashima, M. Ohori, T. Hatano, and M. Tachibana, "Pretreatment neutrophil-to-lymphocyte ratio as an independent predictor of recurrence in patients with nonmetastatic renal cell carcinoma," *Journal of Urology*, vol. 184, no. 3, pp. 873–878, 2010.

[12] I. Bhatti, O. Peacock, G. Lloyd, M. Larvin, and R. I. Hall, "Preoperative hematologic markers as independent predictors of prognosis in resected pancreatic ductal adenocarcinoma: neutrophil-lymphocyte versus platelet-lymphocyte ratio," *The American Journal of Surgery*, vol. 200, no. 2, pp. 197–203, 2010.

[13] P. Ding, X. An, R. Zhang et al., "Elevated preoperative neutrophil to lymphocyte ratio predicts risk of recurrence following curative resection for stage IIA colon cancer," *International Journal of Colorectal Disease*, vol. 25, no. 12, pp. 1427–1433, 2010.

[14] Y. Kishi, S. Kopetz, Y. S. Chun, M. Palavecino, E. K. Abdalla, and J.-N. Vauthey, "Blood neutrophil-to-lymphocyte ratio predicts survival in patients with colorectal liver metastases treated with systemic chemotherapy," *Annals of Surgical Oncology*, vol. 16, no. 3, pp. 614–622, 2009.

[15] K. J. Halazun, M. A. Hardy, and A. A. Rana, "Negative impact of neutrophil-lymphocyte ratio on outcome after liver transplantation for hepatocellular carcinoma," *Annals of Surgery*, vol. 250, no. 1, pp. 141–151, 2009.

[16] M. Aliustaoglu, A. Bilici, M. Seker et al., "The association of pretreatment peripheral blood markers with survival in patients with pancreatic cancer," *Hepato-Gastroenterology*, vol. 57, no. 99-100, pp. 640–645, 2010.

[17] U. U. Tamhane, S. Aneja, D. Montgomery, E.-K. Rogers, K. A. Eagle, and H. S. Gurm, "Association between admission neutrophil to lymphocyte ratio and outcomes in patients with acute coronary syndrome," *American Journal of Cardiology*, vol. 102, no. 6, pp. 653–657, 2008.

[18] B. Azab, M. A. Shariff, R. Bachir, J. P. Nabagiez, and J. T. McGinn Jr., "Elevated preoperative neutrophil/lymphocyte ratio as a predictor of increased long-term survival in minimal invasive coronary artery bypass surgery compared to sternotomy," *Journal of Cardiothoracic Surgery*, vol. 8, no. 193, pp. 1–11, 2013.

[19] B. Azab, M. Zaher, K. F. Weiserbs et al., "Usefulness of neutrophil to lymphocyte ratio in predicting short-and long-term mortality after NonST-elevation myocardial infarction," *American Journal of Cardiology*, vol. 106, no. 4, pp. 470–476, 2010.

[20] O. Sönmez, G. Ertaş, A. Bacaksiz et al., "Relation of neutrophil -to- lymphocyte ratio with the presence and complexity of coronary artery disease: an observational study," *Anadolu Kardiyoloji Dergisi*, vol. 13, no. 7, pp. 662–667, 2013.

[21] L. Guasti, F. Dentali, L. Castiglioni et al., "Neutrophils and clinical outcomes in patients with acute coronary syndromes and/or cardiac revascularisation. A systematic review on more than 34,000 subjects," *Thrombosis and Haemostasis*, vol. 106, no. 4, pp. 591–599, 2011.

[22] M. Sunbul, F. Gerin, E. Durmus et al., "Neutrophil to lymphocyte and platelet to lymphocyte ratio in patients with dipper versus non-dipper hypertension," *Clinical and Experimental Hypertension*, vol. 36, no. 4, pp. 217–221, 2014.

[23] Y. Arbel, A. Finkelstein, A. Halkin et al., "Neutrophil/lymphocyte ratio is related to the severity of coronary artery disease and clinical outcome in patients undergoing angiography," *Atherosclerosis*, vol. 225, no. 2, pp. 456–460, 2012.

[24] B.-J. Park, J.-Y. Shim, H.-R. Lee et al., "Relationship of neutrophil-lymphocyte ratio with arterial stiffness and coronary calcium score," *Clinica Chimica Acta*, vol. 412, no. 11-12, pp. 925–929, 2011.

[25] I. Sari, M. Sunbul, C. Mammadov et al., "Relation of neutrophil-to-lymphocyte and platelet-to-lymphocyte ratio with coronary artery disease severity in patients undergoing coronary angiography," *Kardiologia Polska*, vol. 73, no. 12, pp. 1310–1316, 2015.

[26] K. C. Muhammet, K. E. Mehmet, K. K. Mustafa et al., "Neutrophil to lymphocyte ratio may predict coronary artery disease in geriatric patients," *Acta Medica*, vol. 4, pp. 58–63, 2015.

[27] C. D. Lee, A. R. Folsom, F. J. Nieto, L. E. Chambless, E. Shahar, and D. A. Wolfe, "White blood cell count and incidence of coronary heart disease and ischemic stroke and mortality from cardiovascular disease in African-American and White men and women: atherosclerosis risk in communities study," *American Journal of Epidemiology*, vol. 154, no. 8, pp. 758–764, 2001.

[28] M. Hoffman, A. Blum, R. Baruch, E. Kaplan, and M. Benjamin, "Leukocytes and coronary heart disease," *Atherosclerosis*, vol. 172, no. 1, pp. 1–6, 2004.

28

Alleviating Promotion of Inflammation and Cancer Induced by Nonsteroidal Anti-Inflammatory Drugs

Anthony M. Kyriakopoulos,[1] Markus Nagl,[2] Stella Baliou,[3] and Vasilleios Zoumpourlis[3]

[1] *Nasco AD Biotechnology Laboratory, 11 Sachtouri Str, 18536 Pireus, Greece*
[2] *Division of Hygiene and Medical Microbiology, Medical University of Innsbruck, Schöpfstr. 41, 6020 Innsbruck, Austria*
[3] *National Hellenic Research Foundation, 48 Vas. Konstantinou Av., 11635 Athens, Greece*

Correspondence should be addressed to Anthony M. Kyriakopoulos; rnd@nascoad.com

Academic Editor: Jian-Dong Li

Clinical Relevance. Nonsteroidal Anti-Inflammatory Drugs (NSAIDs) including aspirin are of intensive use nowadays. These drugs exert their activity via the metabolism of arachidonic acid (AA) by cyclooxygenase inhibition. Though beneficial for health in some instances, both unspecific and specific cyclooxygenase inhibitor activity interfere with AA metabolism producing also proinflammatory lipids that may promote cancer. *Materials and Methods.* This review is based on available literature on clinical uses, biochemical investigations, molecular medicine, pharmacology, toxicity, and epidemiology-clinical studies on NSAIDs and other drugs that may be used accordingly, which was collected from electronic (SciFinder, Medline, Science Direct, and ACS among others) and library searches of books and journals. *Results.* Relevant literature supports the notion that NDSAID use may also promote proinflammatory biochemical events that are also related to precancerous predisposition. Several agents are proposed that may be employed in immediate future to supplement and optimize treatment with NSAIDs. In this way serious side effects arising from promotion of inflammation and cancer, especially in chronic NSAID users and high risk groups of patients, could be avoided.

1. Introduction

1.1. Inflammation Route via Arachidonic Acid Metabolism. Inflammation is driven by complex metabolic pathways, with arachidonic acid (AA) as one important molecule of origin. AA metabolism is fundamental for both promotion and inhibition of inflammatory processes. Several enzymes are involved in this regulation of inflammation, cyclooxygenases 1 and 2 [1], lipoxygenases [1], cytochrome P 450 (CYP) epoxygenases and ω-hydroxylases [2], and also the nonenzymatic processes of AA metabolism like the free radical-catalyzed peroxidation [3]. Nonsteroidal Anti-Inflammatory Drugs (NSAIDs) have been designed to decrease above all the classical symptoms of pain and tumefaction, but in the meantime it is known that they cause proinflammatory effects, too. Aspirin targets the COX-1 pathway, whereas the classical NSAIDs target mainly the COX-2 pathway by inhibiting prostaglandin E_2 (PGE_2) formation [4]. The anti-inflammatory effect is due to the inhibition of vasodilatation and to the shortening of mast cell and other immune cells recruitment. Aspirin however acetylates also the COX-2 isoenzyme but due to slight sequence variations this evidently consumes less binding energy for arachidonic acid to become bound and be further metabolized [5].

1.2. Cyclooxygenase (COX) Activity. Early findings on aspirin inhibitory mode of action on prostaglandin (PG) synthesis led to the initial discovery of cyclooxygenase (COX) [6, 7]. This enzyme, now called COX-1, is central to AA catabolism to end up producing PGI_2, also known as prostacyclin, with clear antithrombogenic [8, 9] and cytoprotective to gastric mucosa [10, 11] physiological functions. In 1991, a 64% sequence homologue to COX-1 enzyme was discovered [12, 13] that was inducible in a number of cells to certain proinflammatory stimuli [11] and inhibited in its expression by corticosteroids [7]. This is the enzyme now termed as COX-2. In this area, the variation of severity of side effects caused by different anti-inflammatory drugs including aspirin was puzzling. Particularly, stomach side effects by aspirin led to the development of safer drugs like meloxicam, nimesulide, and etodolac, which are now well accepted as selective COX-2 inhibitors [7]. Although both COX isoenzymes catalyze the oxygenation of arachidonate, COX-2 shows a more diverse substrate selectivity compared to COX-1. For example, COX-2 apart from arachidonic acid oxygenates in the same efficiency 2-arachidonylglycerol (endocannabinoid) [14]. The most evident difference between COX isoenzymes is in their expression in tissue distribution. Unlike COX-1, which is ubiquitous and constitutively expressed throughout the gastrointestinal system, the kidneys, the vascular smooth muscle, and the platelets, COX-2 is constitutively expressed in endothelial cells, brain, and kidneys and is variably induced in its expression by distinct inflammatory stimuli and neoplastic conditions [15, 16]. Unexplained antipyretic and analgesic effects of acetaminophen, phenacetin, and dipyrone, without evident COX-1 or COX-2 inhibition, were made clear by the discovery of yet another COX isoenzyme termed COX-3 that when expressed showed selective inhibition to these agents [17].

1.3. How NSAIDs May Cause Side Effects. NSAIDs, by inhibiting cyclooxygenase enzyme activity, even by different means, may all share to a greater or lesser extent a similar kind of side effects [7]. However, these side effects may be both (a) specific to the NSAID type and (b) cell type specific. Side effects depend on the specific inhibition of prostanoid synthesis due to the agent inducing the COX inhibition and the type of targeted tissue [15]. Prostanoid synthesis alteration contributes to disturbance of homeostasis [7] that may be cell specific, giving an end organ specific toxicity [18–22] (Figure 1).

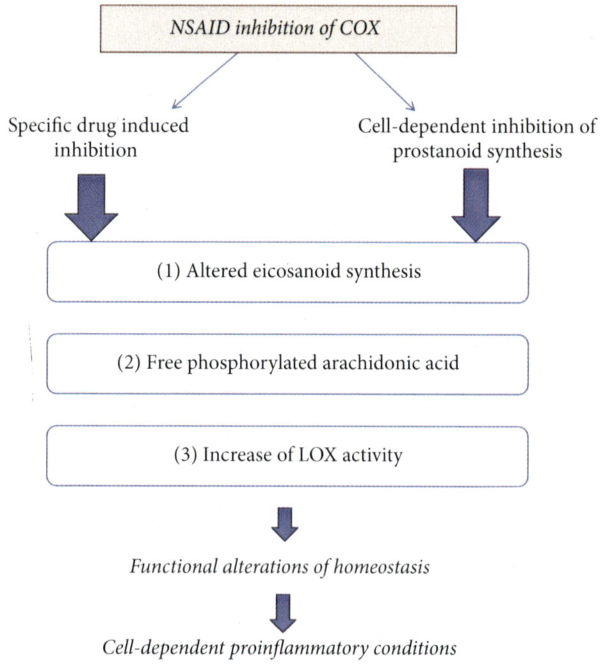

Figure 1: Levels of possible side effects of NSAIDs [18]. Drug- and cell-specific inhibition of COX isoenzymes [15] and respective prostanoids results in alteration of homeostasis [7] and in promotion of proinflammatory conditions [18–22].

1.3.1. The Mechanisms by Which Aspirin Induces Proinflammatory Effects. Acetylation of serine (Ser-530) of COX-1 even by low aspirin concentrations and in a few minutes results in the inhibition of prostaglandin E_2 (PGE_2) formation and the inhibition of platelet function (anticoagulant activity) [23]. This acetylating reaction irreversibly inactivates COX-1 activity [24]. As a consequence, related tissue and blood pressure homeostasis depending on PGE_2 formation may be affected [7, 25]. An example is the kidney normal function that depends on PGE_2 synthesis. Renin is secreted by PGE_2 formation and angiotensin II stimulation is mainly mediated by PGE_2 production by COX-1, but also by COX-2 [25]. Acetylation by aspirin is also occurring on the COX-2 isoform in almost the same manner due to the structural homology between COX-1 and COX-2 isoenzymes. Tyrosine residues (tyr-385) to a greater extent and (tyr-348) to a lesser extent are critical for this acetylation event of COX-2 by aspirin [26]. These tyrosine residues constitute a hydrogen binding network that is critical for the precise positioning and the relative reactivity rendering the closeness of Ser-530 with the acetyl group of aspirin feasible. Arginine 120 (Arg-120) just below Ser-530 in the active sites of COX, however, makes the difference of arachidonic acid binding ability between COX-1 and COX-2 isoenzymes (Figure 2). In the COX-1 case of binding of arachidonic acid, an ionic bond is formed between Arg-120 and the carboxylate of arachidonate. In COX-2 case however, instead of an ionic bond, a hydrogen bond is formed with Arg-120 and arachidonate thus conferring less to the binding energy needed for the molecule to become bound [27, 28]. During the acetylation event in COX-1, the arachidonic acid is irreversibly inhibited from binding when Arg-120 makes the Ser-530 acetylation efficient by forming a weak ionic bond with the carboxylate of aspirin. Conversely, the acetylation event in COX-2 does not irreversibly inhibit its activity but just lowers the arachidonic acid binding ability to the enzyme's active site (Figure 2).

The acetylation event by aspirin, shown to produce also the aspirin-triggered lipotoxins by transcellular (cell-to-cell) interactions [29, 30], is also supported by clinical evidence. Direct clinical evidence shows that among the derived eicosanoids produced by aspirin acetylation are the lipoxin A_4 (LXA_4), which is vasodilatory, and the leukotrienes C_4 and D_4 (LTC_4, LTD_4), which are potent vasoconstrictors. These eicosanoids have been shown to be generated under aspirin treatment in the atherosclerotic lumen of blood vessels [31]. Also, in aspirin intolerance, excessive amounts of LTC_4 have been isolated from nasal secretions and bronchial biopsies [32]. These leukotrienes produced are implicated to severe gastrointestinal [33] and severe cardiovascular side effects [34] as they constitute important mediators of inflammation, ischemia [35], and bronchoconstriction [36].

1.3.2. The Transcellular Biosynthesis of Eicosanoid Derivatives: Crossover Pathways. The transcellular biosynthesis of lipoxins requires interactions between LOX isoenzymes

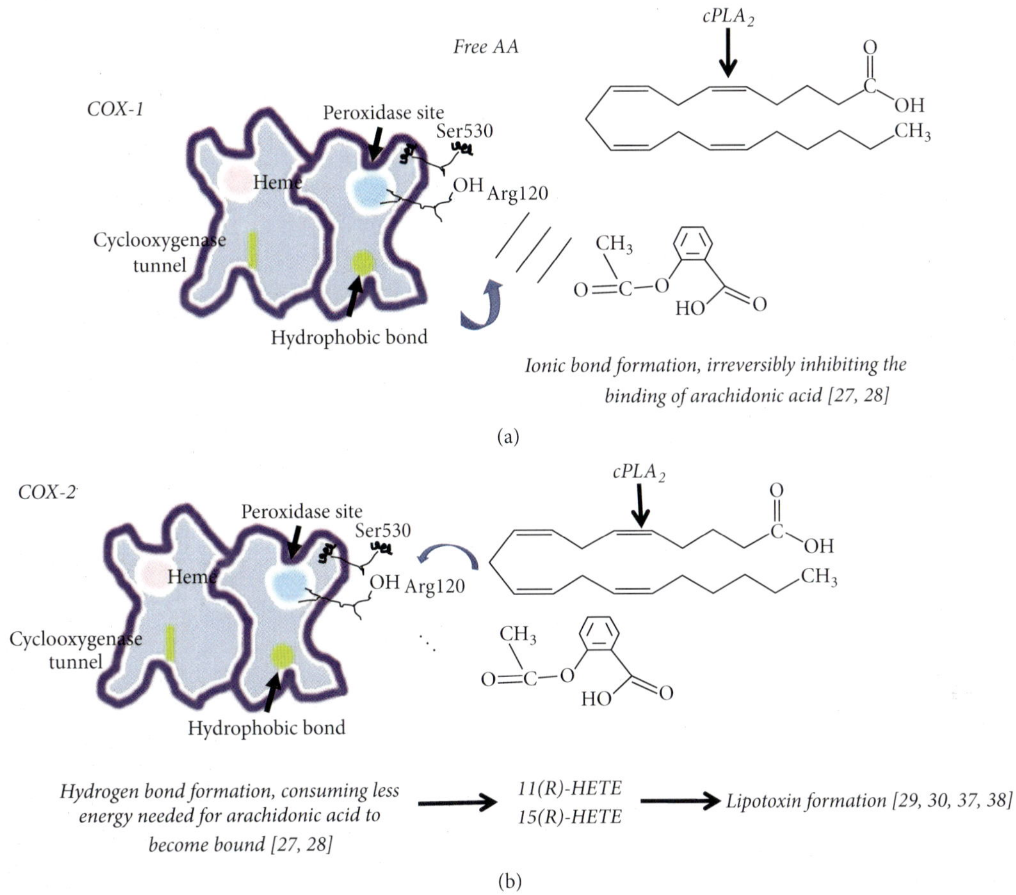

FIGURE 2: (a) Aspirin acetylation of COX-1 irreversibly inhibits arachidonic acid to become bound, whereas (b) acetylation of COX-2 leads to the formation of lipoxins [27–30, 37].

(LOX-LOX interactions) and can promote generation of leukotrienes (LTs) by endothelial cells [37]. When COX-2 is acetylated by aspirin, interaction with 5-lipoxygenase (5-LOX) occurs that triggers the transcellular biosynthesis of 15-R epimers of lipoxins [29, 38]. The derived eicosanoids by the acetylation of COX-2 in close association with 5-LOX are of the type of "S" conformation [39, 40]. Hereby, it has to be emphasized that in all cases arachidonic acid is first transformed to unstable precursor intermediate molecules ending up to many "S" conformations after aspirin treated COX-2 [30, 41]. Therefore, even 15-S-HETE formation cannot be excluded even by aspirin-induced specific 15-R-HETE formation as it may occur also in a nonenzyme dependent fashion [41]. During aspirin-triggered lipoxin synthesis, the precursor LTA_4 (that is also of "S" conformation) may be formed by 5-LOX and serve as substrate for leukotriene synthesis of LTB_4 that is formed prior to LTC_4 and LTD_4 [35] (Figure 3(a)). Apart from the absolute belief of 15-R-HETE being a sole product, as derived by the acetylation of COX-2, the presence of the double dioxygenated product, 5S-12S-DiHETE isolated in vivo, suggests further transcellular metabolic events that show further eicosanoid synthesis by 5- and 12-LOX interactions [31]. Research during that time may have identified generation of byproducts via enzymatic conversion of LTA_4 [30, 42, 43]. Similar latter results indicate the possibility of 5S-15S-DiHETE to be formed in vivo by the acetylated COX-2 activity and 5-LOX-15-LOX interactions having 5S-hydroxy-6E,8Z,11Z,14Z-eicosatetraenoic acid (5-S-HETE) as a substrate [44]. As LOX activity is not inhibited by aspirin, through the unstable intermediate formed by the acetylated COX-2, LOX isoenzymes continue the eicosanoid synthesis to produce active compounds [30, 40]. Further, all S-conformations produced during COX-2 acetylation and interaction with lipoxygenases can be relatively good substrates for 5-hydroxyeicosanoid dehydrogenase (5-HEDH) to produce 5-OXO-ETE [45]. Thus, another important proinflammatory mediator may be also formed (Figure 3(a)). Under oxidative conditions 5-HEDH transforms (5-S-HETE) to 5-OXO-ETE [46] as under normal conditions 5-HEDM is inactive because it requires $NADP^+$ as a cofactor. Under stress conditions, however, NADPH oxidase activity has been described for its serious role in mediating inflammation [47].

5-S-HETE is on its own a potent proinflammatory mediator [48] to induce stress conditions together with potent proinflammatory leukotrienes LTB_4 and the cysteinyl leukotrienes LTC_4 and LTD_4. The metabolic tendency of 5-LOX to produce the 5-OXO-ETE derivative coupled with LTB_4 is important for inflammation and cancer [48, 49],

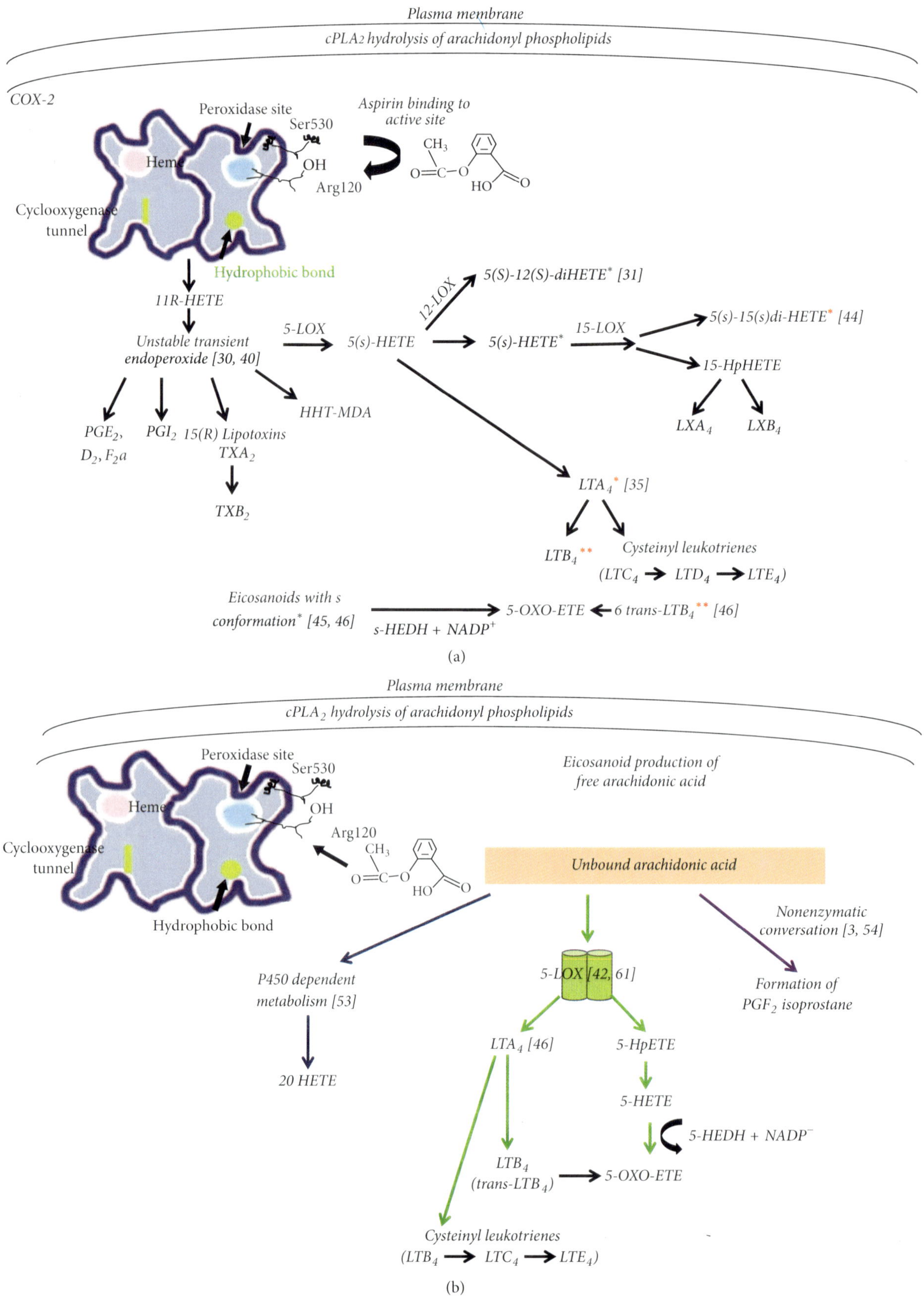

FIGURE 3: Metabolic events that follow acetylation of COX-2 and further transcellular activities: (a) eicosanoid production by crossover pathways of acetylated COX-2 and LOX isoenzymes [31, 35, 37–44]. (b) Eicosanoid production by free arachidonic acid [3, 44–46, 53, 54, 61].

which has not been linked adequately as a serious proinflammatory condition due to NSAID use. The 5-S-HETE metabolite, when accumulating, is a potent neutrophil activator [50]. The 5-OXO-ETE derivative, however, has been shown to be a 100 times more potent neutrophil activator than its precursor [51]. As synthetic 5-OXO-HETE derivatives prove to be even more potent than 5-OXO-ETE, the native derivatives also traced in vivo may be further implicated in the promotion of chronic inflammation and cancer [49, 52]. 5-OXO-HETE acts proinflammatorily via the OXO-ETE receptor that is known to promote eosinophil and other inflammatory cells migration [48]. 5-OXO-ETE is formed in neutrophil microsomes under the presence of $NADP^+$- and Ca^{2+}- dependent translocation of 5-LOX to the nuclear membrane to act on arachidonic acid bound by the nuclear membrane accessory protein 5-LOX activating protein (FLAP). The neutrophil microsomes under reduced conditions prefer, as well as the 5-S-HETE, to produce the 5-OXO-ETE derivative lipid using the 6-transanalogue of LTB_4 as a substrate [46].

Free activated arachidonic acid not bound to COX-2 may be also used by 5-LOX to produce leukotrienes during inflammation in vivo [42]. Furthermore, it may be utilized by the P450 metabolism to produce 20-HETE [53] and by nonenzymatic conversion to form PGF_2 isoprostanes [3, 54] (Figure 3(b)).

2. Materials and Methods

The literature study was conducted from scientific journals and books and electronic sources such as SciFinder, Science Direct, Medline, and Google Scholar, covering the period from January 1945 to the end of December 2016.

3. Results

3.1. Nonaspirin NSAIDs

3.1.1. Traditional NSAID Clinical Side Effects. Traditional NSAIDs during clinical practice vary on the degree of causing vascular side effects. Increased risk is noticed by high doses of diclofenac and ibuprofen due to the increased myocardial infarction events recorded, whereas increased doses of naproxen have substantially smaller risk [55], suggesting differential inhibition of activity of COX-2. Acute myocardial infarction risk is potentiated in patients with coronary artery disease by high and low doses of diclofenac and rofecoxib and other NSAIDs, but not with naproxen even when administered in high doses [34]. The risk for renal disease development is tightly correlated with acetaminophen overuse [56]. Acetaminophen provides a unique example of cell-specific COX inhibition that may negatively affect the prostanoid synthesis in tumor cells by altering the levels of PGE_2 [57, 58]. Upon NSAID inhibition of COX activity by traditional COX-2 inhibitors like diclofenac, an alternate housekeeping COX-1-like activity, of a third COX isoenzyme may be also inhibited by concurrent use of acetaminophen [28]. Also, this drug's specific COX-2-like inhibition may affect homeostatic mechanisms of the central nervous system, the gastrointestinal system, and the renal system [15].

3.1.2. Proinflammatory Mechanisms Caused by Traditional NSAIDs. In general, for traditional nonselective COX inhibitors, the mechanism of drug generated myocardial pathology [34] may be due to prostacyclin and other prostanoid inhibition that depends on the degree of COX-2 inhibition [7]. The constitutive COX-2 isoenzyme that is inhibited plays an important role in the regulation of salt, volume, and blood pressure maintenance [59] by providing the appropriate prostaglandins to regulate the renin-angiotensin system [60]. Apart from prostanoid synthesis diminishment, free hydrolyzed arachidonic acid from c Phospolipase A_2 ($cPLA_2$) may be utilized by LOX isoenzymes to produce increased amounts of proinflammatory leukotrienes [61] and toxic metabolites like 5-S-HETE and 5-OXO-ETE as seen with the aspirin acetylation of COX-2 [45, 46] (Figure 3(b)).

3.2. "More Selective" COX-2 Inhibitors

3.2.1. Proinflammatory Mechanisms by "More Selective" COX-2 Inhibitors. The clear distinction between COX-1 and COX-2 inhibitors cannot be defined fully [62]. The term selective COX-2 inhibitor requires further examination as it is oversimplified and therefore the term "more selective" is used in this article. To identify proinflammatory effects caused by COX-2 more selective inhibitors, the interrelationships between COX-1 and COX-2 catalytic functions have to be taken into account. COX-1 and COX-2 have similar binding sites for NSAIDs other than aspirin that block arachidonic acid metabolism. Naproxen, for example, due to its smaller molecular size occupies easily the hydrophobic COX-1 binding site of arachidonic acid where an isoleucine is at position 523. Celecoxib is a larger molecule that naproxen cannot occupy the COX-1 binding site for arachidonic acid. Instead it occupies in an easier manner the COX-2 binding site where a smaller valine instead of isoleucine is at position 523 [63]. Thus due to small structural differences between the two COX isoenzyme active sites NSAIDs show greater or lower selectivity for COX-1 and COX-2 resulting in greater or lower relative inhibition of arachidonic acid metabolism. Relatively increased inhibition of COX-2 activity results in relative diminishment of prostacyclin inhibition which is a known cardioprotective prostanoid [64]. Recent epidemiologic studies come to directly associate the use of a large number of individual NSAIDs with hospital administration for heart failure [65]. Looking at a different metabolic pathway, more selective COX inhibitory NSAIDs may block the metabolism of 20-HETE to $PGF_{2\alpha}$ and other mediators during P450 metabolism of arachidonic acid thereby resulting in increased accumulation of 20-HETE [53] (Figure 3(b)). 20-HETE has also been shown to be a serious promoter of renal hypertension and to be implicated in an increased risk for renal [33] and cardiovascular diseases [34] such as myocardial infarction, hypertension, and heart failure that have also been observed but in a smaller scale with the administration of nonaspirin traditional NSAIDs [6, 7, 34] (Figure 3(b)). Arachidonic acid that remains not bound and oxygenized by COX isoenzymes may be used by p450 and 5-LOX dependent, as well as enzyme independent, metabolic pathways to produce proinflammatory metabolites [45, 46, 61] like LTB_4, LTC_4, and 5-OXO-ETE as in aspirin acetylation's case (Figure 3(b)).

3.2.2. "More Selective" COX-2 Inhibitor Clinical Side Effects. Withdrawal of rofecoxib (a similar agent to celecoxib with increased vascular side effects) from clinical use is perhaps the best example to account for side effects by a more selective COX-2 inhibitor [53, 66]. Clearly, increased myocardial infarction events are associated with more selective COX-2 inhibitor use although nonselective inhibitors of cyclooxygenase are not excluded from being potent risk factors for the development of cardiovascular episodes [34, 62, 67].

Coadministration of aspirin in clinical practice is recommended for certain groups of patients taking vast amounts of NSAIDs as a thrombolytic agent for cardioprotection [63]. These patients are at increased risk from thrombotic events by taking selective COX-2 inhibitor NSAIDs to treat inflammatory disorders [68]. Guidelines however state that aspirin use may not always be an efficient protection [62]. As for traditional NSAIDs, the more selective COX-2 inhibition may also contribute to a subsequent surplus of arachidonic acid that can be used by lipoxygenases (Figure 3(b)). As already described 5-LOX may be an important mediator enzyme for inflammation and cancer producing more proinflammatory leukotrienes LTC_4 [69], LTB_4 [46, 61, 70], and 5-OXO-ETE [45, 49].

3.3. Hypersensitivity Response. Eosinophils among other stimuli are also driven by LTC_4, which is induced by NSAID use (Figures 3(a) and 3(b)), and are essential mediator cells in the production of allergic inflammation [71]. Various types of NSAIDs are warranted for causing respiratory intolerance [72]. By proinflammatory mediator generation they have been implicated to produce allergic and inflammatory reactions as well as ischemia at the level of lung mucosa leading to asthma [73, 74]. NSAID-induced gastrointestinal injury is mediated by increased LTB_4 synthesis, too. LTB_4 level is elevated in arthritis treated with NSAIDs [75] (Figures 3(a) and 3(b)). Indomethacin may cause acute gastropathy, and the induced overproduction of tumor necrosis factor α (TNFα) has also been implicated in the pathogenesis of disease state [76]. Complementarily, indomethacin to a greater extent than ibuprofen causes renal dysfunctional abnormalities in preterm neonates, and unfortunately both are the drugs of choice for patent ductus arteriosus failure [77]. The immune response in urticaria provides another good example for NSAID driven side effect [78]. Urticaria is the clinical term of a heterogenous group of diseases characterized by wheels and flares of skin's vascular inflammation. Aspirin and other more selective to COX-2 NSAIDs (rofecoxib) and traditional NSAIDs (nimesulide, acetaminophen) cause the aspirin acute intolerant urticaria that in some cases may lead to the aspirin chronic urticaria [79] that has a sound basis of autoimmunity [78]. As it has been shown that in chronic cases of urticaria a specific set of IgE autoantibodies directed against thyroid peroxidase may constitute a novel pathogenetic mechanism, this may be serious for chronic NSAID users [80]. Selective to COX-2 NSAIDs and aspirin have been reported to be implicated in hypersensitivity responses and excess of histamine release, and this may be extended to various hypersensitivity immune disorders [81–83]. However, further studies are needed to investigate the possible IgE elevation in urticaria events that is caused by "more selective" NSAIDs.

4. Discussion

4.1. Alleviating NSAID Associated Proinflammatory Activity. As already described, NSAID side effects occur primarily due to the inhibition of cyclooxygenases that metabolize arachidonic acid and synthesize prostaglandins with beneficial activities under normal conditions [7, 62]. An example of a current therapeutic way to overcome NSAID side effects is the combination of aspirin coadministration in patients receiving "more selective" COX-2 inhibitors in order to avoid thrombotic vascular events, although this may not always be sufficiently protective [62]. Scientific evidence remains to be clarified by large epidemiological and meta-analysis studies to establish safety standards for patients in high risk of developing serious cardiovascular side effects [84]. This process is both time and cost demanding. For example, results from large and recent epidemiologic studies in Europe clarify that heart failure is associated with increased NSAID usage. This increased risk of heart failure is dose dependent and associated with traditional and more selective to COX-2 inhibitors [65]. In all respects, the optimum selection of NSAID coadministration requires deep scientific knowledge to identify the bottom end of prostaglandin synthesis and inhibition with subsequent imbalance of homeostasis (Figure 1).

Better chances to optimize treatment of NSAIDs with relatively high and low COX-2 inhibitory activities can perhaps be conferred by supplementary agents that may interfere with COX in a different manner.

Arachidonic acid hydrolyzed by $cPLA_2$ (phospholipase A_2), if not metabolized by cyclooxygenases, remains an available substrate to be used in other catabolic pathways: (1) the lipoxygenase, (2) the P450 epoxygenase, and (3) the nonenzymatic synthesis leading to isoprostane (Figure 3(b)).

It has been described that by inhibition of COX activity the increase of cysteinyl leukotriene family (CysLT) potent proinflammatory lipid mediators is feasible [63]. Human studies on aspirin intolerance support this hypothesis. When PGE_2 levels are decreased by inhibition of COX-1, altered prostanoid production, combined with increased enzymatic expression like the LTC_4 synthase expression, leads to increased leukotriene synthesis producing the disease state [32, 85, 86].

A way to circumvent proinflammatory leukotrienes (LTB_4 and LTC_4) production by an overwhelming 5-LOX activity may be the already developed specific LOX inhibitors [87, 88]. These may block the undesirable side effects of both LTB_4 and LTC_4 (a cysteinyl derived leukotriene) [89]. Furthermore, the use of selective agonists of cysteinyl leukotriene receptor 1 ($CysLTR_1$) is referred to circumvent leukotriene-associated pathologies probably by inhibition of cytosolic Ca^{2+} [90]. Also the inhibition of CysLTR by other agents may provide suitable pharmacologic activity. The use of either leukotriene biosynthesis inhibitors or leukotriene receptor antagonists [91] may also help to minimize NSAID side effects. Since LTC_4 production is blocked by inactivation of $CysLT_1$ receptor, selective $CysLT_1$ antagonists may be applied [92]. Also, $CysLT_1$ receptor antagonists to reduce eosinophilia may be of therapeutic value [91].

NSAIDs activity as already discussed (Figures 3(a) and 3(b)) may favor 5-LOX to catalyze the formation of LTA_4 and 5-S-hydroperoxy-6,8,11,14-eicosatetraenoic acid (5-HpETE), which is rapidly reduced to 5S-hydroxy-6E,8Z,11Z,14Z eicosatetraenoic acid (5-S-HETE). This metabolic intermediate is oxidized by 5-hydroxyeicosanoid dehydrogenase (5-HEDH) to produce 5-OXO-ETE [46]. 5-HEDH activity is inhibited by 5-hydroxy-fatty acids [45]. Recent advances in the formation of 5-OXO-ETE receptor antagonists [93] may also help to prevent hypersensitivity reactions by COX inhibitors. Conversion of 5-S-HETE into 5-OXO-ETE is highly reversible in the presence of NADPH and alleviation of oxidant conditions. The use of antioxidants may favor restoration of 5-OXO-ETE side effects via the 5-OXO-ETE receptor in asthma, cancer, and cardiovascular conditions [48, 94].

Apart from LOX favored metabolism during COX inhibition, oxidized arachidonic acid may sustain nonenzymatic conversion to form prostaglandin F_2 compounds (PGF_2-isoprostanes). Isoprostanes are very readily formed in biological fluids [3] from oxidized arachidonic acid and through endoperoxide intermediates [54]. Modulation of inflammation by NSAIDs as a natural way of treatment is a very natural way of treatment is by the concurrent prolonged use of naturally derived d-α tocopheryl acetate [95, 96]. Asthmatic and atherosclerotic patients seem to benefit by natural-source d-α-tocopheryl acetate as this is shown to reduce allergen-induced F_2-isoprostane formation [95, 97].

Arachidonic acid, once liberated from membrane phospholipases and not being metabolized further by cyclooxygenases due to NSAID inhibition, may be efficiently metabolized by isoforms of the cytochrome P450 (CYP) family to form 20-hydroxyeicosatetraenoic acid (20-HETE) [98, 99]. 20-HETE promotes coagulation of platelets, thus shortening the time of bleeding, and its synthesis is being increased by rofecoxib, suggesting serious cardiovascular side effects for this drug [53].

In order to identify agents that may inhibit undesired 20-HETE synthesis by NSAID-COX inhibition, the experimental model of spontaneous hypertensive rats provides significant clinical information. Agents that induce heme oxygenase reduce the renal formation of 20-HETE and also decrease hypertension [100, 101]. In clinical research, heme oxygenase inducers are of increasing interest to overcome spontaneous reactions that lead to kidney failure [102].

Heme oxygenase-1 (HO-1), which is expressed in all tissues, receives electrons from NADPH by P450 enzyme fractions due to CRP microsomal protein mediator and P450 protein-to-protein interactions [103]. This may prove to be important clinically, since under severe hypoxia there may be a way to circumvent 5-OXO-ETE accumulation by expenditure of NADPH to $NADP^+$ to reform 5-HETE [104] and to deprive arachidonic acid reserves to form 20-HETE by P450 enzymes at the same time [105] (Figure 6). In this respect, attention is drawn on the induction of HO-1 by naturally derived agents like the endogenous haloamines of taurine, that is, N-chlorotaurine (NCT) and N-bromotaurine (NBrT), also termed as small molecule NSAIDS [106, 107]. These haloamines have been shown to downregulate the production of Cox-2 derived PGE_2 [108] in a way independent of COX-2. NCT exerts its anti-inflammatory activity in rheumatoid arthritis synoviocytes by inhibiting IL-β induced production of PGE_2 by decreasing COX-2 isoenzyme expression leaving COX-1 expression unaltered [109]. However, at lower cytotoxic concentrations both NCT and NBrT decrease PGE_2 synthesis without affecting COX-2 expression [108]. Haloamines of taurine (NBrT and NCT) at present state can be administered locally in cases of cutaneous body cavities and organ infection and inflammation to inactivate microbes, minimize inflammation, and reduce pain and other symptoms [110–113].

Another target for NSAID minimization of side effects on the cardiovascular system may be the maintenance of low levels of nitric oxide (NO) that are essential for cardioprotection [114] (Figure 4). NO at normal levels inhibits thromboxane synthase and activates prostacyclin synthase [115]. LOX activity leading to increased LTB_4 and LTC_4 formation may create a surplus of reactive oxygen species (ROS) and especially superoxide [63]. In such a case, cardioprotective levels of nitric oxide may be consumed by ROS to form peroxynitrite, a prostacyclin synthase inhibitor and thromboxane receptor stimulator [116]. The overall effect caused by more selective COX-2 inhibitors is a low level of prostacyclin and high levels TXA_2 [63], promoting a platelet activating thrombosis event. Restoration of nitric oxide levels is said to be achieved by consumption of certain doses of taurine (2-aminoethanesulfonic acid), which may act as an antioxidant on a diseased vascular state and as a prooxidant in an otherwise normal vasculature being at risk from NSAID use [117]. Also, taurine derivatives NCT and NBrT are known to reduce excessive nitric oxide formation [118]. Curcumin, a natural antioxidant consumption, may also be of help for NSAID users, especially for those being at risk. Curcumin modulates arachidonic acid release from cellular membranes by blocking the hydrolysis event by cytosolic phospholipase A_2, and it inhibits the 5-LO catalytic functions and nitric oxide synthase activity [119]. During COX-1 and COX-2 inhibition by NSAIDs, generation of NO and ROS is not suppressed under inflammatory stimulation, whereas $cPLA_2$ activity is increased under inflammatory conditions. A probable direct synergy with its function with 12- and 15-LOX isoenzymes to produce NO and ROS, via a $cPLA_2$. 12- and 15-LOX pathway are suggested [120]. The use of 12-/15-LOX inhibitors may be beneficial, especially in neurodegenerative diseases where NO activity is a major proinflammatory mediator [120, 121].

Finally, recent scientific effort is focusing on the trials of new cyclooxygenase inhibitors [122] in order to overcome undesirable cyclooxygenase metabolism of arachidonic acid in inflammation and cancer. These compounds have lower

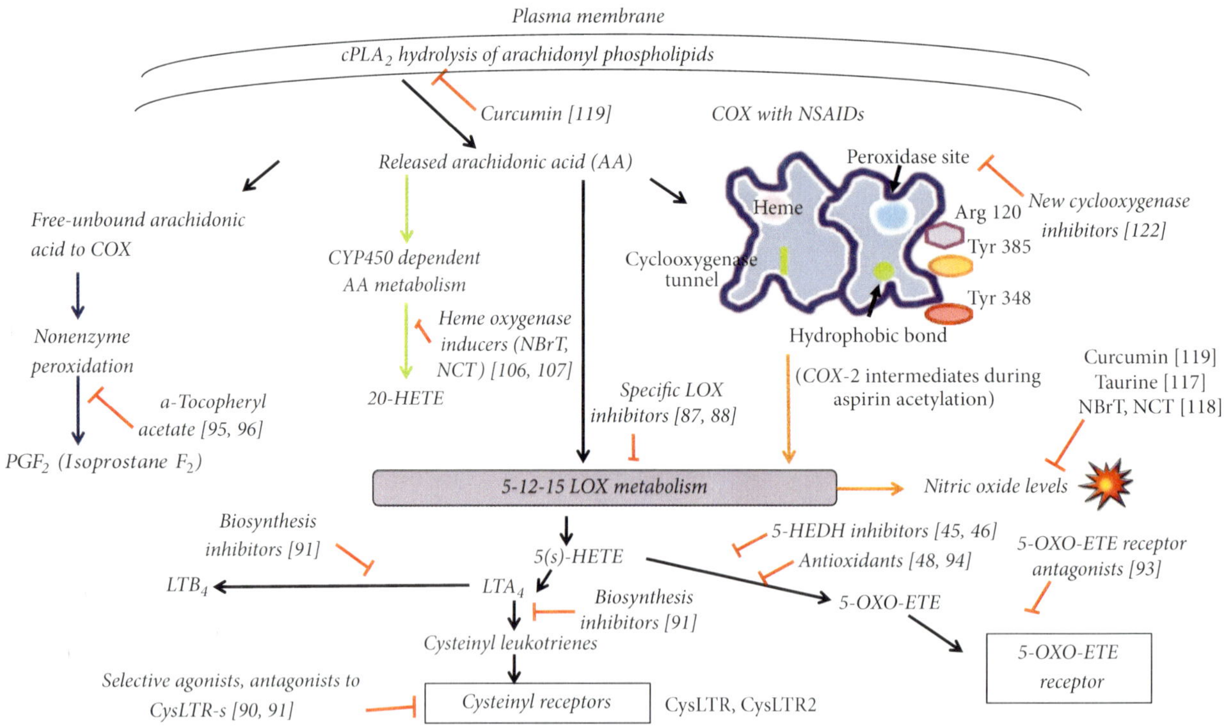

FIGURE 4: Possible target points of supplementary agent's use to alleviate NSAID promotion of proinflammatory and cancerous conditions.

isoform selectivity to COX than the NSAID "more specific" cyclooxygenase inhibitors (coxibs), which may result in reduced side effects.

4.2. NSAIDs and Risk for Cancer

4.2.1. Studies with Clinical Evidence for Cancer Development. Epidemiologic studies provide contradictory results on cancer risk development by NSAIDS that may be due to the cell-specific activity of producing prostanoids and the specificity on COX inhibition by a particular NSAID (Figures 1 and 2 and Table 1).

Subjects using certain types of NSAIDs are being protected from colorectal cancer [123]. Specifically, aspirin users have better protection from the close to rectum and distal to colon cancer development, whereas the nonaspirin NSAID users are being more protected from the proximal to colon cancer development [123–125]. It should be mentioned, however, that anatomic locations in this type of cancer development are also tightly associated with the age, gender, and the race of patients [126]. Some studies indicate that breast cancer development risk is also lowered by NSAID use [127, 128], although this may be a small decrease of relative risk [129]. Moreover, type of NSAID, specific dose, and duration of treatment have not been yet identified [130]. Other studies, however, indicate increased risk for developing breast cancer irrespective of hormonal status (estrogen/progesterone (ER/PR) receptor positive/negative) and that the risk for developing ER/PR (−) breast cancer is raised in long term daily use aspirin users [131, 132]. Traditional NSAID use (diclofenac, etodolac, and meloxicam) is also associated with decreased risk in developing aggressive skin cancers, whereas "more selective" to COX-2 inhibitors were not found to be protective [133, 134]. Also, whilst aspirin and other NSAIDS may protect from developing esophageal and noncardia gastric carcinomas, these are nonprotective for the development of cardia gastric carcinoma [135, 136].

Epidemiological studies are controversial regarding a protective [137] or promoting [138] effect of NSAIDs for prostate cancer. In prostate cancer, genetic variation in the COX-2 gene is associated with increased risk [139]. Epidemiologic studies clearly indicate that acetaminophen and nonaspirin NSAIDs are associated with a significant risk of developing kidney cancer [140, 141]. Complementarily, whilst aspirin and other NSAID users have lower risk for developing hepatocellular carcinoma (HCC) [142, 143], men only gain protection from intrahepatic carcinoma (IHC) by taking aspirin and this did not account for any other NSAID use [142]. Aspirin and other NSAID users are not protected from developing brain tumors and the use of traditional and "more selective" COX inhibitors seems to increase the risk for developing meningiomas [144].

Although epidemiology data on cancer risk by NSAIDs are controversial, by comparison of results important indications may be drawn (Table 1). Inhibition of prostanoid synthesis due to aspirin acetylation on COX isoenzymes, although in a different manner [7, 26], may be protective of a variety of types of cancers. Acetylating of COX by aspirin was found to be protective of prostate cancer development in a subgroup of subjects having specific sequence variations within the COX-2 genome [139]. Also, risk reduction for colorectal cancer

TABLE 1: Cancer risk development from NSAID use as recorded from various epidemiology studies.

Type of cancer	Aspirin	Traditional nonaspirin NSAID	More selective COX-2 inhibitor
Proximal colon*	No effect on risk [123] Decreased risk in women [124]	Reduced risk [123]	No data available (NDA)
Distal colon*	Decreased risk [123] No effect in women [124]	Reduced risk [123]	NDA
Rectum*	Decreased risk [123] No effect in women [124]	No effect on risk [123]	NDA
Nonmelanoma skin cancer (NMSC)	Decreased risk for BCC[a] SCC[b] [133] Slightly decreased risk for BCC SCC [134]	Decreased risk for BCC SCC [133] Slightly decreased risk for BCC SCC [134]	Decreased risk for BCC SCC [133] Stronger decreased risk for BCC SCC [134]
Melanoma skin cancer (MSC)	Slightly decreased risk [133]	Slightly decreased risk [133]	No effect on risk [133]
Breast ER/PR (+)	Highly increased risk by aspirin-only NSAID users [131] No effect on risk [127]	No effect on risk by acetaminophen [131]	Increased risk [131] Decreased risk in HER2+ [127] **
Breast ER/PR (−)	Highly increased risk by aspirin-only NSAID users [131] Increased risk [132]	No effect on risk by acetaminophen [131]	Increased risk [131] Decreased risk in HER2+ [127] **
Brain glioma	No effect on risk [144]	No effect on risk [144]	No effect on risk [144]
Brain meningioma	No effect on risk [144]	Slightly increased risk [144]	Slight increased risk [144]
Hepatocellular Carcinoma (HCC)	Decreases risk [142, 143]	Decreases risk [142]	Decreases risk [142]
Intrahepatic cholangiosarcoma (ICC)	Decreases risk in men [142] No effect on risk in women [142]	No effect on risk by ibuprofen [142]	No effect on risk [142]
Prostate***	No effect on risk [138]	Increased risk with acetaminophen, even stronger for metastatic type [138]	Increased risk, even stronger for metastatic type [138]
Esophageal squamous cell carcinoma (ESCC)	Decreased risk [135, 136]	Slightly decreased risk [135, 136]	Slightly decreased risk [135, 136]
Esophageal adenocarcinoma (EA)	Decreased risk [135, 136]	Slightly decreased risk [135, 136]	Slightly decreased risk [135, 136]
Noncardia gastric carcinoma	Decreased risk [135, 136]	Slightly decreased risk [135, 136]	Slightly decreased risk [135, 136]
Cardia gastric carcinoma	No effect on risk [135, 136]	No effect on risk [135, 136]	No effect on risk [135, 136]

*Anatomic locations are associated with gender, age, and race of patients [126]. **Study indicates decreased risk in special subgroups of patients. ***Genetic predisposition may increase risk [139]. [a]Basal cell carcinoma. [b]Squamous cell carcinoma.

development with aspirin is related only to specific genotypes near the IL-6 genome [145]. Thereby genetic variation seems be an important parameter for the aspirin effect in cancer development. By contrast, aspirin use increases the risk for breast cancer development irrespective of hormonal influence [131]. Cell-dependent prostanoid formation is also another important serious parameter (Figure 1). Any given prostanoid forming cell selects a particular prostanoid as its major product [15]. Brain and mast cells, for example, preferably produce PGD_2, and its formation provides the core for vital homeostasis mechanisms [146, 147].

4.2.2. What Are the Effects of NSAIDs on Cancer? Traditional and "more selective" COX inhibitors preferentially bind on arachidonic acid's active site of respective isoenzymes. The degree to which COX inhibitors cause inhibition of COX-1, COX-2, or COX-3 depends on their selective preference for COX active sites [62, 63]. Under normal conditions, constitutive COX-1 maintains prostacyclin and PGE_2 levels as well as other prostanoids in all tissues, whereas COX-2, when activated in an inducible way (i.e., during inflammation), produces prostacyclin and other prostanoids in most, but not all, organs [15]. From epidemiologic studies it is evident that some groups of subjects benefit from developing certain types of cancer by nonaspirin NSAIDs, for example, nonmelanoma skin cancers [134], whereas the same use of NSAIDs elevates the risk of developing some other types of cancer, for example, in the kidney [141]. The differential inhibition of COX-1, COX-2, and COX-3 isoenzymes results in differential beneficial activities and side effects [15] (Figure 1). For cancer, the situation is even more complicated as it may also depend on both the impact on COX and the subsequent synthesis inhibition of protective prostaglandins.

4.3. Mechanisms of Promotion of Cancer by the AA System and the NSAIDs. PGE_2 association with tumorigenesis has been thoroughly investigated. Measurement of increased amounts of PGE_2 in colorectal cancer has long been implicated to contribute to tumorigenesis [148], where apparently COX-2 and not COX-1 is overexpressed [149], and COX-2 expression is more essential for tumor development in the distal colon [150]. Nowadays, inducible PGE_2 synthesis is implicated in many types of cancers [58, 151]. However, it should always be considered that PGE_2 is a major component of tissue homeostasis under normal conditions [21, 58] and its constitutive synthesis may be impaired by the frequent use of all classes of NSAIDs [7].

Frequent use of NSAIDS leading to depletion of COX activity may favor the metabolism of arachidonic acid by the LOX pathways [15, 63] as discussed. There are several human and animal studies finely reviewed to support this hypothesis [18]. 5- and 12-LOX metabolic pathways are linked to carcinogenesis [152], and altered COX and LOX metabolism of arachidonic acid are a common factor in malignancy [35]. One major metabolite of 5-LOX, the LTB_4, was shown to produce cancer predisposition by activating transcriptional factor NF-kB in hepatoma cells [153]. The cysteinyl leukotrienes (TLC_4, LTD_4, and LTE_4) may also be oversynthesized as increased amounts of LTC_4 and LTD_4 and decreased amounts of PGE_2 are detected in nasal secretions if patients with aspirin intolerance are treated with this medication [154] (Figure 3(a)). LTC_4 induces the phosphorylation of NF-kB p65, activates the complex NF-kB p50-p66 [155], and via the CysLT2 receptor induces the phosphorylation of IkBa by involving protein kinase family enzymes [156]. Aspirin decreases the expression of Bcl-2 by blocking the IL6-IL6R-$STAT_3$ signaling pathway [157]. The decreased expression of Bcl-2 may cause apoptosis by tumor necrosis factor apoptosis-inducing ligand and increased levels of TNFα expressed [158]. However, overproduced TNFα may not function proapoptotically but contribute to cell survival (Figure 5). TNFα bound to the tumor necrosis receptor 1 (TNFR-1), apart from other causalities, recruits TNFR-1-associated death domain protein (TRADD). TRADD in turn has a dual activity. When TRADD recruits the receptor interacting protein kinase- (RIPK-) and Fas-associated death domain protein (FADD), this finally results in apoptosis [159]. However, when TRADD recruits TNF receptor factor 2 (TRAF-2) and FADD, this results in activation of survival transcription factor NF-kB [160–162]. TNF-α also results in activation of the transcription factor AP-1 via the JNK signaling cascade, which subsequently increases cellular proliferation [163].

Furthermore, extensive 5-LOX activity from arachidonic acid accumulating from NSAID inhibition of COX may also lead to increased 5-OXO-ETE formation (Figures 3(a) and 3(b)). This may be of raised interest in oncology studies as 5-OXO-ETE lipid molecules seem to be required for cancer cell proliferation [48]. In prostate cancer cells, for example, 5-OXO-ETE and the 12-LOX metabolism are also important for tumor propagation [48, 88]. Marked expression of 5- and 12-LOX is being detected in prostate neoplasia in contrast to normal and benign epithelia [88]. The platelet 12-LOX overexpression in prostate cancer is also said to be a trigger for angiogenesis and tumor growth by enhancing avβ3 and avβ5 integrin expression [15]. Complementarily, by data drawn from a Gln261Arg polymorphism of the 12-LOX gene meta-analysis study, clearly enough, this polymorphism was shown to be a significant risk factor for increased susceptibility to at least five types of cancer, including prostate cancer, specifically in the Asian population [164].

4.4. Description of New Drugs and Their Possible Use for Alleviation of Cancer Predisposition with NSAIDs. Lipoxygenases are an emerging group of cancer targets as numerous studies indicate that 5-LOX and 15-LOX-1 are associated with the development of cancer via the NF-kB pathway [61]. Treatment with specific LOX inhibitors may be important as therapeutic option in order to overcome LOX overexpression [88]. Looking at the pathway of downstream production of 5-OXO-ETE, as a serious promoter of carcinogenesis, the novel synthesis of 5-OXO-ETE receptor antagonists may be another therapeutic option [93] (Figure 5). Recently we have discovered that the taurine derivative NBrT is a significant proliferative inhibitor leading to cell death among numerous cancer cell lines. Antiproliferative activity is enhanced on PC3 (prostate cancer), A549 (lung cancer), HeLa (cervical cancer), and MDA-MB231 (breast cancer) cell lines, (A. Kyriakopoulos et al. unpublished data). It would be a future interesting model to test the aspirin-induced proliferative ability of these particular cell lines and subsequently the inhibitory effect by the heme oxygenase inducers such as NBrT. The extensive antiproliferative effect on numerous human cancer cell lines by NBrT is in accordance with the recently demonstrated effect of G cycle arrest of glucocorticoid resistant cancer cells and the optimized concurrent anticancer effect of cisplatin with NBrT. NBrT has been considered in studies as a small molecule NSAID as it leads to decreased PGE_2 levels independently of COX expression [106, 108, 165]. As cyclooxygenase [166] and lipoxygenase [61] metabolism have long ago been associated with tumorigenesis, a possible therapeutic intervention with heme oxygenase inducers (including taurine derivatives) may be of significance and should be tested in animal models. Stress conditions that may lead to renal disease [33, 53, 103] (under hypoxic conditions [60]) and possible cancer predisposition enhancement may be circumvented (Figure 6).

5. Conclusion

Only scarce previous studies in the past have been focused on the avoidance of adverse effects of NSAID use [167]. Due to both older and recent research data on proinflammatory effects and cancer development in connection with NSAIDs, selective therapeutic targets and newer agents like the small molecule NSAIDs with an improved benefit-risk ratio become of interest. By all means, a thorough investigation of lipid metabolism under NSAID use is required,

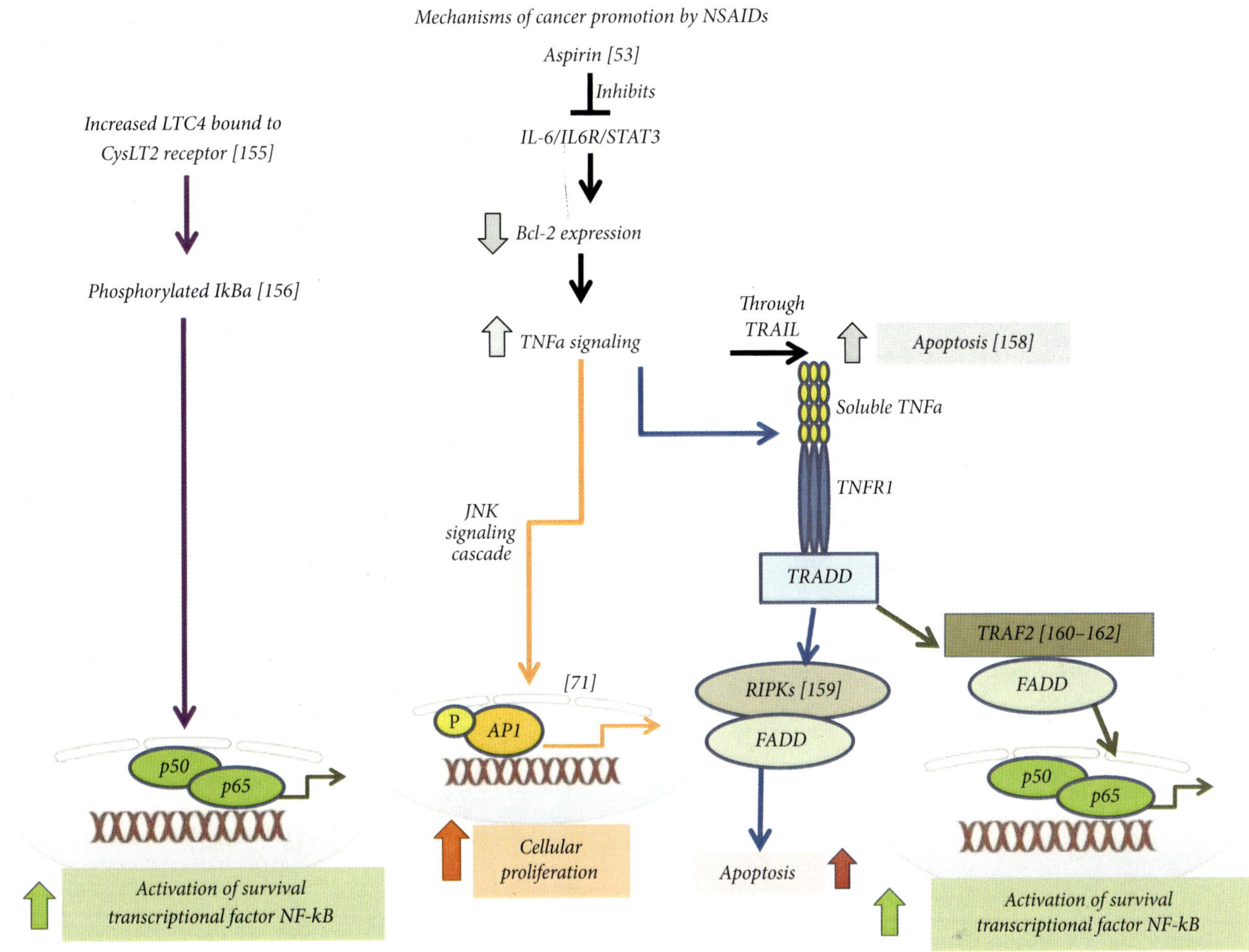

FIGURE 5: Molecular pathways that may contribute to promoting cancer by NSAID use [155–158, 160–163]. LTC_4 and TNF_a may activate transcription factor NF-kB and increase cellular proliferation by concurrent pathways that otherwise induce apoptosis.

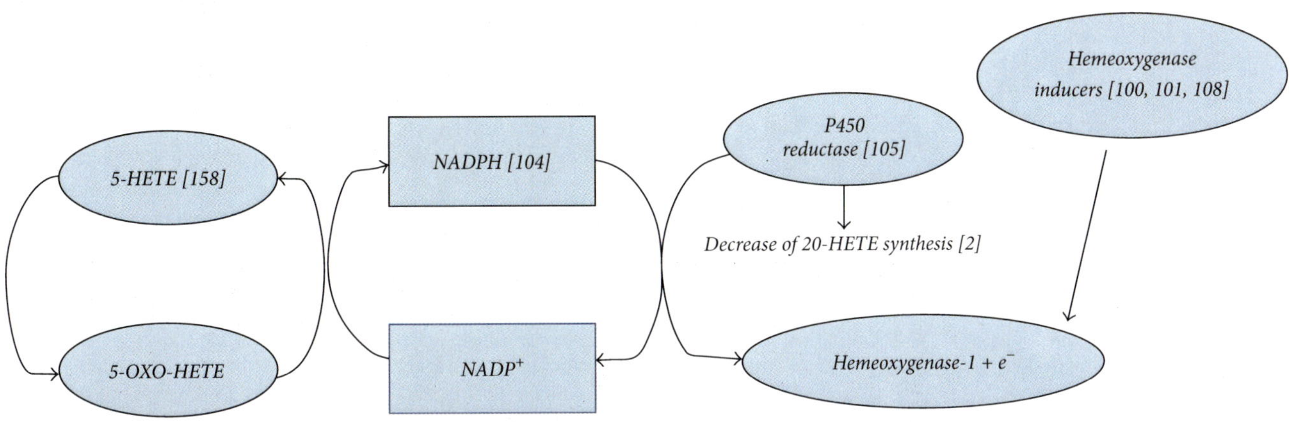

FIGURE 6: Proposed mechanism of heme oxygenase inducer application to overcome accumulation of toxic metabolites [102, 104, 105] induced by NSAIDs. Induction of heme oxygenase by several agents [100, 101, 108] and receival of electrons via P450 [103, 105] may result in decreased formation of 20-HETE and 5-OXO-ETE toxic metabolite accumulation.

and this must be coupled with large scale epidemiological studies to provide valuable clinical information. For example, although accumulated data suggest a protective role of some COX inhibitors in the development of certain types of cancer, the predicted increased risk for other cancers by NSAID use is also equally important. Alterations of AA metabolism by NSAID, prompt further investigating the possible development of inflammation and cancer.

Authors' Contributions

A. M. Kyriakopoulos has written the manuscript with the assistance of M. Nagl. V. Zoumpourlis provided the unpublished cancer data. S. Baliou aided mostly with schematic presentations making her contribution adequate for coauthorship.

Acknowledgments

The authors thank N. Kotsalas MD and I. Panagiotopoulos, MD, for their aid with the schematic presentations and literature research. This manuscript has been solely supported by Nasco AD Biotechnology Laboratory. The authors also thank JPA Medical Co. for sponsorship of publication fees.

References

[1] M. L. Capone, S. Tacconelli, L. Di Francesco, A. Sacchetti, M. G. Sciulli, and P. Patrignani, "Pharmacodynamic of cyclooxygenase inhibitors in humans," *Prostaglandins and Other Lipid Mediators*, vol. 82, no. 1–4, pp. 85–94, 2007.

[2] J. Capdevila, N. Chacos, J. Werringloer, R. A. Prough, and R. W. Estabrook, "Liver microsomal cytochrome P-450 and the oxidative metabolism of arachidonic acid," *Proceedings of the National Academy of Sciences of the United States of America*, vol. 78, no. 9, pp. 5362–5366, 1981.

[3] J. D. Morrow, T. M. Harris, and L. Jackson Roberts II, "Noncyclooxygenase oxidative formation of a series of novel prostaglandins: analytical ramifications for measurement of eicosanoids," *Analytical Biochemistry*, vol. 184, no. 1, pp. 1–10, 1990.

[4] M. Ouellet, D. Riendeau, and M. D. Percival, "A high level of cyclooxygenase-2 inhibitor selectivity is associated with a reduced interference of platelet cyclooxygenase-1 inactivation by aspirin," *Proceedings of the National Academy of Sciences of the United States of America*, vol. 98, no. 25, pp. 14583–14588, 2001.

[5] C. J. Rieke, A. M. Mulichak, R. M. Garavito, and W. L. Smith, "The role of arginine 120 of human prostaglandin endoperoxide H synthase- 2 in the interaction with fatty acid substrates and inhibitors," *Journal of Biological Chemistry*, vol. 274, no. 24, pp. 17109–17114, 1999.

[6] J. R. Vane, "Inhibition of prostaglandin synthesis as a mechanism of action for aspirin-like drugs," *Nature New Biology*, vol. 231, no. 25, pp. 232–235, 1971.

[7] J. R. Vane, "The fight against rheumatism: from willow bark to COX-1 sparing drugs," *Journal of Physiology and Pharmacology*, vol. 51, no. 4, pp. 573–586, 2000.

[8] S. Moncada, R. Gryglewski, S. Bunting, and J. R. Vane, "An enzyme isolated from arteries transforms prostaglandin endoperoxides to an unstable substance that inhibits platelet aggregation," *Nature*, vol. 263, no. 5579, pp. 663–665, 1976.

[9] F. P. Berenger, J.-P. Cano, and P. H. Rolland, "Antithrombogenic endothelial cell defense. Basal characteristics in cultured endothelial cells and modulation by short-term and long-term exposure to isosorbide nitrates," *Circulation Research*, vol. 60, no. 4, pp. 612–620, 1987.

[10] B. J. Whittle, "Inhibition of prostacyclin (PGI2) formation in the rat small-intestine and gastric mucosa by the ulcerogen, indomethacin [proceedings]," *British Journal of Pharmacology*, vol. 64, no. 3, p. 438P, 1978.

[11] B. J. R. Whittle, G. A. Higgs, K. E. Eakins, S. Moncada, and J. R. Vane, "Selective inhibition of prostaglandin production in inflammatory exudates and gastric mucosa," *Nature*, vol. 284, no. 5753, pp. 271–273, 1980.

[12] D. L. Simmons, D. B. Levy, Y. Yannoni, and R. L. Erikson, "Identification of a phorbol ester-repressible v-src-inducible gene," *Proceedings of the National Academy of Sciences of the United States of America*, vol. 86, no. 4, pp. 1178–1182, 1989.

[13] W. Xie, J. G. Chipman, D. L. Robertson, R. L. Erikson, and D. L. Simmons, "Expression of a mitogen-responsive gene encoding prostaglandin synthase is regulated by mRNA splicing," *Proceedings of the National Academy of Sciences of the United States of America*, vol. 88, no. 7, pp. 2692–2696, 1991.

[14] K. R. Kozak, S. W. Rowlinson, and L. J. Marnett, "Oxygenation of the endocannabinoid, 2-arachidonylglycerol, to glyceryl prostaglandins by cyclooxygenase-2," *The Journal of Biological Chemistry*, vol. 275, no. 43, pp. 33744–33749, 2000.

[15] J. Clària, "Cyclooxygenase-2 biology," *Current Pharmaceutical Design*, vol. 9, no. 27, pp. 2177–2190, 2003.

[16] E. Vernieri, I. Gomez-Monterrey, C. Milite et al., "Design, synthesis, and evaluation of new tripeptides as COX-2 inhibitors," *Journal of Amino Acids*, vol. 2013, Article ID 606282, 7 pages, 2013.

[17] N. V. Chandrasekharan, H. Dai, K. L. T. Roos et al., "COX-3, a cyclooxygenase-1 variant inhibited by acetaminophen and other analgesic/antipyretic drugs: cloning, structure, and expression," *Proceedings of the National Academy of Sciences of the United States of America*, vol. 99, no. 21, pp. 13926–13931, 2002.

[18] B. P. Burnett and R. M. Levy, "5-Lipoxygenase metabolic contributions to NSAID-induced organ toxicity," *Advances in Therapy*, vol. 29, no. 2, pp. 79–98, 2012.

[19] A. Bruno, S. Tacconelli, and P. Patrignani, "Variability in the response to non-steroidal anti-inflammatory drugs: mechanisms and perspectives," *Basic & Clinical Pharmacology & Toxicology*, vol. 114, no. 1, pp. 56–63, 2014.

[20] K. L. DeCicco-Skinner, S. J. Nolan, M. M. Deshpande, E. L. Trovato, T. A. Dempsey, and J. S. Wiest, "Altered prostanoid signaling contributes to increased skin tumorigenesis in Tpl2 knockout mice," *PLoS ONE*, vol. 8, no. 2, Article ID e56212, 2013.

[21] M. Nagamachi, D. Sakata, K. Kabashima et al., "Facilitation of Th1-mediated immune response by prostaglandin E receptor EP1," *Journal of Experimental Medicine*, vol. 204, no. 12, pp. 2865–2874, 2007.

[22] M. Sánchez-Borges, F. Caballero-Fonseca, A. Capriles-Hulett, and L. González-Aveledo, "Hypersensitivity reactions to nonsteroidal anti-inflammatory drugs: an update," *Pharmaceuticals*, vol. 3, no. 1, pp. 10–18, 2010.

[23] G. J. Roth, N. Stanford, and P. W. Majerus, "Acetylation of prostaglandin synthase by aspirin," *Proceedings of the National Academy of Sciences of the United States of America*, vol. 72, no. 8, pp. 3073–3076, 1975.

[24] P. Tosco and L. Lazzarato, "Mechanistic insights into cyclooxygenase irreversible inactivation by aspirin," *ChemMedChem*, vol. 4, no. 6, pp. 939–945, 2009.

[25] J. Schnermann, "Cyclooxygenase-2 and macula densa control of renin secretion," *Nephrology Dialysis Transplantation*, vol. 16, no. 9, pp. 1735–1738, 2001.

[26] G. P. Hochgesang Jr., S. W. Rowlinson, and L. J. Marnett, "Tyrosine-385 is critical for acetylation of cyclooxygenase-2 by aspirin," *Journal of the American Chemical Society*, vol. 122, no. 27, pp. 6514–6515, 2000.

[27] C. J. Rieke, A. M. Mulichak, R. M. Garavito, and W. L. Smith, "The role of arginine 120 of human prostaglandin endoperoxide H synthase-2 in the interaction with fatty acid substrates and inhibitors," *The Journal of Biological Chemistry*, vol. 274, no. 24, pp. 17109–17114, 1999.

[28] D. L. Simmons, D. Wagner, and K. Westover, "Nonsteroidal anti-inflammatory drugs, acetaminophen, cyclooxygenase 2, and fever," *Clinical Infectious Diseases*, vol. 31, pp. S211–S218, 2000.

[29] J. Claria and C. N. Serhan, "Aspirin triggers previously undescribed bioactive eicosanoids by human endothelial cell-leukocyte interactions," *Proceedings of the National Academy of Sciences*, vol. 92, no. 21, pp. 9475–9479, 1995.

[30] A. J. Marcus and D. P. Hajjar, "Vascular transcellular signaling," *Journal of Lipid Research*, vol. 34, no. 12, pp. 2017–2031, 1993.

[31] D. A. Brezinski, R. W. Nesto, and C. N. Serhan, "Angioplasty triggers intracoronary leukotrienes and lipoxin A4. Impact of aspirin therapy," *Circulation*, vol. 86, no. 1, pp. 56–63, 1992.

[32] A. P. Sampson, A. S. Cowburn, K. Sladek et al., "Profound overexpression of leukotriene C4 synthase in bronchial biopsies from aspirin-intolerant asthmatic patients," *International Archives of Allergy and Immunology*, vol. 113, no. 1–3, pp. 355–357, 1997.

[33] P. Patrignani, S. Tacconelli, A. Bruno, C. Sostres, and A. Lanas, "Managing the adverse effects of nonsteroidal anti-inflammatory drugs," *Expert Review of Clinical Pharmacology*, vol. 4, no. 5, pp. 605–621, 2011.

[34] C. Varas-Lorenzo, N. Riera-Guardia, B. Calingaert et al., "Myocardial infarction and individual nonsteroidal anti-inflammatory drugs meta-analysis of observational studies," *Pharmacoepidemiology and Drug Safety*, vol. 22, no. 6, pp. 559–570, 2013.

[35] D. Wang and R. N. DuBois, "Eicosanoids and cancer," *Nature Reviews Cancer*, vol. 10, no. 3, pp. 181–193, 2010.

[36] P. M. O'Byrne, "Leukotrienes in the pathogenesis of asthma," *Chest*, vol. 111, no. 2, supplement, pp. 27S–34S, 1997.

[37] H.-E. Claesson and J. Haeggström, "Human endothelial cells stimulate leukotriene synthesis and convert granulocyte released leukotriene A4 into leukotrienes B4, C4, D4 and E4," *European Journal of Biochemistry*, vol. 173, no. 1, pp. 93–100, 1988.

[38] J. Clària, M. H. Lee, and C. N. Serhan, "Aspirin-triggered lipoxins (15-epi-LX) are generated bythe human lung adenocarcinoma cell line (A549) neutrophil interactions and are potent inhibitors of cell proliferation," *Molecular Medicine*, vol. 2, no. 5, pp. 583–596, 1996.

[39] P. Borgeat, M. Hamberg, and B. Samuelsson, "Transformation of arachidonic acid and homo-gamma-linolenic acid by rabbit polymorphonuclear leukocytes. Monohydroxy acids from novel lipoxygenases," *The Journal of Biological Chemistry*, vol. 251, no. 24, pp. 7816–7820, 1976.

[40] P. Borgeat and B. Samuelsson, "Transformation of arachidonic acid by rabbit polymorphonuclear leukocytes. Formation of a novel dihydroxyeicosatetraenoic acid," *The Journal of Biological Chemistry*, vol. 254, no. 8, pp. 2643–2646, 1979.

[41] P. Borgeat and B. Samuelsson, "Arachidonic acid metabolism in polymorphonuclear leukocytes: unstable intermediate in formation of dihydroxy acids," *Proceedings of the National Academy of Sciences*, vol. 76, no. 7, pp. 3213–3217, 1979.

[42] S. Zarini, M. A. Gijón, A. E. Ransome, R. C. Murphy, and A. Sala, "Transcellular biosynthesis of cysteinyl leukotrienes in vivo during mouse peritoneal inflammation," *Proceedings of the National Academy of Sciences of the United States of America*, vol. 106, no. 20, pp. 8296–8301, 2009.

[43] A. Muller, E. Rechencq, C. Kugel et al., "Comparative biological activities of the four synthetic (5,6)-dihete isomers," *Prostaglandins*, vol. 38, no. 6, pp. 635–644, 1989.

[44] S. Mulugeta, T. Suzuki, N. T. Hernandez, M. Griesser, W. E. Boeglin, and C. Schneider, "Identification and absolute configuration of dihydroxy-arachidonic acids formed by oxygenation of 5 S-HETE by native and aspirin-acetylated COX-2," *Journal of Lipid Research*, vol. 51, no. 3, pp. 575–585, 2010.

[45] P. Patel, C. Cossette, J. R. Anumolu et al., "Substrate selectivity of 5-hydroxyeicosanoid dehydrogenase and its inhibition by 5-hydroxy-Delta 6-long-chain fatty acids," *Journal of Pharmacology and Experimental Therapeutics*, vol. 329, no. 1, pp. 335–341, 2009.

[46] W. S. Powell, F. Gravelle, and S. Gravel, "Metabolism of 5(S)-hydroxy-6,8,11,14-eicosatetraenoic acid and other 5(S)-hydroxyeicosanoids by a specific dehydrogenase in human polymorphonuclear leukocytes," *The Journal of Biological Chemistry*, vol. 267, no. 27, pp. 19233–19241, 1992.

[47] L. Qin and F. T. Crews, "NADPH oxidase and reactive oxygen species contribute to alcohol-induced microglial activation and neurodegeneration," *Journal of Neuroinflammation*, vol. 9, article 5, 2012.

[48] W. S. Powell and J. Rokach, "Biochemistry, biology and chemistry of the 5-lipoxygenase product 5-oxo-ETE," *Progress in Lipid Research*, vol. 44, no. 2-3, pp. 154–183, 2005.

[49] G. E. Grant, J. Rokach, and W. S. Powell, "5-Oxo-ETE and the OXE receptor," *Prostaglandins and Other Lipid Mediators*, vol. 89, no. 3-4, pp. 98–104, 2009.

[50] J. T. O'Flaherty, D. Jacobson, and J. Redman, "Mechanism involved in the mobilization of neutrophil calcium by 5-hydroxyeicosatetraenoate," *Journal of Immunology*, vol. 140, no. 12, pp. 4323–4328, 1988.

[51] W. S. Powell, S. Gravel, R. J. MacLeod, E. Mills, and M. Hashefi, "Stimulation of human neutrophils by 5-oxo-6,8,11,14-eicosatetraenoic acid by a mechanism independent of the leukotriene B4 receptor," *Journal of Biological Chemistry*, vol. 268, no. 13, pp. 9280–9286, 1993.

[52] N. W. Snyder, *Investigations of bio-activity, disposition and metabolism of lipids through liquid chromatography mass spectrometry [Ph.D. thesis]*, University of Pennsylvania, 2013, http://repository.upenn.edu/cgi/viewcontent.cgi?article=2087&context=edissertations.

[53] J. Y. Liu, N. Li, J. Yang et al., "Metabolic profiling of murine plasma reveals an unexpected biomarker in rofecoxib-mediated cardiovascular events," *Proceedings of the National Academy of Sciences of the United States of America*, vol. 107, no. 39, pp. 17017–17022, 2010.

[54] J. D. Morrow, K. E. Hill, R. F. Burk, T. M. Nammour, K. F. Badr, and L. J. Roberts II, "A series of prostaglandin F2-like compounds are produced in vivo in humans by a non-cyclooxygenase, free radical-catalyzed mechanism," *Proceedings of the National Academy of Sciences of the United States of America*, vol. 87, no. 23, pp. 9383–9387, 1990.

[55] P. M. Kearney, C. Baigent, J. Godwin, H. Halls, J. R. Emberson, and C. Patrono, "Do selective cyclo-oxygenase-2 inhibitors and traditional non-steroidal anti-inflammatory drugs increase the risk of atherothrombosis? Meta-analysis of randomised trials," *British Medical Journal*, vol. 332, no. 7553, pp. 1302–1305, 2006.

[56] Y.-G. Chen, C.-L. Lin, M.-S. Dai et al., "Risk of acute kidney injury and long-term outcome in patients with acetaminophen intoxication: a nationwide population-based retrospective cohort study," *Medicine*, vol. 94, no. 46, Article ID e2040, 2015.

[57] R. M. Botting, "Mechanism of action of acetaminophen: is there a cyclooxygenase 3?" *Clinical Infectious Diseases*, vol. 31, no. 5, pp. S202–S210, 2000.

[58] M. Nakanishi and D. W. Rosenberg, "Multifaceted roles of PGE2 in inflammation and cancer," *Seminars in Immunopathology*, vol. 35, no. 2, pp. 123–137, 2013.

[59] R. C. Harris, J. A. McKanna, Y. Akai, H. R. Jacobson, R. N. Dubois, and M. D. Breyer, "Cyclooxygenase-2 is associated with the macula densa of rat kidney and increases with salt restriction," *The Journal of Clinical Investigation*, vol. 94, no. 6, pp. 2504–2510, 1994.

[60] R. C. Harris, "Macula densa signalling—a potential role of cyclooxygenase-2 (COX-2)?" *Nephrology Dialysis Transplantation*, vol. 15, no. 10, pp. 1504–1506, 2000.

[61] R. Wisastra and F. J. Dekker, "Inflammation, cancer and oxidative lipoxygenase activity are intimately linked," *Cancers*, vol. 6, no. 3, pp. 1500–1521, 2014.

[62] E. M. Antman, J. S. Bennett, A. Daugherty, C. Furberg, H. Roberts, and K. A. Taubert, "Use of nonsteroidal antiinflammatory drugs: an update for clinicians: a scientific statement from the American heart association," *Circulation*, vol. 115, no. 12, pp. 1634–1642, 2007.

[63] E. M. Antman, D. DeMets, and J. Loscalzo, "Cyclooxygenase inhibition and cardiovascular risk," *Circulation*, vol. 112, no. 5, pp. 759–770, 2005.

[64] R. J. Bing and M. Lomnicka, "Why do cyclo-oxygenase-2 inhibitors cause cardiovascular events?" *Journal of the American College of Cardiology*, vol. 39, no. 3, pp. 521–522, 2002.

[65] A. Arfè, L. Scotti, C. Varas-Lorenzo et al., "Non-steroidal anti-inflammatory drugs and risk of heart failure in four European countries: nested case-control study," *British Medical Journal*, vol. 354, Article ID i4857, 2016.

[66] P. A. Dieppe, S. Ebrahim, R. M. Martin, and P. Jüni, "Lessons from the withdrawal of rofecoxib," *British Medical Journal*, vol. 329, no. 7471, pp. 867–868, 2004.

[67] P. McGettigan and D. Henry, "Cardiovascular risk and inhibition of cyclooxygenase: a systematic review of the observational studies of selective and nonselective inhibitors of cyclooxygenase 2," *The Journal of the American Medical Association*, vol. 296, no. 13, pp. 1633–1644, 2006.

[68] A. Schafer, "My doctor recently recommended that i take low-dose aspirin to minimize the risk of a heart attack or stroke. I routinely take ibuprofen for arthritis pain. Do i need both, and is it safe to combine the two?" *Health News*, vol. 6, p. 10, 2000.

[69] D. Steinhilber, "5-Lipoxygenase: a target for antiinflammatory drugs revisited," *Current Medicinal Chemistry*, vol. 6, no. 1, pp. 71–85, 1999.

[70] S. Poulin, C. Thompson, M. Thivierge et al., "Cysteinyl-leukotrienes induce vascular endothelial growth factor production in human monocytes and bronchial smooth muscle cells," *Clinical and Experimental Allergy*, vol. 41, no. 2, pp. 204–217, 2011.

[71] K. D. Stone, C. Prussin, and D. D. Metcalfe, "IgE, mast cells, basophils, and eosinophils," *Journal of Allergy and Clinical Immunology*, vol. 125, no. 2, supplement 2, pp. S73–S80, 2010.

[72] G. Grigiene, J. Norkuniene, and V. Kvedariene, "The time delay between drug intake and bronchospasm for nonsteroidal antiinflammatory drugs sensitive patients," *World Allergy Organization Journal*, vol. 3, no. 12, pp. 266–270, 2010.

[73] C. Alvarez, M. M. Amaral, C. Langellotti, and M. Vermeulen, "Leukotriene C4 prevents the complete maturation of murine dendritic cells and modifies interleukin-12/interleukin-23 balance," *Immunology*, vol. 134, no. 2, pp. 185–197, 2011.

[74] S. Poulin, C. Thompson, M. Thivierge et al., "Cysteinyl-leukotrienes induce vascular endothelial growth factor production in human monocytes and bronchial smooth muscle cells," *Clinical & Experimental Allergy*, vol. 41, no. 2, pp. 204–217, 2011.

[75] N. Hudson, M. Balsitis, S. Everitt, and C. J. Hawkey, "Enhanced gastric mucosal leukotriene B4 synthesis in patients taking non-steroidal anti-inflammatory drugs," *Gut*, vol. 34, no. 6, pp. 742–747, 1993.

[76] L. Santucci, S. Fiorucci, M. Giansanti, P. M. Brunori, F. M. Di Matteo, and A. Morelli, "Pentoxifylline prevents indomethacin induced acute gastric mucosal damage in rats: role of tumour necrosis factor alpha," *Gut*, vol. 35, no. 7, pp. 909–915, 1994.

[77] K. Allegaert, J. de Hoon, A. Debeer, and M. Gewillig, "Renal side effects of non-steroidal anti-inflammatory drugs in neonates," *Pharmaceuticals*, vol. 3, no. 2, pp. 393–405, 2010.

[78] D. C. Napoli and T. M. Freeman, "Autoimmunity in chronic urticaria and urticarial vasculitis," *Current Allergy and Asthma Reports*, vol. 1, no. 4, pp. 329–336, 2001.

[79] R. Asero, "Chronic urticaria with multiple NSAID intolerance: is tramadol always a safe alternative analgesic?" *Journal of Investigational Allergology and Clinical Immunology*, vol. 13, no. 1, pp. 56–59, 2003.

[80] Y. S. Shin, D. Suh, E. Yang, Y. Ye, and H. Park, "Serum specific IgE to thyroid peroxidase activates basophils in aspirin intolerant urticaria," *Journal of Korean Medical Science*, vol. 30, no. 6, pp. 705–709, 2015.

[81] C. W. Hsieh, J. W. Lee, E. C. Liao, and J. J. Tsai, "A disease marker for aspirin-induced chronic urticaria," *International Journal of Molecular Sciences*, vol. 15, no. 7, pp. 12591–12603, 2014.

[82] M. Venturini Díaz, S. San Juan De La Parra, and N. Segura Arazuri, "Selective immediate hypersensitivity to etoricoxib," *Journal of Investigational Allergology and Clinical Immunology*, vol. 18, no. 6, pp. 485–487, 2008.

[83] S. Altrichter, H.-J. Peter, D. Pisarevskaja, M. Metz, P. Martus, and M. Maurer, "IgE mediated autoallergy against thyroid peroxidase—a novel pathomechanism of chronic spontaneous urticaria?" *PLoS ONE*, vol. 6, no. 4, Article ID e14794, 2011.

[84] W. B. White, "Cardiovascular effects of the cyclooxygenase inhibitors," *Hypertension*, vol. 49, no. 3, pp. 408–418, 2007.

[85] A. S. Cowburn, K. Sladek, J. Soja et al., "Overexpression of leukotriene C4 synthase in bronchial biopsies from patients with aspirin-intolerant asthma," *The Journal of Clinical Investigation*, vol. 101, no. 4, pp. 834–846, 1998.

[86] M. Varghese and R. F. Lockey, "Aspirin-exacerbated asthma," *Allergy, Asthma and Clinical Immunology*, vol. 4, no. 2, pp. 75–83, 2008.

[87] C. Pergola and O. Werz, "5-Lipoxygenase inhibitors: a review of recent developments and patents," *Expert Opinion on Therapeutic Patents*, vol. 20, no. 3, pp. 355–375, 2010.

[88] M. Matsuyama, R. Yoshimura, M. Mitsuhashi et al., "Expression of lipoxygenase in human prostate cancer and growth reduction by its inhibitors," *International Journal of Oncology*, vol. 24, no. 4, pp. 821–827, 2004.

[89] J. Martel-Pelletier, D. Lajeunesse, P. Reboul, and J.-P. Pelletier, "Therapeutic role of dual inhibitors of 5-LOX and COX, selective and non-selective non-steroidal anti-inflammatory drugs," *Annals of the Rheumatic Diseases*, vol. 62, no. 6, pp. 501–509, 2003.

[90] C. Shimbori, N. Shiota, and H. Okunishi, "Effects of montelukast, a cysteinyl-leukotriene type 1 receptor antagonist, on the pathogenesis of bleomycin-induced pulmonary fibrosis in mice," *European Journal of Pharmacology*, vol. 650, no. 1, pp. 424–430, 2011.

[91] E. Lee, T. Robertson, J. Smith, and S. Kilfeather, "Leukotriene receptor antagonists and synthesis inhibitors reverse survival in eosinophils of asthmatic individuals," *American Journal of Respiratory and Critical Care Medicine*, vol. 161, no. 6, pp. 1881–1886, 2000.

[92] P. Montuschi and M. L. Peters-Golden, "Leukotriene modifiers for asthma treatment," *Clinical and Experimental Allergy*, vol. 40, no. 12, pp. 1732–1741, 2010.

[93] V. Gore, P. Patel, C.-T. Chang et al., "5-Oxo-ETE receptor antagonists," *Journal of Medicinal Chemistry*, vol. 56, no. 9, pp. 3725–3732, 2013.

[94] K.-R. Erlemann, J. Rokach, and W. S. Powell, "Oxidative stress stimulates the synthesis of the eosinophil chemoattractant 5-oxo-6,8,11,14-eicosatetraenoic acid by inflammatory cells," *The Journal of Biological Chemistry*, vol. 279, no. 39, pp. 40376–40384, 2004.

[95] A. Hoskins, J. L. Roberts II, G. Milne, L. Choi, and R. Dworski, "Natural-source d-α-tocopheryl acetate inhibits oxidant stress and modulates atopic asthma in humans in vivo," *Allergy*, vol. 67, no. 5, pp. 676–682, 2012.

[96] P. Reddanna, M. Krishna Rao, and C. Channa Reddy, "Inhibition of 5-lipoxygenase by vitamin E," *FEBS Letters*, vol. 193, no. 1, pp. 39–43, 1985.

[97] L. J. Roberts II, J. A. Oates, M. F. Linton et al., "The relationship between dose of vitamin E and suppression of oxidative stress in humans," *Free Radical Biology and Medicine*, vol. 43, no. 10, pp. 1388–1393, 2007.

[98] J. M. Lasker, W. B. Chen, I. Wolf, B. P. Bloswick, P. D. Wilson, and P. K. Powell, "Formation of 20-hydroxyeicosatetraenoic acid, a vasoactive and natriuretic eicosanoid, in human kidney. Role of CYP4F2 and CYP4A11," *The Journal of Biological Chemistry*, vol. 275, no. 6, pp. 4118–4126, 2000.

[99] D. Sacerdoti, A. Gatta, and J. C. McGiff, "Role of cytochrome P450-dependent arachidonic acid metabolites in liver physiology and pathophysiology," *Prostaglandins and Other Lipid Mediators*, vol. 72, no. 1-2, pp. 51–71, 2003.

[100] D. Sacerdoti, B. Escalante, N. G. Abraham, J. C. Mcgiff, R. D. Levere, and M. L. Schwartzman, "Treatment with tin prevents the development of hypertension in spontaneously hypertensive rats," *Science*, vol. 243, no. 4889, pp. 388–390, 1989.

[101] R. D. Levere, P. Martasek, B. Escalante, M. L. Schwartzman, and N. G. Abraham, "Effect of heme arginate administration on blood pressure in spontaneously hypertensive rats," *Journal of Clinical Investigation*, vol. 86, no. 1, pp. 213–219, 1990.

[102] K. A. Nath, G. Balla, G. M. Vercellotti et al., "Induction of heme oxygenase is a rapid, protective response in rhabdomyolysis in the rat," *Journal of Clinical Investigation*, vol. 90, no. 1, pp. 267–270, 1992.

[103] A. L. M. Spencer, I. Bagai, D. F. Becker, E. R. P. Zuiderweg, and S. W. Ragsdale, "Protein/protein interactions in the mammalian heme degradation pathway: heme oxygenase-2, cytochrome P450 reductase, and biliverdin reductase," *Journal of Biological Chemistry*, vol. 289, no. 43, pp. 29836–29858, 2014.

[104] Y. Higashimoto, H. Sakamoto, S. Hayashi et al., "Involvement of NADPH in the interaction between heme oxygenase-1 and cytochrome P450 reductase," *The Journal of Biological Chemistry*, vol. 280, no. 1, pp. 729–737, 2005.

[105] R. J. Roman, "P-450 metabolites of arachidonic acid in the control of cardiovascular function," *Physiological Reviews*, vol. 82, no. 1, pp. 131–185, 2002.

[106] S. Logotheti, N. Khoury, S. A. Vlahopoulos et al., "N-bromotaurine surrogates for loss of antiproliferative response and enhances cisplatin efficacy in cancer cells with impaired glucocorticoid receptor," *Translational Research*, vol. 173, pp. 58–73.e2, 2016.

[107] P. P. N. Rao, S. N. Kabir, and T. Mohamed, "Nonsteroidal anti-inflammatory drugs (NSAIDs): progress in small molecule drug development," *Pharmaceuticals*, vol. 3, no. 5, pp. 1530–1549, 2010.

[108] R. Olszanecki, M. Kurnyta, R. Biedroń, P. Chorobik, M. Bereta, and J. Marcinkiewicz, "The role of heme oxygenase-1 in down regulation of PGE2 production by taurine chloramine and taurine bromamine in J774.2 macrophages," *Amino Acids*, vol. 35, no. 2, pp. 359–364, 2008.

[109] E. Kontny, W. Maśliński, and J. Marcinkiewicz, "Anti-inflammatory activities of taurine chloramine: implication for immunoregulation and pathogenesis of rheumatoid arthritis," *Advances in Experimental Medicine and Biology*, vol. 526, pp. 329–340, 2003.

[110] W. Gottardi and M. Nagl, "N-chlorotaurine, a natural antiseptic with outstanding tolerability," *Journal of Antimicrobial Chemotherapy*, vol. 65, no. 3, pp. 399–409, 2010.

[111] W. Gottardi, D. Debabov, and M. Nagl, "N-chloramines: a promising class of well-tolerated topical antiinfectives," *Antimicrobial Agents and Chemotherapy*, vol. 57, no. 3, pp. 1107–1114, 2013.

[112] C. Kim and Y.-N. Cha, "Taurine chloramine produced from taurine under inflammation provides anti-inflammatory and cytoprotective effects," *Amino Acids*, vol. 46, no. 1, pp. 89–100, 2014.

[113] J. Marcinkiewicz and E. Kontny, "Taurine and inflammatory diseases," *Amino Acids*, vol. 46, no. 1, pp. 7–20, 2014.

[114] S. P. Jones and R. Bolli, "The ubiquitous role of nitric oxide in cardioprotection," *Journal of Molecular and Cellular Cardiology*, vol. 40, no. 1, pp. 16–23, 2006.

[115] M. L. Wade and F. A. Fitzpatrick, "Nitric oxide modulates the activity of the hemoproteins prostaglandin I2 synthase and thromboxane A2 synthase," *Archives of Biochemistry and Biophysics*, vol. 347, no. 2, pp. 174–180, 1997.

[116] M. Bachschmid, S. Thurau, M.-H. Zou, and V. Ullrich, "Endothelial cell activation by endotoxin involves superoxide/NO-mediated nitration of prostacyclin synthase and thromboxane receptor stimulation," *The FASEB Journal*, vol. 17, no. 8, pp. 914–916, 2003.

[117] F. S. Bircan, B. Balabanli, N. Turkozkan, and G. Ozan, "Effects of taurine on nitric oxide and 3-nitrotyrosine levels in spleen during endotoxemia," *Neurochemical Research*, vol. 36, no. 11, pp. 1978–1983, 2011.

[118] E. Park, M. R. Quinn, C. E. Wright, and G. Schuller-Levis, "Taurine chloramine inhibits the synthesis of nitric oxide and the release of tumor necrosis factor in activated RAW 264.7 cells," *Journal of Leukocyte Biology*, vol. 54, no. 2, pp. 119–124, 1993.

[119] J. Hong, M. Bose, J. Ju et al., "Modulation of arachidonic acid metabolism by curcumin and related β-diketone derivatives: effects on cytosolic phospholipase A_2, cyclooxygenases and 5-lipoxygenase," *Carcinogenesis*, vol. 25, no. 9, pp. 1671–1679, 2004.

[120] D. Y. Chuang, A. Simonyi, P. T. Kotzbauer, Z. Gu, and G. Y. Sun, "Cytosolic phospholipase A2 plays a crucial role in ROS/NO signaling during microglial activation through the lipoxygenase pathway," *Journal of Neuroinflammation*, vol. 12, article 199, 2015.

[121] G. C. Brown, "Mechanisms of inflammatory neurodegeneration: INOS and NADPH oxidase," *Biochemical Society Transactions*, vol. 35, no. 5, pp. 1119–1121, 2007.

[122] S. K. Sharma, B. J. Al-Hourani, M. Wuest et al., "Synthesis and evaluation of fluorobenzoylated di- and tripeptides as inhibitors of cyclooxygenase-2 (COX-2)," *Bioorganic and Medicinal Chemistry*, vol. 20, no. 7, pp. 2221–2226, 2012.

[123] E. H. Ruder, A. O. Laiyemo, B. I. Graubard, A. R. Hollenbeck, A. Schatzkin, and A. J. Cross, "Non-steroidal anti-inflammatory drugs and colorectal cancer risk in a large, prospective cohort," *American Journal of Gastroenterology*, vol. 106, no. 7, pp. 1340–1350, 2011.

[124] A. Mahipal, K. E. Anderson, P. J. Limburg, and A. R. Folsom, "Nonsteroidal anti-inflammatory drugs and subsite-specific colorectal cancer incidence in the Iowa Women's Health Study," *Cancer Epidemiology Biomarkers & Prevention*, vol. 15, no. 10, pp. 1785–1790, 2006.

[125] W. E. Smalley and R. N. DuBois, "Colorectal cancer and nonsteroidal anti-inflammatory drugs," *Advances in Pharmacology*, vol. 39, pp. 1–20, 1997.

[126] R. L. Nelson, T. Dollear, S. Freels, and V. Persky, "The relation of age, race, and gender to the subsite location of colerectal carcinoma," *Cancer*, vol. 80, no. 2, pp. 193–197, 1997.

[127] T. Dierssen-Sotos, I. Gómez-Acebo, M. de Pedro et al., "Use of non-steroidal anti-inflammatory drugs and risk of breast cancer: the Spanish Multi-Case-Control (MCC) study," *BMC Cancer*, vol. 16, article 660, 2016.

[128] R. E. Harris, K. K. Namboodiri, and W. B. Farrar, "Nonsteroidal antiinflammatory drugs and breast cancer," *Epidemiology*, vol. 7, no. 2, pp. 203–205, 1996.

[129] S. A. Khuder and A. B. Mutgi, "Breast cancer and NSAID use: a meta-analysis," *British Journal of Cancer*, vol. 84, no. 9, pp. 1188–1192, 2001.

[130] A. Agrawal and I. S. Fentiman, "NSAIDs and breast cancer: a possible prevention and treatment strategy," *International Journal of Clinical Practice*, vol. 62, no. 3, pp. 444–449, 2008.

[131] S. Friis, L. Thomassen, H. T. Sørensen et al., "Nonsteroidal anti-inflammatory drug use and breast cancer risk: a Danish cohort study," *European Journal of Cancer Prevention*, vol. 17, no. 2, pp. 88–96, 2008.

[132] S. F. Marshall, L. Bernstein, H. Anton-Culver et al., "Nonsteroidal anti-inflammatory drug use and breast cancer risk by stage and hormone receptor status," *Journal of the National Cancer Institute*, vol. 97, no. 11, pp. 805–812, 2005.

[133] S. A. Johannesdottir, E. T. Chang, F. Mehnert, M. Schmidt, A. B. Olesen, and H. T. Saørensen, "Nonsteroidal anti-inflammatory drugs and the risk of skin cancer: a population-based case-control study," *Cancer*, vol. 118, no. 19, pp. 4768–4776, 2012.

[134] D. Reinau, C. Surber, S. S. Jick, and C. R. Meier, "Nonsteroidal anti-inflammatory drugs and the risk of nonmelanoma skin cancer," *International Journal of Cancer*, vol. 137, no. 1, pp. 144–153, 2015.

[135] D. C. Farrow, T. L. Vaughan, P. D. Hansten et al., "Use of aspirin and other nonsteroidal anti-inflammatory drugs and risk of esophageal and gastric cancer," *Cancer Epidemiology Biomarkers and Prevention*, vol. 7, no. 2, pp. 97–102, 1998.

[136] W. H. Wang, J. Q. Huang, G. F. Zheng, S. K. Lam, J. Karlberg, and B. C. Wong, "Non-steroidal anti-inflammatory drug use and the risk of gastric cancer: a systematic review and meta-analysis," *CancerSpectrum Knowledge Environment*, vol. 95, no. 23, pp. 1784–1791, 2003.

[137] A. C. Vidal, L. E. Howard, D. M. Moreira, R. Castro-Santamaria, G. L. Andriole, and S. J. Freedland, "Aspirin, NSAIDs, and risk of prostate cancer: results from the REDUCE study," *Clinical Cancer Research*, vol. 21, no. 4, pp. 756–762, 2015.

[138] T. Veitonmäki, T. J. Murtola, L. Määttänen et al., "Prostate cancer risk and nonsteroidal antiinflammatory drug use in the Finnish prostate cancer screening trial," *British Journal of Cancer*, vol. 111, no. 7, pp. 1421–1431, 2014.

[139] K. Shahedi, S. Lindström, S. L. Zheng et al., "Genetic variation in the COX-2 gene and the association with prostate cancer risk," *International Journal of Cancer*, vol. 119, no. 3, pp. 668–672, 2006.

[140] T. K. Choueiri, Y. Je, and E. Cho, "Analgesic use and the risk of kidney cancer: a meta-analysis of epidemiologic studies," *International Journal of Cancer*, vol. 134, no. 2, pp. 384–396, 2014.

[141] E. Cho, G. Curhan, S. E. Hankinson et al., "Prospective evaluation of analgesic use and risk of renal cell cancer," *Archives of Internal Medicine*, vol. 171, no. 16, pp. 1487–1493, 2011.

[142] J. L. Petrick, V. V. Sahasrabuddhe, A. T. Chan et al., "NSAID use and risk of hepatocellular carcinoma and intrahepatic cholangiocarcinoma: the liver cancer pooling project," *Cancer Prevention Research*, vol. 8, no. 12, pp. 1156–1162, 2015.

[143] V. V. Sahasrabuddhe, M. Z. Gunja, B. I. Graubard et al., "Nonsteroidal anti-inflammatory drug use, chronic liver disease, and hepatocellular carcinoma," *Journal of the National Cancer Institute*, vol. 104, no. 23, pp. 1808–1814, 2012.

[144] F. J. Bannon, M. A. O'Rorke, L. J. Murray et al., "Non-steroidal anti-inflammatory drug use and brain tumour risk: a case-control study within the Clinical Practice Research Datalink," *Cancer Causes and Control*, vol. 24, no. 11, pp. 2027–2034, 2013.

[145] H. Nan, C. M. Hutter, Y. Lin et al., "Association of aspirin and NSAID use with risk of colorectal cancer according to genetic variants," *JAMA*, vol. 313, no. 11, pp. 1133–1142, 2015.

[146] K. Tanaka, K. Ogawa, K. Sugamura, M. Nakamura, S. Takano, and K. Nagata, "Cutting edge: differential production of prostaglandin D2 by human helper T cell subsets," *The Journal of Immunology*, vol. 164, no. 5, pp. 2277–2280, 2000.

[147] I. R. Jowsey, A. M. Thomson, J. U. Flanagan et al., "Mammalian class Sigma glutathione S-transferases: catalytic properties and

tissue-specific expression of human and rat GSH-dependent prostaglandin D2 synthases," *Biochemical Journal*, vol. 359, no. 3, pp. 507–516, 2001.

[148] B. Rigas, I. S. Goldman, and L. Levine, "Altered eicosanoid levels in human colon cancer," *The Journal of Laboratory and Clinical Medicine*, vol. 122, no. 5, pp. 518–523, 1993.

[149] W. Kutchera, D. A. Jones, N. Matsunami et al., "Prostaglandin H synthase 2 is expressed abnormally in human colon cancer: evidence for a transcriptional effect," *Proceedings of the National Academy of Sciences of the United States of America*, vol. 93, no. 10, pp. 4816–4820, 1996.

[150] M. Nakanishi, A. Menoret, T. Tanaka et al., "Selective PGE_2 suppression inhibits colon carcinogenesis and modifies local mucosal immunity," *Cancer Prevention Research*, vol. 4, no. 8, pp. 1198–1208, 2011.

[151] N. Markosyan, E. P. Chen, V. N. Ndong et al., "Deletion of cyclooxygenase 2 in mouse mammary epithelial cells delays breast cancer onset through augmentation of type 1 immune responses in tumors," *Carcinogenesis*, vol. 32, no. 10, pp. 1441–1449, 2011.

[152] G. P. Pidgeon, J. Lysaght, S. Krishnamoorthy et al., "Lipoxygenase metabolism: roles in tumor progression and survival," *Cancer and Metastasis Reviews*, vol. 26, no. 3-4, pp. 503–524, 2007.

[153] Y. Zhao, W. Wang, Q. Wang, X. Zhang, and L. Ye, "Lipid metabolism enzyme 5-LOX and its metabolite LTB4 are capable of activating transcription factor NF-κB in hepatoma cells," *Biochemical and Biophysical Research Communications*, vol. 418, no. 4, pp. 647–651, 2012.

[154] C. Picado, "Aspirin intolerance and nasal polyposis," *Current Allergy and Asthma Reports*, vol. 2, no. 6, pp. 488–493, 2002.

[155] K. S. Lee, S. R. Kim, H. S. Park et al., "Cysteinyl leukotriene upregulates IL-11 expression in allergic airway disease of mice," *Journal of Allergy and Clinical Immunology*, vol. 119, no. 1, pp. 141–149, 2007.

[156] C. Thompson, A. Cloutier, Y. Bossé et al., "Signaling by the cysteinyl-leukotriene receptor 2: involvement in chemokine gene transcription," *Journal of Biological Chemistry*, vol. 283, no. 4, pp. 1974–1984, 2008.

[157] H. Raza, A. John, and S. Benedict, "Acetylsalicylic acid-induced oxidative stress, cell cycle arrest, apoptosis and mitochondrial dysfunction in human hepatoma HepG2 cells," *European Journal of Pharmacology*, vol. 668, no. 1-2, pp. 15–24, 2011.

[158] K. M. Kim, J. J. Song, J. Y. An, Y. T. Kwon, and Y. J. Lee, "Pretreatment of acetylsalicylic acid promotes tumor necrosis factor-related apoptosis-inducing ligand-induced apoptosis by down-regulating BCL-2 gene expression," *The Journal of Biological Chemistry*, vol. 280, no. 49, pp. 41047–41056, 2005.

[159] V. Baud and M. Karin, "Signal transduction by tumor necrosis factor and its relatives," *Trends in Cell Biology*, vol. 11, no. 9, pp. 372–377, 2001.

[160] S. Q. Zhang, A. Kovalenko, G. Cantarella, and D. Wallach, "Recruitment of the IKK signalosome to the p55 TNF receptor: RIP and A20 bind to NEMO (IKKgamma) upon receptor stimulation," *Immunity*, vol. 12, no. 3, pp. 301–311, 2000.

[161] A. Devin, A. Cook, Y. Lin, Y. Rodriguez, M. Kelliher, and Z. Liu, "The distinct roles of TRAF2 and RIP in IKK activation by TNF-R1: TRAF2 recruits IKK to TNF-R1 while RIPmediates IKK activation," *Immunity*, vol. 12, no. 4, pp. 419–429, 2000.

[162] A. Devin, Y. Lin, S. Yamaoka, Z. Li, M. Karin, and Z. Liu, "The α and β subunits of IκB kinase (IKK) mediate TRAF2-dependent IKK recruitment to tumor necrosis factor (TNF) receptor 1 in response to TNF," *Molecular and Cellular Biology*, vol. 21, no. 12, pp. 3986–3994, 2001.

[163] D. N. Chadee, T. Yuasa, and J. M. Kyriakis, "Direct activation of mitogen-activated protein kinase kinase kinase MEKK1 by the Ste20p homologue GCK and the adapter protein TRAF2," *Molecular and Cellular Biology*, vol. 22, no. 3, pp. 737–749, 2002.

[164] D. Shan, K. Shen, J. Zhu et al., "The polymorphism (Gln261Arg) of 12-lipoxygenase and cancer risk: a meta-analysis," *International Journal of Clinical and Experimental Medicine*, vol. 8, no. 1, pp. 488–495, 2015.

[165] A. Kyriakopoulos, S. Logotheti, J. Marcinkiewicz, and M. Nagl, "N-chlorotaurine and N-bromotaurine combination regimen for the cure of valacyclovir-unresponsive herpes zoster comorbidity in a multiple sclerosis patient," *International Journal of Medical and Pharmaceutical Case Reports*, vol. 7, no. 2, pp. 1–6, 2016.

[166] W. Dempke, C. Rie, A. Grothey, and H.-J. Schmoll, "Cyclooxygenase-2: a novel target for cancer chemotherapy?" *Journal of Cancer Research and Clinical Oncology*, vol. 127, no. 7, pp. 411–417, 2001.

[167] J. M. Scheiman and C. E. Hindley, "Strategies to optimize treatment with NSAIDs in patients at risk for gastrointestinal and cardiovascular adverse events," *Clinical Therapeutics*, vol. 32, no. 4, pp. 667–677, 2010.

Permissions

All chapters in this book were first published in IJI, by Hindawi Publishing Corporation; hereby published with permission under the Creative Commons Attribution License or equivalent. Every chapter published in this book has been scrutinized by our experts. Their significance has been extensively debated. The topics covered herein carry significant findings which will fuel the growth of the discipline. They may even be implemented as practical applications or may be referred to as a beginning point for another development.

The contributors of this book come from diverse backgrounds, making this book a truly international effort. This book will bring forth new frontiers with its revolutionizing research information and detailed analysis of the nascent developments around the world.

We would like to thank all the contributing authors for lending their expertise to make the book truly unique. They have played a crucial role in the development of this book. Without their invaluable contributions this book wouldn't have been possible. They have made vital efforts to compile up to date information on the varied aspects of this subject to make this book a valuable addition to the collection of many professionals and students.

This book was conceptualized with the vision of imparting up-to-date information and advanced data in this field. To ensure the same, a matchless editorial board was set up. Every individual on the board went through rigorous rounds of assessment to prove their worth. After which they invested a large part of their time researching and compiling the most relevant data for our readers.

The editorial board has been involved in producing this book since its inception. They have spent rigorous hours researching and exploring the diverse topics which have resulted in the successful publishing of this book. They have passed on their knowledge of decades through this book. To expedite this challenging task, the publisher supported the team at every step. A small team of assistant editors was also appointed to further simplify the editing procedure and attain best results for the readers.

Apart from the editorial board, the designing team has also invested a significant amount of their time in understanding the subject and creating the most relevant covers. They scrutinized every image to scout for the most suitable representation of the subject and create an appropriate cover for the book.

The publishing team has been an ardent support to the editorial, designing and production team. Their endless efforts to recruit the best for this project, has resulted in the accomplishment of this book. They are a veteran in the field of academics and their pool of knowledge is as vast as their experience in printing. Their expertise and guidance has proved useful at every step. Their uncompromising quality standards have made this book an exceptional effort. Their encouragement from time to time has been an inspiration for everyone.

The publisher and the editorial board hope that this book will prove to be a valuable piece of knowledge for researchers, students, practitioners and scholars across the globe.

List of Contributors

Kassandra Weber
Diabetic Cardiovascular Disease Center,Washington University School of Medicine, St. Louis, MO 63110, USA
Department ofMedicine, Washington University School of Medicine, St. Louis, MO 63110, USA

Joel D. Schilling
Diabetic Cardiovascular Disease Center,Washington University School of Medicine, St. Louis, MO 63110, USA
Department ofMedicine, Washington University School of Medicine, St. Louis, MO 63110, USA
Department of Pathology and Immunology,Washington University School of Medicine, St. Louis, MO 63110, USA

Leila Shahbaznejad
Children's Medical Center, Pediatrics Center of Excellence, Tehran, Iran
Department of Pediatrics, Mazandaran University of Medical Sciences, Sari, Iran

Fatemeh Tahghighi
Children's Medical Center, Pediatrics Center of Excellence, Tehran, Iran
Department of Pediatrics, Tehran University of Medical Sciences, Tehran, Iran

Sayed-Reza Raeeskarami, Raheleh Assari and Vahid Ziaee
Pediatric Rheumatology Research Group, Rheumatology Research Center, Tehran University of Medical Sciences, Tehran, Iran
Department of Pediatrics, Tehran University of Medical Sciences, Tehran, Iran

Yahya Aghighi
Department of Pediatrics, Tehran University of Medical Sciences, Tehran, Iran

Abbas Shakoori and Hamidreza Azhideh
Department of Medical Genetics, Tehran University of Medical Sciences, Tehran, Iran

Tõnu Jõgi, Madis Joonsalu and Markus Vardja
1Hematology and Oncology Clinic, Department of Radiotherapy and Oncological Therapy, Tartu University Hospital, 51003 Tartu, Estonia

Jana Jaal
Hematology and Oncology Clinic, Department of Radiotherapy and Oncological Therapy, Tartu University Hospital, 51003 Tartu, Estonia
Faculty of Medicine, University of Tartu, 50411 Tartu, Estonia

Marju Kase
Hematology and Oncology Clinic, Department of Radiotherapy and Oncological Therapy, Tartu University Hospital, 51003 Tartu, Estonia
East-Tallinn Central Hospital, Center of Oncology, 10138 Tallinn, Estonia

Ave Minajeva, Mikk Saretok, Aidi Adamson, Jelizaveta Junninen and Tõnis Metsaots
Faculty of Medicine, University of Tartu, 50411 Tartu, Estonia

Toomas Asser
Faculty of Medicine, University of Tartu, 50411 Tartu, Estonia
Neurology Clinic, Department of Neurosurgery, Tartu University Hospital, 51014 Tartu, Estonia

Si-Wei Zhu
RayBiotech, Inc., Guangzhou 510600, China

Zhizhou Kuang, Shuhong Luo and Ruo-Pan Huang
RayBiotech, Inc., Guangzhou 510600, China
RayBiotech, Inc., 3607 Parkway Lane, Norcross, GA 30092, USA
South China Biochip Research Center, Guangzhou 510600, China

Jarad J. Wilson
RayBiotech, Inc., 3607 Parkway Lane, Norcross, GA 30092, USA

Jun-ichi Nagao, Shojiro Ikezaki, Sonoko Tasaki, Yuka Narita and Tamaki Cho
Section of Infection Biology, Department of Functional Bioscience, Fukuoka Dental College, Fukuoka 814-0193, Japan

Marie Hashimoto
Section of Infection Biology, Department of Functional Bioscience, Fukuoka Dental College, Fukuoka 814-0193, Japan

Section of Image Diagnosis, Department of Diagnostics and General Care, Fukuoka Dental College, Fukuoka 814-0193, Japan

Yoshihiko Tanaka
Section of Infection Biology, Department of Functional Bioscience, Fukuoka Dental College, Fukuoka 814-0193, Japan
Advanced Science Research Center, Fukuoka Dental College, Fukuoka 814-0193, Japan

Kenji Yuasa
Section of Image Diagnosis, Department of Diagnostics and General Care, Fukuoka Dental College, Fukuoka 814-0193, Japan

Ken-ichi Arita-Morioka
Advanced Science Research Center, Fukuoka Dental College, Fukuoka 814-0193, Japan

Amnon Altman
Division of Cell Biology, La Jolla Institute for Allergy and Immunology, La Jolla, CA 92037, USA

Bérengère Tanné, Stéphane Bernier and Nancy Dumais
Département de Biologie, Facultédes Sciences, Université de Sherbrooke, Sherbrooke, QC, Canada J1K 2R1

Lusine Khondkaryan
Group of Cell Technologies, Institute of Molecular Biology, National Academy of Sciences, Yerevan, Armenia

David Poghosyan
Laboratory of Molecular and Cellular Immunology, Institute of Molecular Biology, National Academy of Sciences, Yerevan, Armenia

Sona Margaryan and Gayane Manukyan
Laboratory of Molecular and Cellular Immunology, Institute of Molecular Biology, National Academy of Sciences, Yerevan, Armenia
Russian-Armenian (Slavonic) University, Yerevan, Armenia

Akinobu Takaki and Kazuhide Yamamoto
Department of Gastroenterology and Hepatology, Okayama University Graduate School of Medicine, Dentistry, and Pharmaceutical Sciences, 2-5-1 Shikata-cho, Kita-ku, Okayama 700-8558, Japan

Takahito Yagi
Department of Gastroenterological Surgery Transplant and Surgical Oncology, Okayama University
Graduate School ofMedicine, Dentistry, and Pharmaceutical Sciences, 2-5-1 Shikata-cho, Kita-ku, Okayama 700-8558, Japan

Archana Mootha, Sankari Malaiappan, N. D. Jayakumar, Sheeja S. Varghese and Julie Toby Thomas
Department of Periodontics, Saveetha Dental College and Hospitals, No. 162, Poonamallee High Road,Velappanchavadi, Chennai 600077, India

Sami Aldaham
College of Medicine, Al-Imam Mohammad Ibn Saud Islamic University (IMSIU), Riyadh 11432, Saudi Arabia

Janet A. Foote
Mel & Enid Zuckerman College of Public Health, University of Arizona, Tucson, AZ 85724, USA

Iman A. Hakim
Mel & Enid Zuckerman College of Public Health, University of Arizona, Tucson, AZ 85724, USA
Arizona Cancer Center, University of Arizona, Tucson, AZ 85724, USA

H.-H. Sherry Chow
Arizona Cancer Center, University of Arizona, Tucson, AZ 85724, USA

Vikas Sarangal, Jagriti Bhatia and Dharmveer S. Arya
Department of Pharmacology, All India Institute of Medical Sciences, New Delhi 110029, India

Mahaveer Golechha
Department of Pharmacology, All India Institute of Medical Sciences, New Delhi 110029, India
Public Health Foundation of India, New Delhi 110070, India

Shreesh Ojha
Department of Pharmacology andTherapeutics, Faculty ofMedicine&Health Sciences, UAE University, Al Ain, UAE

Lyubomir A. Dourmishev, Dimitrina V. Guleva and Ljubka G. Miteva
Department of Dermatology and Venereology, Medical University-Sofia, Bulgaria

Darshna Yagnik
Department of Natural Sciences, School of Science and Technology, Middlesex University,The Burroughs, London NW4 4BT, UK

Rodrigo G. Rosique, Marina J. Rosique and Jayme A. Farina Junior
Division of Plastic Surgery, Department of Surgery and Anatomy, Ribeirão Preto School of Medicine, University of São Paulo, Avenida Bandeirantes 3900, 14048-900 Ribeirão Preto, SP, Brazil

Runkuan Yang
Department of Intensive Care Medicine, Tampere University Hospital, University of Tampere, 10 Biokatu, 33014 Tampere, Finland
Department of Critical Care Medicine, University of Pittsburgh Medical School, 3550 Terrace Street, Pittsburgh, PA 15261, USA
Department of Emergencies and Critical Care, Oslo University Hospital, 4950 Nydalen, 0424 Oslo, Norway

Jyrki Tenhunen
Department of Intensive Care Medicine, Tampere University Hospital, University of Tampere, 10 Biokatu, 33014 Tampere, Finland
Department of Surgical Science, Anesthesiology and Intensive Care Medicine, Uppsala University, 751 85 Uppsala, Sweden

Tor Inge Tonnessen
Department of Emergencies and Critical Care, Oslo University Hospital, 4950 Nydalen, 0424 Oslo, Norway
Institute of Clinical Medicine, University of Oslo, Blindern, 0316 Oslo, Norway

Marta Imamura and Linamara Rizzo Battistella
Clinical Research Center, Institute of Physical Medicine and Rehabilitation, University of São Paulo School of Medicine, Rua Jandiatuba, 580 Vila Andrade, 05716-150 São Paulo, SP, Brazil

Fábio Marcon Alfieri
Clinical Research Center, Institute of Physical Medicine and Rehabilitation, University of São Paulo School of Medicine, Rua Jandiatuba, 580 Vila Andrade, 05716-150 São Paulo, SP, Brazil
São Paulo Adventist University Center, Estrada de Itapecerica, 5859 Jardim IAE, 05858-001 São Paulo, SP, Brazil

Fernando Ezquerro
University of São Paulo School of Medicine, Avenida Dr. Arnaldo, 455 Cerqueira César, 01246903 São Paulo, SP, Brazil

Lucy Vilas Boas and Tania Regina Tozetto-Mendoza
Tropical Hematology Laboratory, Institute of Tropical Medicine of São Paulo and Medical Research Laboratory, LIM 52,University of São Paulo, Avenida Dr. Arnaldo, 455 Cerqueira C´esar, 01246903 São Paulo, SP, Brazil

Janini Chen
Institute of Physical Medicine and Rehabilitation, University of São Paulo School of Medicine, Rua Domingo de Soto 100,Vila Mariana, 04116-030 São Paulo, SP, Brazil

Levent Özçakar
Department of PhysicalMedicine and Rehabilitation, Hacettepe University Medical School, Hacettepe University Faculty of Medicine, Sıhhiye, 06100 Ankara, Turkey

Lars Arendt-Nielsen
Center for Sensory-Motor Interaction, School of Medicine, Aalborg University, Fredrik Bajers Vej 7, Building D3,9220 Aalborg E, Denmark

Aurora Moen
National Institute of Occupational Health, 0033 Oslo, Norway
Department of Physical Medicine and Rehabilitation, Oslo University Hospital, 0424 Oslo, Norway

Johannes Gjerstad
National Institute of Occupational Health, 0033 Oslo, Norway
Department of Physical Medicine and Rehabilitation, Oslo University Hospital, 0424 Oslo, Norway
Department of Molecular Biosciences, University of Oslo, 0371 Oslo, Norway

Cecilie Røe
Department of Physical Medicine and Rehabilitation, Oslo University Hospital, 0424 Oslo, Norway
Faculty of Medicine, University of Oslo, 0316 Oslo, Norway

Anne-Li Lind and Torsten Gordh
Department of Surgical Sciences, Uppsala University, 751 85 Uppsala, Sweden

Måns Thulin
Department of Statistics, Uppsala University, 751 20 Uppsala, Sweden

Masood Kamali-Moghaddam
Department of Immunology, Genetics and Pathology, Science for Life Laboratory, Uppsala University, 751 85 Uppsala, Sweden

Mark Farrugia and Byron Baron
Centre for Molecular Medicine and Biobanking, Faculty of Medicine and Surgery, University of Malta, Msida MSD 2080, Malta

Abidullah Khan, Iqbal Haider, Maimoona Ayub and Mohammad Humayun
KTH, Peshawar, Pakistan

Daniel Pitz Jacobsen and Fred Haugen
National Institute of Occupational Health, Oslo, Norway

Aurora Moen and Johannes Gjerstad
National Institute of Occupational Health, Oslo, Norway
Department of Biosciences, University of Oslo, Norway

Andressa Coope, Lívia Bitencourt Pascoal, Francesca Aparecida Ramos da Silva, José Diego Botezelli, Maria de Lourdes Setsuko Ayrizono, Michel Gardere Camargo, Cilene Bicca Dias, João José Fagundes and Raquel Franco Leal
IBD Research Laboratory, Surgery Department, University of Campinas (UNICAMP), Medical School, Campinas, SP, Brazil

Marciane Milanski and Mariana Portovedo
Laboratory of Metabolic Disorders, Faculty of Applied Sciences, University of Campinas (UNICAMP), Campinas, SP, Brazil

Núria Planell
Department of Gastroenterology and Bioinformatics Platform, CIBER-EHD, Barcelona, Spain

Moerbono Mochtar, Alamanda Murasmita, M. Eko Irawanto, Indah Julianto and Harijono Kariosentono
Dermatovenerology Department, Sebelas Maret University, Dr. Moewardi General Hospital, Surakarta, Indonesia

Fajar Waskito
Dermatovenerology Department, Gadjah Mada University, Dr. Sardjitó General Hospital, Yogyakarta, Indonesia

Mitsuaki Moriyama, Ayano Hashimoto, Hideyo Satoh, Kenji Kawabe, Mizue Ogawa, Katsura Takano and Yoichi Nakamura
Laboratory of Integrative Physiology in Veterinary Sciences, Osaka Prefecture University, Izumisano, Osaka, Japan

Krzysztof Laudanski, Toby Steinberg and Arpit Patel
Department of Anesthesiology and Critical Care, University of Pennsylvania, Philadelphia, PA 19104, USA

Michael Stentz
Department of Anesthesiology and Intensive Care, Emory University, Atlanta, GA 30322, USA

Matthew DiMeglio and William Furey
Philadelphia College of Osteopathic Medicine, Philadelphia, PA 19131, USA

Ditte Søvsø Gundelund Nielsen, Marlene Fredborg and Stig Purup
Department of Animal Science, Aarhus University, Blichers Allé 20, 8830 Tjele, Denmark

Vibeke Andersen
Hospital of Southern Jutland, 6200 Aabenraa, Denmark
Institute of Regional Health Research and Institute of Molecular Medicine, University of Southern Denmark, 5000 Odense, Denmark

E. Tsitoura and I. Lasithiotaki
School of Medicine, Laboratory of Molecular and Cellular Pneumonology, University of Crete, Heraklion, Crete, Greece

K. Karagiannis, A. Proklou and K. M. Antoniou
School of Medicine, Laboratory of Molecular and Cellular Pneumonology, University of Crete, Heraklion, Crete, Greece
Department of Respiratory Medicine, University Hospital of Heraklion, Heraklion, Crete, Greece

D. Moraitaki and N. Tzanakis
Department of Respiratory Medicine, University Hospital of Heraklion, Heraklion, Crete, Greece

C. Kalpadaki
Department of Haematology, University Hospital of Heraklion, Heraklion, Crete, Greece

I. Sperelakis and G. Kontakis
Department of Orthopedics, University Hospital of Heraklion, Heraklion, Crete, Greece

Kamal Sharma and Alap K. Patel
Department of Cardiology, U. N. Mehta Institute of Cardiology and Research Centre, Ahmedabad, Gujarat, India

Komal H. Shah and Ashwati Konat
Department of Research, U. N. Mehta Institute of Cardiology and Research Centre, Ahmedabad, Gujarat, India

Anthony M. Kyriakopoulos
Nasco AD Biotechnology Laboratory, 11 Sachtouri Str, 18536 Pireus, Greece

Markus Nagl
Division of Hygiene and Medical Microbiology, Medical University of Innsbruck, Sch¨opfstr. 41, 6020 Innsbruck, Austria

Stella Baliou and Vasilleios Zoumpourlis
National Hellenic Research Foundation, 48 Vas. Konstantinou Av, 11635 Athens, Greece

Index